Springer Specialist Surgery Series

Series Editor

J.S.P. Lumley
London, UK

Each volume in this series covers the core information required for study and daily practice. Written in a concise and readable style by experts in the field from around the world, the books describe established procedures and give the reader a grounding within the discipline. The series provides an excellent point of reference to the topics that its covers.

More information about this series at http://www.springer.com/series/4162

Nadey Hakim • Mehmet Haberal
Daniel Maluf
Editors

Transplantation Surgery

Second Edition

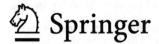

Editors
Nadey Hakim
Imperial College London
London
UK

Mehmet Haberal
Başkent University
Ankara
Turkey

Daniel Maluf
University of Virginia Medical Center
Charlottesville, VA
USA

Springer Specialist Surgery Series
ISBN 978-3-030-55246-6   ISBN 978-3-030-55244-2   (eBook)
https://doi.org/10.1007/978-3-030-55244-2

This Springer imprint is published by the registered company Springer Nature Switzerland AG
The registered company address is: Gewerbestrasse 11, 6330 Cham, Switzerland

Foreword

It is like a fairy tale! Or at least a beautiful epic, a truly significant page in the history of medicine, a staggering scene in which several actors come into play, both fundamentalists and clinical practitioners, eager to place all these new developments at the disposal of those suffering from ill health.

Everyone is passionate about their work, be it providing new knowledge or perfecting new therapeutic methods.

Man has always been fascinated by the possibility of replacing a damaged organ with a healthy one. Several attempts have been made over the centuries, and some miracles have been reported, such as those of Saint Damien and Saint Come as illustrated by Fra Angelico.

The modern saga, however, started more modestly on the mouse. It is on the mouse that the first tissue group was discovered; yet the study of human tissue groups could only be carried out on a human. One human must be subjected to the thousands of tests that have enabled us to unravel the extraordinary complexity of the HLA system.

Organ transplantation has developed in stages. The first was almost singularly marked by renal transplantation assisted by histocompatibility. Had we fully comprehended the chance that there exists only one major tissue complex?

Then, the resounding crash of cymbals! The discovery of a powerful immunosuppressant which freed the surgeons from the immediate restraint of strict compatibility (even though this plays a part in long-term survival). So, boldness permitting, heart, liver, lungs, pancreas and, of course, multi-organ transplants are now possible. Transplantation has therefore become a daily therapy as a result of the number of amazing surgical feats carried out by these clinical practitioners. It is, however, unfortunately curbed by a shortage of organs and thousands of patients still await the benefits it can bring.

Will we know how to respond to this expectation? Will xenotransplantation be the next stage?

Finally, do not forget those individuals who have been given the chance to survive as a result of a marrow or, even better, haematopoietic transplant. Here compatibility recaptures its rights.

This book, edited by world transplantation experts, will be an indispensable tool for new generations involved in transplantation.

Jean Dausset
Prix Nobel

Foreword

What do you need to look for and find when you are in search of a book on transplantation? The first element in the quest is to consider the editors who have constructed the topics, sought out authors and compiled the book into a readable and cohesive whole. In this volume, we cannot ask for better than Nadey Hakim, Mehmet Haberal, and Daniel Maluf. They are experts not only in their field but also in communicating their knowledge. Prof Haberal is the current President of the Transplantation Society amongst his many responsibilities and is a surgeon's surgeon. He has brought modern transplantation surgical practices to Turkey, the Middle East and widely across the globe through his relentless travel, teaching, publishing and research. Prof Hakim is a true renaissance man, just as at home with a scalpel, a sculptor's chisel and a musical instrument, each used with exquisite delicacy and skill. Impacting the field of transplantation through the World Surgical Society just as he has through his practice in London and through Europe. Daniel Maluf started medical training in Argentina and is now practising in Virginia where he combines skills and interests at the surgical table and at the laboratory bench in genomics. The provenance for the book is outstanding.

The second important element of a useful and readable book is to have a series of great authors marshalled to provide the breadth of the field from their individual expert perspectives. The list of authors is a 'dream team' of contributors from whom you will learn the details of the expanding clinical practice of organ transplantation from the kidney and liver to the heart and lung. You will read not only the details of the surgical techniques, but also the relevant immunology and the ways in which we can manipulate the immune system to bring so many people back from the brink of death due to end-stage organ failure. You will read of the sciences of organ preservation, histocompatibility matching, anaesthetic management, early post-transplantation care, the concerns about selecting the right patients, long-term issues with cancer and the science of immunobiology that backs up the clinical programs of immunosuppression. The length and breadth of the field is carried through chapters on bone marrow transplantation and the complexities of composite allografts which challenge both the surgeon with the multiple surgical connections needed and the physician who must prevent rejection of the multiple different tissues involved.

Taking the reader into the near future, the chapters on liver perfusion and robotic transplantation provide details on what is here today in a few specialised research centres. Finally, the reader will head into the evaluation of the next major impact on organ availability in a chapter on the realities and practicalities of xenotransplantation.

This wonderful compilation of knowledge on the evolution of clinical transplantation will remind those of us in the field how far we have travelled and surprise us about facets we are less familiar with. It will take the reader who is unfamiliar with this modern medical miracle through the details of how this has happened and perhaps persuade them to take up the scalpel or stethoscope to provide the community with the next generation of expertise.

Nadey Hakim
Imperial College London
London, UK

Jeremy Chapman
The Transplantation Society
Sydney, NSW, Australia

Contents

Organ Transplantation: A Historical Perspective

Justin Barr, J. Andrew Bradley, and David Hamilton

AIMS of Chapter

1. To provide a historical overview of the modern era of organ transplantation
2. To chart the major scientific and clinical advances
3. To highlight key events and individuals involved in early failures and successes

1.1 Introduction

Organ transplantation is simultaneously the most exciting and the most challenging field of surgery. Generations of humans have dreamt about the possibility of trading body parts, but accomplishing that goal required decades of research to assemble the technical and scientific competence necessary to succeed. Today, surgeons have the ability to take a patient dying from end-organ failure and replace that organ, granting the recipient a new lease on life—a transformation hitherto unachievable. But we are far from reaching perfection as the immunologic challenges of rejection and social conundrums over proper allocation of limited organs demand continued investigation. In this short chapter, we briefly review the history of the field. Exploring this evolution, the key figures and discoveries that pushed the discipline forward, and the socio-cultural implications thereof, we hope to provide some historical context for the subsequent chapters in the book and, perhaps, some inspiration to take the next step forward.

1.2 Early History of Organ Transplantation

The idea of switching body parts among individuals—even between humans and animals—is as old as civilization, with ancient stories featuring chimeric monsters and preternatural beings. Roman physicians Celsus and Galen both discuss methods of replacing lost tissue, and the Indian doctor Sushruta famously developed techniques to replace the human nose that were later copied by Europeans like sixteenth century surgeon Gaspare -Tagliacozzi [1]. Jesus Christ replaced the ear of a servant, and the patron saints of surgery, Cosmas and Damian, reportedly transplanted the diseased leg of a sexton with that from a Moor who had

J. Barr (✉)
Duke University Department of Surgery, Durham, NC, USA
e-mail: justin.barr@duke.edu

J. A. Bradley
Surgery and Head of the Department, University of Cambridge, Cambridge, UK
e-mail: jab52@cam.ac.uk

D. Hamilton
Alexandria, MN, USA

Fife, UK
https://www.Davidhamiltonstandrews.com

© Springer Nature Switzerland AG 2021
N. Hakim et al. (eds.), *Transplantation Surgery*, Springer Specialist Surgery Series,
https://doi.org/10.1007/978-3-030-55244-2_1

Fig. 1.1 Cosmas and Damian, patron saints of medicine, were credited with posthumous cures, including the transplantation of a leg. Photo shows the Aspe of the Basilic of Sts. Cosmas and Damian, with a mosaic portraying Peter (white robes at Christ's left hand) presenting Damien and Paul presenting Cosmas to heaven (right)

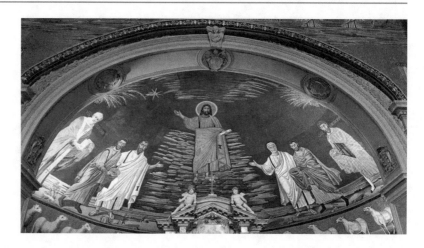

died several days earlier (see Fig. 1.1) [2]. As historian Thomas Schlich points out, these examples reflect examples of plastic surgery—external body parts with external function—yet they nonetheless evidence an early and persistent interest in the field [3].

Organ transplant per se began in the late nineteenth century. Earlier advances like anesthesia and antiseptic surgery enabled longer, safer operations. As medicine moved beyond neo-humoralism, it began to focus on organs and their specific physiological purpose. This shift in understanding disease created the fundamental intellectual conditions necessary to start modern transplantation: as doctors increasingly understood the purpose of specific organs, the idea of replacing missing or malfunctioning ones appeared the logical solution. The thyroid became the prototypical organ in the pre-World War II era—and for decades the most commonly transplanted one. Surgeons like Theodor Kocher were becoming increasingly skilled at removing the thyroid for conditions like goiter, but in a time before facile hormone replacement, the lethal effects of total thyroidectomies quickly became apparent. Replacing some thyroid tissue seemed an appropriate solution. In July 1883, Kocher implanted part of a thyroid into a man's neck, performing the first modern organ transplantation [4].

The concept quickly expanded from thyroids to other organs. Surgeons implanted adrenal glands for Addison's disease (1887), portions of the pancreas to cure diabetes (1894), ovaries for infertility (1895), and parathyroids for hypocalcemia (1907) [4]. Charles-Éduard Brown-Séquard famously inaugurated testicular extract transplantation to rejuvenate men in the 1880s; by 1889, over 12,000 physicians reported using his therapy [5].

Surgeons expanded this concept from glandular tissue to solid organs like the kidney. In France, Mathieu Jaboulay transplanted a pig kidney into the antecubital fossa of one patient and a goat kidney into another patient [6]. In Berlin, Germany, Ernst Unger and then Sconstadt had transplanted kidneys taken from a monkey into patients [7]. Yu Yu Voronoy in 1936 [8] performed the world's first human to human kidney transplantation operation. The recipient chosen by Voronoy was a 26-year-old female who had been admitted to hospital in a semicomatose state after purposely ingesting 4 grams of mercuric chloride (then a popular method of suicide). The donor kidney was obtained from an elderly male who had died after a head injury and was blood group incompatible with the recipient. The operation was carried out under local anaesthetic; the donor kidney was placed in the thigh with anastomosis of the renal artery and vein to the femoral vessels, leaving the ureter to drain cutaneously (Fig. 1.2). Unfortunately, the graft never functioned, and the recipient died 2 days later.

Voronoy's efforts focused attention on two problems that have challenged the field of organ transplantation: technical and immunological. Whereas the aforementioned thyroid and other glands could obtain sufficient blood supply by

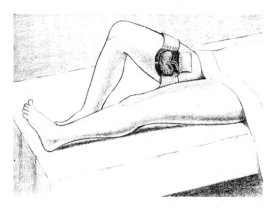

Fig. 1.2 Voronoy's illustration of his, the first human kidney allograft, carried out in Kiev in 1933 using the thigh location

diffusion, larger organs like the kidney required surgical connections between blood vessels. The field of vascular surgery was developing contemporaneously, and surgeons around the world proposed various mechanisms to connect arteries and veins [9]. Most famously, in 1902 Alexis Carrel articulated his triangulation method for sewing vessels together, which Voronoy used in his cases [10]. In 1912, Carrel received the Nobel Prize in medicine for this technique. Carrel immediately recognized the potential for his method to facilitate solid organ transplantation [11]. By 1905, he was already performing kidney transplants in animals, experiments he soon extended to other organs [12]. He established the technical foundations for the field and consistently succeeded auto-transplanting organs around the body, but his allografts universally failed. "From a surgical point of view, the problem of grafting is solved," declared Carrel in an interview. "Whether it ever will be viewed from the angle of compatible organs, I cannot tell. Perhaps someday—perhaps never" [13].

Despite failing scientifically, organ transplantation attracted great popular interest in the late nineteenth and early twentieth centuries. The popularity of H.G. Well's contemporary novel The Island of Dr. Moreau (1896) and references to Mary Shelly's Frankenstein (1818) exposed societal fears of the potential implications of surgically trading body parts [14, 15]. But most of the attention was laudatory. Newspaper articles

closely followed the experiments and praised the accomplishments of the surgeons. Carrel received hundreds of letters from patients beseeching him to try his transplantation on them, willing to risk their own death, if necessary [12]. Unlike many scientific achievements that remain forever ensconced in the ivory tower, organ transplantation was widely known and broadly supported throughout Europe and the United States in this era. This fame did not correlate with clinical success: essentially all these early transplants failed.

Two forms of organ transplantation that did succeed wildly were skin grafts and blood transfusions. Skin grafting was the second most popular operation in the United States in the 1920s (appendectomies were first), used for burns, trauma, and wound coverage [16]. Blood—which for hundreds of years doctors removed from sick patients—took on new meaning in the late nineteenth century with the demise of the humoral system and the (slow) recognition of the importance of blood in treating shock [17]. Prone to clotting when removed from the body, early blood transfusions required direct donor-to-recipient connections of blood vessels. The process became safer with the discovery of blood types by Karl Landsteiner in 1900, although cross-matching did not become common until after World War I. With the advent of sodium citrate in 1915, stored blood and eventually blood banks developed [18].

Many of the social issues that bedevil the transplant community today first appeared at the turn of the century. How do you convince people to donate? Is it ethical to pay donors? What are the implications of trans-racial transplant, or of taking tissue from persecuted minorities? Should children be able to donate? How did various religions interpret the notions of giving or receiving a body part? Society struggled to address these issues in 1910, but the answers they created largely endured, albeit with much debate, into the present. Today, skin grafts and blood transfusions have become so routinized that neither physicians nor society at large considers them organ transplants, but in their day, they commanded the same excitement and potential as the kidney surgeries of Murray and heart operations of Barnard.

1.3 The Science of Immunology

Moving forward in transplantation required understanding why the host's body rejected the implanted organ and then devising strategies to keep that from happening. Coincident with the germ theory of disease, novel ideas about how the body fought off infections developed [19]. Élie Metchnikoff famously observed phagocytosis and from this experience derived the cellular system of immunity. At the same time, Paul Ehrlich identified the general properties of what we now know are antibodies, a discovery that led to cures for hitherto fatal diseases like diphtheria and laid the foundation for the humoral theory of immunity. Metchnikoff and Ehrlich were jointly awarded the Nobel Prize in 1908 for their work in immunology. Almroth Wright helped unify the cellular and humoral theories into a single system through the opsonins that he identified and named (opsonin derives from Greek: to prepare for eating).

Slowly, scientists recognized that these same mechanisms attacked not only bacteria but also any tissue that induced an inflammatory reaction, including that which surgeons transplanted. In 1912, for example, Georg Schöone observed that second transplants in the same host failed more rapidly than did the first, implying an immune response [20]. James Murphy realized the importance of lymphoid tissue in rejecting organs. While some early efforts around radiation and cytotoxic chemicals like benzol adumbrated the promise of immunosuppression, it had no clinical relevance, and following the cataclysmic effects of World War I, research in the field largely ceased.

Given the widely accepted therapeutic potential of transplantation, why did efforts stop? Neither scientists nor surgeons had achieved their desired results; Carrel's admission of defeat—coming from one of the most famous doctors in the world—clearly put a damper on field. But slow progress in later eras did not have a similarly arresting effect. Simultaneously, establishing different arenas in surgery, particularly on the gastrointestinal tract, pulled attention away from experimental fields like transplant surgery. Crucially, Europe after World War I was shattered, impoverished, and struggling to re-build, lacking the time, energy, money, and infrastructure to delve deeply into medical investigation.

These years also represent a transition period for medical science. Before World War I, most experiments were relatively inexpensive, and private charities funded the majority of research. After World War II, government agencies like the National Institutes of Health in the United States poured billions of dollars into laboratories. But the years between the wars represent a time when science was becoming increasingly resource-intensive without well-established mechanisms of providing those resources, stymieing work in disciplines like transplantation.

Renewed investigation into immunology after World War II launched the modern era of transplant surgery. Here, British scientist Peter Medawar played a central role. Medawar's interest in the subject occurred by chance when he was a young postgraduate experimental biologist in Oxford. A Royal Air Force bomber had crashed in North Oxford near his home, and one of the injured was an airman who received extensive burns. Medawar was invited by a colleague, Dr. J.F. Barnes, to see whether he had any new suggestions for how the patient's limited amount of healthy skin might be used to cover the burns. Medawar was intrigued by the repeated failure of non-autogenous skin grafts in these patients and took it upon himself to find out the reason why grafts were rejected and what, if anything, could be done to prevent rejection from occurring.

With the aid of a grant from the Medical Research Council, Medawar traveled to Glasgow to study skin grafting at the Burns Unit at Glasgow Royal Infirmary. There, he teamed up with Tom Gibson, a gifted plastic surgeon who was also interested in skin graft rejection. Shortly after Medawar's arrival in Glasgow, a young woman was admitted to the ward with severe burns after falling onto an open gasfire. Gibson grafted the woman's burns with a series of small "pinch" skin grafts taken from her brother, and Medawar proceeded to study the fate of the skin grafts by taking biopsies of them for histological examination. As expected, the grafts were destroyed after some days. When a second set of grafts from the same donor was applied 2 weeks later, these were destroyed even more quickly. This so-called 'second set' phenomenon was taken as clear evidence that the rejection response was due to actively acquired immunity and not to a nonspecific inflammatory reaction. Medawar and Gibson published their findings in the Journal of Anatomy in 1943 [21] (Fig. 1.3). They concluded that an as yet unidentified antibody was responsible. After returning to Oxford, Medawar undertook detailed studies on the rejection of skin grafts in the rabbit [22]. For the first time, convincing evidence was obtained that the variation between unrelated individuals was such that transplantation inevitably led to graft rejection. Medawar reasoned that because sensitization to a graft from one donor did not usually sensitize the recipient to a graft from a different donor animal, a number of different genes must be responsible for provoking graft rejection. Medawar's work made it clear that successful grafting between unrelated individuals would require effective suppression of the recipient's immune system (Fig. 1.4).

THE FATE OF SKIN HOMOGRAFTS IN MAN

By T. GIBSON* AND P. B. MEDAWAR, *Mr Clark's Surgical Unit and the Department of Pathology, Glasgow Royal Infirmary*

Fig. 1.3 Title of Gibson and Medawar's classic report in the *Journal of Anatomy* 1943 on the human "second set" response, which together with Medawar's experimental extension of the work, signaled the start of the modern era of transplantation immunology. Reused with Permission from Springer

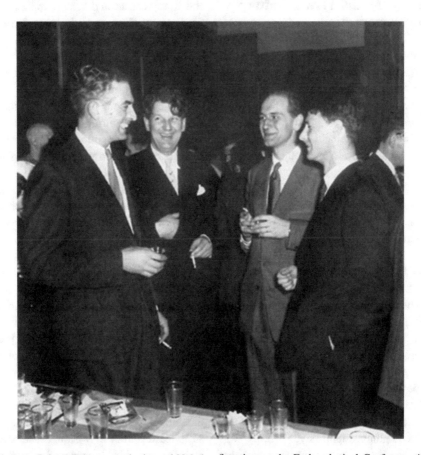

Fig. 1.4 Sir Peter Brian Medawar, zoologist and Nobel Prize winner, established in the 1940s that "actively acquired immunity" was the basis of allograft rejection. His later work with steroids and tolerance encouraged hopes that the immunological barrier to survival of human organ transplants might be breached. He is seen here on the left, meetin Milan Hasek (second from right) for the first time at the Embryological Conference in Brussels, 1955. Hasek was. Czechoslovakian immunologist who described tolerance induction in chickens. British immunologist Leslie Brent stands far right. From J Ivanyi, "Milan Hasek and the Discovery of Immunological Tolerance," *Nature Reviews Immunology* 3 (2003): 591–7. Used with permission

While debates confronted the relative roles of humoral or cellular immunity, there was now widespread acceptance that immunological mechanisms were the cause of graft rejection, and that it was an active, biological process. Immunological rejection was viewed as an inevitable consequence of organ transplantation. Still, no effective way of preventing rejection was known, despite some early research involving steroids and radiation. The view of the experimentalists, and nearly all clinicians, in the early 1950s was that little was to be gained by attempting kidney transplantation in humans until further progress had been made in the laboratory.

1.4 The Beginning of the Modern Era of Kidney Transplantation

The pessimistic view of the experimentalists did not prevent a number of enthusiastic surgeons in both North America and France from attempting kidney transplantation in humans. These operations had minimal, if any, clinical benefit to the recipients, but they did elucidate the many challenges inherent to organ transplantation and thus paved the way for future success. On 17 June 1950, R.H. Lawler, a surgeon at the Presbyterian Hospital in Chicago, removed the diseased left kidney from a 44-year-old woman with polycystic disease and replaced it with a healthy kidney taken from a blood group compatible female donor who had died from bleeding esophageal varices [23]. It was not possible to determine the extent to which the transplanted kidney produced urine since the recipient's native right kidney still functioned. The operation attracted considerable interest, mostly of a negative nature, from both the medical profession and the public. Lawler did not carry out any further kidney transplants, but his single case stimulated surgeons in France to begin human kidney transplantation. Even though no effective immunosuppressive therapy was then available, French clinicians reasoned that the impaired immunity that was known to accompany kidney failure might be sufficient to allow graft survival, especially if supplementary corti-

costeroids were given. The early French kidney transplants were performed at the Centre Medico-Chirurgical Foch and at the Hôpital Necker by three separate medical teams [24–26].

On 12 January 1951, Charles Dubost and his team transplanted a kidney, obtained from an executed prisoner, into a 44-year-old female with renal failure due to chronic pyelonephritis. Meanwhile, another surgical team, which included Marceau Servelle and his colleague Rougeulle, transplanted the other kidney from the same donor into a 22-year-old female with hypertensive nephropathy. Both recipients died of advanced uremia within a few days. In these, and in later cases performed by the French pioneers, the transplanted kidneys were placed in the iliac fossa, with anastomoses of the renal to the iliac vessels and restoration of the urinary tract. Rene Küss and his team carried out the third transplant in the French series on 30 January 1951. Although some degree of early graft function was obtained, the patient died 1 month later—another failure.

French surgeons performed a further five kidney transplants during 1951. All failed, but one deserves special mention since it was the first living related kidney transplant: the recipient was a 16-year-old boy who had ruptured a kidney during a fall. Doctors controlled the life-threatening hemorrhage with an emergent nephrectomy only to discover the boy had a congenital solitary kidney. His mother, in a brave attempt to save the life of her son, insisted that one of her own kidneys should be used for transplantation. After careful consideration, the medical team, comprising Jean Hamburger and Louis Michon, acceded to her wish. They performed the operation at the Hôpital Necker on Christmas Eve 1952. The transplanted organ initially functioned well, but tragically after 22 days the graft rejected and the recipient died.

Meanwhile, attempts at human kidney transplantation were also taking place in North America at centers in Boston, Cleveland, Chicago and Toronto. The largest and best documented series of transplants were those carried out in Boston at the Peter Bent Brigham Hospital by David Hume between 1951 and 1953.

The presence in the Brigham Hospital during the early 1950s of one of the few, newly available artificial kidneys stimulated the development of transplantation there. The artificial kidney had been developed by Wilhelm Kolff in German-occupied Holland during the Second World War [27]. The modified machine in Boston attracted large numbers of patients with kidney disease to the Brigham. It allowed the temporary support of renal function for some patients both before and after transplantation. Renal dialysis in the peri-transplant period was particularly important in the 1950s since the donor kidneys usually incurred significant ischemic injury prior to implantation. It was first used in a transplant carried out by Dr. Scola at the nearby Springfield Hospital, which failed. Although the early kidney machine proved effective for temporary renal support, it was not a practicable solution for long-term dialysis. The machine was cumbersome and difficult to use, and each dialysis session required recannulation of an artery and vein. It was not until 1960, when Belding Scribner developed the Scribner shunt, that permanent vascular access and hence long-term dialysis became feasible.

The next eight kidney transplants in Boston were performed at the Brigham Hospital. Frances Moore chaired the department of surgery at the Brigham and, given his interest in human metabolism generally, strongly supported the transplant program. John Merrill was an internist and a central figure in the transplant team. Like many other interested clinicians of the time, Merrill had visited Paris to observe first-hand the techniques of the French pioneers. Interestingly, the American surgeons chose, unlike the French, to site their kidney grafts in the upper thigh of the recipient and to allow the ureter to drain to the skin surface. The early Boston transplants were mostly, but not all, blood group compatible, and some of the recipients received treatment with corticosteroids. As with the early French transplants, graft rejection proved insurmountable; the results were generally poor. Some of the kidney grafts survived a surprisingly long time, and one notable success gave rise to a glimmer of hope: the patient was a 26-year-old South American doctor who, on 11 February 1953, received a kidney graft from a donor who had died during an open-heart operation (another new and hazardous area of surgery). After a period of time, during which support of the recipient by the artificial kidney machine was needed, the graft began to function satisfactorily. However, after 6 months severe hypertension had developed, graft function declined rapidly, and the patient died. The failure of the graft in this case was attributed not to immunologic rejection but to hypertension. Hume and colleagues documented in detail the first nine transplants of the Boston series in their classic paper of 1955 [28]. Their manuscript not only described with accuracy the histopathological features of graft rejection but also suggested that recurrence of the original renal disease in the graft could be a problem. Furthermore, they showed that removing the recipient's native kidneys may help to avoid hypertensive damage to the graft (Fig. 1.5).

The lack of any long-term success in either France or North America was disappointing to the transplant teams involved and seemed to support the widely held view that the genetic individuality in humans was such that, as in the animal studies, immunologic rejection was inevitable. The broader surgical community did not show a great deal of interest in these early attempts at transplantation and indeed evinced some hostility, but invaluable technical expertise in the kidney transplant procedure had been acquired by those involved. As with Carrel's animal studies in the early 1900s, vascular anastomosis and urinary drainage of the graft had been shown to present no particular technical problem. The challenge was biological.

1.5 Renal Transplantation Between Identical Twins

Physicians first succeeded in organ transplantation by going around the problem of immunological rejection rather than solving it. The first kidney transplant that was successful in the long-term took place towards the end of 1954 when the Boston transplant team encountered the opportunity to transplant kidneys between identi-

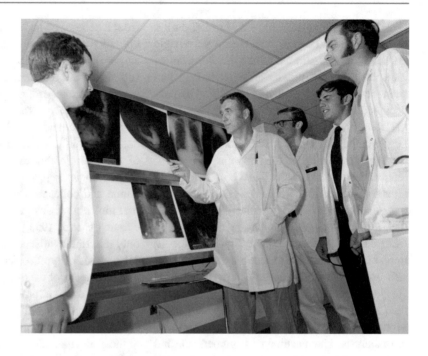

cal twins, thereby avoiding any risk of graft rejection [29]. The recipient was a 23-year-old man who had recently been diagnosed with chronic renal failure and was referred to the Brigham Hospital for treatment with the newly acquired artificial kidney machine. Fortuitously, the patient had an identical twin brother. After careful consideration by the transplant team, they decided to transplant the recipient with a kidney from his healthy twin. Identical twins were known to accept each other's skin grafts permanently [30], and to ensure that the brothers were genetically identical, skin grafts were exchanged prior to kidney transplantation. These were not rejected, and so the operation proceeded. On 23 December 1954, the donor kidney was removed by Hartwell Harrison, a urologist, and the recipient operation was performed synchronously by Joseph Murray, the plastic surgeon who had taken over David Hume's responsibilities at the Brigham (Nobel Laureate 1991). On this occasion, the American surgeons followed the lead of their French colleagues and placed the kidney transplant in the iliac fossa retroperitoneally, with anastomosis of the donor renal artery to the internal iliac artery, the renal vein to the iliac vein and the ureter to the bladder. No attempt was made to

cool the kidney after removal from the donor, nor was intravascular flush performed before transplantation. Nevertheless, good graft function was obtained within a few days, and both the donor and recipient made a full recovery. The recipient later married one of his nurses, became a father, and lived for over 20 years with a functioning graft until he died from coronary artery disease.

The first twin kidney transplant was soon followed by successful kidney transplants between identical twins in Boston, Oregon, Paris and Toronto. Unfortunately, one of the kidney donors in the Boston twin series turned out to have multiple renal arteries, and after transplantation, the graft failed for technical reasons. Thereafter, the use of aortography in the donor to establish the anatomy of the renal vasculature was introduced to avoid repetition of this tragic situation. The demonstration that human kidney transplantation could be achieved with technical success when no immunological barrier existed was undoubtedly an important milestone in the history of transplantation and attracted considerable publicity. There had been concern by some that a kidney graft might be physiologically incapable of providing adequate long-term renal function. The success of the twin transplants proved such fears unfounded. However, although the twin transplants provided a clear demonstration of the potential of organ transplantation as a major new therapy, they did not solve the problem of immune rejection—and there were only so many patients suffering from kidney disease lucky enough to have a healthy twin. Advancing the field required further research.

1.6 Developments in Transplant Immunology

Although during the mid-1950s the immunological barrier to transplantation between unrelated individuals seemed insuperable, a number of very important developments were occurring in the laboratory that were to lead to a major advance in the field of transplant immunology. Medawar's earlier studies had already laid the foundations for the future, and in the early 1950s Billingham, Brent and Medawar made their landmark observations on the induction of neonatal tolerance [31, 32] (Fig. 1.6). The initial stimulus for Medawar's work on tolerance was the observation that skin grafts exchanged between non-identical cattle twins were not, contrary to expectation, rejected. The explanation for this apparent paradox became clear when Medawar and his colleagues

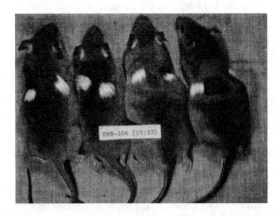

Fig. 1.6 Billingham, Brent and Medawar induced tolerance experimentally in the early 1950s. Image shows results of their famous skin grafts on mice made immunologically tolerant in utero. From *Philosophical Transactions of the Royal Society, Series B, 1956.* Used with permission from the Royal Society

came across a monograph by F.M. Burnet and F. Fenner on the production of antibodies [33] and learned, through this, of the work of Ray Owen. While at the University of Wisconsin, Owen had shown that dizygotic cattle twins were chimeric with respect to their circulating red blood cells because the twins shared a common placenta and had communication between their chorionic vessels [34]. Medawar's group went on to show that adult mice could be made tolerant to skin grafts if, as embryos or neonates, they were injected intraperitoneally with donor strain lymphoid cells. For his work on immunological tolerance, Medawar was awarded the Nobel Prize in 1960. Although induction of transplant tolerance by this approach was not practical in humans, its success in the laboratory meant that there was increasing confidence that transplant immunologists would soon solve the problem of graft rejection in the clinic. Such was the attractiveness of this powerful method of suppression that other approaches, notably the use of steroids, were disregarded. Future laboratory work in the 1950s focused almost exclusively on the concept of transplant tolerance; little interest was shown in developing non-specific ways of suppressing the immune response even though these were soon to open the way to successful human organ transplantation.

During the 1950s, unequivocal evidence that cell-mediated immunity was responsible for graft rejection emerged. Until then, transplant immunology was dominated by the idea that humoral immunity was all-important in mediating allograft rejection. Medawar's early studies had already questioned the role of antibody in graft rejection, but it was the experiments of Avrion Mitchison that firmly established the role of cellular immunity as an important effector mechanism in transplantation (Fig. 1.7). Mitchison, while working as a PhD student in Oxford, showed that lymphoid cells—not serum—transferred immunity to allogeneic tumors in the mouse [35]. The following year Billingham, Brent and Medawar showed that lymphoid cells were also responsible for rejecting skin allografts in mice, and they used the term "adoptively acquired immunity" to describe the phenomenon

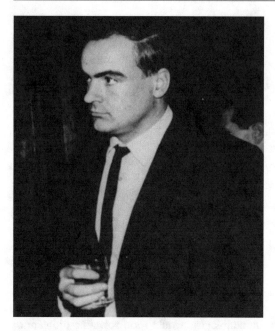

Fig. 1.7 N. Avrion Mitchison, who encouraged the view that cellular mechanisms rather than antibody were the cause of allograft rejection

[36]. These studies, along with the work of James Gowans and others on the circulation of lymphocytes, signaled the importance of "cellular immunology" to rejection [37–39]. The crucial role of the thymus gland in cell mediated immunity and graft rejection was established by J.F.A.P. Miller in the early 1960s. Miller showed that mice that had been thymectomized during the neonatal period became profoundly depleted of lymphocytes and as a result were not able to reject skin allografts [40]. By the end of the 1960s, the phenotypic and functional division of lymphocytes into T and B cell lines was well established.

The 1950s and early 1960s were, therefore, a period of rapid growth in understanding of the immunology of graft rejection, and for a detailed account the reader is referred to the volume by Leslie Brent (who later worked with one of the editors of this book Nadey Hakim) which provides a full and insightful account of the history of transplantation immunology [41]. Although these advances in the laboratory would later contribute to the successful development of kidney transplantation by enabling specific, designed medications to control the immune-

response, in the short term, empirical use of nonspecific immunosuppressive drugs by innovative and bold clinicians proved the critical next step.

1.7 Towards Success in the Clinic

The next step in the evolution of kidney transplantation was the use of whole-body irradiation in an attempt to attenuate the graft rejection response. The arrival of the atomic bomb at the end of World War II and the threat it posed of mass destruction had stimulated much research into the detrimental effects of irradiation. Experiments had shown that animals given an otherwise lethal dose of irradiation could be rescued by an allogeneic bone marrow transplant. Following recovery, the chimeric animals readily accepted a skin graft from the donor of the bone-marrow, suggesting that this approach might have clinical application.

In 1958, the Boston transplant team began to use irradiation in an attempt to prolong the survival of kidney allografts in their patients. Two patients were given whole-body irradiation and donor bone-marrow, and a further ten patients received sublethal irradiation alone. Overall, the results were very poor, and all but one of the recipients died within a month of transplantation [42, 43]. Simultaneously across the ocean, French transplanters also began to use irradiation in an attempt to prevent kidney allograft rejection. They performed 25 such transplants using living related donors, and although the patients did badly, they too had one long-term survivor [44]. Irradiation was also used to a limited extent elsewhere in Europe. Despite the occasional success, it became increasingly apparent that whole-body irradiation was not a satisfactory method for preventing graft rejection. Unless large doses of radiation were given it was ineffective, and when high doses were used, the incidence of serious side effects was far too high.

The way forward in transplantation lay instead with the use of chemical agents to suppress the immune response of the recipient. A breakthrough in the search for an immunosuppressive compound came with the realization that anti-cancer agents were immunosuppressive. Robert

Schwartz and William Damashek in Boston had become interested in the effects of new agents on immunity during their work on the use of anti-cancer compounds to ablate the bone marrow of leukemic patients prior to bone-marrow transplantation. In 1959, Schwartz and Damashek showed that non-myeloablative doses of the purine analog 6-mercaptopurine were effective in reducing the antibody response to human serum albumin in rabbits [45]. The following year, they reported that administration of 6-mercaptopurine prolonged the survival of skin allografts in the rabbit [46]. Roy Calne, then a surgical trainee at the Royal Free Hospital in London, heard of this work and went on to demonstrate that 6-mercaptopurine also prolonged kidney allograft survival in the dog [47]. Independently, Zukoski and Hume working in Richmond, Virginia made the same observation [48].

Calne then traveled to Boston in order to undertake further research with Joseph Murray. On the way there he stopped off to visit George Hitchings and Trudy Elion at the Burroughs Wellcome Research Laboratories, and they provided him with a further supply of 6-mercaptopurine, together with a number of analogs of the parent compound, one of which was azathioprine (Figs. 1.8 and 1.9). In Boston, Calne and Murray demonstrated that azathioprine, like 6-mercaptopurine, prolonged the survival of canine kidney allografts [49]. The results obtained in the dog with azathioprine and 6-mercaptopurine, although better than those obtained with radiation, were far from perfect. Most of the animals died from infection or rejection, although there were some long-term successes. Similarly, patients given purine analogues did poorly, and, with few exceptions, rejected their organs soon after transplant [44, 50, 51].

While purines alone failed, the combination of purines with steroids proved effective. This advance, like many other developments in transplantation, was based to a large extent on empiricism: there were no preexisting experimental data to suggest that the combination would offer any synergistic benefit. Willard Goodwin at the University College of Los Angeles had added large doses of prednisolone to nitrogen mustard and successfully reversed rejection in a patient

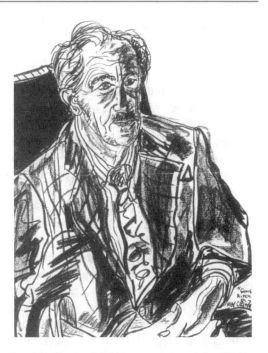

Fig. 1.8 George Hitchings as portrayed by Sir Roy Calne. Hitchings gave azathioprine to Calne for experimental study and later for successful use in human patients in Boston in the early 1960s. By courtesy of Roy Calne

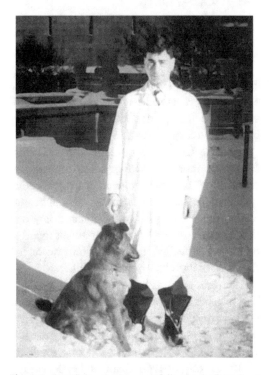

Fig. 1.9 Roy Calne as a research fellow at the Peter Bent Brigham Hospital, Boston, pictured with one of the first dogs (Lollipop) in which azathioprine was used successfully to prolong kidney allograft survival

with a kidney allograft [52]. Independently, Thomas Starzl, at the University of Colorado in Denver, gave large doses of prednisolone as a temporary measure to treat acute rejection in recipients of live donor kidney transplants who were receiving azathioprine as baseline immunosuppression [53]. The results from Denver were particularly impressive using the combined regimen, and the majority of treated patients showed prolonged graft survival to an extent hitherto unprecedented. The logical next step involved using steroids as part of the baseline therapy (instead of relying on them to rescue patients from rejection). The use of azathioprine and steroids was quickly adopted with success by Hume in Richmond, Murray in Boston, Woodruff in Edinburgh and by the French pioneers. As news of success spread, a large number of new kidney transplant units were established during the mid-1960s, and azathioprine and steroids became the standard immunosuppressive therapy.

1.8 Other Early Immunosuppression Strategies: Anti-Lymphocyte Antibody Therapy

Throughout the 1960s and 1970s, azathioprine and steroids remained the mainstay of immunosuppressive therapy for kidney transplantation, but several other approaches aimed at inhibiting lymphocyte activity were examined in an attempt to produce more effective or selective immunosuppression. Topical irradiation of the graft, total lymphoid irradiation and various surgical manipulations such as thymectomy, splenectomy and thoracic duct drainage were all tried but found to be either ineffective, overly problematic or too risky for routine clinical use [54–58].

However, one new approach that did prove to be a valuable addition to existing therapy was anti-lymphocyte globulin. Anti-lymphocyte serum had been shown to be effective in prolonging the survival of skin grafts in rodents during the early 1960s [59, 60]. In 1966, Starzl and colleagues in Denver reported on the use of a horse anti-lymphocyte globulin (ALG) preparation as an adjunct to

azathioprine and steroids in patients receiving a kidney transplant [61]. Thereafter, many other kidney transplant centers began using ALG to treat steroid resistant acute rejection, and some centers used it alongside azathioprine and steroids as baseline immunosuppression [62]. The increased immunosuppression provided by anti-lymphocyte antibody therapy also contributed to the early successes in heart and in liver transplants.

1.9 Histocompatibility Antigens, the Development of Tissue Typing, and the Advent of Organ Sharing

Rejection proved less problematic when the surgeons understood how to match donors and recipients. The importance of histocompatibility antigens in determining the fate of an allograft was readily apparent from the pioneering studies of mouse immunogenetics in the 1940s by Peter Gorer (Fig. 1.10) and George Snell. The discovery of human histocompatibility antigens (HLA) in the late 1950s can be attributed to three independent studies, namely by Jean Dausset in Paris, (he wrote the foreword of the first editor of this book) Rose Payne at Stanford and Jon Van Rood in Leiden. Dausset, who was awarded the Nobel Prize in 1983 alongside Snell and Benaceraf, identified the first leukocyte antigen [63]. Around the same time, Payne and Van Rood showed that sera obtained from multiparous women often contained agglutinating antibodies which reacted with leukocytes from their husbands and children and could be used as tools to identify different groups of leukocyte antigens [64, 65].

Progress in defining the human histocompatibility antigens by this serological approach was greatly facilitated by a regular series of International HLA workshops. The first of these workshops took place in 1964 at Durham, North Carolina, and was organized by Bernard Amos of Duke University. The second workshop took place the following year in Leiden, Holland, and further workshops were held biannually thereafter. These meetings allowed exchange of different antisera from around the world, sharing of

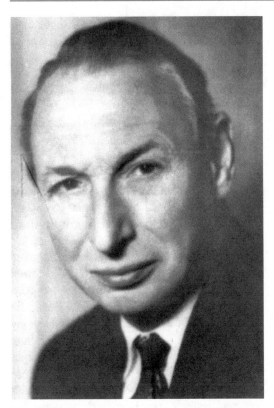

Fig. 1.10 Peter Gorer, the Guy's Hospital pathologist, demonstrated the first transplantation alloantibody in mice in 1936, and working with Snell later at Bar Harbour in 1946, the two agreed on the importance of the H2 region in mouse histocompatibility. Image from: Biographical Memoires of the Fellows of the Royal Society, vol. 7 (1961): 95–109

methodology and the establishment of a standardized nomenclature for HLA.

As kidney transplant activity expanded rapidly during the 1960s, there was widespread expectation by many of those involved that the problems of graft rejection could, to a large extent, be overcome by achieving a close tissue match between the donor and recipient. It was clear from studies in the mouse that histocompatibility antigens were critical determinants of graft rejection, and it was thought probable that histocompatibility antigens were also important determinants of graft rejection in humans. Kidney transplants between genetically related individuals were known to fare better than kidneys transplanted from unrelated donors. However, some grafts from unrelated donors did surprisingly well, possibly, it was thought, through fortuitous sharing of histocompatibility antigens.

Dausset began exploring the clinical implications of histocompatibility matching in 1962, collaborating with Felix Rapaport. Under the guidance of John Converse at the New York Medical Center, Rapaport had developed an interest in experimental skin grafting in humans. Working initially in New York and then in France, Rapaport and Dausset performed multiple skin grafts between both related and unrelated volunteers and showed convincingly that the serologically detected HLA antigens on leukocytes did indeed influence the fate of skin grafts [66, 67]. When the relatively crude antisera which were then available were used to determine tissue types in patients who had received a kidney transplant, the results suggested that matching of donor and recipient for the known tissue types might also benefit kidney graft survival [68, 69].

However, hopes that close matching of donor and recipient would confer a major benefit on kidney graft survival received a serious setback in 1970 when Paul Terasaki presented controversial data to a meeting of the Transplantation Society. His analysis demonstrated that cadaver kidneys poorly matched for HLA-A and HLA-B often did well. Conversely, some grafts that were apparently well matched did badly [70]. Terasaki's disappointing message to the transplant community led to the termination of his NIH research grant. Fortunately, his laboratory prospered through income arising from the sale of his novel microtest tissue typing trays.

Although the benefits of tissue typing had fallen short of expectations, it was generally accepted that cadaveric kidneys well matched for HLA-A and –B fared better than their poorly matched counterparts. A further significant advance in tissue typing came in 1978 when Alan Ting and Peter Morris in Oxford showed the importance of matching HLA-DR in cadaveric kidney transplantation [71]. Despite these convincing data, clinicians remained divided on the extent to which the relatively modest advantage in graft survival afforded by a well-matched graft justified the disadvantages of waiting for the right organ.

In addition to defining the role of HLA matching in kidney transplantation, tissue typing laboratories were quick to realize the importance of performing the lymphocytotoxic crossmatch test prior to kidney transplantation. In 1966, Kissmeyer-Nielson in the Danish city of Aarhus described two cases in which sensitized recipients rejected their kidney grafts immediately after transplantation. He termed the phenomenon hyperacute rejection and suggested that preformed antibodies directed against the graft were directly responsible for graft destruction [72]. Other laboratories reported similar cases, and the lymphocytotoxic crossmatch rapidly became a routine part of the pretransplant work-up [73, 74].

Because preformed cytotoxic antibodies were known to have a detrimental effect on allograft survival, there was understandable surprise when, in 1972, Gerhard Opelz, on behalf of Terasaki and his colleagues, presented data from a large retrospective study suggesting that patients who had received blood transfusions prior to renal transplantation actually had better allograft survival than their nontransfused counterparts [75]. Smaller studies from other centers had already hinted at the paradoxical effect of blood transfusion on kidney allograft survival, [76, 77] and the findings of Opelz were soon confirmed by others. As a result, renal transplant units adopted a policy of deliberate blood transfusion prior to listing patients for transplantation. This policy persisted until the early 1980s when the improved graft survival resulting from the use of the recently introduced immunosuppressive drug cyclosporine minimized any additional benefit from blood transfusion.

As the potential benefit of HLA matching became apparent in the late 1960s, enthusiastic tissue typers began to establish organ sharing schemes in order to optimize the opportunity for achieving well-matched transplants. Sharing both relied on and stimulated investigation in organ preservation (next section). Initial efforts were *ad hoc*, local affairs. Terasaki coordinated a group in Los Angeles in 1967; another alliance arose in Boston in 1968. Formally founded in 1969, the Eurotransplant Organization formed to organize exchanges across the continent. In the United States, the Southeastern Organ Procurement Foundation, initially between Duke and the Medical College of Virginia, evolved into the United Network for Organ Sharing (UNOS) that sets policy and coordinates transplants around the country.

1.10 Advances in Organ Preservation

Studies into methods for preserving organs during transplantation started at the beginning of the twentieth century with the experiments of Alexis Carrel who, before transplanting animal organs, flushed them with a physiologically balanced solution at room temperature [78]. Carrel envisioned storerooms of organs that surgeons could readily access and implant in patients. He later pioneered various methods to preserve body parts such as cryotherapy, tissue culture techniques, and, with aviator Charles Lindbergh, organ perfusion pumps [12, 79, 80]. While these technologies—particularly tissue culture—had a profound effects on biological science and vascular surgery, they did not significantly influence the trajectory of organ transplantation.

The modern era of organ preservation began in the late 1950s, delayed by the idea that flushing organs was dangerous. During experimental studies of canine liver transplantation, surface cooling of the liver had been found to reduce hypoxic damage [81]. Thomas Starzl and colleagues improved on this observation by advocating infusion of chilled Ringer's lactate solution into the portal vein of the canine liver [82]. During the early attempts at kidney transplantation, no attempt was made to cool the donor kidney, although it was sometimes flushed to prevent intravascular clots from forming. The practice of flushing human kidneys with chilled perfusate after their removal from the donor was not adopted until the early 1960s [83]. Before tissue-matching became common, organs rarely left a single hospital, moving from one operatory to another. With the prolonged ischemic times inherent in transferring organs around the country, hypothermic flushes had increased importance in preserving function.

In the later 1960s, Geoffrey Collins introduced a new cold flush solution, which provided much better results than those achieved previously using physiologically balanced electrolyte solutions. It was a major advance in organ preservation [84]. Collins' solution had a composition that approximated intracellular fluid (high potassium and low sodium) and thus limited the degree of cell swelling that occurred during hypothermic storage. Around the same time, Fred Belzer and his colleagues in Wisconsin popularized an alternative approach to cold storage based on continuous hypothermic perfusion of kidneys with cryoprecipitated plasma [85].

1.11   Early Attempts at Heart Transplantation

In the entire history of transplantation, the event that undoubtedly attracted the most public interest took place at the Groote Schuur Hospital in Cape Town, South Africa. On 3 December 1967, Christiaan Barnard, a 45-year-old cardiac surgeon, performed the world's first human heart transplant and overnight became a household name [86]. The recipient was a 54-year-old greengrocer. He had severe coronary artery disease and had developed a ventricular aneurysm after a myocardial infarct. Heart transplantation seemed to be the only possible way of saving his life. The opportunity to proceed with the operation presented itself when a 25-year-old female was admitted to the hospital with fatal injuries after accidentally being run over by a car while crossing the road. A few hours after her admission to hospital, cardiac activity ceased, she was declared dead and her heart was removed for transplantation. The heart transplant operation was, to the jubilation of the transplant team, a technical success. In an attempt to prevent graft rejection, the recipient was given chemical immunosuppression in the form of azathioprine and cortisone, together with a course of radiotherapy directed at the newly transplanted heart. The patient made good progress and gradually began to mobilize. Sadly, however, pulmonary infection developed a few days later, and mechanical ventilation was needed. Eighteen days after the transplant, the recipient died.

The events at the Groote Schuur created phenomenal media interest. The lay media elevated Barnard to the status of medical superstar, and his achievement was portrayed as one of the major advances of the twentieth century. Within the international transplant community, however, news that the operation had taken place in South Africa came as a surprise. Cardiac surgeons elsewhere, especially in North America, had been working methodically in animal models towards the goal of heart transplantation. Everyone recognized the first attempt was imminent; no one expected it to take place in Cape Town. The operation was not without controversy, and many in the field thought that Barnard's initial success deflected due recognition from North American pioneers, notably Richard Lower and Norman Shumway (Fig. 1.11), on whose experimental work the transplant surgery had depended [87].

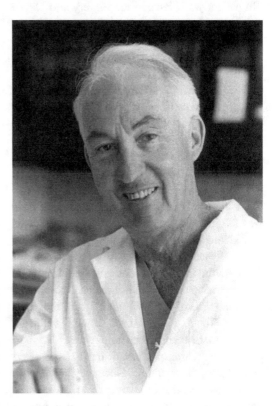

Fig. 1.11 Norman Shumway patiently developed human heart transplantation in the 1970s, prior to its general reintroduction later. By courtesy of Stanford University

In 1966, Barnard had visited several North American centers in preparation for his attempt at human heart transplantation. To learn more about immunosuppression he visited David Hume, the Boston surgeon who had since moved to Richmond, Virginia. Barnard also visited Norman Shumway in Palo Alto, whom he knew from working together under C. Walt Lillehei at the University of Minnesota. By 1967, Lower and Shumway were ready to perform a human heart transplant, but they believed that the best results would come from a brain-dead donor with a beating heart—something not considered to be possible in the United States under existing legislation.

Although Barnard performed the first human transplant, he was not the first person to attempt to place a new heart in a patient. James Hardy, at Jackson University Medical Center in Mississippi, had planned to perform a human cardiac transplant operation 4 years earlier [88]. A 68-year-old patient was prepared for surgery and placed on cardiopulmonary by-pass. The operation was to be carried out using a donor heart from a previously identified dying patient. After starting the recipient operation, arrangements to use the planned donor had to be abandoned. Since, by this stage, the recipient was on cardiopulmonary bypass, death was inevitable unless an alternative source for a donor heart could be identified immediately. The surgical team had performed large numbers of heart transplants in animal models, and they decided to give the patient a donor heart obtained from a chimpanzee. This was the first time a cardiac xenograft had been placed into a human. During the procedure it was apparent that the donor organ was incapable of fulfilling the mechanical demands required of it, and the transplant was an immediate failure.

At the time of the first human heart transplant in Cape Town, a number of surgical teams in North America and elsewhere were poised to attempt heart transplantation and had prepared carefully for the operation. Once they heard news of Barnard's operation, they proceeded quickly with their own cases. The world's second human heart transplant occurred on 7 December 1967 and was undertaken by Dr. Adrian Kantrowitz of Maimonides Medical Center, New York. The transplant, in which recipient and donor were both neonates, was unsuccessful, and the patient died several hours after surgery [89].

Barnard carried out a second heart transplant soon after his first case. The recipient was a 58-year-old white dentist, and the donor was a 24-year-old man who had died from cerebral hemorrhage. It was notable, given the apartheid present in South Africa, that the donor was of mixed race. The transplant operation was performed on 2 January 1968, and this time the recipient survived for over 18 months. Four days after the second transplant in Cape Town, Norman Shumway and his team started their clinical heart transplant program. Their first patient was a middle-aged man with chronic myocarditis who unfortunately died 2 weeks after transplantation.

In the months following the world's first human heart transplant, over one hundred heart transplants were carried out around the world. The transplant centers involved, in addition to those already mentioned, included units in Houston (Denton Cooley and Michael DeBakey), Richmond (Richard Lower) and Paris (Christian Cabrol). Although there were occasional successes, most of the recipients died in the days and weeks after their transplant; a mood of deep disappointment prevailed.

Because of the high failure rate, enthusiasm for heart transplantation waned, and by the early 1970s most centers had discontinued their heart transplant programs. Shumway's team at Stanford and Barnard's group in Cape Town were amongst the few centers that continued to perform the operation, [90] and both made important contributions to the field. For example, a serious problem after heart transplantation was the difficulty in diagnosing graft rejection before it led to irreversible deterioration in the recipient. The demonstration by Philip Caves in the mid-1970s that early rejection could be diagnosed by transjugular endomyocardial biopsy was therefore a significant step forward [91]. Another innovation in heart transplantation was the so-called supplementary or piggyback heart transplant. This procedure was first performed by Barnard and, between 1974 and 1977, he carried out a number of heterotopic or supplementary heart transplant operations in which the recipient's own heart was left in situ and the donor anastomosed to it. The technique was subsequently taken up by other centers, which used it occasionally with some success [92].

1.12 Brain Death

Heart transplants, alongside new intensive care units featuring ventilators and other advanced technology, prompted discussion over the definition of death. Previously, kidneys and other organs came from either living donors or individual whose hearts had stopped beating—a traditional understanding of death in Western Society. For hearts in particular, surgeons recognized the importance of limiting ischemic time. In these same years, patients in ICUs were being kept "alive" on machines where they had a heart beat but no neurological activity. Irreversible brain-death (le coma dépassé) had been described in 1959 by French neurologists but was infrequently diagnosed [93]. Transplants were rare enough—most hospitals did not perform the operation at all—that the notion of removing organs from a beating-heart donor was inconceivable at that time. As transplants became more common and the importance of short ischemic time more important, the plausibility and potential value of such a practice increased. 1966 marked the first time organs were removed from a brain dead donor, immediately raising complex ethical questions.

In 1968, Harvard Medical School created the Ad Hoc Committee Brain Death in an effort to address some of the issues surrounding ICU care. Initiated prior to Barnard's landmark case and its ensuing attention, the panel was chaired by anesthesiologist-ethicist Henry K. Beecher and included transplant surgeon Joseph Murray [94]. Published in JAMA, their joint statement explicitly tried to avoid linking brain death to organ procurement, although many doctors and lay people quickly drew a connection between the two. The definition, undergoing some alteration, slowly spread around the United States and later the western world. In the UK, criteria for the diagnosis of brainstem death were published in 1976, [95] and in the late 1970s the use of heart-beating donors became routine. This greatly improved the quality of the organs procured and was particularly important for ensuring retrieval of viable donor hearts and livers.

The conceptualization of brain death has not been as widely accepted in many Asian countries such as China, India, and Japan. The vast majority of nations have recently passed laws legalizing the practice, but strong cultural moves link life to a beating heart. As a result, around 90% of livers in Asia come from living donors (compared to under 1% in the US) [96]. While this cultural variation has made heart transplants less common, it has simultaneously catalyzed new techniques in liver donation, particularly in regards to living donor, split-liver transplantation.

1.13 The First Attempts at Lung and Heart-Lung Transplantation

Surgeons quickly moved from the heart to other thoracic organs. Demikhov in the Soviet Union had attempted experimental heart and lung transplantation in dogs during the 1940s, but most of the animals died within a few hours of surgery [97]. Twenty years later, Lower and colleagues, using cardiopulmonary bypass, demonstrated that dogs could survive for several days after combined cardiopulmonary transplantation [98]. In 1968, Denton Cooley in Houston performed the world's first heart-lung transplant, but the patient, an infant, died within the first 24 hours [99]. During the 1970s, there were isolated attempts at heart-lung transplantation at other centers, including Cape Town, but there was no long-term success.

The first human lung transplantation was undertaken on 11 June 1963 by James Hardy and his team in Jackson, Mississippi [100]. The recipient was a 58-year-old man who had been sentenced to death for committing murder. Whilst incarcerated in the State Penitentiary, the prisoner, whose general medical condition was very poor, had been found to have a carcinoma of the lung. He agreed to undergo lung transplantation and, on the basis of this agreement, his original sentence of death was commuted. At the operation, his left lung, containing the carcinoma, was excised, but the tumor had already spread outside the confines of the lung. Nevertheless, he was given a single-lung transplant from a patient who had died after a myocardial infarct. The pulmonary veins and arteries of the donor and recipient were anastomosed, as was the main bronchus. Although the graft functioned initially, the recipient's condition deteriorated and he died in renal failure after 18 days. Over the next few years, Hardy and several other groups carried out occasional single-lung or lobe transplants, but none of the patients survived beyond the first few weeks [101]. Dehiscence of the bronchial anastomosis during the early post-transplant period was a major cause of mortality.

The first human lung transplant patient to survive beyond the first month was a young Belgian miner who had developed respiratory failure due to advanced silicosis. Fritz Derom, in Ghent, performed the operation in 1968, transplanting a single-lung from a donor who had died following a cerebrovascular accident [102]. The recipient received azathioprine, prednisolone and antilymphocyte serum. He made a good recovery but died about 10 months later. John Haglin and colleagues in Minnesota carried out the first double-lung transplant in 1970, but it also was not successful.

1.14   Early Attempts at Transplantation of the Liver

The first attempts at human liver transplantation took place in Denver in the early 1960s and were performed by Thomas Starzl. Before moving to Denver in 1961 as associate professor of surgery, Starzl had worked in Chicago. There he had developed an experimental liver transplant program in the dog and had pioneered the use of veno-venous bypass during the anhepatic phase

of the operation. He had also devised the use of cold flush of the donor liver to accelerate cooling and thus improve preservation. After arriving in Denver, Starzl initially concentrated on kidney transplantation, performing a series of living donor kidney transplants using a combination of azathioprine and steroids to prevent rejection. Then on 1 March 1963, he undertook the world's first human liver transplant. The recipient was a 3-year-old boy who had biliary atresia, and the donor was another child who had died during open-heart surgery. The operation proved more formidable than had been expected, not least because of coagulopathy, and unfortunately the child died in the operating theater [103]. Starzl undertook a second liver transplant in May 1963. This time the recipient was an adult with hepatocellular carcinoma who survived for only 3 weeks after the procedure. Subsequent liver transplants suffered a similar fate, and by 1964 a decision had been made to suspend the liver transplant program in Denver. The Boston surgeons, who had considerable experience in experimental liver work, also performed an unsuccessful human liver transplant operation during this time.

Three years later, in 1967, Starzl restarted liver transplantation. The recipients were initially infants and children and, in contrast to the earlier series, ALG was included in the immunosuppressive therapy. The first seven recipients in the series all survived the operation, and although four died in the ensuing months, three children lived longer [104]. Meanwhile, liver transplantation was also being undertaken in Europe. Roy Calne, who had become Professor of Surgery in Cambridge, carried out the first European liver transplant in 1968 and was, together with Starzl, a major pioneer in this area. Calne subsequently formed a fruitful partnership with Roger Williams, a hepatologist at Kings College Hospital in London. In 1968, European liver transplant programs also started in Groningen and in Hanover. Overall, however, the results of liver transplantation throughout the 1970s were disappointing, and there were relatively few long-term survivors. Only a handful of enthusiastic centers maintained active liver transplant programs during this period.

1.15   Early Attempts at Pancreas Transplantation

Attempts to treat diabetes in man by transplanting fragments of pancreas date back to the latter part of the last century, but transplantation of a vascularized organ graft was not undertaken until 1966. Richard Lillehei in Minneapolis led the team responsible and developed the method of transplanting the entire pancreas along with the duodenum—a technique analogous to that currently used. The recipients in Lillehei's series had diabetic nephropathy and were usually given a simultaneous kidney and pancreas transplant. Lillehei and his team had a modest degree of success. Their results, reported in their classic paper, included a patient whose graft survived for over 1 year [105]. A small number of pancreas transplants were undertaken subsequently in other centers, but the procedure remained fraught with technical complication, related predominantly to leakage of exocrine secretions from the duct, and there was little enthusiasm for the procedure amongst diabetologists. By the late 1970s, attention had focused on segmental rather than whole organ grafts. Various procedures had been advocated for dealing with the exocrine component of the graft. These included injection of neoprine into the duct to destroy the exocrine tissue as proposed by Jean-Michel Dubernard in Lyon. Other centers experimented with islet-cell transplants, which precluded the need for the recipient to undergo a major surgery. As beta-islet cells comprise only 1–2% of the pancreas, isolating them in sufficient quantity has proven challenging, as have efforts to maintain enough of them in the host to stave off diabetes [106]. Although the number of transplants gradually increased during the 1970s, most of these were performed by a relatively small number of enthusiastic centers, most notably David Sutherland's group in Minneapolis.

1.16   Modern Immuno-suppression: Calcineurin Inhibitors

The introduction of cyclosporine into clinical practice at the end of the 1970s was the most significant advance in immunosuppressive therapy since azathioprine became available in 1963. Cyclosporine was discovered during routine screening of fungal extracts at the Sandoz laboratories in Basle and proved to have potent anti-lymphocytic activity [107]. Jean-François Borel, a scientist at Sandoz, demonstrated the in vivo immunosuppressive properties of the new drug (designated 24–556) initially in the mouse and then in other animal species [108]. Borel presented his findings on cyclosporine at the Spring 1976 meeting of the British Society of Immunology. David White, a young immunologist from Roy Calne's department in Cambridge, was in the audience and arranged to have some of the new agent sent to Cambridge. When the Cambridge group tested the agent, they found it was remarkably effective at prolonging allograft survival in rodents and dogs; initially, it appeared to be free from adverse side effects [109, 110]. This success in preclinical studies gave Calne and colleagues the confidence to carry out pilot studies in the clinic. They found that cyclosporine was indeed a potent immunosuppressive drug and used it as the only agent in cadaveric renal transplantation. However, somewhat unexpectedly, it caused significant side effects, especially nephro- and hepatotoxicity, neither of which had been predicted from animal studies [111, 112]. Early experience of cyclosporine in Boston and other European transplant centers was also rather disappointing because of major side effects and, for a short time, the future of the new drug seemed in doubt. However, Tom Starzl in Denver also obtained a supply of the new drug and, in contrast to the Cambridge team who used cyclosporine alone, Starzl used the agent together with steroids in kidney graft recipients whereupon he obtained excellent results [113]. In retrospect, it became clear that the dose of cyclosporine used in most of the early clinical studies had been excessive, and this accounted for many of the adverse side effects seen. Large multicenter trials in North America and Europe subsequently affirmed the effectiveness of cyclosporine. By the mid-1980s it had become the mainstay of immunosuppressive therapy in organ transplantation [114, 115].

The late 1980s and early 1990s saw a number of further developments in organ transplantation. Scientists in Japan [116] discovered a novel fungal metabolite designated FK506 (tacrolimus). Starzl's group demonstrated its efficacy as an immunosuppressive agent in 1989 [117]. Ironically, Roy Calne in Cambridge had tested the ability of FK506 to prolong the survival of canine kidney allograft but had abandoned the drug because of the severe side effects it produced at high doses. However, clinical studies in Pittsburgh by Starzl showed it to be a potent immunosuppressive agent with an acceptable side effect profile, and it quickly replaced cyclosporine in the clinical armamentarium. While technically not a calcineurin inhibitor, sirolimus functioned similarly by blocking mTOR [118]. Discovered in the soil of Rapa Nui (hence the trade name Rapamycin or Rapamune) in the 1970s, it was initially classified as an anti-fungal agent until the success of tacrolimus stimulated investigation into its immunosuppressive potential. A series of large trials in both Europe in the United States in the 1990s proved its efficacy and safety, and the drug entered routine use [119].

1.17 The Modern Era of Organ Transplantation

These more advanced immunosuppressive regimens launched the modern era of organ transplantation. Cyclosporine not only improved the results of kidney transplantation but also had a decisive influence on the development of heart, lung, liver and pancreas transplantation: the operations succeeded often enough to move beyond the realm of experiment and into regular clinical practice. This transition was most evident in the field of heart transplantation. Shumway's team in Stanford had been one of the only centers to maintain an active heart transplant program throughout the 1970s, and when they used cyclosporine, the one-year patient survival improved from around 40% to 70%. Using cyclosporine-based immunosuppression, Shumway and Ritz carried out four combined heart–lung transplants in 1981, and although one patient died, the other three recipients survived for periods ranging from 2 to 4 years. Successful cases of single-lung transplantation were also reported, most notably from Toronto [120]. As a result of the improved success in thoracic organ transplantation, the number of hospitals in Europe and North America performing those operations proliferated [121]. Similar improvements in the results of hepatic and pancreas transplantation were also achieved with cyclosporine, leading to a dramatic increase in the number of centers undertaking these procedures.

The improvement in the results of organ transplantation during the 1980s was not due exclusively to superior immunosuppression. There were also refinements in patient selection, surgical technique and postoperative management. For example, in the case of liver transplantation, increasing experience gradually led to improvements in technique, a reduction in biliary complications and problems from coagulopathy. The use of "split" and "cut down" techniques allowed the implantation of adult donor livers in pediatric recipients. In the case of pancreata, the wheel turned full circle in the 1990s when transplantation of the whole organ together with the duodenum once again became the standard technique, with drainage of the exocrine secretions into the bladder or small intestine. For the heart, total artificial implants have not lived up to their purported potential, but ventricular assist devices have definitely proven their value in a series of trials as both bridges to transplant and as effective treatments for patients in severe heart failure who do not qualify to receive an organ [122].

Organ preservation has also improved significantly. The late 1980s witnessed a significant step forward with the invention of the University of Wisconsin (UW) solution by Belzer's laboratory. The new solution was initially developed with a view to improving the preservation of pancreas grafts, [123] but Neville Jamieson and coworkers in Belzer's laboratory showed that it dramatically extended the safe preservation time for canine liver transplantation [124]. Although also useful for kidney preservation, UW solution had its largest impact on liver transplantation, where it extended the safe storage of livers from 6 to 24 h.

Lately, the field has returned to exploring perfusion pumps, not only for their potential to preserve organs during ischemic time but also to improve their baseline function. The underlying idea dates back to Carrel and Lindbergh, and many North American kidney transplant centers adopted machine perfusion of kidneys during the 1970s. However, the added complexity of machine perfusion and the lack of major advantages over simple cold storage led to a decline in its popularity in the 1970s. Most centers abandoned it, reverting instead to simple cold flush with UW and storage in ice.

More recently, ex-vivo perfusion has returned to prominence—and not just in kidneys but in livers, lungs, and hearts as well [125–127]. These inchoate interventions remain under investigation as teams at different institutes experiment with various formulae for the nutrient bath and debate whether to rely on hypothermic or normothermic temperatures, but head-to-head comparisons with standard, cold ischemia demonstrate the potential of the technology. Critically, new perfusion modalities not only do a better job preserving tissue during ischemic time but actually improve the functionality of marginal organs otherwise unsuitable for transplant [127, 128]. In so doing, they have the potential to expand exponentially the number of available organs, helping address the long-standing, seemingly unsolvable issue of lengthy waitlists.

The deeply troubling issue of too few organs has led to innovative attempts to redress the shortage. A renewed emphasis on live donors have helped [129]. More recently, programs have tried to maximize their potential even when a willing donor and specific recipient do not match by setting up kidney exchange programs [130]. Envisioned in 1986, the idea has been adopted in multiple countries and, utilizing complex com-puter algorithms, been expanded to create "daisy-chains" of over a dozen participants. While often providing recipients with well-matched, fresh organs, paired-donor programs only add about 400 organs to the pool each year in the US, helping but not solving the problem. Donation after circulatory death represents another option to increase the supply. Prior to the acceptance of brain death in the late 1960s and early 1970s, all organs came from patients who had suffered cardiac arrests, but this modality fell from favor given the comparative ease and superior quality of organs obtained from brain dead individuals. In 1993, the first year UNOS began tracking that category, only 41 DCD organs were procured in the United States. As demand continued to increase and preservation technology improved, doctors looked to expand the pool of potential donors by returning to donation after cardiac death. In 2019, American surgeons procured 2130 DCD organs, a 50-fold increase over 15 years [131]. Most recent studies have demonstrated outcomes similar to other deceased donors [132].

The benefits of calcineurin inhibitors materially changed the field of organ transplantation, but progress over the last few decades has slowed: while episodes of acute rejection have fallen significantly, long-term graft survival has not changed appreciably. New biologics promise to end that stalemate. When in 1975 George Kohler and Caesar Milstein developed monoclonal antibodies, [133] there were high hopes that such agents would provide potent new tools for manipulating the immune response during human organ transplantation. The first such antibody to be used in transplantation was OKT3, a mouse monoclonal antibody directed against the CD3 molecule on human T cells. The efficacy of this antibody in treating kidney allograft rejection was initially documented in a pilot study of 10 patients in 1981 [134] and then confirmed subsequently in a randomized clinical trial [135]. OKT3 was undoubtedly a useful new immunosuppressive drug, but monoclonal antibodies did not initially have the impact on clinical transplantation that many had expected, at least partly due to its activating effects on T cells leading to cytokine release syndrome in some patients.

The last 20 years have seen rapid developments with these modalities. Calne developed an anti-CD-54 antibody, alemtuzumab (campath), that effectively depletes lymphocytes and more transiently depletes B cells and monocytes. Multiple studies have demonstrated its efficacy as induction therapy with reduced rates of rejection [136, 137]. Lately, surgeon-scientists have tried using biologics like imlifidase, tocilizumab, and bortezomib to de-sensitize patients who could otherwise never find a matching organ; early results are promising [138–140].

Increasingly, scientists are looking to the potential of biologicals as part of an as-yet aspirational strategy to achieve tolerance [141]. Groups at MGH, Stanford, and Northwestern have tried inducing mixed chimerism, which has mostly succeeded in HLA-matched donor-recipient pairs, although remains limited by questions of durability and the significant risks of graft versus host disease. Other efforts, including the multi-national European "One Study," are examining potential of regulatory T cells in suppressing the immune system and inducing tolerance [142]. Teams have also explored the potential of co-stimulatory blockade with agents like belatacept, which inhibits T-cell activation. Phase III trials demonstrated outcomes in EBV positive patients that were superior to traditional triple therapy and, for the first time since cyclosporine, have increased the overall half-life of kidney grafts [143, 144]. Other efforts, like those around drugs such as carfilzomib, center on controlling B and plasma cells. Work remains ongoing, but the role of biologics in immunosuppression and, perhaps, the holy grail of tolerance, seems certain to increase.

1.18 New Plastic Transplants

The field of transplantation started with Cosmas and Damien replacing a diseased leg; the profession has returned to such roots with recent accomplishments in limb, face, and genitalia attachments. The world's first arm transplant, taking surgery into a realm previously occupied only by science fiction, was carried out at the Edouard Herriot Hospital in Lyon, France on 23 September 1998. The international team included Jean Michel Dubernard (Lyon), Earl Owen (Sydney), Nadey Hakim (London), Marco Lanzetta (Milan), Hari Kapila (Sydney), Guillaume Herzberg (Lyon) and Marwan Dawahra (Lyon). It took 13 hours to attach the hand and forearm of a 48-year-old man from New Zealand who had his arm severed below the elbow in an accident with a circular saw in 1984. Since that first transplant dozens of others have been performed, one of them being a double arm transplant again performed in Lyon by the same team [145, 146]. The success of these cases demonstrated the possibilities of vascularized composite allografts and prompted further work.

On 7 November 2005, Dubernard led a large, multi-disciplinary team in performing the first face transplant on Isabelle Dinoire, a woman whose pet dog had macerated her face, biting off her nose, lips, chin, and cheeks [147, 148]. This operation attracted global media attention. While most other transplants were hidden (kidney, etc) or non-identifying (hand), the highly personal nature of the human face introduced questions about the psychological effects of the transplant. In a 2012 interview, Dinoire admitted, "when I look in the mirror, I see a mixture of the two [of us]. The donor is always with me," although she insisted that only her face, not her personality had changed [149]. The first grafts were partial, but by 2010, full-face transplants—including facial bones—had been completed. Over the last 12 years, surgeons around the world have performed 40 face transplants of increasingly complexity, generally with good cosmetic and functional results [150]. It remains a complex procedure, both technically and medically. The vast majority of recipients have suffered at least one episode of acute rejection, and more than a third have developped infections, demonstrating the challenge of balancing immunosuppresion.

More recently, efforts have expanded into penile transplants. In 2006, Weilie Hu led a team at Guangzhou General Hospital that grafted a penis onto a 44 year man who had suffered a traumatic amputation that made micturition difficult, fornication impossible, and caused severe mental distress [151]. Unfortunately, the recipient and his wife were unable to tolerate the graft psychologically, requiring a transplant penectomy on post-operative day 14, a result that led to some criticism for poor patient selection. A South African team consisting Frank Graewe, André van der Merwe, and Rafique Moosa performed the first lasting penile transplant on a 21 year-old victim of a botched circumcision, with good results in 2014 [152]. Given the commonality of improvised explosive devices in Iraq and Afghanistan causing severe pelvic trauma, interest in the procedure has increased, with mainstream media coverage of penis transplants in wounded veterans [153].

These soft tissue grafts raise interesting ethical issues. Surgery in general, and especially transplant surgery with its mandatory immunosuppressive regimen, carries significant risks to the patient. Indeed, Dinoire, the patient who received the first face transplant, died 11 years after her index operation from cancer likely attributable to her suppressed immune system. Any decision to operate must establish benefits that outweigh those risks. In such a calculus, heart, liver, and kidney transplants clearly provide life-sustaining therapy [154]. The value of a hand or a penis is more questionable—one can certainly live without them. That both surgeons and patients feel comfortable accepting the risks of surgery and immunosuppression for non-lifesaving transplants indicates just how far the field has come since its inception in the 1950s.

1.19 Xenotransplantation and Future Directions

Xenotransplanation has been "just around the corner" for over a century, but techniques in gene therapy and research in genetic tolerance make it appear more realistic than ever. The idea of placing animal parts in humans has obvious appeal, eliminating the clinical, ethical, financial, and social problems of acquiring human organs. The idea of mixing tissue of different species dates at least to the Greek mythological Chimera, and various attempts of attaching animal parts to

human bodies appear sporadically through the literature. After surgeons demonstrated the ability of immunosuppression to allow unrelated human-to-human transplants, Keith Reemtsma, noting the lack of suitable human donors for his end-stage uremic patients and not having access to hemodialysis, turned to primates for organs. In 1963, he implanted kidneys from rhesus monkeys into two of his patients at Tulane in New Orleans; both rejected the kidney and subsequently died [155]. Multiple other teams from around the world attempted similar procedures; none achieved long-term success [156]. In 1984, a young child in California was born with a hypoplastic left heart. Given the high mortality of the Norwood procedure and the improbability of acquiring a human organ, Leonard Bailey elected to implant the heart of a female baboon into Baby Fae. Despite Bailey's work on xenotransplantation in the laboratory and the promise of new drugs like cyclosporin, Baby Fae died from rejection 21 days later [157]. The interspecies immunogenicity overpowered contemporary therapies. Investigative efforts continued with great promise but generally poor results.

New research in genetic medicine has overcome some of the earlier problems. In particular, Crispr-Cas9 technology empowers scientists to modify the fundamental genetic code of organisms, reducing cross-species differences. Pharmaceutical and start-up companies around the world have latched onto this technology, breeding litters of genetically altered pigs designed to produce organs compatible with humans [158]. In December 2018, Matthias Längin and his team publishing exciting results in *Nature* that demonstrated pig hearts supporting the life of baboons for up to 945 days (when they were euthanized) [159]. Critically, success depended on the use of organ perfusion pumps and specific medications to reduce cardiac hypertrophy (temsirolimus), again highlighting the importance of integrating multiple avenues of research when pushing the boundaries of science. Xenotransplantation is the future of transplant surgery—and perhaps, as Shumway often intimated, it always will be. But recent discoveries and work in genetic medicine hold particular promise, and the next edition of this chapter will likely recount clinical trials of pig hearts in human bodies.

1.20 Conclusion

Over half a century has now passed since Peter Medawar established the scientific basis for transplantation, and during this time the field has made remarkable progress. Transplantation of abdominal and thoracic organs is now commonplace. Many major hospitals have renal transplant programs, and most large regional centers also have programs for transplantation of the liver, pancreas, heart and lung. These organ transplant operations no longer attract special interest within the hospital in which they are undertaken and are not considered to be particularly newsworthy by the media. The most important key to success was undoubtedly the development of effective immunosuppressive therapy such that the loss of organ grafts from acute rejection is now relatively uncommon. One year graft survival rates after solid organ transplantation hover around 90%. However, many grafts continue to fail in the longer term due to chronic rejection. The demonstration of immunological tolerance by Medawar in the 1950s raised hopes that a clinically applicable strategy for inducing transplant tolerance might be developed in due course. Such an approach would prevent graft rejection and eliminate the problems of infection and malignancy that occur with non-specific immunosuppressive therapy. Recent developments in molecular biology have undoubtedly brought the prospect of tolerance, the Holy Grail of transplantation, a little nearer, but much work remains to be done. Similarly, although transgenic technology has raised hopes for the success of xenotransplantation, major obstacles remain to be overcome before this can be introduced into the clinic. Transplantation has come a long way since the first tentative steps with kidney transplantation in the 1950s, but there is still a considerable distance to go before these problems are surmounted.

1.21 Questions

1. With what miracle are Saints Cosmas and Damian credited?
2. Who performed the first ever human to human kidney transplant operation?
3. What surgical technique did Mathieu Jaboulay and Alexis Carrel describe?
4. What is the "second set" phenomenon? Who developed the first dialysis machine?
5. Who developed the first dialysis shunt?
6. Where and when was the first long-term successful kidney transplant performed?
7. Who was Joseph Murray? What is the historical relevance of the Boston identical twin kidney transplants?
8. In which countries were most of the pioneering kidney transplants performed during the 1950s?
9. What important points did the classical 1955 paper by David Hume and colleagues make?
10. What major advance did Geoffrey Collins make to organ transplantation?
11. Who made the landmark observation on the induction of neonatal tolerance?
12. Which was the first drug shown to prolong survival of skin allografts in the rabbit?
13. To whom is the discovery of HLA contributed?
14. Who showed the importance of matching for HLA-DR in cadaveric kidney transplant?
15. Where was the first cadaveric xenograft performed?
16. Who performed the world's first heart-lung transplant?
17. Who performed the first human lung transplant, who survived beyond the first month?
18. When, where, and by whom was performed the world's first human liver transplant?
19. Who led the team who performed the world's first human pancreas transplant?

References

1. Hamilton D. A history of organ transplantation: from ancient legends to modern practice. Pittsburgh: University of Pittsburgh Press; 2012.

2. Rinaldi E. The first homoplastic limb transplant according to the legend of saint Cosmas and Saint Damian. Ital J Orthop Traumatol. 1987;13:393–406.
3. Schlich T. How gods and saints became transplant surgeons. Hist Sci. 1995;33(101):311–31.
4. Schlich T. The origins of organ transplantation: surgery and laboratory science, 1880–1930. Rochester: University of Rochester Press; 2010.
5. Hamilton D. The monkey gland affair. London: Chatto & Windus; 1986.
6. Jaboulay M. Greffe de reins au pli du coude par soudures arterielles et veineuses. Lyon Med. 1906;107(39):575–83.
7. Winkler EA. Ernst Unger: a pioneer in modern surgery. J Hist Med Allied Sci. 1982;37(3):269–86.
8. Hamilton D, Reid W. Obstetrics. Yu. Yu. Voronoy and the first human kidney allograft. Surg Gyencol Obstet. 1984;159(3):289–94.
9. Barr J. Surgical repair of the arteries in war and peace. Rochester: University of Rochester Press; 2019.
10. Carrel A. La technique opératoire des anastomoses vasculaires et de la transplantation des viscères. Lyon Med. 1902;98:859–64.
11. Carrel A. The transplantation of organs. A preliminary communication. J Am Med Assoc. 1905;45(22):1645–6.
12. Hamilton D. The first transplant surgeon: the flawed genius of Nobel prize winner, Alexis Carrel. London: World Scientific Press; 2017.
13. Pendray E. Twelve men who changed the world. Georgetown archives, carrel collection, box 44.
14. Turney J. Frankenstein's footsteps: science, genetics and popular culture. New Haven: Yale University Press; 1998.
15. Lederer SE. Frankenstein: penetrating the secrets of nature. New Brunswick, NJ: Rutgers University Press; 2002.
16. Lederer SE. Flesh and blood: organ transplantation and blood transfusion in twentieth century America. New York: Oxford University Press; 2008.
17. Pelis K. Taking credit: the Canadian Army medical corps and the British conversion to blood transfusion in WWI. J Hist Med Allied Sci. 2001;56(3):238–77.
18. Swanson KW. Banking on the body: the market in blood, milk, and sperm in modern America. Cambridge: Harvard University Press; 2014. p. 333.
19. Silverstein AM. A history of immunology. Saint Louis: Elsevier Science; 2012.
20. Schöne G. Die Heteroplastische und Homöoplastiche transplantation. Berlin: Springer; 1912.
21. Gibson T, Medawar PB. The fate of skin homografts in man. J Anat. 1943;77:299–310.
22. Medawar PB. The behaviour and fate of skin autografts and skin homografts in rabbits: a report to the war wounds Committee of the Medical Research Council. J Anat. 1944;78:176–99.
23. Lawler RH, West JW, McNulty PH, Clancy EJ, Murphy RP. Homotransplantation of the kidney in the human: supplemental report of a case. J Am Med Assoc. 1951;147(1):45–6.
24. Dubost C, Oeconomos N, Nenna A, Milliez P. Results d'une tentative de greffe rénale. Bulletins et Memoires de la Societe Medicale des Hospitaux de Paris. 1951;67:1372–82.
25. Kuss R, Teinturier J, Milliez P. Quelques essais de greffe de rein chez l'homme. Mem Acad Chir. 1951;77:755–68.
26. Michon L, Hamburger J, Oeconomos N, Delinotte P, Richet G, Vaysse J, et al. Une tentative de transplantation renale chez l'homme. Aspects medicaux et biologiques Presse Medical. 1953;1501(61):1419–23.
27. Peitzman SJ. Dropsy, dialysis, transplant: a short history of failing kidneys. Baltimore: The Johns Hopkins University Press; 2007.
28. Hume DM, Merrill JP, Miller BF, Thorn GW. Experiences with renal homotransplantation in the human: report of nine cases. J Clin Invest. 1955;34(2):327–82.
29. Merrill JP, Murray JE, Harrison JH, Guild WR. Successful homotransplantation of the human kidney between identical twins. J Am Med Assoc. 1956;160(4):277–82.
30. Brown JB. Homo grafting of skin: with report of success in identical twins. Surgery. 1937;1(4):558–63.
31. Billingham RE, Brent L, Medawar PB. Actively acquired tolerance of foreign cells. Nature. 1953;172:603–6.
32. Billingham RE, Brent L, Medawar PB. Quantitative studies on tissue transplantation immunity. III. Actively acquired tolerance. Philos Trans Royal Soc Lond B Biol Sci. 1956;239:357–414.
33. Burnet FM, Fenner F. The production of antibodies. 2nd ed. Melbourne: Macmillan; 1949.
34. Owen RD. Immunogenetic consequences of vascular anastomoses between bovine twins. Science. 1945;102(2651):400–1.
35. Mitchison NA. Passive transfer of transplantation immunity. Nature. 1953;171(4345):267–8.
36. Billingham RE, Brent L, Medawar PB. Quantitative studies on tissue transplantation immunity. II. The origin, strength and duration of actively and adoptively acquired immunity. Proc R Soc Lond. 1954;143(910):58–80.
37. Gowans J. The effect of the continuous re-infusion of lymph and lymphocytes on the output of lymphocytes from the thoracic duct of unanaesthetized rats. Br J Exp Pathol. 1957;38(1):67–81.
38. Terasaki P. Identification of the type of blood-cell responsible for the graft-versus-host reaction in chicks. Development. 1959;7(3):394–408.
39. McGregor D, McCullagh P, Gowans JL. The role of lymphocytes in antibody formation I. Restoration of the haemolysin response in X-irradiated rats with lymphocytes from normal and immunologically tolerant donors. Proc R Soc Lond B. 1967;168(1012):229–43.
40. Miller JFAP. Effect of neonatal thymectomy on the immunological responsiveness of the mouse. J Proc Royal Soc. 1962;156(964):415–28.

41. Brent LB. A history of transplantation immunology. San Diego: Academic; 2005.

42. Murray JE, Merrill JP, Dammin GJ, Dealy JB Jr, Alexandre GW, Harrison JH. Kidney transplantation in modified recipients. Ann Surg. 1962;156(3):337–55.

43. Merrill JP, Murray JE, Harrison JH, Friedman EA, Dealy JB Jr, Dammin G. Successful homotransplantation of the kidney between nonidentical twins. N Engl J Med. 1960;262(25):1251–60.

44. Kuss R, Legrain M, Mathe G, Nedey R, Camey M. Homologous human kidney transplantation: experience with six patients. Postgrad Med J. 1962;38(443):528–31.

45. Schwartz R, Dameshek W. Drug-induced immunological tolerance. Nature. 1959;183(4676):1682–3.

46. Schwartz R, Dameshek W, Donovan J. The effects of 6-mercaptopurine on homograft reactions. J Clin Invest. 1960;39(6):952–8.

47. Calne R. The rejection of renal homografts. Inhibition in dogs by 6-mercaptopurine. Lancet. 1960;1(7121):417–8.

48. Zukoski C, Lee H, Hume D. The effect of 6-mercaptopurine on renal homograft survival in the dog. Surg Gyencol Obstet. 1961;112:707–14.

49. Calne RY, Alexandre G, Murray J. A study of the effects of drugs in prolonging survival of homologous renal transplants in dogs. Ann N Y Acad Sci. 1962;99(3):743–61.

50. Hopewell J, Calne RY, Beswick I. Three clinical cases of renal transplantation. Br Med J. 1964;1(5380):411–3.

51. Murray JE, Merrill JP, Harrison JH, Wilson RE, Dammin G. Prolonged survival of human-kidney homografts by immunosuppressive drug therapy. N Engl J Med. 1963;268(24):1315–23.

52. Goodwin WE, Kaufman JJ, Mims MM, Turner RD, Glassock R, Goldman R, et al. Human renal transplantation. I, clinical experiences with six cases of renal homotransplantation. J Urol. 1963;89(1):13–24.

53. Starzl TE, Marchioro TL, Waddell WR. The reversal of rejection in human renal homografts with subsequent development of homograft tolerance. Surg Gyencol Obstet. 1963;117:385–95.

54. Starzl TE, Marchioro TL, Talmage DW, Waddell WR. Splenectomy and thymectomy in human renal homotransplantation. Proc Soc Exp Biol Med. 1963;113(4):929–32.

55. Tilney N, Murray J, editors. Thoracic duct fistula in human being renal transplantation. Surgical forum. 1966.

56. Franksson C, Blomstrand R. Drainage of the thoracic lymph duct during homologous kidney transplantation in man. Scand J Urol Nephrol. 1967;1(2):123–31.

57. Hume D, Lee H, Williams GM, White H, Ferre J, Wolf J, et al. Comparative results of cadaver and related donor renal homografts in man, and immunologic implications of the outcome of second and paired transplants. Ann Surg. 1966;164(3):352–97.

58. Myburgh JA, Smit JA, Meyers AM, Botha JR, Browde S, Thomson PD. Total lymphoid irradiation in renal transplantation. World J Surg. 1986;10(3):369–80.

59. Woodruff M, Anderson N. Effect of lymphocyte depletion by thoracic duct fistula and administration of antilymphocytic serum on the survival of skin homografts in rats. Nature. 1963;200(4907):702.

60. Monaco AP, Wood ML, Gray J, Russell PS. Studies on heterologous anti-lymphocyte serum in mice: II. Effect on the immune response. J Immunol. 1966;96(2):229–38.

61. Starzl TE, Marchioro TL, Porter K, Iwasaki Y, Cerilli GJ. The use of heterologous antilymphoid agents in canine renal and liver homotransplantation and in human renal homotransplantation. Surg Gyencol Obstet. 1967;124(2):301–18.

62. Najarian JS, Simmons RL, Condie RM, Thompson EJ, Fryd DS, Howard RJ, et al. Seven years' experience with antilymphoblast globulin for renal transplantation from cadaver donors. Ann Surg. 1976;184(3):352–68.

63. Dausset J. Iso-leuco-anticorps. Acta Haematol. 1958;20(1–4):156–66.

64. Payne R, Rolfs MR. Fetomaternal leukocyte incompatibility. J Clin Invest. 1958;37(12):1756–63.

65. Van Rood J, Van Leeuwen A, Eernisse J. Leucocyte antibodies in sera of pregnant women. Vox Sang. 1959;4:427–44.

66. Dausset J, Rapaport F, Colombani J, Feixoold N. A leucocyte group and its relationship to tissue histocompatibility in man. Transplantation. 1965;3(6):701–5.

67. Dausset J, Rapaport F, Ivanyi D, Collombani J. Tissue alloantigens and transplantation. In: Histocompatibility testing. Copenhagen: Munksgaard; 1965. p. 63–72.

68. Terasaki P, Vredevoe D, Porter K, Mickey MA, Marchioro T, Faris T, et al. Serotyping for homotransplantation V. Evaluation of a matching scheme. Transplantation. 1966;4(6):688–99.

69. Vredevoe D, Mickey M, Goyette D, Magnuson N, Terasaki P. Serotyping for Homotransplantation. Viii. Grouping of antisera from various laboratories into five groups. Ann N Y Acad Sci. 1966;129(1):521–8.

70. Mickey M, Kreisler M, Albert E, Tanaka N, Terasaki P. Analysis of HL-A incompatibility in human renal transplants. Tissue Antigens. 1971;1(2):57–67.

71. Ting A, Morris P. Matching for B-cell antigens of the HLA-DR series in cadaver renal transplantation. Lancet. 1978;311(8064):575–7.

72. Kissmeyer-Nielsen F, Olsen S, Petersen VP, Fjeldborg O. Hyperacute rejection of kidney allografts, associated with pre-existing humoral antibodies against donor cells. Lancet. 1966;288(7465):662–5.

73. Williams GM, Hume DM, Hudson RP Jr, Morris PJ, Kano K, Milgrom F. Hyperacute renal-homograft rejection in man. N Engl J Med. 1968;279(12):611–8.

74. Starzl TE, Lerner RA, Dixon FJ, Groth CG, Brettschneider L, Terasaki PI. Shwartzman reaction after human renal homotransplantation. N Engl J Med. 1968;278(12):642–8.

75. Opelz G. Effect of blood transfusions on subsequent kidney transplants. Transpl Proc. 1973;5:253–9.

76. Michielson P. Hemodialyse et Transplatation Renale. Eur Dial Trans Assoc Proc. 1966;3:162.

77. Morris P, Ting A, Stocker J. Leukocyte antigens in renal transplantation. 1. The paradox of blood transfusions in renal transplantation. Med J Aust. 1968;2(24):1088–90.

78. Carrel A. Results of the transplantation of blood vessels, organs and limbs. J Am Med Assoc. 1908;51(20):1662–7.

79. Radin J. Life on ice: a history of new uses for cold blood. Chicago: University of Chicago Press; 2017.

80. Landecker H. Culturing life: how cells became technologies. Cambridge: Harvard University Press; 2010.

81. Moore FD, Smith LL, Burnap TK, Dallenbach FD, Dammin GJ, Gruber UF, et al. One-stage homotransplantation of the liver following total hepatectomy in dogs. Plast Reconstr Surg. 1959;23(1):103–6.

82. Starzl TE, Kaupp HA Jr, Brock DR, Lazarus RE, Johnson RV. Reconstructive problems in canine liver homotransplantation with special reference to the postoperative role of hepatic venous flow. Surg Gyencol Obstet. 1960;111:733–43.

83. Starzl TE, Holmes JH. Experience in renal transplantation. Philadelphia: Saunders; 1980.

84. Collins G, Bravo-Shugarman M, Terasaki P. Kidney preservation for transportation: initial perfusion and 30 hours' ice storage. Lancet. 1969;294(7632):1219–22.

85. Belzer F, Ashby BS, Dunphy JE. 24-hour and 72-hour preservation of canine kidneys. Lancet. 1967;290(7515):536–9.

86. Barnard C. The operation. A human cardiac transplant: an interim report of a successful operation performed at Groote Schuur hospital, Cape Town. S Afr Med J. 1967;41:1271–4.

87. Lower R, Shumway N. Studies on orthotopic homotransplantation of the canine heart. Surg Forum. 1960;11:18–9.

88. Hardy JD, Chavez CM, Kurrus FD, Neely WA, Eraslan S, Turner MD, et al. Heart transplantation in man: developmental studies and report of a case. J Am Med Assoc. 1964;188(13):1132–40.

89. McRae D. Every second counts: the race to Transplant the first human heart. New York: Berkley Books; 2007.

90. Griepp RB, Stinson EB, Dong E, Clark DA, Shumway NE. Hemodynamic performance of the transplanted human heart. Surgery. 1971;70(1):88–96.

91. Caves PK, Stinson EB, Billingham M, Shumway NE. Percutaneous transvenous endomyocardial biopsy in human heart recipients: experience with a new technique. Ann Thorac Surg. 1973;16(4):325–36.

92. David C. Christiaan Barnard: the surgeon who dared. England: Fonthill Media; 2017.

93. Mollaret P, Goulon M. Le coma de' passe (m_moire preliminaire). Rev Neurol. 1959;101:3–15. 116-39

94. Beecher HK. A definition of irreversible coma: report of the ad hoc committee of the harvard medical school to examine the definition of brain death. J Am Med Assoc. 1968;205(6):337–40.

95. Diagnosis of brain death. Statement issued by the honorary secretary of the conference of medical royal colleges and their faculties in the United Kingdom on 11 October 1976. Br Med J. 1976;2(6045): 1187.

96. Lo CM. Deceased donation in Asia: challenges and opportunities. Liver Transpl. 2012;18(S2):S5–7.

97. Demikhov V. Some essential points of the techniques of transplantation of the heart, lungs and other organs. Experimental transplantation of vital organs. Moscow: Medgiz State Press for Medical Literature; 1960.

98. Lower RR, Stofer RC, Hurley EJ, Shumway NE. Complete homograft replacement of the heart and both lungs. Surgery. 1961;50(5):842–5.

99. Cooley DA, Bloodwell RD, Hallman GL, Nora JJ, Harrison GM, Leachman RD. Organ transplantation for advanced cardiopulmonary disease. Ann Thorac Surg. 1969;8(1):30–46.

100. Hardy JD, Webb WR, Dalton ML, Walker GR. Lung homotransplantation in man: report of the initial case. J Am Med Assoc. 1963;186(12):1065–74.

101. Montefusco CM, Veith FJ. Lung transplantation. Surg Clin North Am. 1986;66(3):503–15.

102. Derom F, Barbier F, Ringoir S, Versieck J, Rolly G, Berzsenyi G, et al. Ten-month survival after lung homotransplantation in man. J Thoac Cardiovasc Surg. 1971;61(6):835–46.

103. Starzl TE. The puzzle people: memoirs of a transplant surgeon. Pittsburgh: University of Pittsburgh Press; 1992.

104. Starzl TE, Groth CG, Brettschneider L, Penn I, Fulginiti VA, Moon JB, et al. Orthotopic homotransplantation of the human liver. Ann Surg. 1968;168(3):392–415.

105. Kelly W, Lillehei R, Merkel F, Idezuki Y, Goetz F. Alltransplantation of the pancreas and duodenum along with the kidney in diabetic nephropathy. Surgery. 1967;61(6):827–37.

106. Downing R. Historical review of pancreatic islet transplantation. World J Surg. 1984;8(2): 137–42.

107. Dreyfus M, Haerri E, Hoffman H, Kobel H. Cyclosporin A and C, new metabolites from trichoderma polysporum. Eur J Appl Microbiol. 1976;3(1):125–33.

108. Borel JF, Feurer C, Gubler H, Stähelin H. Biological effects of cyclosporin a: a new antilymphocytic agent. Agents Action. 1994;43(3–4):179–86.

109. Kostakis A, White D, RJIMS C. Prolongation of rat heart allograft survival by cyclosporin A. Int Res Commun Sys Med Sci. 1977;5(280):5l.

110. Calne R, White D. Cyclosporin A—a powerful immunosuppressant in dogs with renal allografts. Int Res Commun Syst Med Sci. 1977;5:595.

111. Calne R, Thiru S, McMaster P, Craddock G, White D, Evans D, et al. Cyclosporin a in patients receiving renal allografts from cadaver donors. Lancet. 1978;312(8104):1323–7.

112. Calne R, Rolles K, Thiru S, McMaster P, Craddock G, Aziz S, et al. Cyclosporin a initially as the only immunosuppressant in 34 recipients of cadaveric organs: 32 kidneys, 2 pancreases, and 2 livers. Lancet. 1979;314(8151):1033–6.

113. Starzl TE, Richard Weil SI III, Klintmalm G, Schröter GP, Koep LJ, Iwaki Y, et al. The use of cyclosporin A and prednisone in cadaver kidney transplantation. Surg Gyencol Obstet. 1980;151(1):17–26.

114. Group EMT. Cyclosporin in cadaveric renal transplantation: one-year follow-up of a multicentre trial. Lancet. 1983;322(8357):986–9.

115. Group CMTS. A randomized clinical trial of cyclosporine in cadaveric renal transplantation. N Engl J Med. 1983;309(14):809–15.

116. Kino T, Hatanaka H, Miyata S, Inamura N, Nishiyama M, Yajima T, et al. FK-506, a novel immunosuppressant isolated from a Streptomyces. J Antibiot. 1987;40(9):1256–65.

117. Starzl TE, Fung J, Venkataramman R, Todo S, Demetris A, Jain A. FK 506 for liver, kidney, and pancreas transplantation. Lancet. 1989;334(8670):1000–4.

118. Napoli KL, Taylor PJ. From beach to bedside: history of the development of sirolimus. Ther Drug Monit. 2001;23(5):559–86.

119. Morath C, Arns W, Schwenger V, Mehrabi A, Fonouni H, Schmidt J, et al. Sirolimus in renal transplantation. Nephrol Dial Transplant. 2007;22(Suppl 8):viii61–viii5.

120. Group TLT. Unilateral lung transplantation for pulmonary fibrosis. N Engl J Med. 1986;314(18):1140–5.

121. Morris PJ, Tilney NL. Progress in transplantation, vol. 2. Edinburgh: Churchill Livingstone; 1985.

122. McKellar S. Artificial hearts the allure and ambivalence of a controversial medical technology. Baltimore: Johns Hopkins University Press; 2017.

123. Wahlberg J, Love R, Landegaard L, Southard J, Belzer F. Successful 72 hours' preservation of the canine pancreas. Transplant Proc. 1987;19:1337–8.

124. Jamieson NV, Sundberg R, Lindell S, Claesson K, Moen J, Vreugdenhil PK, et al. Preservation of the canine liver for 24-48 hours using simple cold storage with UW solution. Transplantation. 1988;46(4):517–22.

125. Steen S, Sjöberg T, Pierre L, Liao Q, Eriksson L, Algotsson L. Transplantation of lungs from a non-heart-beating donor. Lancet. 2001;357(9259):825–9.

126. Ardehali A, Esmailian F, Deng M, Soltesz E, Hsich E, Naka Y, et al. Ex-vivo perfusion of donor hearts for human heart transplantation (PROCEED II): a prospective, open-label, multicentre, randomised non-inferiority trial. Lancet. 2015;385(9987):2577–84.

127. Barbas AS, Goldaracena N, Dib MJ, Selzner M. Ex-vivo liver perfusion for organ preservation: recent advances in the field. Transplant Rev. 2016;30(3):154–60.

128. Fildes JE, Archer LD, Blaikley J, Ball AL, Stone JP, Sjöberg T, et al. Clinical outcome of patients transplanted with marginal donor lungs via ex vivo lung perfusion compared to standard lung transplantation. Transplantation. 2015;99(5):1078–83.

129. Gabolde M, Moulin AM. French response to 'Innovation': the return of the living donor organ transplantation. In: Stanton J, editor. Innovations in health and medicine: diffusion and resistance in the twentieth century. New York: Routledge; 2002. p. 188–208.

130. Mierzejewska B, Durlik M, Lisik W, Baum C, Schroder P, Kopke J, et al. Current approaches in national kidney donation programs. Annals of Transplant. 2013;18:112–24.

131. UNOS. Donors recovered in the U.S. by Donor type. Available from: https://optn.transplant.hrsa.gov/data/view-data-reports/national-data/.

132. Steinbrook R. Organ donation after cardiac death. N Engl J Med. 2007;357(3):209–13.

133. Köhler G, Milstein C. Continuous cultures of fused cells secreting antibody of predefined specificity. Nature. 1975;256(5517):495–7.

134. Cosimi AB, Burton RC, Colvin RB, Goldstein G, Delmonico FL, Laquaglia MP, et al. Treatment of acute renal allograft rejection with OKT3 monoclonal antibody. Transplantation. 1981;32(6):535–9.

135. Group OMTS. A randomized clinical trial of OKT3 monoclonal antibody for acute rejection of cadaveric renal transplants. N Engl J Med. 1985;313(6):337–42.

136. Calne R, Moffatt SD, Friend PJ, Jamieson NV, Bradley JA, Hale G, et al. Campath IH allows low-dose cyclosporine monotherapy in 31 cadaveric renal allograft recipients. Transplantation. 1999;68(10):1613–6.

137. Knechtle SJ, Fernandez LA, Pirsch JD, Becker BN, Chin LT, Becker YT, et al. Campath-1H in renal transplantation: the University of Wisconsin experience. Surgery. 2004;136(4):754–60.

138. Lonze BE, Tatapudi VS, Weldon EP, Min ES, Ali NM, Deterville CL, et al. IdeS (Imlifidase): a novel agent that cleaves human IgG and permits successful kidney transplantation across high-strength donor-specific antibody. Ann Surg. 2018;268(3):488–96.

139. Kwun J, Burghuber C, Manook M, Iwakoshi N, Gibby A, Hong JJ, et al. Humoral compensation after

bortezomib treatment of allosensitized recipients. J Am Soc Nephrol. 2017;28(7):1991–6.

140. Vo AA, Choi J, Kim I, Louie S, Cisneros K, Kahwaji J, et al. A phase I/II trial of the interleukin-6 receptor–specific humanized monoclonal (tocilizumab)+ intravenous immunoglobulin in difficult to desensitize patients. Transplantation. 2015;99(11):2356–63.

141. Ezekian B, Schroder PM, Freischlag K, Yoon J, Kwun J, Knechtle SJ. Contemporary strategies and barriers to transplantation tolerance. Transplantation. 2018;102(8):1213–22.

142. Baum CE, Mierzejewska B, Schroder PM, Khattar M, Stepkowski S. Optimizing the use of regulatory T cells in allotransplantation: recent advances and future perspectives. Expert Rev Clin Immunol. 2013;9(12):1303–14.

143. Vincenti F, Rostaing L, Grinyo J, Rice K, Steinberg S, Gaite L, et al. Belatacept and long-term outcomes in kidney transplantation. N Engl J Med. 2016;374(4):333–43.

144. Kirk AD, Guasch A, Xu H, Cheeseman J, Mead SI, Ghali A, et al. Renal transplantation using belatacept without maintenance steroids or calcineurin inhibitors. Am J Transplant. 2014;14(5): 1142–51.

145. Dubernard J-M, Owen E, Herzberg G, Lanzetta M, Martin X, Kapila H, et al. Human hand allograft: report on first 6 months. Lancet. 1999;353(9161):1315–20.

146. Dickenson D, Hakim NS. Ethical issues in limb transplants. Postgrad Med J. 1999;75:513–5.

147. Devauchelle B, Badet L, Lengelé B, Morelon E, Testelin S, Michallet M, et al. First human face allograft: early report. Lancet. 2006;368(9531): 203–9.

148. Dubernard J-M, Lengelé B, Morelon E, Testelin S, Badet L, Moure C, et al. Outcomes 18 months after the first human partial face transplantation. N Engl J Med. 2007;357(24):2451–60.

149. Lanchin M. Isabelle dinoire: life after the world's first face transplant. BBC Magazine. 2012, 27 November.

150. Rifkin WJ, David JA, Plana NM, Kantar RS, Diaz-Siso JR, Gelb BE, et al. Achievements and challenges in facial transplantation. Ann Surg. 2018;268(2):260–70.

151. Hu W, Lu J, Zhang L, Wu W, Nie H, Zhu Y, et al. A preliminary report of penile transplantation. Eur Urol. 2006;50(4):851–3.

152. Bateman C. World's first successful penis transplant at Tygerberg hospital. S Afr Med J. 2015;105(4):251–2.

153. Grady D. 'Whole Again': Vet Mained by an I.E.D. Receives a transplanted penis. New York Times. 2018 24 April 2018; Sect. Science.

154. Rana A, Gruessner A, Agopian VG, Khalpey Z, Riaz IB, Kaplan B, et al. Survival benefit of solid-organ transplant in the United States survival benefit of solid-organ transplant survival benefit of solid-organ transplant. JAMA Surg. 2015;150(3):252–9.

155. Reemtsma K, McCracken BH, Schlegel JU, Pearl M. Heterotransplantation of the kidney: two clinical experiences. Science. 1964;143(3607):700–2.

156. Reemtsma K. Renal heterotransplantation from nonhuman primates to man. Ann N Y Acad Sci. 1969;162(1):412–8.

157. Bailey LL, Nehlsen-Cannarella SL, Concepcion W, Jolley WB. Baboon-to-human cardiac xenotransplantation in a neonate. J Am Med Assoc. 1985;254(23):3321–9.

158. Zhang S. Genetically engineered pigs grow organs for people. The Atlantic 2017.

159. Längin M, Mayr T, Reichart B, Michel S, Buchholz S, Guethoff S, et al. Consistent success in life-supporting porcine cardiac xenotransplantation. Nature. 2018;564(7736):430–3.

Tissue Typing, Crossmatching and the Allocation of Deceased Donor Kidney Transplants

2

William R. Mulley, Fiona Hudson, and Darren Lee

2.1 Introduction

The field of tissue typing and crossmatching has undergone extensive growth over the last 20 years with increasing refinement in the definition of Human Leukocyte Antigens (HLA) and an increased understanding of the immunologically important parts of HLA molecules. At the same time, advances in techniques for the detection of anti-HLA antibodies in recipients have become increasingly sensitive and sophisticated. Currently, the interpretation of crossmatch data is frequently beyond the grasp of the general nephrologist and

can require considerable input from a specialised tissue typing scientist [1]. Amongst this, deceased donor kidneys remain scarce, relative to demand, with novel strategies for determining the best allocation method emerging.

This chapter describes modern tissue typing, crossmatching and deceased donor organ allocation methodologies relevant to kidney transplantation.

2.1.1 Tissue Typing

In transplantation, tissue typing refers to the determination of an individual's HLA profile. The HLA typing of a potential donor and recipient are then compared to assess for matches and mismatches. Mismatched donor HLA are considered the major antigenic targets for a recipient's immune responses that result in graft rejection. Additionally, knowledge of donor-recipient HLA mismatches together with the anti-HLA antibody profile of the recipient, allows assessment of the immunological risk of rejection involved with that pairing. Tissue typing techniques are divided into serological and molecular methods with the latter becoming increasingly complex over time [2].

2.1.1.1 Serological Tissue Typing

Serological typing was the initial method for determining HLA expression. It can be performed by agglutination or lymphocytotoxicity with the latter preferred. This technique employs

W. R. Mulley (✉)
Department of Nephrology, Monash Medical Centre, Clayton, Victoria, Australia

Centre for Inflammatory Diseases,
Department of Medicine, Monash University,
Clayton, Victoria, Australia
e-mail: William.Mulley@monashhealth.org

F. Hudson
Victorian Transplantation and Immunogenetic Service, Australian Red Cross Blood Service, West Melbourne, Victoria, Australia
e-mail: FHudson@redcrossblood.org.au

D. Lee
Department of Renal Medicine, Eastern Health, Box Hill, Victoria, Australia

Eastern Health Clinical School, Monash University, Clayton, Victoria, Australia

Department of Nephrology, Austin Health, Heidelberg, Victoria, Australia
e-mail: Darren.Lee@easternhealth.org.au

© Springer Nature Switzerland AG 2021
N. Hakim et al. (eds.), *Transplantation Surgery*, Springer Specialist Surgery Series,
https://doi.org/10.1007/978-3-030-55244-2_2

lymphocytes, which are easily accessed via peripheral blood sampling. T cells are a reliable, numerous, robust source for HLA class I typing, whilst B cells are required for HLA class II typing. Serological typing techniques rely on well-defined panels of known antisera (anti-HLA antibodies) to assign antigen specificity. Multiple antisera are incubated with lymphocytes. After a period of incubation, rabbit complement is added to the test system. The cells are then stained with an ethidium bromide-acridine orange dye. When the cell has been lysed by antibody binding and complement activation, the cells appear red; cells that remain intact appear green. Knowing the specificity of the antisera which resulted in cell lysis allows determination of an individual's serological tissue type (HLA antigen expression). However, this technique has numerous limitations [3, 4]. HLA typing by serological techniques give low resolution results, identifying the antigen family, but not functional allelic differences within the antigen family. Many antisera used for serological typing purposes were also cross-reactive across multiple HLA antigens, often making interpretation difficult. Serological techniques are also unable to reliably define HLA typing for low expression antigens such as DPB1 and C [2]. The strengths of serological typing include its capacity to be performed quickly and its clinical validity in only detecting antigens which are expressed, as opposed to molecular typing which can determine encoded HLA which may not be expressed [2].

2.1.2 Molecular Tissue Typing

Serological typing methods have now largely been replaced by molecular based techniques, which can better define the complexity of the HLA system. These methods seek to describe the HLA profile of an individual through an assessment of their DNA at the chromosomal level. Molecular typing has evolved from techniques which analyse fragments of DNA amplified by polymerase chain reaction (PCR) (Sequence Specific Oligonucleotide (SSO) and Sequence Specific Primers (SSP) techniques) to current state of the art complete direct sequencing techniques, "Next Generation Sequencing". Through examining DNA sequences in HLA coding regions, it has become apparent that there is a great deal of polymorphism within HLA serotypes [5]. This means that HLA proteins expressed by different individuals may have the same serotype but potentially important differences in the coding sequence and hence structure which were unable to be detected by serological techniques.

Molecular typing has resulted in a substantial increase in the number of recognised Class I and Class 2 HLA alleles which as of April 2018 number 17 939 (https://www.ebi.ac.uk/ipd/imgt/hla/stats.html). This complexity is reflected in the nomenclature system for HLA which has developed to account for allelic variations within antigen groups.

The concurrent development of HLA sequencing techniques, advanced HLA antibody identification using Luminex Single Antigen bead technology and modelling of the HLA molecule has led to the identification of immunogenic subunits on the HLA molecule that provide targets for alloantibody development, termed epitopes [6–8].

2.2 Epitopes

Anti-HLA antibodies do not bind the entire HLA molecule. They are not large enough and many parts of HLA are not immunogenic [8]. Epitopes are regions of HLA that interact with antibodies and are therefore the antigenic subunits of HLA (Fig. 2.1) [10, 11]. Through three-dimensional studies, the epitopes of each HLA allele have been described. Epitopes are defined by amino acid differences on the HLA molecule that are accessible by alloantibodies. These epitopes may be shared by multiple antigens at a single HLA locus or shared between different loci [8]. This principle was previously demonstrated by the cross-reactive nature of many antigens detected using serological typing methods [12]. Due to the cross-reactive nature of the HLA antigens, HLA typing for all loci from both donor and recipient is required to accurately define epitope matching.

Because HLA alloantibodies react against epitopes, rather than specific HLA proteins, a single

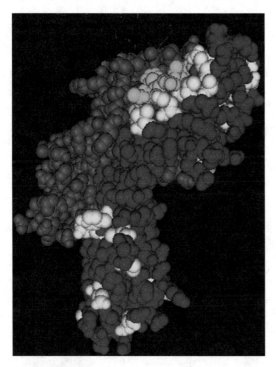

Fig. 2.1 Topography of HLA-DR [9]. This three-dimensional model of HLA DR highlights in yellow, the areas of the HLA protein (epitopes) which are capable of interacting with anti HLA antibodies. Not all parts of the HLA protein are immunogenic

HLA transplant mismatch may stimulate antibodies reactive with multiple HLA proteins where antigens share the same mismatched epitopes. Determining HLA mismatches at the antigen level does not provide sufficient information to fully evaluate HLA compatibility, whereas epitope mismatches provide a more complete matching picture. Epitope analysis has been applied to transplant cohorts and demonstrated an effect of increased epitope mismatching on clinical outcomes in lung and kidney transplantation [13, 14].

2.2.1   Crossmatching

The purpose of crossmatching is to detect preformed antibodies in the recipient that are specific for a potential donor. Transplantation across a positive crossmatch is associated with an increased risk of antibody mediated rejection (AMR) which can result in: immediate graft loss

due to hyperacute rejection with graft thrombosis and infarction, acute AMR with significant graft injury or mild AMR which may be subclinical but with chronic graft injury and scarring [15]. Crossmatching techniques can be functional assays, such as the complement dependent cytotoxicity assay (CDC crossmatch) or antibody binding assays without a functional readout, such as the flow crossmatch or antigen coated bead assays [1]. The different crossmatch methodologies have differing sensitivities to detect antibody, with the CDC crossmatch the least sensitive assay and antigen coated bead assays the most sensitive. As the sensitivity of the assay increases however, debate regarding the clinical relevance of a positive result also increases.

2.2.1.1 The CDC Crossmatch

The CDC crossmatch was developed by Terasaki and colleagues in the 1960s [16, 17]. It is a functional assay which measures the degree of complement dependent cell lysis of donor lymphocytes when mixed with recipient serum. Lymphocytes, separated into T and B cell subsets, are incubated with recipient serum and complement. If donor specific antibody (DSA) is present, it binds HLA molecules present on donor lymphocyte cell surfaces. If the antibody is capable of activating complement, cell lysis ensues (Fig. 2.2). The read out from the CDC crossmatch is the proportion of lymphocytes lysed in the assay. A scoring range of 1–8 is commonly used with 1 representing a negative result with <20% cell lysis and a score of 8 representing >80% of cells lysed, with scores of 2, 4 and 6 representing increasing degrees of cell lysis.

The sensitivity of the CDC crossmatch can be increased by adding anti-human globulin (AHG) to the assay. Multiple AHG's bind each DSA attached to donor lymphocytes increasing the number of Fc receptors available to activate complement. Therefore, addition of AHG will result in an increased likelihood that a low level DSA will generate a positive crossmatch. While for strongly positive crossmatches, the strength of the DSA can be further elicited by performing crossmatches with serial dilutions of recipient serum. If the crossmatch becomes negative after

Fig. 2.2 The CDC crossmatch [1]. Recipient serum potentially containing donor specific anti-HLA antibodies is added to donor T or B lymphocytes, along with complement (**a**). If donor-specific antibodies are not present, no lysis occurs, and the result is deemed negative (**b**). If donor-specific anti-HLA antibodies bind to the lymphocytes and then activate complement, cell lysis will occur, and the crossmatch result will be deemed positive (**c**). The proportion of lysed cells is assessed, and the crossmatch is graded a being weakly, moderately or strongly positive

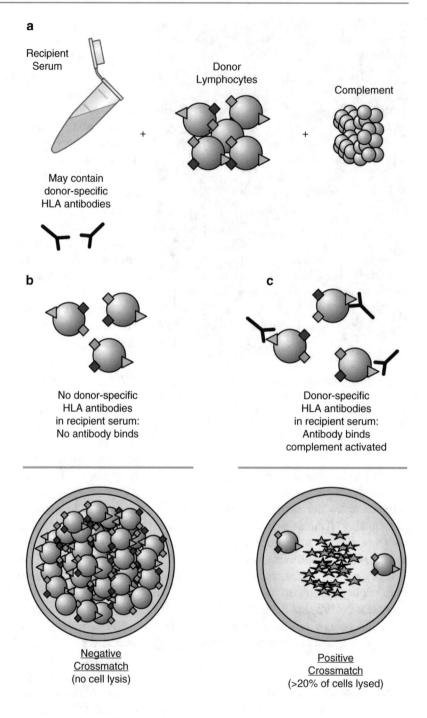

one or two dilutions it implies a lesser DSA strength or avidity than one that remains positive after multiple dilutions. This may guide the potential to desensitise the patient for transplantation.

The differential expression of class I and II HLA by T and B cells provides further information regarding the antigenic target of the DSA. T-cells express class I but little class II and therefore a positive T-cell crossmatch suggests there are one or more DSA directed against class I. B-cells express both class I and II hence a positive B-cell crossmatch suggests the antibodies present are directed against class I or II or both. Furthermore, B-cells express class I to a greater extent than T-cells, making it possible for a low level DSA against class I to generate a negative T-cell crossmatch but a positive B-cell crossmatch [18].

A positive crossmatch may be falsely positive. This is more common in B-cell crossmatching where up to 50% are considered false positives [19]. False positives are commonly due to interfering substances such as autoantibodies of the IgM subclass. These can be neutralised by adding the chemical, Dithiotheritol (DTT) to the assay to reduce the disulphide bonds in IgM. Hence a positive crossmatch which becomes negative after the addition of DTT is thought to have been a false positive. Importantly, a control reaction should also be included when using DTT to account for the dilutional effect of adding DTT, rather than its effects on negating IgM. If the DTT and the dilution control well are both negative in the setting of a positive non-diluted crossmatch, this implies the presence of a weak DSA. CDC crossmatches can be negative in the setting of a DSA if: the DSA is at a low level; the DSA does not activate complement; or if donor lymphocytes express minimal HLA of the type the DSA is directed against e.g. HLA-C antigens.

A true positive CDC crossmatch is interpreted as meaning that there are one or more donor specific antibody/ies present in recipient serum which can bind donor lymphocytes and activate complement. A positive T-cell crossmatch has long been considered a contraindication to transplantation due to a substantial risk of hyperacute rejection [16, 20]. A positive B-cell CDC crossmatch does not carry the same predictive value but certainly prompts the search for further information to quantify the risk of rejection [19, 21]. Generally, this is undertaken with flow and virtual crossmatching.

2.2.1.2 The Flow Crossmatch

Flow crossmatching is performed with similar initial substrates to the CDC crossmatch [22]. Donor T and B lymphocytes are mixed with recipient serum to allow binding of DSA if present. Bound DSA is detected by the addition of a fluorescein tagged capture antibody directed against human immunoglobulin. The degree of DSA binding is measured by the amount of fluorescence detected on a flow cytometer (Fig. 2.3). Therefore, a negative flow crossmatch is one in which there is no fluorescence detected, implying that there is no DSA present, while a positive flow crossmatch generates a fluorescent signal. The intensity of the fluorescence can be used to stratify the strength of the DSA. This intensity is measured in how many channel shifts of fluorescence the reaction generates compared with a negative control.

The advantage of a flow crossmatch over a CDC crossmatch is that it is more sensitive for DSA and therefore can detect weaker DSA than can the CDC crossmatch [23]. Additionally, the DSA subclass can be determined by adding an isotype specific capture antibody such as anti-IgG or anti-IgM. The major advantage of CDC over flow crossmatching is the functional readout of the CDC, as for it to be positive the DSA needs to be able to activate complement. Flow crossmatching does not have a functional readout and the DSA needs only to bind lymphocytes for the assay to be positive. The increased sensitivity and the lack of a functional element to the readout means that a positive flow crossmatch is less predictive of hyperacute or accelerated antibody mediated rejection than a CDC crossmatch. However, flow crossmatching can be used to stratify the risk of rejection on the basis of the number of channel shifts seen. Some transplanting units use a channel shift threshold to guide the suitability of a potential transplant donor-recipient pairing or to judge the efficacy of a pre-transplant desensitisation protocol [24, 25].

As with CDC crossmatching, a positive T-cell flow crossmatch implies the presence of one or

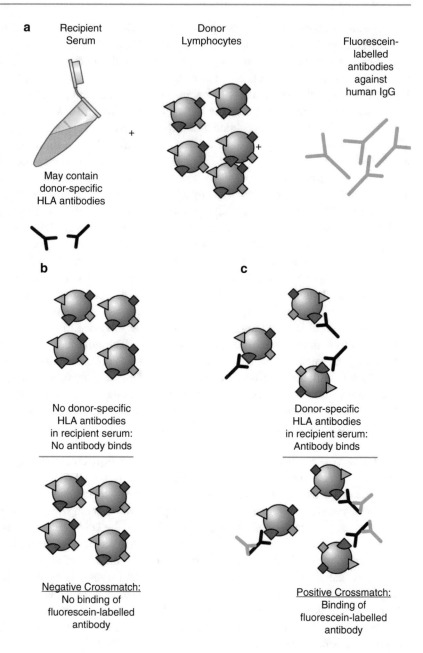

Fig. 2.3 The flow crossmatch [1]. Recipient serum potentially containing donor-specific anti-HLA antibodies is added to donor T or B lymphocytes, along with fluorescein-labelled antibodies against human IgG (**a**). If donor-specific antibodies are not present, no binding occurs, and the result is deemed negative (**b**). If donor-specific anti-HLA antibodies bind to the lymphocytes, these can then bind the fluorescein-labelled antihuman IgG antibody, and this will be detectable by flow cytometry (**c**). The strength of the fluorescence can be measured and expressed as 'channel shifts' above the control sample

more DSA directed against class I HLA, while a positive B-cell crossmatch implies one or more DSA against class I, class II or both. Hence the B-cell flow crossmatch sums the total binding of all anti-HLA DSA providing a measure of the cumulative DSA load a potential transplant pairing bears. In this way the B-cell flow crossmatch may be the most useful assay of the two [24, 25].

2.2.1.3 The Virtual Crossmatch

Virtual crossmatching has emerged over the last decade and is rapidly replacing CDC and flow crossmatching in many transplant situations [26]. The technology employs screening for HLA antibodies using beads coated with HLA antigens [27]. The beads are mixed with recipient serum and a fluorescent capture antibody is added to the assay. A specialised flow cytometer is used to detect any bead which fluoresces while also determining the specificity of the bead on the basis of the bead colour. Each bead is coloured specifically (shades of red) to identify the HLA antigens on its surface. The strength of the antibody is determined by the degree of fluorescence of the bead measured as the mean fluorescence intensity (MFI). Therefore, the assay determines the specificity and the strength of the anti-HLA antibody (Fig. 2.4).

The beads can be coated with a single HLA-antigen or with several antigens. The latter test is used as a screening tool to detect the presence of any anti-HLA Abs. If this is negative, further testing with single antigen beads is not necessary. While single antigen beads are used to specifically define which anti-HLA antibody is present, in some centres the screening beads are not used as the single antigen beads are thought to be more sensitive. The beads are separated into HLA Class I and Class II sets. Each set contains approximately 100 beads.

The virtual crossmatch requires identification of the specificity of anti-HLA antibodies by single antigen bead testing. The other half of the equation is the donor HLA, which is determined by tissue typing. Donor HLA is compared with the anti-HLA antibody profile of the recipient. A positive virtual crossmatch is the situation wherein an antibody, specific for one or more of the donor's HLA is detected. The MFI of the DSA provides a guide to the risk of rejection associated with proceeding with the transplant. MFI values vary between laboratories and even within the same laboratory, between assays, therefore they are not directly comparable. In general, however, a low level DSA has an MFI <2000, intermediate 2001–8000 and strong >8000.

The best-known bead assay is the Luminex assay (One Lambda, Canoga, CA, USA). While this technology has been very useful in determining immunological risk in transplantation, there are some well described limitations to consider. Firstly, not all HLA types are represented on the bead sets as there are a finite number of beads in

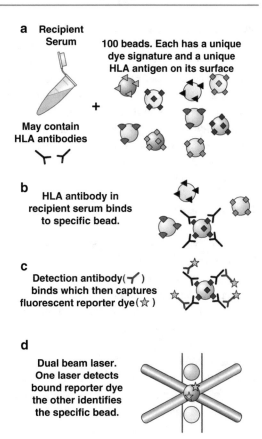

Fig. 2.4 The virtual crossmatch [1]. Recipient serum potentially containing anti- HLA antibodies is added to a mixture of synthetic beads. Each bead is coated with a set of antigens (screening beads) or with a single antigen (single antigen beads). A unique dye signature specifies the identity of each bead (**a**). If anti-HLA antibodies are present, they will bind to the appropriate bead (**b**). A detection antibody carrying a reporter dye binds the anti-HLA antibody (**c**). Dual laser capture allows simultaneous detection of the reporter dye and the bead specificity to identify which anti-HLA antibodies are present (**d**). A profile of antibodies can thus be identified in the recipient and compared with the known HLA identity of any potential donor, allowing a prediction of the crossmatch result

the sets. This means that DSA directed against an HLA that is not represented on the bead panel will be missed. This is especially problematic for rare donor HLA types. Secondly, some HLA antigens on the beads are prone to denaturation which can lead to non-specific antibody binding and false positive results [28]. Additional issues include that, like flow crossmatching, the assay does not have a functional output and that due to its increased sensitivity for DSA, many potentially successful transplants may be cancelled due to concerns about rejection risk. The former issue has been partially addressed by the C1q assay which detects antibodies capable of activating complement. C1q positive DSA are reported to be more predictive of AMR and graft loss than C1q -ve DSA, however this finding is not universal as reviewed by Tait [28].

2.2.1.4 Clinical Uses of Crossmatching

Assessing the Degree of HLA Sensitisation: Panel Reactive Antibodies

Crossmatching techniques can be used to assess a prospective transplant recipient's breadth of sensitisation to HLA antigens. The CDC crossmatch technique has been used for this purpose for many years. Multiple CDC crossmatches are performed simultaneously with T and B lymphocytes isolated from numerous blood donors and serum from a potential transplant recipient. Each crossmatch is against a single donor. The proportion of donors for which the recipients serum generates a positive crossmatch is termed the panel reactive antibody (PRA). A PRA of 80% means that the recipient has anti-HLA antibodies that react with 80% of the population. This assumes that blood donors are representative of the broader community in terms of HLA type. Patients who have been sensitised to HLA through pregnancy, blood transfusions or previous transplantation can have PRAs of 100%.

More recently, delineation of the individual HLA antibodies present in the sera of prospective recipients by single antigen beads has allowed a calculated PRA to be generated. The antibodies present are compared against the frequency of expression of HLA in the population to calculate the proportion of potential donors the recipient would have a positive virtual crossmatch against. The MFI that a virtual crossmatch is considered positive can be set arbitrarily at any level e.g. 2000, 5000 or 8000.

HLA antibody screening is routinely repeated while patients are on the waiting list. The serum which generates the highest PRA for a patient is termed their peak PRA while the PRA using their most recent serum is termed their current PRA. The degree of HLA sensitisation of a potential transplant recipient has implications for the likelihood of the patient receiving a transplant, as many deceased donor kidney allocation systems do not make positive CDC crossmatch offers. Hence, patients with very high PRA (99%) will be eligible for transplantation from only one in every 100 donors. Determining the degree of HLA sensitisation of patients therefore, allows clinicians the opportunity to counsel patients about their likelihood of receiving a transplant in a timely fashion. Broadly sensitised patients typically wait longer for a transplant than non-sensitised patients and may need to accept a kidney from a donor to whom they have one or more DSA [29]. Some transplant services offer desensitisation programmes to highly sensitised patients while on the waiting list, in order to reduce their current anti-HLA antibody profile [30]. This increases their prospects of a negative crossmatch, using current serum, with a greater proportion of donors.

Determining the Immunological Risk of a Transplant Pairing

For any living or deceased donor kidney transplant pairing, crossmatching can provide a guide to the immunological/rejection risk involved. Rejection due to antibodies can occur immediately causing loss of the kidney due to thrombosis, hyperacute rejection or can occur in a less acute or even chronic fashion. Overall, recipients with DSA (positive virtual crossmatch) have a shorter expected duration of graft survival compared with those without DSA [31]. However, not all DSA positive transplants will result in hyperacute rejection. The risk of hyperacute rejection can be stratified by crossmatching. If the CDC crossmatch is positive, the risk of hyperacute rejection is very high. In this case the flow and virtual crossmatches will also be positive, unless the CDC crossmatch is a false positive. A negative CDC crossmatch with positive flow and virtual crossmatches implies a lower level DSA or a DSA which does not activate complement and portends a lower risk of hyperacute rejection. Proceeding with a transplant in this situation is not uncommon and is generally undertaken with a desensitisation protocol to further reduce the risk of rejection. If the CDC and flow crossmatches are negative but the virtual crossmatch reveals a low level DSA, the risk of hyperacute rejection is negligible. A desensitisation protocol is still commonly employed as the risk of some form of AMR is still increased relative to DSA negative transplants.

Crossmatching can also be used to guide the timing of transplantation for a recipient sensitised to their intended living donor. Protocols to reduce the crossmatch to negative or at least an acceptable level have been described. Generally, these employ antibody removal techniques such as plasma exchange or immunoadsorption to remove DSA while preventing rebound of the antibodies with immunosuppressive medications [20]. Crossmatches are repeated during the desensitisation programme until they become negative or within a target range and then the transplant is undertaken. Commonly a negative CDC crossmatch or a flow crossmatch below a predetermined number of channel shifts is the trigger for proceeding.

2.2.1.5 Cellular Crossmatching

The techniques discussed above relate to preformed antibodies which might react with a specific donor's HLA. They do not measure primed cellular responses to donor antigens. Attempts to measure donor specific cellular reactivity have been made. The most studied technique is the Enzyme-Linked ImmunoSpot (ELISPOT) assay. This assay mixes donor and recipient leukocytes and measures the degree of recipient cellular responses through the production of proinflammatory cytokines such as interferon-gamma [32, 33]. There are correlations between those with strong donor specific ELISPOT responses and increased graft rejection with variations depending on recipient ethnicity and induction regimens [32, 33]. Further validation is required before cel-

lular crossmatching is extended to routine clinical use.

2.2.2 Allocation of Deceased Donor Kidneys for Transplantation

The number of patients awaiting a kidney transplant exceeds the number of kidneys available from deceased donors. Therefore, a system is required to determine how to allocate this scarce resource among those on waiting lists. Multiple allocation protocols are possible, they vary between jurisdictions and evoke much debate. The guiding ethical principles for allocation of donor kidneys include equity and utility [34]. Equity dictates that there should be fair and equal access for all while utility promotes allocation on the basis of achieving the greatest benefit. Allocation protocols have been devised predominantly by transplant clinicians, with some arguing that this may not be appropriate as donor organs are a public resource and therefore their allocation should be determined by the broader community [34]. Interestingly, a recent study of community attitudes to organ allocation arrived at themes supportive of balancing equity and utility [35]. While these principles are clearly important, they do not always move together, therefore a compromise must be met. Waiting time is generally used to represent equity principles with those waiting the longest being prioritised in allocation while to meet utility principles, younger recipient age and greater HLA matching are prioritised. The following section will review factors that can be included in allocation algorithms and how various current allocation systems are structured around the world, summarised in Table 2.1.

2.2.2.1 Principles of Allocation: Equity and Fairness Versus Utility

To achieve the balance between utility and equity, a priority point system exists as the backbone of most allocation systems, where points are awarded for factors considered of

Table 2.1 Factors considered in deceased donor kidney allocation internationally

	United States	United Kingdom	Euro transplant	Australia	Canada
Longevity matching	+ Young to Young: Low KDPI to low EPTS	+ Young to Young: Scoring to minimise donor-recipient age difference	+ Old to Old: ESP	– (To be implemented)	+ Young to Young (varies amongst provinces)
HLA mismatch A/B/DR importance Zero mismatch	+ DR only +	+ (especially in young recipients) DR>B +	+ (except in ESP) DR=B=A Graded	+ Varies amongst states +	– (in most provinces) – Varies amongst provinces
Waiting time on dialysis	+	From listing date	+	+	+
Highly sensitised cPRA criteria	+ ≥99%	+ ≥85%	+ >85% (Acceptable Mismatch)	+ >80% (1/6 or 2/6 HLA MM) ≥50% (0/6 HLA MM)	+ ≥95%
Prior living kidney donor	+	+	+	Varies amongst states	+
Racial minority: Blood group B	A2 and A2B donor prioritisation	O donors allocated	–	–	–
Paediatric priority	+	+	+	+	+
Medical urgency	+	Paediatric patients only	+	Varies amongst states	+

importance. For instance, in the new Kidney Allocation System (KAS) in the United States (US), 4 points are awarded for a prior living organ donor who has now developed kidney failure (equity and fairness), 2 points for a zero HLA DR mismatch donor kidney (utility) and 1 point for each year spent on dialysis (equity and fairness) [36]. A prior living donor will therefore be allocated a donor kidney ahead of a zero HLA DR mismatched recipient who has recently commenced on dialysis and a patient on dialysis for 3 years, but not one on dialysis not for 5 years. In addition to the priority point system, a proportion of donor kidneys may be preferentially allocated to a subgroup of waitlisted patients considered best suited. An example is for the 20% of patients with the longest predicted patient survival to be prioritised for the allocation of the 20% of kidneys with the longest predicted graft survival in the new US KAS to maximise utility.

2.3 Utility

2.3.1 Longevity Matching

There is a clear survival benefit from transplantation compared with remaining on dialysis after the early post-transplant period [37]. This benefit extends to older recipients with medical comorbidities despite a more prolonged period of increased early mortality risk, which is attenuated by having a living donor transplant [38]. However, older patients are also less likely to have a living kidney donor option [39]. Therefore, in an increasingly aging population, the demand for deceased donor kidneys will continue to grow. In general, older kidney transplant recipients are more likely to have shorter patient survival and more likely to die with a functioning graft compared with younger recipients. Therefore, unrestricted allocation of kidneys from younger donors (with longer predicted graft survival) to older recipients would result in a loss of graft life years due to a shorter predicted life expectancy of the recipient. Conversely, transplanting kidneys from older donors (with shorter predicted graft survival) to young recipients will not result in maximum benefit relative to a younger donor kidney [40], and it means that the recipient will return to the waiting list sooner, placing further demand on the donor pool. Avoiding transplanting younger donor kidneys into older recipients has been modelled to increase overall graft life years and cost savings [41, 42]. Various allocation polices internationally have implemented strategies to optimise this aspect of utility, with the term "longevity matching" used to describe models matching the life expectancy of donor organs with the life expectancy of recipients. In general, younger kidneys with longer graft survival are either preferentially allocated to younger recipients with longer estimated survival or restricted from being allocated to older recipients with shorter estimated survival.

2.3.1.1 Facilitating "Young to Young" and Avoiding "Young to Old"

In addition to the paediatric bonus (discussed later), some jurisdictions preferentially allocate younger kidneys to younger recipients. In the United Kingdom (UK), a large donor-recipient age difference leads to a deduction in points for the potential recipient. In effect, kidneys from younger donors are more likely to be allocated to younger than older recipients [43]. Although variations exist in different provinces of Canada, kidneys from younger donors (age ≤ 35) are preferentially allocated to recipients aged ≤ 55 years, for instance in the allocation algorithm of British Columbia, to restrict kidneys with longer graft survival being transplanted into older recipients [44].

2.3.1.2 Facilitating "Old to Old"

The Eurotransplant program is an international collaboration amongst Germany, the Netherlands, Austria, Belgium, Luxembourg, Slovenia, Croatia and Hungary. In addition to the conventional Eurotransplant Kidney Allocation System (ETKAS), non-sensitised patients aged ≥ 65 years are eligible for the Eurotransplant Senior Program (ESP) to receive kidneys from donors aged ≥ 65 years. The allocation of the ESP is based solely on dialysis waiting time and favours local allocation to reduce cold ischaemic time. Since implementation of the ESP, patients have had decreased waiting times with a reduction in rates of delayed graft function. The 1-year and 5-year patient survival was 86 and 60% in ESP (mean age 67.7 years) compared with 90 and 74% in recipients aged 60–64 years (mean age 63.6 years) [45]. Although older recipients receiving kidney transplants from older donors have a higher (especially early) mortality risk, they still benefit long-term compared with waitlisted patients, as demonstrated in the United States (US) [38]. Therefore, this is considered an effective allocation system. However, a recent review in the Netherlands (a member of Eurotransplant) concluded that older recipients may not benefit from receiving kidneys from older (≥ 65 years) donors (old-to-old) [46]. From the commencement of dialysis, compared with waitlisted patients, old-to-old recipients had similar 5-year mortality from donation after brain death (DBD) donors (60.4% versus 61.3%) but higher mortality from donation after circulatory death (DCD) donors (64.5%). This contrasts with the 5-year mortality risk of approximately 50% for older recipients of young DBD and DCD kidneys. While allocation of older donor kidneys to carefully selected older recipients represents optimised utility of organs and may benefit these patients, it does pose additional risks to this susceptible group compared with receiving kidneys from younger donors.

2.3.1.3 Kidney Donor Profile Index (KDPI) and Estimated Post-Transplant Survival (EPTS)

The most significant and novel change in the US Kidney Allocation System (KAS) implemented since December 2014 was longevity matching. This was based on continuous scores of predicted

Table 2.2 Factors consider in Kidney Donor Performance Index (KDPI) and Estimated Post Transplant Survival (EPTS)

KDPI	EPTS
Age	Age
Height	Dialysis time
Weight	Prior organ transplant status
Ethnicity	Diabetes status
Hypertension	
Diabetes	
Cause of death	
Serum creatinine	
Hepatitis C status	
Donation after circulatory death	

post-transplant patient survival and graft survival by Estimated Post-Transplant Survival (EPTS)[46] and Kidney Donor Profile Index (KDPI) [47] respectively. The scores are based on four recipient and 10 donor characteristics respectively (Table 2.2). Although this approach replaces the dichotomous stratification of recipient and donor age in the abovementioned allocation policies, the EPTS and KDPI scores remain heavily influenced by age. In the new KAS, the 20% of waitlisted patients with the longest (EPTS score ≤20%) are prioritised for the 20% of kidneys with the longest estimated graft survival (KDPI ≤20%). As a result, younger donor kidneys are preferentially allocated to younger recipients. A similar approach is planned to be implemented in Australia where currently there is no longevity matching in the allocation system.

Unlike the ESP, kidneys from older donors with higher KDPI are not preferentially allocated to older patients with higher EPTS. However, accepting these kidneys may benefit older patients compared with waiting for a lower EPTS kidneys which are prioritised to younger patients with lower EPTS. Prior to the KAS changes, older patients (>50 years) with a median wait time of ≥33 months were shown to have an increased short-term mortality risk but better long-term survival if they accepted higher KDPI (71–80%, 81–90% and 91–100%) donor kidneys compared to those who waited longer on dialysis for a lower KDPI kidney [48]. This was supported by a further study which demonstrated that older recipients (>60 years) experienced a

lower mortality risk beyond the first post-transplant year when accepting kidneys with a KDPI >85%, compared with waitlisted controls [49].

It is worth noting that both KDPI and EPTS scores, similar to any prediction models, do not predict graft and patient outcomes respectively with certainty. C-statistic is a recognised measure of how well a risk score predicts the actual outcome. A c-statistic of 0.5 is no better than flipping a coin while 1.0 predicts the outcome with absolute precision. For KDPI, the average c-statistic is only 0.62, which represents only modest predictive power for graft outcome. It improves to 0.78 (considered good discriminatory power) when comparing donors from the highest and lowest 20% of estimated graft survival, supporting its use in risk stratification for the purpose of allocation [50]. There is, however, a concern of the labelling effect of high KDPI kidneys resulting in their increased discard rates and therefore compromising overall utility by decreasing the transplant rate [51, 52]. Similarly, the c-statistic for EPTS is 0.69 [53], which has been externally validated in a cohort from Australia and New Zealand [54]. This suggests that although longevity matching may not be precise for each individual donor-recipient pair, the use of EPTS and KDPI should improve the utility of the scarce resource of donor kidneys. Efforts should be made to reduce unnecessary discard of high KDPI kidneys which may still benefit some recipients with higher EPTS.

2.3.2 HLA Matching

Even with contemporary immunosuppression, each additional HLA A, B or DR mismatch is associated with a decrease in graft survival [55]. As illustrated in Fig. 2.5a, there is an approximate 10% difference in 5-year graft survival between 0 and 6 HLA A+B+DR mismatches while the difference between 3 and 4 HLA mismatches is minimal. Similarly, there is a 14% difference in 20-year graft survival between 0 and 6 mismatches with a median survival of 18.3 and 12.7 years respectively (Fig. 2.5b), whereas there is no difference

Fig. 2.5 (a) Five-year graft survival by HLA matching [56]. (b) Twenty-year graft survival by HLA matching [57]

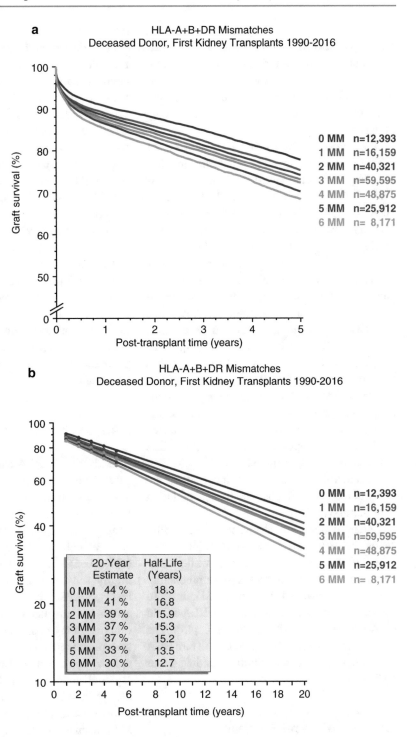

between 3 and 4 mismatches. In addition, those with a poorly matched graft are more likely to become broadly sensitised to HLA, reducing their prospect of re-transplantation. Therefore, incorpo-rating HLA matching into allocation algorithms to maximise utility seems sensible. However, its emphasis varies in different jurisdictions as it com-petes with equity and fairness against those who have waited longer on dialysis, those with rare HLA typing and HLA-homozygous patients. Most allocation policies prioritising HLA matching involve organ sharing across regions, and sometimes countries, resulting in increased cold ischaemic time and the need to re-balance the exchange of organs.

The Eurotransplant Kidney Allocation System (ETKAS) places the most emphasis on HLA matching. Points are awarded for the absence of each HLA A, B or DR mismatch. In contrast, HLA matching is not considered in most Canadian provinces, and there is no national sharing of well-matched donor kidneys. Most jurisdictions prioritise national sharing of zero-mismatched kidneys including the UK, US and Australia. Otherwise, there is a trend to place less emphasis on HLA matching globally. Apart from zero HLA A+B+DR mismatch, points are only awarded for DR matching in the US [36]. In the UK, HLA-DR matching is ranked higher than HLA-B matching while HLA-A matching is no longer considered [43]. In addition, points for the recipient's age are combined with HLA matching to prioritise younger patients for well-matched grafts [43]. This approach aims to minimise HLA sensitisation and improve access to re-transplantation for younger recipients who are likely to require more than one transplant during their lifetime [58].

Certain patients are disadvantaged in an allocation system that favours HLA matching. Ethnic minorities have less common HLA while HLA-homozygous individuals have a lower probability of receiving a lower HLA-mismatched kidney. To address this, points are awarded for HLA-B and HLA-DR homozygosity in the UK [43]. The ETKAS awards points for patients with rare HLA as they have a lower probability of finding a 0 or 1 HLA-mismatched donor.

2.4 Equity and Fairness

2.4.1 Waiting Time

Waiting time is the most widely accepted factor for equity and fairness in deceased donor kidney allocation. Most allocation policies calculate waiting time from the commencement of dialysis regardless of when the patient was waitlisted. In contrast, waiting time starts from the time of activation on the waiting list in the UK [43]. The US originally adopted a similar approach to the UK. However, since 2014, one of the changes to the US KAS was to award waiting time points based on time spent on dialysis to avoid inequalities for those with reduced access to the waiting list [36]. Even in the contemporary era, time on dialysis is a strong predictor for post-transplant mortality [59, 60]. While 13,501 patients received a deceased donor kidney transplant in the US in 2016, 4830 patients died on the waiting list, and a further 4411 patients became too sick to receive a transplant and were removed from the list [61]. Therefore, a fair kidney allocation system needs to avoid a minority of patients waiting longer than others and developing dialysis related complications which could render them no longer transplantable.

2.4.2 Sensitisation

Sensitisation to HLA can be induced by events such as previous organ transplants, pregnancies and blood transfusions. Some patients may therefore develop anti-HLA antibodies against a high percentage of potential donors expressed as the calculated panel reactive antibody (cPRA). Different allocation policies define highly sensitised patients (HSP) by different levels of cPRA (Table 2.1). HSP have limited access to transplantation and without prioritisation, they may miss an opportunity to receive a transplant from an immunologically compatible donor. To facilitate transplantation in HSP, regional and/or national sharing of organs is often required. Most highly sensitised programs prioritise allocation of kidneys based on avoidance of unacceptable antigens defined by solid phase assays (where patients have pre-formed antibodies against donor HLA). In contrast, allocation through the Eurotransplant Acceptable Mismatch program is based on defining acceptable antigens by the lack of antibody reactivity in CDC assays using cells expressing a single HLA and eplet analysis using HLAMatchmaker [7]. Compared with the regular ETKAS, such an approach employed by the Acceptable Mismatch program resulted in superior 10-year death-censored graft survival (72.8% vs 62.4%), only marginally inferior to non-sensitised patients (74.8%) [62].

HSP, many of whom had previous transplants, have inferior graft survival. Patients with a PRA of >50% have a 10-year graft survival of 55.5% compared with 72.4% for those with a PRA of 0% [63]. Patients with repeat transplants also have inferior graft survival compared with those with first transplants (Fig. 2.6). Therefore, equity for HSP to receive a kidney transplant competes with the principle of utility of the limited resource of donor organs. Furthermore, some argue that prioritisation of HSP for re-transplantation ahead of those who have not yet been given a first transplant is against the principle of equity and fairness [65]. Clearly, this is a difficult ethical dilemma, and a balance needs to be struck to avoid excessive prioritisation and unacceptable reduction in graft years for HSP.

2.4.3   Prior Living Kidney Donors

Living kidney donors facilitate timely (often pre-emptive) transplantation and superior patient and graft survival over deceased donors. They alleviate the demand for deceased donor organs [66]. Despite its relative safety, there is a small but increased risk of end-stage kidney disease compared with healthy non-donors [67, 68]. It only seems fair therefore, that any disadvantage to their health from their act of altruism should be offset. To that end, many allocation policies incorporate prioritisation for prior living kidney donors.

2.4.4   Blood Group

In most jurisdictions, kidneys are allocated to blood group identical (rather than compatible) waitlisted recipients, with the exceptions of prioritisation for HSP and zero HLA A+B+DR mismatch. This is to avoid the imbalance of the universally compatible blood group O donor kidneys being allocated to non-O recipients. As evident in the original Eurotransplant Senior

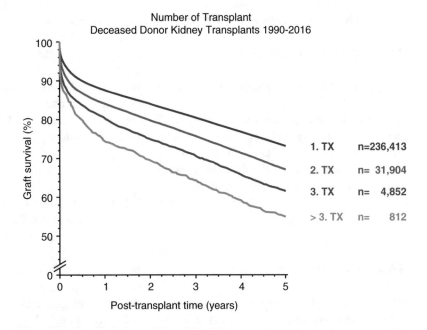

Fig. 2.6 Graft survival by transplant number [64]

Number of Transplant
Deceased Donor Kidney Transplants 1990-2016

1. TX   n=236,413
2. TX   n= 31,904
3. TX   n= 4,852
> 3. TX   n=   812

Program (ESP) in Germany where O kidneys were allocated to all compatible blood groups, blood group O patients had longer waiting times and were more likely to accumulate on the waiting list compared with non-O patients [69].

Allocation of kidneys by identical blood type, however, contributes to the ethnic minorities being disadvantaged in their access to transplantation. Blood group B is represented by ethnic minorities in 71.4% (including 44% black, 13.8% Asian and 11.6% Hispanic) compared to 50.2% in blood group A in the US [70]. They have reduced access to deceased donor kidneys and longer waiting time due to the higher percentage of waitlisted patients of ethnic minorities compared to that of the donor pool from the general population [71, 72]. To address this, blood group B (but not A or AB) candidates are eligible to receive O donor kidneys in the UK. Given the long-term success of transplanting A2 and A2B kidneys into blood group B recipients (who often have persistently low anti-A titres) [70], for US transplant programs with specific consents, A2 and A2B donor kidneys are prioritised to pre-consented B candidates. This initiative increased the transplant rate in B candidates from the participating Donation Service Areas (DSA), demonstrating graft survival comparable to B recipients of B kidneys [73].

2.5 Medical Urgency and Needs

2.5.1 Inadequate Dialysis

For patients with inadequate dialysis without options for further dialysis access, kidney transplantation becomes an urgent lifesaving treatment. Most allocation policies consider patients under such circumstances as medical urgency to be allowed prioritisation. Where there is more than one kidney transplant program in the same region, agreement from other transplant programs is generally required.

2.5.2 Paediatric Bonus

Priority for paediatric patients is widely accepted in most allocation policies due to the detrimental impact of dialysis and unique benefits of transplantation for growth [74] and cognitive development [75]. Donor kidneys of higher quality are often coupled with the paediatric bonus. The intention is to improve the utility of graft years for paediatric recipients with longer expected survival, while minimising sensitisation for future re-transplantation. Share-35 was an initiative to preferentially offer young deceased donors (<35 years old) to paediatric patients (<18 years old), implemented in 2005 in the US. Although it doubled the number of transplants from young deceased donors, the majority of these were 5 or 6 HLA A+B+DR mismatched kidneys. In addition, the proportion of paediatric living kidney transplants decreased from 55 to 35%, an unintended consequence [76].

Paediatric patients usually require re-transplantation. To avoid broad HLA sensitisation from receiving deceased donor kidneys with high HLA mismatches, different strategies have been employed. In the new KAS, paediatric patients receive 1 point if the donor has a KDPI <35%, while 3–4 points (depending on the age of the patient) are awarded if a zero HLA mismatched donor kidney is offered [36]. In the UK, zero mismatched and well-matched (no DR mismatches) kidneys are prioritised to paediatric recipients [43]. Alternatively, rather than promoting HLA matching in a minority of paediatric recipients, the Royal Children's Hospital in Australia established prospective exclusions of donors with HLA associated with high eplet mismatches for each individual patient. This approach significantly lowered class 2 eplet mismatches to reduce the risk of broad sensitisation while still allowing timely access to transplantation [77].

2.5.3 Changes to the Kidney Allocation System (KAS) in the United States

In December 2014, the United States implemented several amendments to the KAS. The key changes, their goals, whether achieved or not, are outlined in Table 2.3. The changes aimed to pro-

Table 2.3 Key changes, goals and consequences in the Kidney Allocation System in the United States

Key changes	Goals	Consequences
Low KDPI (≤20%) donor kidneys preferentially allocated to low EPTS (≤20%) candidates	Longevity matching to avoid wasted graft years (Utility)	• Donor-recipient age mismatch >30 years decreased from 21.1 to 16.3% • Recipients aged ≥65 receiving KDPI 0–20% kidneys decreased from 3.2 to 1.1% • Recipients aged ≤40 receiving KDPI 0-20% kidneys increased from 7.1 to 12.8% • Recipients aged 18-34 increased from 8.8 to 12.8% • Recipients aged ≥65 decreased from 22.9 to 18.1%
Broader sharing of kidneys to highly sensitised candidates with cPRA ≥99% Stepwise priority points for cPRA ≥20%	To increase access to transplantation for highly sensitised patients (Equity and fairness)	• Recipients with cPRA ≥99% increased by 4-fold from 2.4 to 13.4% (after bolus effect: from peak of 14.8 to 12.1%)
Points for waiting time from dialysis initiation rather than activation on waiting list	To avoid disadvantaging patients with reduced access to early referral for transplantation (Equity and fairness)	• Recipients with ≥10 years of dialysis vintage increased from 4.3 to 10.9% (after bolus effect: from peak of 13.1 to 7.9%)
Blood group A_2 and A_2B kidneys preferentially allocated to blood group B candidates	To reduce waiting time for blood group B candidates with longer waiting time than blood group A candidates (Equity and fairness)	• A_2/A_2B donor kidneys to B recipients increased from 0.2 to 1.0% • No increase in blood group B recipients • No decrease in blood group A recipients
Broader sharing of kidneys with high KDPI (>85%)	To reduce discard rate of high KDPI kidneys which may still benefit some recipients (Utility)	• No increase in use of kidneys with KDPI ≥85% • Marginal increase in discard rate from 18.5 to 19.4%

mote both utility and equity. These included (1) longevity matching by preferentially allocating lower KDPI kidneys to lower EPTS patients, (2) broader sharing of kidneys for HSP, (3) awarding points for waiting time from dialysis initiation to compensate disadvantaged patients (often ethnic minorities) for being referred late for transplantation, (4) allocation of blood group A2 and A2B kidneys to B candidates, and (5) broader sharing of high KDPI kidneys to reduce discard rate and increase utilisation [36]. Some of the goals were achieved comparing pre-KAS and the first year post-KAS, including reducing donor-recipient age mismatch and increasing transplant rates for HSP and those with long dialysis waiting time, with a bolus effect [78]. However, no increase in transplant rates for blood group B recipients was observed due to the low uptake of A2 and A2B donor kidneys for these patients. There was also no increase in the use of high KDPI kidneys. In fact, there was a marginal increase in discard rate.

As a result of broader sharing of organs, cold ischaemic times (CIT) increased from 17.0 to 17.9 h, with the percentage of transplants with a CIT >24 h increasing from 18.2 to 21.3%. Delayed graft function also increased from 24.4 to 29.2% across all CIT categories. It has been suggested that this may relate to transplanting patients with longer dialysis vintage. Although the 6-month graft survival has remained similar, longer follow-up is required to ensure that the changes to KAS have not resulted in reduced graft survival [78]. Some argue that these changes may not have achieved the desired goals and led to unintended consequences [65]. For instance, HSP with cPRA ≥99% may have been "overcompensated" in the current KAS. As a perfect kidney allocation system is unlikely to exist, the new changes to KAS have fulfilled many of their goals to optimise utility and equity. However, monitoring for possible undesired consequences is crucial to facilitate potential revisions of KAS in the future.

References

1. Mulley WR, Kanellis J. Understanding crossmatch testing in organ transplantation: a case-based guide for the general nephrologist. Nephrology (Carlton). 2011;16(2):125–33.
2. Althaf MM, El Kossi M, Jin JK, Sharma A, Halawa AM. Human leukocyte antigen typing and cross-match: a comprehensive review. World J Transplant. 2017;7(6):339–48.
3. Otten HG, Tilanus MG, Barnstijn M, van Heugten JG, de Gast GC. Serology versus PCR-SSP in typing for HLA-DR and HLA-DQ: a practical evaluation. Tissue Antigens. 1995;45(1):36–40.
4. Woszczek G, Borowiec M, Mis M, Gorska M, Kowalski ML. Comparison of serological and molecular (PCR-SSP) techniques of HLA-DR typing in clinical laboratory routine. Ann Transplant. 1997;2(1):39–42.
5. International HapMap C. A haplotype map of the human genome. Nature. 2005;437(7063): 1299–320.
6. Duquesnoy RJ. A structurally based approach to determine HLA compatibility at the humoral immune level. Hum Immunol. 2006;67(11):847–62.
7. Duquesnoy RJ, Askar M. HLAMatchmaker: a molecularly based algorithm for histocompatibility determination. V. Eplet matching for HLA-DR, HLA-DQ, and HLA-DP. Hum Immunol. 2007;68(1):12–25.
8. Tambur AR, Claas FH. HLA epitopes as viewed by antibodies: what is it all about? Am J Transplant. 2015;15(5):1148–54.
9. Duquesnoy RJ. HLAmatchmaker. 2018. http://www.epitopes.net/publications.html.
10. Duquesnoy RJ, Marrari M. HLAMatchmaker: a molecularly based algorithm for histocompatibility determination. II. Verification of the algorithm and determination of the relative immunogenicity of amino acid triplet-defined epitopes. Hum Immunol. 2002;63(5):353–63.
11. MacCallum RM, Martin AC, Thornton JM. Antibody-antigen interactions: contact analysis and binding site topography. J Mol Biol. 1996;262(5):732–45.
12. Starzl TE, Eliasziw M, Gjertson D, et al. HLA and cross-reactive antigen group matching for cadaver kidney allocation. Transplantation. 1997;64(7):983–91.
13. Walton DC, Hiho SJ, Cantwell LS, et al. HLA matching at the eplet level protects against chronic lung allograft dysfunction. Am J Transplant. 2016;16(9):2695–703.
14. Wiebe C, Pochinco D, Blydt-Hansen TD, et al. Class II HLA epitope matching-A strategy to minimize de novo donor-specific antibody development and improve outcomes. Am J Transplant. 2013;13(12):3114–22.
15. Gloor J, Cosio F, Lager DJ, Stegall MD. The spectrum of antibody-mediated renal allograft injury: implications for treatment. Am J Transplant. 2008;8(7):1367–73.
16. Patel R, Terasaki PI. Significance of the positive crossmatch test in kidney transplantation. N Engl J Med. 1969;280(14):735–9.
17. Terasaki PI, McClelland JD. Microdroplet assay of human serum cytotoxins. Nature. 1964;204:998–1000.
18. Pellegrino MA, Belvedere M, Pellegrino AG, Ferrone S. B peripheral lymphocytes express more HLA antigens than T peripheral lymphocytes. Transplantation. 1978;25(2):93–5.
19. Le Bas-Bernardet S, Hourmant M, Valentin N, et al. Identification of the antibodies involved in B-cell crossmatch positivity in renal transplantation. Transplantation. 2003;75(4):477–82.
20. Stegall MD, Gloor J, Winters JL, Moore SB, Degoey S. A comparison of plasmapheresis versus high-dose IVIG desensitization in renal allograft recipients with high levels of donor specific alloantibody. Am J Transplant. 2006;6(2):346–51.
21. Pollinger HS, Stegall MD, Gloor JM, et al. Kidney transplantation in patients with antibodies against donor HLA class II. Am J Transplant. 2007;7(4):857–63.
22. Garovoy MR RM, Bigos M, Perkins H, Colombe, BFN, Salvatierra O. Flow cytometry analysis: a high technology crossmatch technique facilitating transplantation. Transplant Proc. 1983;XV:1939–1944.
23. Karpinski M, Rush D, Jeffery J, et al. Flow cytometric crossmatching in primary renal transplant recipients with a negative anti-human globulin enhanced cytotoxicity crossmatch. J Am Soc Nephrol. 2001;12(12):2807–14.
24. Burns JM, Cornell LD, Perry DK, et al. Alloantibody levels and acute humoral rejection early after positive crossmatch kidney transplantation. Am J Transplant. 2008;8(12):2684–94.
25. Stegall MD, Diwan T, Raghavaiah S, et al. Terminal complement inhibition decreases antibody-mediated rejection in sensitized renal transplant recipients. Am J Transplant. 2011;11(11):2405–13.
26. Bielmann D, Honger G, Lutz D, Mihatsch MJ, Steiger J, Schaub S. Pretransplant risk assessment in renal allograft recipients using virtual crossmatching. Am J Transplant. 2007;7(3):626–32.
27. Tait BD, Hudson F, Cantwell L, et al. Review article: Luminex technology for HLA antibody detection in organ transplantation. Nephrology (Carlton). 2009;14(2):247–54.
28. Tait BD. Detection of HLA antibodies in organ transplant recipients – triumphs and challenges of the solid phase bead assay. Front Immunol. 2016;7:570.
29. Cecka JM, Kucheryavaya AY, Reinsmoen NL, Leffell MS. Calculated PRA: initial results show benefits for sensitized patients and a reduction in positive crossmatches. Am J Transplant. 2011;11(4):719–24.
30. Jordan SC, Choi J, Vo A. Kidney transplantation in highly sensitized patients. Br Med Bull. 2015;114(1):113–25.
31. Lefaucheur C, Loupy A, Hill GS, et al. Preexisting donor-specific HLA antibodies predict outcome

in kidney transplantation. J Am Soc Nephrol. 2010;21(8):1398–406.

32. Augustine JJ, Siu DS, Clemente MJ, Schulak JA, Heeger PS, Hricik DE. Pre-transplant IFN-gamma ELISPOTs are associated with post-transplant renal function in African American renal transplant recipients. Am J Transplant. 2005;5(8):1971–5.

33. Hricik DE, Augustine J, Nickerson P, et al. Interferon gamma ELISPOT testing as a risk-stratifying biomarker for kidney transplant injury: results from the CTOT-01 multicenter study. Am J Transplant. 2015;15(12):3166–73.

34. Gutmann T, Land W. The ethics of organ allocation: the state of debate. Transplant Rev (Orlando). 1997;11(4):191–207.

35. Tong A, Jan S, Wong G, et al. Patient preferences for the allocation of deceased donor kidneys for transplantation: a mixed methods study. BMC Nephrol. 2012;13:18.

36. Israni AK, Salkowski N, Gustafson S, et al. New national allocation policy for deceased donor kidneys in the United States and possible effect on patient outcomes. J Am Soc Nephrol. 2014;25(8):1842–8.

37. Wolfe RA, Ashby VB, Milford EL, et al. Comparison of mortality in all patients on dialysis, patients on dialysis awaiting transplantation, and recipients of a first cadaveric transplant. N Engl J Med. 1999;341(23):1725–30.

38. Gill JS, Schaeffner E, Chadban S, et al. Quantification of the early risk of death in elderly kidney transplant recipients. Am J Transplant. 2013;13(2):427–32.

39. Karim A, Farrugia D, Cheshire J, et al. Recipient age and risk for mortality after kidney transplantation in England. Transplantation. 2014;97(8):832–8.

40. Schold JD, Meier-Kriesche HU. Which renal transplant candidates should accept marginal kidneys in exchange for a shorter waiting time on dialysis? Clin J Am Soc Nephrol. 2006;1(3):532–8.

41. Lim WH, Chang S, Chadban S, et al. Donor-recipient age matching improves years of graft function in deceased-donor kidney transplantation. Nephrol Dial Transplant. 2010;25(9):3082–9.

42. Meier-Kriesche HU, Schold JD, Gaston RS, Wadstrom J, Kaplan B. Kidneys from deceased donors: maximizing the value of a scarce resource. Am J Transplant. 2005;5(7):1725–30.

43. NHS Blood and Transplant. NHS Blood and transplant. Kidney transplantation: deceased donor organ allocation (POLICY POL186/9). 2017. https://nhsbtdbe.blob.core.windows.net/umbraco-assets-corp/6522/pol186-kidney-transplantation-deceased-donor-organ-allocation.pdf. Accessed 19 May 2018.

44. British Columbia Transplant. British Columbia transplant. Clinical guidelines for kidney transplantation. 2017. http://www.transplant.bc.ca/Documents/Health%20Professionals/Clinical%20guidelines/Clinical%20Guidelines%20for%20Kidney%20Transplantation.pdf. Accessed 20 May 2018.

45. Frei U, Noeldeke J, Machold-Fabrizii V, et al. Prospective age-matching in elderly kidney transplant recipients--a 5-year analysis of the eurotransplant senior program. Am J Transplant. 2008;8(1):50–7.

46. Peters-Sengers H, Berger SP, Heemskerk MB, et al. Stretching the limits of renal transplantation in elderly recipients of grafts from elderly deceased donors. J Am Soc Nephrol. 2017;28(2):621–31.

47. Organ Procurement and Transplantation Network. Organ procurement and transplantation network, a guide to calculating and interpreting the kidney donor profile index (KDPI). 2016. https://optn.transplant.hrsa.gov/media/1512/guide_to_calculating_interpreting_kdpi.pdf. Accessed 20 May 2018.

48. Massie AB, Luo X, Chow EK, Alejo JL, Desai NM, Segev DL. Survival benefit of primary deceased donor transplantation with high-KDPI kidneys. Am J Transplant. 2014;14(10):2310–6.

49. Jay CL, Washburn K, Dean PG, Helmick RA, Pugh JA, Stegall MD. Survival benefit in older patients associated with earlier transplant with high KDPI kidneys. Transplantation. 2017;101(4):867–72.

50. Rao PS, Schaubel DE, Guidinger MK, et al. A comprehensive risk quantification score for deceased donor kidneys: the kidney donor risk index. Transplantation. 2009;88(2):231–6.

51. Bae S, Massie AB, Luo X, Anjum S, Desai NM, Segev DL. Changes in discard rate after the introduction of the kidney donor profile index (KDPI). Am J Transplant. 2016;16(7):2202–7.

52. Stewart DE, Garcia VC, Aeder MI, Klassen DK. New insights into the alleged kidney donor profile index labeling effect on kidney utilization. Am J Transplant. 2017;17(10):2696–704.

53. Organ Procurement and Transplantation Network. Organ Procurement and Transplantation Network. A guide to calculating and interpreting the estimated post-transplant survival (EPTS) score used in the kidney allocation system (KAS). 2014. https://optn.transplant.hrsa.gov/media/1511/guide_to_calculating_interpreting_epts.pdf. Accessed 20 May 2018.

54. Clayton PA, McDonald SP, Snyder JJ, Salkowski N, Chadban SJ. External validation of the estimated post-transplant survival score for allocation of deceased donor kidneys in the United States. Am J Transplant. 2014;14(8):1922–6.

55. Williams RC, Opelz G, McGarvey CJ, Weil EJ, Chakkera HA. The risk of transplant failure with HLA mismatch in first adult kidney allografts from deceased donors. Transplantation. 2016;100(5):1094–102.

56. Collaborative Transplant Study. K-21101-0218. 2018. http://www.ctstransplant.org/public/graphics/archive.shtml.

57. Collaborative Transplant Study. K-21103-0218. 2018. http://www.ctstransplant.org/public/graphics/archive.shtml.

58. Gralla J, Tong S, Wiseman AC. The impact of human leukocyte antigen mismatching on sensitization rates and subsequent retransplantation after first graft failure in pediatric renal transplant recipients. Transplantation. 2013;95(10):1218–24.

59. Haller MC, Kainz A, Baer H, Oberbauer R. Dialysis vintage and outcomes after kidney transplantation: a retrospective cohort study. Clin J Am Soc Nephrol. 2017;12(1):122–30.

60. Helantera I, Salmela K, Kyllonen L, Koskinen P, Gronhagen-Riska C, Finne P. Pretransplant dialysis duration and risk of death after kidney transplantation in the current era. Transplantation. 2014;98(4):458–64.

61. Hart A, Smith JM, Skeans MA, et al. OPTN/SRTR 2016 annual data report: kidney. Am J Transplant. 2018;18(Suppl 1):18–113.

62. Heidt S, Haasnoot GW, van Rood JJ, Witvliet MD, Claas FHJ. Kidney allocation based on proven acceptable antigens results in superior graft survival in highly sensitized patients. Kidney Int. 2018;93(2):491–500.

63. Opelz G, Collaborative TS. Non-HLA transplantation immunity revealed by lymphocytotoxic antibodies. Lancet. 2005;365(9470):1570–6.

64. Collaborative Transplant Study. K-11101-0218. 2018. http://www.ctstransplant.org/public/graphics/archive.shtml.

65. Klintmalm GB, Kaplan B. The kidney allocation system claims equity: it is time to review utility and fairness. Am J Transplant. 2017;17(12):2999–3000.

66. Australia and New Zealand Dialysis and Transplant Registry. Australia and New Zealand dialysis and transplant registry. Transplantation. [Internet]. 2016. http://www.anzdata.org.au/anzdata/AnzdataReport/40thReport/c07_transplant_2016_v1.0_20180509.pdf. Accessed 19 May 2018.

67. Mjoen G, Hallan S, Hartmann A, et al. Long-term risks for kidney donors. Kidney Int. 2014;86(1):162–7.

68. Muzaale AD, Massie AB, Wang MC, et al. Risk of end-stage renal disease following live kidney donation. JAMA. 2014;311(6):579–86.

69. Liefeldt L, Budde K, Glander P. Accumulation of elderly ESRD patients with blood group O on the waiting list. Transpl Int. 2011;24(10):e83–4.

70. Bryan CF, Cherikh WS, Sesok-Pizzini DA. A2/A2 B to B renal transplantation: past, present, and future directions. Am J Transplant. 2016;16(1):11–20.

71. Hurst FP, Sajjad I, Elster EA, et al. Transplantation of A2 kidneys into B and O recipients leads to reduction in waiting time: USRDS experience. Transplantation. 2010;89(11):1396–402.

72. Rudge C, Johnson RJ, Fuggle SV, Forsythe JL. Kidney, pancreas advisory group UKTNHSBT. Renal transplantation in the United Kingdom for patients from ethnic minorities. Transplantation. 2007;83(9):1169–73.

73. Williams WW, Cherikh WS, Young CJ, et al. First report on the OPTN national variance: allocation of A2/A2 B deceased donor kidneys to blood group B increases minority transplantation. Am J Transplant. 2015;15(12):3134–42.

74. Nissel R, Brazda I, Feneberg R, et al. Effect of renal transplantation in childhood on longitudinal growth and adult height. Kidney Int. 2004;66(2):792–800.

75. Hartmann H, Hawellek N, Wedekin M, et al. Early kidney transplantation improves neurocognitive outcome in patients with severe congenital chronic kidney disease. Transpl Int. 2015;28(4):429–36.

76. Agarwal S, Oak N, Siddique J, Harland RC, Abbo ED. Changes in pediatric renal transplantation after implementation of the revised deceased donor kidney allocation policy. Am J Transplant. 2009;9(5):1237–42.

77. Kausman JY, Walker AM, Cantwell LS, Quinlan C, Sypek MP, Ierino FL. Application of an epitope-based allocation system in pediatric kidney transplantation. Pediatr Transplant. 2016;20(7):931–8.

78. Stewart DE, Kucheryavaya AY, Klassen DK, Turgeon NA, Formica RN, Aeder MI. Changes in deceased donor kidney transplantation one year after KAS implementation. Am J Transplant. 2016;16(6):1834–47.

The Immunobiology of Transplant Rejection and Acceptance

3

John P. Vella and Amjad Mehboob

3.1 Introduction

The immune system normally functions to mitigate infectious and neoplastic risk. In the absence of immunosuppression, the transplantation of allogeneic tissue constitutes a challenge as allorecognition triggers injurious effector mechanisms culminating in graft destruction. This chapter will focus on innate immunity, the basic mechanisms of allorecognition, co-stimulation, T cell amplification, effector mechanisms, and antibody production.

3.1.1 Immune Response to Transplanted Tissue

To adequately understand the response to transplanted tissue, it is helpful and important to review the general immune response. The immune system can be divided into two core components (see Table 3.1). Innate immune system is nonspecific and non-adaptive while the adaptive immune system is antigen specific and exhibits memory, or secondary, immune responses.

J. P. Vella (✉) · A. Mehboob
Maine Medical Center, Tufts University
School of Medicine, Portland, ME, USA
e-mail: vellajp@mmc.org

3.2 The Innate Immune System

Innate immunity refers to the nonspecific natural immune system that involves macrophages, dendritic cells, neutrophils, NK (natural killer) cells, cytokines, toll-like receptors, and complement components. Innate immune system provides immediate albeit incomplete protection against intruders and, at best, has only short-term memory.

3.3 Role of Innate Immune System in Allograft Rejection

How the innate immune system recognizes allogeneic non-self is incompletely understood. It has long been established that cells of the innate immune system do not directly participate in allorecognition. Rather, NK cells respond to inflammatory ligands released by dying cells [1, 2]. These inflammatory ligands include uric acid and nuclear protein high-mobility group box 1, among others. Such mediators are allograft nonspecific and relate more to hypoxic injury and signal through innate pattern recognition receptors [3, 4]. Such receptors include Toll-like receptors and various components of the inflammasome, all of which also participate in the recognition of microbes.

NK cells are activated by stimulatory ligands such as the MHC I- related proteins MICA and

© Springer Nature Switzerland AG 2021
N. Hakim et al. (eds.), *Transplantation Surgery*, Springer Specialist Surgery Series,
https://doi.org/10.1007/978-3-030-55244-2_3

Table 3.1 Comparison of Innate and Adaptive Immunity

Innate immunity	Adaptive immunity
Non-specific	Specific
Involves physical and chemical barriers, macrophages, phagocytic leukocytes, dendritic and NK cells	Involves B and T lymphocytes
No memory cells	Involves generation of "memory cells" against specific antigens for future enhanced response
Respond to any foreign antigen	Responds to a specific antigen
Inherited	Can't be inherited
Faster response	Slower response
Activation of alternative and lectin pathways	Classical pathway

MICB which have been detected in solid organ allografts as well as the absence of inhibitory signals delivered by self-MHC [5]. However such stimulatory signals are generally insufficient for complete activation of NK cells as is seen after a viral infection [6]. Interestingly, studies on T and B cell deficient RAG −/− (recombination-activating gene) mice have shown that a specific alloimmune response to allogenic non-self was mounted independent of NK cells [7]. The findings provide direct evidence that monocytes mediate a response to allogeneic non-self, a function not previously attributed to them, and suggest the presence of mismatching at loci unlinked to MHC. The allo-determinants for these loci unlinked to MHC may be polymorphic genes that are outside the MHC as Polymorphic Ig Domain containing genes that are expressed in cells of the innate immune system in mice and humans [8]. Recently a study [9] on the innate response of $Rag2^{-/-}\gamma c^{-/-}$ mice, which lack T, B, and NK cells, to grafts from allogeneic showed that donor polymorphism in the gene encoding signal regulatory protein alpha (SIRPα) is a key modulator of the recipients innate allorecognition response.

3.4   The Adaptive Immune System

The adaptive immune system recognizes non-self-antigens to initiate immune responses. Unlike the innate immune system, which func-

tions based on the identification of general threats, adaptive immunity is activated by exposure to pathogens or alloantigens, and uses immunological memory to learn about the threat and enhance the immune response accordingly. Adaptive immunity is often lifelong. In general terms, the adaptive immune response is slower to respond to threats and infections than the innate immune response, which is primed and ready to combat threats at all times.

Adaptive immune responses are triggered when APCs activate antigen-specific T cells within secondary lymphoid organs leading to effector cell generation and their migration to the allograft where they mediate rejection. The majority of effector T cells eventually undergoes apoptosis and the few that survive become long-lived memory T cells that endanger the survival of a subsequent organ transplant.

3.4.1   Cells of the Adaptive Immune System

The adaptive immune system mainly relies on *T cells* and *B cells*. Both T cells and B cells are lymphocytes that are derived from bone marrow derived multipotent hematopoietic stem cells.

3.4.1.1 T Cells
Naïve T cells are formed in the bone marrow, and then migrate to the thymus (hence the name "T cell") in order to mature. While in the thymus, the developing T cells start to express T cell receptors (TCRs), and either CD4 or CD8 receptors.

Unlike antibodies, which can bind to antigens directly, T cell receptors can only recognize antigens that are bound to Major Histocompatibility Complex class 1 (MHCI) or class 2 (MHCII). These MHC molecules are membrane-bound surface receptors on professional antigen-presenting cells, such as dendritic cells and macrophages. CD4 and CD8 play a role in T cell recognition and activation. Class 1 MHC molecule present peptide antigens to CD8-positive T cells while MHC class-II Molecules presents antigen to CD4-positive T cells.

T cells undergo two selection processes:

1. Positive selection ensures MHC restriction by testing the ability of MHC-I and MHC-II to distinguish between self and non-self-proteins. In order to pass the positive selection process, cells must be capable of binding only self-MHC molecules. If these cells bind non-self-molecules instead of self-MHC molecules, they fail the positive selection process and are eliminated by apoptosis.

2. Negative selection tests for self-tolerance. Negative selection tests the binding capabilities of CD4 and CD8 specifically. For example, T cells only bind to self-MHC molecules presenting a foreign antigen. If a T cell binds to a self-MHC molecule that isn't presenting an antigen, or alternately, binds to a self-MHC molecule presenting self-antigen, it will fail negative selection and be eliminated by apoptosis. These two selection processes mitigate autoimmunity risk.

The end result of positive and negative selection includes: Helper T cells, Cytotoxic T cells, and T regulatory cells.

3.4.1.2 Helper T Cells

T helper (Th) cells are divided into two main populations: Type 1 (Th1) and Type 2 (Th2) cells. A third T-cell subset (T helper cells Type 17) has also been identified. These cells are involved in early response to pathogens, in autoimmunity and tissue inflammation.

3.4.1.3 Type 1 Helper Cells

Th1 cells produce interleukin (IL)-2, gamma-interferon (IFN-gamma) and tumor necrosis factor-beta and are involved in delayed type hypersensitivity reactions. In addition, they are the main cells involved in acute allograft rejection.

3.4.1.4 Type 2 Helper Cells

Th2 cells express IL-4, IL-5, IL-6, IL-10 and IL-13 and provide help for B-cell production of antibody, and particularly IgE response (parasitic infections). This IgE response is mediated by IL-4 which acts as a growth factor for B cells

antibody production while directly inhibiting the T cell maturation into Th1 pathway.

3.4.1.5 Cytotoxic T Cells

Cytotoxic T Cells express CD8 and are principally involved in the killing of tumor and virally infected cells. Activation of Cytotoxic T cells involves interactions between molecules on the surface of cytotoxic T cells and APC's. The first signal is interaction between peptide bound MHC class 1 molecule on APC and the TCR on CD8+ T cells. The second signal is interaction between CD28 molecule on T-cell and either CD80 or CD 86 (also called B7–1 and B7–2) on APC. Activation of cytotoxic T cells leads to killing of the infected cells by either delivering a "lethal hit" or alternatively by inducing apoptosis. After activation, CD8+ T cells release cytoxins, perforins, granzyme B, and granulysin. Through the action of perforin, granzymes enter the cytoplasm of the target cell and their serine protease function triggers the interleukin-1-beta converting enzyme (ICE) mediated protease pathway that eventually lead to cell death. This pathway is critically important for eradication of microbial infection. A second way to induce "activation-induced cell death is by utilizing the FAS pathway [10–13]. When a cytoxic T cell is activated it starts to express the surface protein FAS ligand (FasL) (Apo1L)(CD95L), which can bind to Fas (Apo1) (CD95) molecules expressed on the target cell. Engagement of Fas with FasL allows for recruitment of the death-induced signaling complex (DISC) which comprises activated caspases leading to cleavage of death substrates such as lamin A, lamin B1, lamin B2, PARP (poly ADP ribose polymerase), and DNA-PKcs (DNA-activated protein kinase) [14].The final result is apoptosis of the cell that expressed FAS. The FAS pathway is of importance in limiting T-cell proliferation in response to antigenic stimulation. Cell-mediated cytotoxicity has been shown to play an important role in acute, although not chronic, allograft rejection [15].

The diagnostic utility of measurement on mRNA encoding cytotoxic attack proteins granzyme B and perforin in urine specimens obtained from renal allograft recipients, has been investigated and reported that mRNA levels of perforin and granzyme B were significantly higher in the urinary cells obtained from renal allograft recipients with a biopsy confirmed episode of acute rejection than in the patients without an episode of acute rejection. Analysis involving the receiver-operating-characteristic curve demonstrated that acute rejection can be predicted with a sensitivity of 83% and a specificity of 83% using perforin mRNA levels, and with a sensitivity of 79% and a specificity of 77% using granzyme B mRNA levels [16]. Similarly, reverse transcriptase-polymerase chain reaction (RT-PCR) has been used to identify intrarenal expression of cytotoxic attack molecules (granzyme B and perforin) and immunoregulatory cytokines (IL-2, IL-4, IL-10, IFN-gamma, and TGF-beta 1) in human renal allograft biopsies. Molecular analyses revealed that intragraft display of mRNA encoding granzyme B, IL-10 or IL-2 is a correlate of acute rejection, and intrarenal expression of TGF beta 1 mRNA, of chronic rejection [17].

3.4.1.6 T Regulatory Cells

Regulatory T cells (Tregs) play a pivotal role in regulating other cells in the immune system. Tregs mediate their regulatory function through multiple soluble and cell surface markers. The most widely used markers for Tregs are (see Fig. 3.1): CD25, cytotoxic T lymphocyte-associated antigen 4 (CTLA-4), glucocorticoid-induced tumor necrosis factor receptor family-related gene (GITR), lymphocyte activation gene-3 (LAG-3) and forkhead/winged-helix transcription factor box P3 (Foxp3) [18–20]. However accumulating evidence suggests that these markers are not strictly Treg-specific. For example, CTLA-4/TCR interactions with their co stimulatory ligands on APC's and CD25 with IL-2 involvement leads to production of soluble messengers TGF-beta, IL-10 and adenosine (Fig. 3.1) which in turn suppresses activation, proliferation and cytokine production of CD4+ T cells. CD8+ T cells and are thought to suppress B cells and dendritic cells [21, 22]. Tregs impact immune responses to self-antigens, allergens, and commensal microbiota as well as immune responses to infectious agents and tumors. In addition, T regulatory cells by distinguishing between self and non-self-molecules, play an important role in reducing the risk of auto immune diseases. When regulatory T cells (Tregs) emerged as a mechanism in control of autoimmunity [23, 24], considerable interest focused on their role in organ transplantation and their potential for cell-based therapy. Such studies often incorporate forkhead box P3 (FOXP3), a forkhead-winged helix transcription factor expressed on the X chromosome, important in the development and function of Tregs. Such studies [25–27] were facilitated by the discovery of Foxp3 loss-of-function mutations in humans

Fig. 3.1 Regulatory T cell receptors and activation

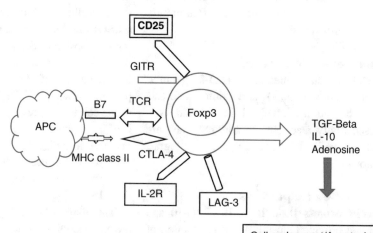

leading to a severe multi-organ autoimmune and inflammatory disorder IPEX (Immune dysregulation, Polyendocrinopathy, Enteropathy, X-Linked) and a similarly devastating widespread lesions in a mouse mutant strain, *scurfy*. Thus demonstrating the importance of FOXP3 in cells which regulate self-tolerance. The majority of Foxp3-expressing regulatory T cells are found within the major histocompatibility complex (MHC) class II restricted CD4-expressing (CD4+) population and express high levels of the interleukin-2 receptor alpha chain (CD25) [28].

3.4.2 Role of Tregs in Experimental Allograft Tolerance

In the past decade numerous reports have revealed the importance of Tregs in the promotion of transplant tolerance in animal models of heart, kidney, and skin transplantation [29–31]. In a mouse model of liver transplantation, recent studies have demonstrated the critical role that Tregs play in the establishment of tolerance [32, 33]. The presence of Tregs was increased in the periphery and in the tolerant graft from day 5 after transplantation to day 100. The increased number of Tregs was associated with the heightened expression of Tregs effector molecules (TGF-b and CTLA4) and IL-4 production. Treatment of tolerant mice with Tregs-depleting anti-CD25 antibodies resulted in acute allograft rejection, which was associated with a reduced Tregs/T effector cell ratio, decreased production of IL-4, and increased production of IL-10 and IL-2. Furthermore, anti-CD25 antibody–treated mice displayed reduced numbers of apoptotic alloreactive T cells, and suggesting that Tregs mediate their activity through the induction of apoptosis of activated T cells. The engagement of CTLA4 was found to be important for the induction of spontaneous tolerance in a mouse model of liver transplantation and treatment with antibodies to CTLA4 prevented the induction of tolerance. The anti-CTLA4 antibody treatment was associated with the increased activity of donor-specific T cells and natural killer cells in both the liver and the spleen. Furthermore, blocking

CTLA4 with antibodies led to the protection of alloreactive T cells from apoptosis, and this suggests that the Tregs effector molecule mediates its tolerogenic effect by killing the target cells in the tolerant graft and the periphery [33].

Monitoring the expression of Tregs effector molecules has been used experimentally to predict tolerance and rejection. The expression of a panel of Tregs effector genes with a novel multiplex real-time polymerase chain reaction platform (GeXP analysis system, Beckman Coulter) in murine models of rapamycin-induced cardiac tolerance, spontaneous hepatic tolerance, and cardiac rejection has been analyzed [34]. The increased expression of fibrinogen-like protein 2, killer cell lectin-like receptor G1, and Foxp3 was found to be associated with tolerance in both tolerant cardiac and liver allografts, whereas in rejected cardiac grafts, the increased expression of CD25, granzyme B, and interferon-c was associated with rejection.

3.5 Mechanisms of Allograft Rejection

Allorecognition is the first step of a series of complex events that leads to T-cell activation, antibody production, and allograft rejection. Donor antigen can be recognized directly or indirectly by T cells.

In the direct pathway, recipient T-cells recognize intact allogeneic HLAs expressed by donor APC (Antigen Presenting Cells). In the indirect pathway, T-cells recognize donor MHC peptides presented by recipient APC (Fig. 3.2). The direct and indirect pathways are well understood in organ transplantation. The direct pathway is very important in the immediate post-transplant period. Without appropriate immunosuppression, a strong and effective alloimmune response ensues, due to the high number of recipient T-cells that will recognize the graft antigens and leading to acute rejection. While the indirect pathway of allorecognition may also participate in acute rejection, it is usually predominant in the late onset of rejection, and especially chronic rejection. As long as the allograft is present in the host, the recipient APCs

Fig. 3.2 Direct and
indirect pathway of T
cell activation

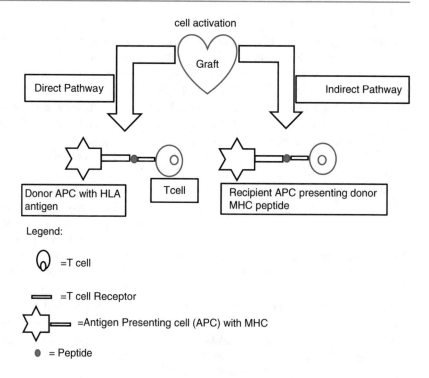

can pick up the alloantigen shed from the graft initiating the alloimmune response.

3.5.1 Three-Signal Model of T-Cell Activation

The key process of allograft rejection is the T-cell activation. The most common sited mechanism of T cell activation includes interaction of two cells (Dendritic and T cells) and involves 3 signals (Fig. 3.3).

3.5.1.1 Signal One (Recognition)

During an immune response, extracellular antigen is endocytosed and processed by the endoplasmic reticulum before translocating back to the cell surface in the context of self MHC. In the lymph nodes, the antigen peptides are presented by MHC-class II molecules present on APC's to naïve T-cells for activation. The initiation of intracellular signaling (signal 1) is transduced through the TCR-CD3 complex. CD3, formerly a target of OKT3, a now discontinued murine monoclonal formerly used to treat severe rejection episodes [35].

3.5.1.2 Signal Two (Co-stimulatory Signals)

The second co-stimulatory signal depends on the receptor-ligand interactions between T-cells and APCs (signal 2). Numerous co-stimulatory pathways have been described and blockage of these pathways can lead to antigen-specific inactivation or death of T-cell [36]. The best-studied ones are the CD28-CD 80 and CD154-CD40 pathways. CD28 and CD154 are expressed on T-cells, and their ligands B7 and CD40 are expressed on APCs. CD28 has two ligands, B7–1 (CD80) and B7–2 (CD86). T-cells also express cytotoxic T-lymphocyte associated antigen-4 (CTLA-4) only when they are activated as compared with to CD28 which is present on T-Cells in resting state. CTLA-4 is homologous to CD28 and has a higher affinity than CD28 to bind B7. However, when CTLA-4 binds B7 (both CD80 and CD86), it produces an inhibitory signal resulting in Tc anergy. CTLA-4-Ig (belatacept) is a novel immunosuppressive medication, which is a recombinant fusion protein that contains the extracellular domain of soluble CTLA4 combined with an immunoglobulin G1 (IgG1) heavy chain [36]. CTLA4Ig is a competitive inhibitor of CD28

Fig. 3.3   3 Signal model
of allo-recognition

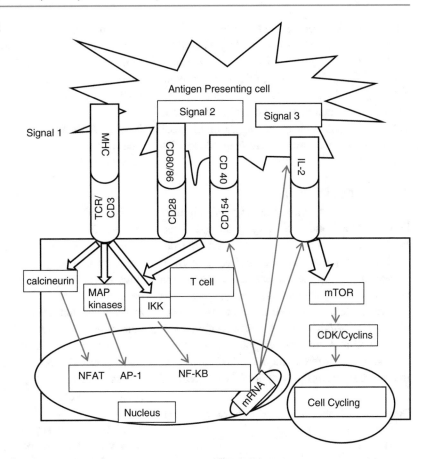

binding, resulting in T-cell anergy in vitro. In addition, the importance of CTLA-4 can be emphasized by observation of development of lymphoproliferative disease in genetically engineered mouse in which gene for CTLA-4 has been knocked down. Similarly, exacerbation of autoimmune disease by administration of anti-CTLA-4 monoclonal antibodies is another practical illustration that the CTLA-4 induced signal play an important role in the activation of T cells.

The other best studied co stimulatory pathways is the interaction between CD40 and its ligand CD40L (CD 154). CD40, a member of the tumor necrosis factor (TNF) receptor superfamily, is expressed on B cells and other APCs, including dendritic cells while CD40 ligand, CD40L (CD154), is expressed early on activated T cells. CD154-CD40 inhibition has also been shown to prevent allograft rejection in animal models, including anti-CD154 antibody and molecules that target CD40.

The combination of signal 1 and 2 activates three downstream signal transduction pathways: the calcium-calcineurin pathway, the RAS-mitogen activated protein kinase pathway, and the IKK-nuclear factor κB (NF-κB) pathway. These three pathways further activate transcription factors including the nuclear factor of activated T cells, activated protein-1, and NF-κB, respectively. Several new molecules and cytokines including CD25, CD154, interleukin (IL)-2, and IL-15 are subsequently expressed.

3.5.1.3 Signal Three- Proliferation

IL-2 and IL-15 deliver growth signals through the mammalian target of rapamycin pathway and phosphoinositide-3-kinase pathway, which subsequently trigger the T-cell cycle and proliferation. The fully activated T-cells undergo clonal expansion and produce a large number of cytokines and effector T-cells, which eventually produce CD8$^+$ T-cell mediated cytotoxicity, help macrophage-induced delayed type hypersensitivity response (by CD4+Th1), and help B cells for antibody production (by CD4+Th2). A subset of activated T-cells becomes the alloantigen-specific memory T-cells. For Th1 and Th2 differentiation, initiation of signal three requires the presence of IFN-gamma and IL-4 respectively. Dendritic cell and naive Th cells are unable to produce IFN-gamma or IL-4 themselves.

3.5.1.4 T Cell Migration

Naïve T cells and central memory cells circulate between blood and secondary lymphoid tissue. Leukocyte trafficking is critical for immunosurveillance purposes. This migration pattern is guided mainly by the cell surface expression of specific homing molecules, such as selectins, integrins, and chemokine receptors. (See Table 3.2). Activation of naïve lymphocytes occurs within secondary lymphoid tissue. Upon activation and differentiation, marked changes in the homing behavior of lymphocytes are observed

Table 3.2 Adhesion molecules involved in T cells migration

Steps in T cell migration	Adhesions molecules
Rolling	Selectin mediated (L, E and P selectins)
Triggering	Chemokine mediated (CCR1, CCR3 and CCR5)
Firm adhesion	Integrin mediated (ICAM-1, VCAM-1)
Transmigration	PECAM and integrin mediated

as a direct result of changes in the cell surface expression of homing molecules. The interactions between these molecules and their ligands or receptors triggers a sequential and coordinated series of events which summarized in Fig. 3.4.

3.5.1.5 Rolling

The rolling step is mediated by selectins, a closely related family of Ca (2+)-dependent lectins (L, E and P selectins, respectively). They are found on leukocytes, inflamed vascular endothelial cells and platelets. L-selectin is expressed constitutively on leukocytes. The interaction between selectins and its ligand are loose, reversible, and occur in settings of shear flow. Because rolling precedes (and appears to be essential for) the integrin-mediated firm arrest before extravasation in response to inflammatory or infectious stimuli, inhibition of selectin function has potential for anti-inflammatory therapy, but also presents some significant challenges because of the complexity of the processes involved.

3.5.1.6 Triggering

Leukocyte activation or triggering is mediated by chemokines which are produced by both leukocytes and endothelial cells. Chemokines, are a family of chemotactic cytokines that signal through G-protein-coupled receptors, play critical roles in regulating the leukocyte recruitment cascade. The signals basically convert the loose selectin mediated rolling into integrin mediated

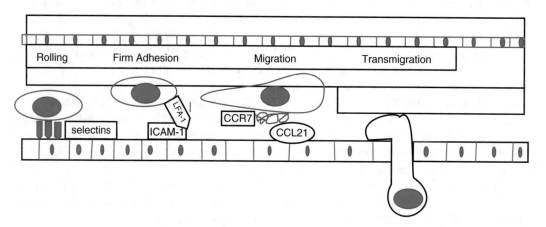

Fig. 3.4 Steps in extravasation of T cells

leukocyte-endothelial adhesions. Chemokines can be transported and immobilized on the surface of vascular endothelial cells, where they activate leukocyte subsets expressing specific receptors. These include chemokine receptor 1 (CCR1), CCR2, CXCR3, and CCR5. These receptors are predominantly expressed during an allograft rejection. CCR5 which is a high affinity receptor for chemokines has been shown to play a significant role in leukocyte trafficking in transplanted allografts in animal models and clinical observations [37]. In addition, much work has been done to characterize the chemokines expressed in the rejection of heart allografts. The specific chemokines found to be important for lymphocyte trafficking in rejecting heart grafts include CXCL9 (MIG), CXCL10 (IP-10), and CXCL11 (I-TAC) [38]. Neutralizing chemokines or blocking their receptors has been shown to prolong graft survival and prevent graft infiltration in animal models [39, 40]. Chemokines can also direct migration of adherent cells across the endothelium, and control segregation of cells into specific microenvironments within tissues. The regulated expression of chemokines and their receptors is a critical determinant for homing of specialized lymphocyte subsets, and controls both tissue and inflammation-specific immune processes.

3.5.1.7 Firm Adhesion

Firm adhesion of leukocytes to the endothelium is induced by chemokine stimulations and high-affinity integrin activation. The resulting integrin conformation change after activation can lead to as much as a 10,000-fold affinity increase of lymphocyte function-associated antigen-1 (LFA-1) to its ligand ICAM-1 [41]. In addition to LFA-1, Very late antigen-4 (VLA-4) ligation of endothelial vascular cell adhesion molecule-1 (VCAM-1) also provides the principal interaction leading to adhesion.

3.5.1.8 Transmigration

The final and less well understood step in the homing cascade is transmigration. Though traditionally thought of as the passage of the lymphocyte between endothelial cells (paracellular), it is

becoming more apparent that lymphocytes can also migrate directly through endothelial cells (transcellular) [42]. This process is mediated predominantly by the platelet endothelial cell adhesion molecule (PECAM). Migration along the endothelium is primarily dictated by chemokine signals that direct cell chemotaxis via chemotactic gradients. In addition, both β1 and β2 integrins are also thought to be involved in these processes via interaction with endothelial junction integrin ligands such as JAM-B and JAM-A, respectively [43].

3.5.1.9 B Cells

There are two lineages of B-cells; B1 cells are part of innate immune system and develop during fetal and perinatal life; B2 cells are part of the adaptive immune system and develop during post-natal life.

3.5.1.10 B Cell Development

B1 cells are self-renewing and form part of 'Natural Memory'. B2 cells are formed from pluripotent hematopoietic stem cells that mature in bone marrow. At this time IgM is expressed, forming B cell receptor (BCR). These naive B cells move into spleen and differentiate into follicular or marginal zone B cells.

3.5.1.11 B Cell Activation

B cells are activated by antigen stimulation. They undergo extrafollicular differentiation to plasma cells when the B cell has high affinity for that specific antigen. In contrary, if the affinity is low for the antigen, cells enter the germinal centers and undergo affinity maturation through a process of somatic hypermutation of the BCR. This ultimately leads to differentiation into either memory B cells or plasma cells. The purpose of this intense regulation is to ensure that the initial response against a specific antigen should be mounted by plasma cells which carry the highest binding capacity for that specific antigen. T helper cells facilitate B-cell activation either through intimate membrane contact involving a variety of receptors and ligands (such as CD40:CD154) or through the secreted soluble cytokines (such as IL-4). In a transplant, HLA antibodies formed against donor HLA antigens is a major cause for allograft rejection and premature graft failure. Allograft injury is mediated either by activating the complement cascade [complement-dependent cytotoxicity (CDC)] or *via* Fc receptor on natural killer (NK) cells, neutrophils, and eosinophils (antibody-dependent cellular cytotoxicity).

3.5.1.12   B Cell Signaling

Differentiation of naïve B lymphocytes into effector cells (plasma and memory cells) starts with engagement of cytokine receptors by specific ligands. This activates Janus Kinase signal transducer and activator of transcription (STAT) signaling pathways [44, 45]. Four JAK and seven STAT proteins have been identified. IL-21 predominantly activates STAT 1 and STAT 3 in human B cells and has been identified as a potent regulator of B cell differentiation [46, 47]. In vitro and In vivo studies on inactivating STAT 3 mutations dramatically reduced the ability of IL-21 to induce differentiation of Naïve B cells into plasma and memory cells [48]. In contrast STAT 1 deficiency has no effect on the differentiation of naïve B cells. Tofacitinib (CP690550) a novel JAK 3 inhibitor, is an immunosuppressive agent that appears to selectively reduce natural killer- and T- cell subsets. This agent is FDA approved for treatment of Rheumatoid arthritis and psoriatic arthropathy. Unfortunately, clinical trials in kidney transplantation revealed efficacy and safety concerns halting development for this indication [49].

3.6   MHC: Major Histocompatibility Complex

The principal target of the alloimmune response are the major histocompatibility complex (MHC, described in more details in Chap. 2) molecules expressed on the surface of donor cells (allo-MHC). In humans, these MHC molecules are called human leukocyte antigens (HLA) and they are located on the short arm of chromosome 6. Each parent provides a haplotype (a linked set of MHC genes) to each offspring in Mendelian co-dominant inheritance. The protein products of the MHC have been classified into three classes;

Class I, II and III Molecules. Class I and II proteins are integral components of the immune system whose primary role is the presentation of peptide antigen to T cell receptor.

Class I molecules (HLA-A, -B, and -C) are composed of a polymorphic heavy chain (α chain, 44 kDa) and a non-polymorphic light chain ($\beta2$ macroglobulin, 12 kDa). They are expressed on all nucleated cells and generally present endogenous small antigens (typically 9–11 amino acids), such as viruses and self-protein fragments to CD8[+] T cells. The CD8-positive cells then subsequently induce cell lysis (by inducing apoptosis or actively killing cells by cytotoxic proteins).

Class II molecules (HLA-DP, −DQ, and -DR) are composed of alpha and beta heterodimers. They are constitutively expressed only on professional antigen-presenting cells (APC), including dendritic cells, macrophages, and B-cells. Their expression is upregulated on epithelial and vascular endothelial cells after exposure to pro-inflammatory cytokines. Class II molecules present relatively larger antigens (12–28 amino acids), derived from extracellular proteins to CD4[+] T-cells. The degree of HLA mismatch between donor and recipient plays a role in determining the risk of chronic rejection and graft loss. HLA-A, -B, and -DR (3 pairs, 6 antigens) are traditionally used for typing and matching before kidney or pancreas transplant. HLA-Cw, -DP, and -DQ are now increasingly typed and used in many transplant centers. For kidney transplants, long-term graft survival is best in HLA-identical living related kidney transplants [50].

Class III molecules includes several components of complement system (i.e. C2, C4a, C4b, Bf) and inflammatory cytokines, tumor necrosis factor, two heat shock proteins (HSP) etc. They are not membrane proteins and have no role in Ag presentation. MHC Class III molecules are not structurally related to class I and class II molecules.

3.6.1   Minor Histocompatibility Antigens

Minor histocompatibility antigens (MiHA) are small endogenous peptides that occupy the antigen-binding site of donor MHC molecules.

Their importance in transplantation is best described when donor and recipients share identical MHC types, such as HLA matched, nonidentical twin siblings, and yet still are at rejection risk in the absence of immunosuppression. The prototypic minor histocompatibility antigen, the male or H-Y antigen, is derived from a group of proteins encoded on the Y chromosome. Alloresponses to this antigen may explain reduced long-term graft survival observed in male-to-female donations. They are generally recognized by $CD8^+$ cytotoxic T-cells in the context of self-MHC, which leads to graft rejection. In bone marrow transplant, MiHA play an important role in graft-*vs*-host disease in patients who have received HLA-matched cells. MHC class 1 related chain A and B (MICA and MICB) antigens are surface glycoproteins with functions related to innate immunity. Antibodies against MICA and/or MICB can cause antibody-mediated rejection (AMR) and graft loss [51].

Other reported antibodies causing graft rejection include anti-angiotensin-II type 1(AT1) receptor antibodies (activating IgG antibodies) that have been implicated in causing allograft rejection and hypertension. Affected patients might benefit from removal of AT_1-receptor antibodies or from pharmacologic blockade of AT_1 receptors, anti-glutathione S-transferase T1, and anti-endothelial antibodies. Anti-endothelial antibody can be detected by using donor monocytes for crossmatch. Some minor transplant antigens may come from mitochondrial proteins and enzymes. As our knowledge in transplant immunology advances, there will likely be more alloreactive and autoreactive antibodies to uncover.

3.6.2 ABO Blood Group Antigens

ABO blood group antigens consist of oligosaccharides which is expressed on red blood cells, epithelial cells, lymphocytes, platelets and vascular endothelial cells. Patients with different blood groups differ with respect to their antigen density on erythrocytes. Compared to blood group A1 and blood group B individuals, blood group A2 recipients, (20% of blood group A Caucasians) have

relatively low level expression (30–50%) on the surface of erythrocytes, thus explaining the reduced immunogenic potential of organs from blood group A2 donors. Of interest, anti-A/B antibodies are formed upon contact with gut bacteria during early infancy. Naturally occurring anti-A/B antibodies are predominantly of the IgM class but especially in blood group O individuals they also consist of IgG and IgA class. The pathogenic importance of anti-A/B antibodies in solid organ transplantation is well known. These preformed antibodies cause hyper acute rejection. Thus, ABO compatibility between donor and recipient are essential for organ transplantation. Desensitization protocols to remove the preformed hemagglutinin A and/or B from recipient circulation have been used for ABO incompatible kidney transplants [52, 53]. The rhesus factor and other red cell antigens are of minimal relevance to organ transplant, as they are not expressed on endothelium.

Disclosures
Dr. Vella discloses research contracts with:
Bristol Myers Squib and Astellas
There are no off-label discussions of any medications in this manuscript.
Manuscript Instructions: 15–20 pages, 5–6 tables, 3–5 Figures. No restrictions on number of references
Bibliography style: Springer Vancouver with numbered citations
Target Date of Submission: 7/31/2018

References

1. Gallucci S, Lolkema M, Matzinger P. Natural adjuvants: endogenous activators of dendritic cells. Nat Med. 1999;5(11):1249–55.
2. Kono H, Rock KL. How dying cells alert the immune system to danger. Nat Rev Immunol. 2008;8(4):279–89.
3. Chen CJ, Kono H, Golenbock D, Reed G, Akira S, Rock KL. Identification of a key pathway required for the sterile inflammatory response triggered by dying cells. Nat Med. 2007;13(7):851–6.
4. Tsung A, Klune JR, Zhang X, Jeyabalan G, Cao Z, Peng X, et al. HMGB1 release induced by liver ischemia involves toll-like receptor 4 dependent reactive oxygen species production and calcium-mediated signaling. J Exp Med. 2007;204(12):2913–23.
5. Hankey KG, Drachenberg CB, Papadimitriou JC, Klassen DK, Philosophe B, Bartlett ST, et al. MIC expression in renal and pancreatic allografts. Transplantation. 2002;73(2):304–6.

6. Kitchens WH, Uehara S, Chase CM, Colvin RB, Russell PS, Madsen JC. The changing role of natural killer cells in solid organ rejection and tolerance. Transplantation. 2006;81(6):811–7.

7. Zecher D, van Rooijen N, Rothstein DM, Shlomchik WD, Lakkis FG. An innate response to allogeneic nonself mediated by monocytes. J Immunol. 2009;183(12):7810–6.

8. Barclay AN, Brown MH. The SIRP family of receptors and immune regulation. Nat Rev Immunol. 2006;6(6):457–64.

9. Dai H, Friday AJ, Abou-Daya KI, Williams AL, Mortin-Toth S, Nicotra ML, et al. Donor SIRPalpha polymorphism modulates the innate immune response to allogeneic grafts. Sci Immunol. 2017;2(12):eaam6202.

10. Brunner T, Mogil RJ, LaFace D, Yoo NJ, Mahboubi A, Echeverri F, et al. Cell-autonomous Fas (CD95)/Fas-ligand interaction mediates activation-induced apoptosis in T-cell hybridomas. Nature. 1995;373(6513):441–4.

11. Dhein J, Walczak H, Baumler C, Debatin KM, Krammer PH. Autocrine T-cell suicide mediated by APO-1/(Fas/CD95). Nature. 1995;373(6513):438–41.

12. Ju ST, Panka DJ, Cui H, Ettinger R, El-Khatib M, Sherr DH, et al. Fas(CD95)/FasL interactions required for programmed cell death after T-cell activation. Nature. 1995;373(6513):444–8.

13. Russell JH, Rush B, Weaver C, Wang R. Mature T cells of autoimmune lpr/lpr mice have a defect in antigen-stimulated suicide. Proc Natl Acad Sci U S A. 1993;90(10):4409–13.

14. Bakshi RK, Cox MA, Zajac AJ. Cytotoxic T lymphocytes. In: Mackay IR, Rose NR, Diamond B, Davidson A, editors. Encyclopedia of medical immunology: autoimmune diseases. New York, NY: Springer; 2014. p. 332–42.

15. Forbes RD, Zheng SX, Gomersall M, Al-Saffar M, Guttmann RD. Evidence that recipient CD8+ T cell depletion does not alter development of chronic vascular rejection in a rat heart allograft model. Transplantation. 1994;57(8):1238–46.

16. Li B, Hartono C, Ding R, Sharma VK, Ramaswamy R, Qian B, et al. Noninvasive diagnosis of renal-allograft rejection by measurement of messenger RNA for perforin and granzyme B in urine. N Engl J Med. 2001;344(13):947–54.

17. Suthanthiran M. Molecular analyses of human renal allografts: differential intragraft gene expression during rejection. Kidney Int Suppl. 1997;58:S15–21.

18. Abbas AK, Benoist C, Bluestone JA, Campbell DJ, Ghosh S, Hori S, et al. Regulatory T cells: recommendations to simplify the nomenclature. Nat Immunol. 2013;14(4):307–8.

19. Nocentini G, Riccardi C. GITR: a modulator of immune response and inflammation. Adv Exp Med Biol. 2009;647:156–73.

20. Schaer DA, Murphy JT, Wolchok JD. Modulation of GITR for cancer immunotherapy. Curr Opin Immunol. 2012;24(2):217–24.

21. Roncarolo MG, Gregori S, Battaglia M, Bacchetta R, Fleischhauer K, Levings MK. Interleukin-10-secreting type 1 regulatory T cells in rodents and humans. Immunol Rev. 2006;212:28–50.

22. Kitani A, Chua K, Nakamura K, Strober W. Activated self-MHC-reactive T cells have the cytokine phenotype of Th3/T regulatory cell 1 T cells. J Immunol. 2000;165(2):691–702.

23. Kim JM, Rasmussen JP, Rudensky AY. Regulatory T cells prevent catastrophic autoimmunity throughout the lifespan of mice. Nat Immunol. 2007;8(2):191–7.

24. Sakaguchi S, Sakaguchi N, Shimizu J, Yamazaki S, Sakihama T, Itoh M, et al. Immunologic tolerance maintained by CD25+ CD4+ regulatory T cells: their common role in controlling autoimmunity, tumor immunity, and transplantation tolerance. Immunol Rev. 2001;182:18–32.

25. Brunkow ME, Jeffery EW, Hjerrild KA, Paeper B, Clark LB, Yasayko SA, et al. Disruption of a new forkhead/winged-helix protein, scurfin, results in the fatal lymphoproliferative disorder of the scurfy mouse. Nat Genet. 2001;27(1):68–73.

26. Bennett CL, Christie J, Ramsdell F, Brunkow ME, Ferguson PJ, Whitesell L, et al. The immune dysregulation, polyendocrinopathy, enteropathy, X-linked syndrome (IPEX) is caused by mutations of FOXP3. Nat Genet. 2001;27(1):20–1.

27. Wildin RS, Ramsdell F, Peake J, Faravelli F, Casanova JL, Buist N, et al. X-linked neonatal diabetes mellitus, enteropathy and endocrinopathy syndrome is the human equivalent of mouse scurfy. Nat Genet. 2001;27(1):18–20.

28. Fontenot JD, Rasmussen JP, Williams LM, Dooley JL, Farr AG, Rudensky AY. Regulatory T cell lineage specification by the forkhead transcription factor foxp3. Immunity. 2005;22(3):329–41.

29. Wood KJ, Sakaguchi S. Regulatory T cells in transplantation tolerance. Nat Rev Immunol. 2003;3(3):199–210.

30. Kang SM, Tang Q, Bluestone JA. CD4+CD25+ regulatory T cells in transplantation: progress, challenges and prospects. Am J Transplant. 2007;7(6):1457–63.

31. Li W, Carper K, Zheng XX, Kuhr CS, Reyes JD, Liang Y, et al. The role of Foxp3+ regulatory T cells in liver transplant tolerance. Transplant Proc. 2006;38(10):3205–6.

32. Li W, Kuhr CS, Zheng XX, Carper K, Thomson AW, Reyes JD, et al. New insights into mechanisms of spontaneous liver transplant tolerance: the role of Foxp3-expressing CD25+CD4+ regulatory T cells. Am J Transplant. 2008;8(8):1639–51.

33. Li W, Zheng XX, Kuhr CS, Perkins JD. CTLA4 engagement is required for induction of murine liver transplant spontaneous tolerance. Am J Transplant. 2005;5(5):978–86.

34. Xie L, Ichimaru N, Morita M, Chen J, Zhu P, Wang J, et al. Identification of a novel biomarker gene set with sensitivity and specificity for distinguishing between allograft rejection and tolerance. Liver Transpl. 2012;18(4):444–54.

35. Norman DJ. Mechanisms of action and overview of OKT3. Ther Drug Monit. 1995;17(6):615–20.
36. Larsen CP, Pearson TC, Adams AB, Tso P, Shirasugi N, Strobert E, et al. Rational development of LEA29Y (belatacept), a high-affinity variant of CTLA4-Ig with potent immunosuppressive properties. Am J Transplant. 2005;5(3):443–53.
37. Abdi R, Tran TB, Sahagun-Ruiz A, Murphy PM, Brenner BM, Milford EL, et al. Chemokine receptor polymorphism and risk of acute rejection in human renal transplantation. J Am Soc Nephrol. 2002;13(3):754–8.
38. El-Sawy T, Fahmy NM, Fairchild RL. Chemokines: directing leukocyte infiltration into allografts. Curr Opin Immunol. 2002;14(5):562–8.
39. Hancock WW, Lu B, Gao W, Csizmadia V, Faia K, King JA, et al. Requirement of the chemokine receptor CXCR3 for acute allograft rejection. J Exp Med. 2000;192(10):1515–20.
40. Miura M, Morita K, Kobayashi H, Hamilton TA, Burdick MD, Strieter RM, et al. Monokine induced by IFN-gamma is a dominant factor directing T cells into murine cardiac allografts during acute rejection. J Immunol. 2001;167(6):3494–504.
41. Shimaoka M, Takagi J, Springer TA. Conformational regulation of integrin structure and function. Annu Rev Biophys Biomol Struct. 2002;31:485–516.
42. Carman CV, Sage PT, Sciuto TE, de la Fuente MA, Geha RS, Ochs HD, et al. Transcellular diapedesis is initiated by invasive podosomes. Immunity. 2007;26(6):784–97.
43. Ley K, Laudanna C, Cybulsky MI, Nourshargh S. Getting to the site of inflammation: the leukocyte adhesion cascade updated. Nat Rev Immunol. 2007;7(9):678–89.
44. Akira S. Functional roles of STAT family proteins: lessons from knockout mice. Stem Cells. 1999;17(3):138–46.
45. Shuai K, Liu B. Regulation of JAK-STAT signalling in the immune system. Nat Rev Immunol. 2003;3(11):900–11.
46. Ozaki K, Spolski R, Feng CG, Qi CF, Cheng J, Sher A, et al. A critical role for IL-21 in regulating immunoglobulin production. Science. 2002;298(5598):1630–4.
47. Pene J, Gauchat JF, Lecart S, Drouet E, Guglielmi P, Boulay V, et al. Cutting edge: IL-21 is a switch factor for the production of IgG1 and IgG3 by human B cells. J Immunol. 2004;172(9):5154–7.
48. Asao H, Okuyama C, Kumaki S, Ishii N, Tsuchiya S, Foster D, et al. Cutting edge: the common gamma-chain is an indispensable subunit of the IL-21 receptor complex. J Immunol. 2001;167(1):1–5.
49. Vincenti F, Silva HT, Busque S, O'Connell PJ, Russ G, Budde K, et al. Evaluation of the effect of tofacitinib exposure on outcomes in kidney transplant patients. Am J Transplant. 2015;15(6):1644–53.
50. Takemoto SK, Terasaki PI, Gjertson DW, Cecka JM. Twelve years' experience with national sharing of HLA-matched cadaveric kidneys for transplantation. N Engl J Med. 2000;343(15):1078–84.
51. Zou Y, Stastny P, Susal C, Dohler B, Opelz G. Antibodies against MICA antigens and kidney-transplant rejection. N Engl J Med. 2007;357(13):1293–300.
52. Klein C BD. HLA and ABO sensitization and desensitization in renal transplantation. UpToDate [Internet], 2013. Available from: http://www.uptodate.com/contents/hla-and-abo-sensitization-and-desensitization-in-renal-transplantation
53. Montgomery RA. Renal transplantation across HLA and ABO antibody barriers: integrating paired donation into desensitization protocols. Am J Transplant. 2010;10(3):449–57.

Immune Tolerance

4

Jeevan Kumar Shrestha

4.1 Introduction

The state of lack or downregulation of immune response to specific antigens is immune tolerance. It can be also defined as immunological unresponsiveness to an antigen due to previous exposure to the same antigen. It is different from immunosuppression and immunodeficiency as it is an active antigen-dependent process in response to an antigen. The individual immune system is usually tolerant of self-antigens (cells, tissues, and organs). When the state of tolerance is disturbed, it causes autoimmune disease and food allergy. There are several checkpoints in the human body which delete the lymphocytes active against self-antigens. It is also normal to have self-reactive lymphocytes in the body in an anergic state which cannot damage self-antigens. The regulatory immune cells circulate through the body and maintain tolerance which also turns the immune response off once the task is done.

Immune tolerance can be broken naturally or artificially (X-rays, drug treatments, and exposure to cross-reactive antigens). When the immune system fails to recognize self-antigens, then it starts to attack its own cells, tissues, and organs which cause autoimmune disease. Some of the autoimmune diseases are common like type 1 diabetes, multiple sclerosis, lupus, and rheumatoid arthritis, while others are rare and difficult to diagnose. The genetic inheritance, infections, drugs, and other environmental factors influence autoimmune disease.

4.2 History

During the 1940s, Burnet stated the importance of distinguishing "self" and "non-self" for the protection of organisms against infection. Later, he postulated that antigens encountered during the immature stage of the immune system can tolerate the relevant lymphocytes [1]. In support of Burnet's ideas, Medawar found that a significant proportion of mice were fully tolerant as skin graft at the young adult stage was not rejected after the late embryonic stage or neonate mice were injected with a cell suspension of another strain of mice [2]. In 1960, both of them were awarded Nobel prize in Physiology and Medicine for the discovery of acquired immunological tolerance.

4.3 Cellular Mechanisms of Tolerance

The diversity created by V(D)J rearrangement may generate approximately 10^{14} distinct BCRs on the surface of immature B cells that may

J. K. Shrestha (✉)
National Chung-Hsing University, Taichung, Taiwan
e-mail: jeevan@smail.nchu.edu.tw

© Springer Nature Switzerland AG 2021
N. Hakim et al. (eds.), *Transplantation Surgery*, Springer Specialist Surgery Series,
https://doi.org/10.1007/978-3-030-55244-2_4

Fig. 4.1 Mechanisms of immune response and immune tolerance by the lymphocytes once exposed to antigens [3, 4]. (**a**) proliferation and differentiation lymphocyte occurs which produces an immune response. (**b**) death of lymphocyte occurs by apoptosis. (**c**) lymphocytes remain unreactive (**d**) rearrangement of the receptors of lymphocyte occurs which no longer responds to antigens

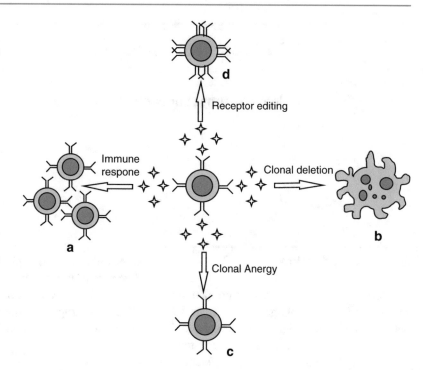

contain self-reactive BCRs which can be tolerized by at least four mechanisms: Anergy, Clonal Deletion, Suppressor Cells (Regulatory cells) and Receptor Editing (Fig. 4.1) [5].

1. **Clonal Deletion**

It is the mechanism that controls the development and expansion of self-reactive lymphocytes that may cause autoimmune disease. Antigen receptor stimulation or failure to produce membrane-bound antigen receptors causes the elimination of lymphocyte progenitors. It occurs centrally during the differentiation of T-cells and B-cells and peripherally even later.

T-cells require the random rearrangement of genes and expression of antigen receptors (TCR) for the maturation in the thymus. In addition, T-cell may lack the functional CD4 or CD8 co-receptors to recognize the MHC-peptide complex which leads to the suppression of T-cell differentiation, thus T-cell death occurs. The expression of both CD4 and CD8 co-receptors and the presence of high-affinity MHC bound peptide also leads to T-cell death [6]. The minor change in the antigen may

raise the affinity of antigenic peptides and results in autoimmune disease [7].

B-cells require the rearrangement of B-cell receptors (BCR) during the maturation, and failure to rearrange will lead to the death of B-cells. When BCR is not stimulated after transportation into the primary lymphoid organs like lymph and spleen, B-cell death occurs. Once stimulated, the lack of helper signal from Helper T-cells or cytokines also cause B-cell death. Unlike T-cells, mature B-cells may also undergo deletion. Mutation of BCR after antigenic activation causes the reduced antigen receptors (BCRs) which have signaling with complement receptor CD21. In this case, stimulation of B-cell by an antigen without a complement causes B-cell deletion [6]. Clonal deletion of B-cell is not complete as some B-cells with self-reactive BCR may undergo receptor editing and avoid clonal deletion [8].

Molecular mimicry has suggested that microorganisms are capable of developing antigenic determinants resembling the host antigen and avoid recognition and elimination by the host. Hyaluronic acid covering of Beta hemolytic *Streptococci* resembles the hyaluronic acid in the joint fluid of human which make them partially tolerant [7]. Also, the cross-reaction of antigenic epitopes of microorganisms and antigen present in the body may result in injurious immune response and subsequent autoimmune disease.

2. **Clonal Anergy**

The mechanism of silencing in which lymphocytes are inactivated after exposure to antigen and remain in the hyporesponsive state for a long time. When lymphocytes encounter an antigen, the negative gene regulation for Interleukin-2 (IL-2) starts inside the cell by which cells cannot produce IL-2 [9]. Clonal anergy may cause autoimmune diseases such as systemic lupus erythematosus and type 1 diabetes [10].

T-cell anergy falls into two categories viz. growth arrest state and in vivo anergy (adaptive tolerance). In the growth arrest state, the activation is incomplete which occurs in previously activated T-cells. It is maintained by the Ras/MAP kinase pathway and can be reversed by IL-2 or anti-OX40 signaling [11]. In in vivo anergy, the activation occurs in the naïve T-cells in the surrounding with low costimulation and high co-inhibition which can be reversed with the absence of antigen [11]. B-cell anergy occurs with the reduced life span of T-cells, it's altered migration and anatomical localization and inability to interact with helper T cells to create immune response [10].

The activation of lymphocytes needs a different signal from an antigen and another source. When the lymphocyte lacks the signal from other various sources, it results in intolerance. The contribution of genetic reprogramming to the tolerance cannot be neglected. Elevated intracellular free Calcium ions up-regulate the transcription of the Nuclear Factor of Activated T-cells (NFAT) which play a critical role to inactivate T-cells without the signal from sources other than antigen [12].

3. **Suppressor Cells**

Suppressor cells (Regulatory cells) are able to transfer the properties to inhibit the immune response from tolerized individuals to other individuals in an antigen-specific manner. According to the study in mice, the removal of natural $CD4^+CD25^+$ T regulatory cells (Treg) at day 3 of their life or transfer of Regulatory T-cells (Tregs) deficient T-cells result in widespread autoimmune disease [13]. The IL-10 secreting Tr1 cells [14] and the TGF-β secreting Th3 cells [15] also cut-off the proliferation and cytokine secretion of effector T cells.

It has been reported that that Human Gamma Globulin (HGG)-fed macrophages cannot signal spleen cells from HGG-tolerant animals to produce initiator cells. Also, the capacity of normal animals to produce initiator cells has been inhibited when the spleen cells from tolerant animals and normal animals are mixed. These facts suggest that suppressor cells affect the immunological action of other antigens presented by the same macrophages [16].

4. **Receptor Editing**

The recognition of the antigen by the receptors on the surface of B-cells is important for the immune response. Immunoglobulin heavy (IgH) chain and immunoglobulin light (IgL) chain forms B-cell receptors (BCRs) which will be unique in each cell [17]. Some of the B-cells may act against "self" antigens which is a kind of autoimmune disease. About 50% of developing B cells are considered to be initially self-reactive [18] and receptor editing of B-cells is the principal mechanism that maintains tolerance [19].

BCRs specificity is altered predominantly through secondary Vκ → Jκ light (L)-chain rearrangements. The alternation of the variable region of heavy (H)-chains by the insertion of a V_H gene segment rarely cause V_HDJ_H rearrangement [5]. The secondary gene rearrangement of the H-chain or L-chain gene enhances the cross-linking of BCRs. The extensive cross-linking of BCRs leads to low or no affinity to the surrounding antigens. This is achieved by the reactivation of the recombination machinery and re-expression of Recombination Activating Gene-1 (RAG-1) and Recombination Activating Gene-2 (RAG-

2) proteins [20]. In this way, receptor editing removes the autoreactive B-cells.

Rearrangements at several steps, recombination arrest, positive selection of single-positive (CD4+ or CD8+) αβT cells, and migration into medulla occur during the development of T-cells. Low-affinity signal by recognition of particular peptide-MHC complex is required for the cessation of recombination and the beginning of the positive selection. When such a requirement is not fulfilled, double-positive (CD4+CD8+) thymocytes with complete antigen receptors may recombine and results in the altered receptor specificity [17].

The receptor editing rescue autoreactive B cells from deletion. This action depends on the availability of multiple joining light chain gene segments as a substrate for secondary immunoglobulin light chain gene rearrangement and is independent of the affinity of the autoantigen [19]. However, extravagant receptor editing can result in the generation of B cells containing autoreactive BCRs [21].

4.4   Sites of Tolerance Induction

The induction of immune tolerance consists of mainly two coordinated mechanisms: the deletion of autoreactive lymphocytes in the central lymphoid organs before maturity and their suppression in the periphery after escaping the deletion [22]. These two mechanisms of tolerance are called central tolerance and peripheral tolerance respectively.

1. **Central Tolerance**

     T-cell precursors originate in the bone marrow and migrate to thymus. These cells fail to express CD4 and CD8 cell markers at the beginning known as a double negative. Later, proliferation and maturation acquire both CD4 and CD8 markers referred to as double positive. During the process, T-cells acquire TCR which varies from non-reactive to highly reactive. The survival or death of these T-cells depends upon the clonal selection.

Clonal selection occurs to prevent the immune response against self-antigens. Positive selection occurs to T-cells expressing TCR which does not respond to self-MHC complex and dies [23]. About 95% of T-cells are deleted by neglect and a small proportion of T-cells that respond to self-MHC complex with mild avidity will undergo maturation into CD4+ or CD8+ single-positive stage [24]. So, the clonal deletion is the principal and also the default mechanism of central tolerance when receptor editing fails.

Then, the developing thymocytes undergo negative selection in which T-cells responding to self MHC with high avidity are deleted by apoptosis [25]. Strong TCR ligation stimulates the rapid onset of Fas-dependent apoptosis of naïve T-cells [26]. Then, T-cells are exposed to a broad range of self-MHC complex and deleted if they respond [27]. Co-stimulation of the antigen-presenting cells (APC) and CD28 provides the signal for subsequent negative selection [28].

2. **Peripheral Tolerance**

     In addition to central tolerance, peripheral tolerance acts to maintain immune tolerance. Many self-antigens are not exposed to T-cells in the thymus and it requires an additional mechanism to induce tolerance to those antigens. After positive and negative selection, the mature T-cells are released into peripheral circulation and secondary lymphoid organs, where they are deleted if they respond with mild avidity to self-MHC complex [24].

     A small number of self-antigens down-regulates the TCR of self-reactive CD8+ cells and induce tolerance [29]. The clonal deletion in the periphery is due to apoptosis after the activation of the Fas/FasL pathway and the Bim dependent mitochondrial pathway [30]. It involves the regulatory T-cells (Treg) like CD4+ which express both high-affinity IL-2 receptor (CD25) and transcription factor Foxp3 [31]. The depletion of CD4+CD25+ CD4+ T-cells leads to the development of autoimmunity in many organs which confirm that these cells are required for peripheral tolerance [32].

T-cells' immune response depends upon the capability of the immune system to differentiate naïve T-cells into helper (Th1 and Th2 cells) effector T-cells that cross regulate each other. Th-1 T cells produce IL-2 and IFN-y whereas Th-2 T cells produce IL-4, IL-5, IL-10, and TGF-l3. IL-10 and TGF-13 are associated with immunosuppressive activities [33]. TGF-13 also regulates oral tolerance. The formation of T-cells effector cells in CD4$^+$ and CD8$^+$ compartment contributes to the peripheral immune tolerance [33].

4.5 Immune Tolerance and Transplantation

The immune system is the main barrier to transplantation failure. The induction of tolerance can reduce the risk of chronic rejection. There are three ways to induce tolerance during transplantation such as matching, non-specific immunosuppression, and induction of transplantation tolerance [34]. One-fourth of the siblings have a chance of matching Human Leukocyte Antigen (HLA) with the transplant recipient which determines the success or failure of transplantation. It has been successfully applied in kidney and bone marrow transplantation and accepted for partial liver and lung transplantation in children. Non-specific immunosuppression is achieved with drugs like steroids, antimetabolites, and monoclonal antibodies.

The immunosuppressive drugs increase the risk of infection, renal failure, cardiovascular diseases, and malignancies. In the case of organ or cell transplantation, immune tolerance is the specific unresponsiveness of the immune cells to the donor graft by maintaining normal immune response to other antigens in the absence of immunosuppression. The host must have a certain degree of allogeneic tolerance before transplantation. T-cells play a role in allograft rejection, graft failure, or graft vs host disease (GVHD) [24]. The thymus plays a central role in transplantation tolerance.

As the shortage of allogenic organs is obvious, the use of xenografts is needed but the immune response against xenografts is even stronger. The induction of tolerance at both humoral and cellular level can overcome the immune response and can be applied for xenotransplantation [35]. Although various approaches have successfully induced tolerance to mice, mixed chimerism is the most advanced approach in higher animals.

4.5.1 Mixed Chimerism and Transplantation Tolerance

It is a state in which hematopoietic stem cells (HSC) of donor and recipient co-exists at a certain level to be detected by standard technique [36]. The transfer of HSC can confer tolerance to any cells or organs of the same donor. The HSC supply circulating T-cells and Dendritic cells (DCs) progenitors in thymus which delete the host T-cells reactive to the donor graft [37]. The Graft Versus Host (GVH) reactivity drives the expansion of donor T-cells which ultimately delete host T-cells. Specific deletion of T-cells with donor reactive TCR occurs in the periphery. Although it is not the major mechanism, it creates donor-specific hyporesponsiveness [38].

As long as the host contains T-cells reactive to donor graft, the risk of developing Graft Versus Host Disease (GVHD) still remains [39]. Its incidence and severity can be correlated with HLA mismatch [40]. Mixed chimerism is preferred over full chimerism because of the higher risk of developing GVHD in full chimerism [41]. Nevertheless, full chimerism has reduced immune competence [42].

References

1. Mackay IR. The 'Burnet era' of immunology: origins and influence. Immunol Cell Biol. 1991;69:301–5.
2. Simpson E. Medawar's legacy to cellular immunology and clinical transplantation: a commentary on Billingham, Brent, and Medawar's (1956) 'Quantitative studies on tissue transplantation immunity. III Actively acquired tolerance'. Philos Trans R Soc Lond B Biol Sci. 2015;370:20140382.
3. Chackerian B, Peabody DS. Factors that govern the induction of long-lived antibody responses. Viruses. 2020;74:1–10.

4. Milojevic D, Nguyen KD, Wara D, Mellins ED. Regulatory T cells and their role in rheumatic diseases: a potential target for novel therapeutic development. Pediatr Rheumatol. 2008;6:1–13.
5. Kelsoe G. Heavy-chain receptor editing unbound. Proc Natl Acad Sci U S A. 2015;112:2297–8.
6. Russell JH. Clonal deletion. In: Delves P, Roitt I, editors. Encyclopedia of immunology. 2nd ed. Oxford: Elsevier; 1998. p. 569–73.
7. Rose NR. Molecular mimicry and clonal deletion: a fresh look. J Theor Biol. 2015;375:71–6.
8. Prak ETL, Monestier M, Eisenberg RA. B cell receptor editing in tolerance and autoimmunity. Ann N Y Acad Sci. 2011;1217:96–121.
9. Becker JC, Brabletz T, Kirchner T, Conrad CT, Bröcker EB, Reisfeld RA. Negative transcriptional regulation in anergic T cells. Proc Natl Acad Sci U S A. 1995;92:2375–8.
10. Cambier JC, Gauld SB, Merrell KT, Vilen BJ. B-cell anergy: from transgenic models to naturally occurring anergic B cells? Nature reviews. Immunology. 2007;7:633–43.
11. Schwartz RH. T cell anergy. Annu Rev Immunol. 2003;21:305–34.
12. Yarkoni Y, Getahun A, Cambier JC. Molecular underpinning of B-cell anergy. Immunol Rev. 2010;237:249–63.
13. Sakaguchi S, Sakaguchi N, Asano M, Itoh M, Toda M. Immunologic self-tolerance maintained by activated T cells expressing IL-2 receptor alpha-chains (CD25). Breakdown of a single mechanism of self-tolerance causes various autoimmune diseases. J Immunol. 1995;155:1151–64.
14. Groux H, O'Garra A, Bigler M, Rouleau M, Antonenko S, de Vries JE, Roncarolo MG. A CD4+ T-cell subset inhibits antigen-specific T-cell responses and prevents colitis. Nature. 1997;389:737–42.
15. Weiner HL. Induction and mechanism of action of transforming growth factor-beta-secreting Th3 regulatory cells. Immunol Rev. 2001;182:207–14.
16. Segal S, Tzehoval E, Feldman M. Immunological tolerance: high-dose antigen-induced suppressor cells from tolerant animals inactivate antigen-presenting macrophages. Proc Natl Acad Sci U S A. 1979;76:2405–9.
17. Nemazee D. Receptor editing in lymphocyte development and central tolerance. Nat Rev Immunol. 2006;6:728–40.
18. Wardemann H, Yurasov S, Schaefer A, Young JW, Meffre E, Nussenzweig MC. Predominant autoantibody production by early human B cell precursors. Science. 2003;301:1374–7.
19. Halverson R, Torres RM, Pelanda R. Receptor editing is the main mechanism of B cell tolerance toward membrane antigens. Nat Immunol. 2004;5:645–50.
20. Zou YR, Grimaldi C, Diamond B. B cells. In: Budd RC, Gabriel SE, IB MI, O'Dell JR, editors. Kelley and Firestein's textbook of rheumatology. 10th ed. Philadelphia, PA: Elsevier; 2017. p. 207-30e3.
21. Mauri C, Reddy V, Blair PA. B cell activation and B cell tolerance. In: Mackay IR, editor. The autoimmune diseases. 5th ed. Boston: Academic Press; 2014. p. 147–58.
22. Griesemer AD, Sorenson EC, Hardy MA. The role of the thymus in tolerance. Transplantation. 2010;90:465–74.
23. Blackman M, Yagüe J, Kubo R, Gay D, Coleclough C, Palmer E, Kappler J, Marrack P. The T cell repertoire may be biased in favor of MHC recognition. Cell. 1986;47:349–57.
24. Alpdogan O, van den Brink MRM. Immune tolerance and transplantation. Semin Oncol. 2012;39:629–42.
25. Ramsdell F, Fowlkes BJ. Clonal deletion versus clonal anergy: the role of the thymus in inducing self tolerance. Science. 1990;248:1342–8.
26. Kishimoto H, Sprent J. Strong TCR ligation without costimulation causes rapid onset of Fas-dependent apoptosis of naive murine CD4+ T cells. J Immunol. 1999;163:1817–26.
27. Kappler JW, Roehm N, Marrack P. T cell tolerance by clonal elimination in the thymus. Cell. 1987;49:273–80.
28. Page DM, Kane LP, Allison JP, Hedrick SM. Two signals are required for negative selection of CD4+CD8+ thymocytes. J Immunol. 1993;151:1868–80.
29. Ferber I, Schonrich G, Schenkel J, Mellor AL, Hammerling GJ, Arnold B. Levels of peripheral T cell tolerance induced by different doses of tolerogen. Science. 1994;263:674–6.
30. Mueller DL. Mechanisms maintaining peripheral tolerance. Nat Immunol. 2009;11:21.
31. Hori S, Nomura T, Sakaguchi S. Control of regulatory T cell development by the transcription factor Foxp3. Science. 2003;299:1057–61.
32. Sakaguchi S, Fukuma K, Kuribayashi K, Masuda T. Organ-specific autoimmune diseases induced in mice by elimination of T cell subset. I. Evidence for the active participation of T cells in natural self-tolerance; deficit of a T cell subset as a possible cause of autoimmune disease. J Exp Med. 1985;161:72–87.
33. Renz H, Herz U. Immune mechanisms of peripheral tolerance. Nutr Res. 1998;18:1327–33.
34. Sachs DH. Mixed chimerism as an approach to transplantation tolerance. Clin Immunol. 2000;95:S63–S8.
35. Sykes M. Immune tolerance: mechanisms and application in clinical transplantation. J Intern Med. 2007;262:288–310.
36. Leventhal J, Abecassis M, Miller J, Gallon L, Ravindra K, Tollerud DJ, King B, Elliott MJ, Herzig G, Herzig R, Ildstad ST. Chimerism and tolerance without GVHD or engraftment syndrome in HLA-mismatched combined kidney and hematopoietic stem cell transplantation. Sci Transl Med. 2012;4:124ra28.
37. Tomita Y, Khan A, Sykes M. Role of intrathymic clonal deletion and peripheral anergy in transplantation tolerance induced by bone marrow transplantation in mice conditioned with a nonmyeloablative regimen. J Immunol. 1994;153:1087.

38. Zuber J, Sykes M. Mechanisms of mixed chimerism-based transplant tolerance. Trends Immunol. 2017;38:829–43.
39. Pasquini M, Wang Z, Horowitz MM, Gale RP. Current uses and outcomes of hematopoietic cell transplants for blood and bone marrow disorders. Clin Transpl. 2013;2013:187–97.
40. Ferrara JLM, Levine JE, Reddy P, Holler E. Graft-versus-host disease. Lancet. 2009;373:1550–61.
41. Sykes M, Sheard MA, Sachs DH. Graft-versus-host-related immunosuppression is induced in mixed chimeras by alloresponses against either host or donor lymphohematopoietic cells. J Exp Med. 1988;168:2391–6.
42. Singer A, Hathcock KS, Hodes RJ. Self recognition in allogeneic radiation bone marrow chimeras. A radiation-resistant host element dictates the self specificity and immune response gene phenotype of T-helper cells. J Exp Med. 1981;153:1286–301.

Donation After Circulatory Death

5

James P. Hunter, Bernadette Haase,
and Rutger J. Ploeg

5.1 Introduction

The development of donation after circulatory death (DCD) donor programmes across mainland Europe, the United Kingdom and the United States has significantly increased transplant rates in the past 20 years. DCD donation is an excellent example of international collaboration that has allowed the transplant community to push the boundaries of medicine by combining science and technology to the benefit of patients. DCD donor programmes are underpinned by complex regulations, legislation, ethical issues, retrieval logistics and surgical techniques. This chapter aims to provide an overview of DCD organ donors, DCD programmes including organ retrieval and their outcomes following transplantation.

J. P. Hunter (✉)
Nuffield Department of Surgical Sciences, University of Oxford, Oxford, UK

University Hospitals Coventry & Warwickshire NHS Trust, Coventry, UK
e-mail: james.hunter@nds.ox.ac.uk

B. Haase
The Dutch Transplant Foundation,
Leiden, The Netherlands
e-mail: b.haase@transplantatiestichting.nl

R. J. Ploeg
Nuffield Department of Surgical Sciences, University of Oxford, Oxford, UK

Oxford University Hospitals NHS Foundation Trust, Oxford, UK
e-mail: rutger.ploeg@nds.ox.ac.uk

5.2 History

In the beginning of transplantation only kidneys from living donors or donors after cardiac death, the so called Non-Heart Beating Donors (NHBD) were used. The first NHBD was reported in 1933 in the Ukraine [1]. However, this transplant failed immediately, due to ischaemic damage caused by a prolonged period between cessation of the circulation and procurement of the organ. Subsequent improvements in retrieval technique of kidneys from asystolic donors reduced the ischaemic time period, resulting in successful transplantations. In 1968 the concept of brain death and the criteria for the diagnosis of brain death based on the Harvard criteria was introduced and became widely accepted. This resulted in a replacement of NHBD by donation after brain death donors (DBD). However, it became clear that the available number of brain death donors could not meet the increasing demand of kidneys for transplantation. To address this shortage NHBD programmes were restarted in the 1990s in an attempt to enlarge the deceased donor pool. In the early days NHB donors could only provide kidneys, and liver, pancreas and cardiothoracic organ procurement was not until later. Together with the reintroduction of the NHB donors there was a need to develop guidelines to address ethical, legal, organizational and technical aspects of the programme.

© Springer Nature Switzerland AG 2021
N. Hakim et al. (eds.), *Transplantation Surgery*, Springer Specialist Surgery Series,
https://doi.org/10.1007/978-3-030-55244-2_5

In Europe, the term non-heart beating donor (NHBD) was used to describe an organ donor after cardiorespiratory arrest, in order to distinguish from the brain death donor. In 1995 the first International NHBD workshop was organized by Gauke Kootstra in Maastricht, in which surgeons, nephrologist, ethicists and policymakers participated to agree upon the term non-heart beating donor as a formal description of a donor after cardiorespiratory arrest. In addition, this meeting established the first classification of the NHB donor into four categories, to determine criteria for the establishment of death (Table 5.1) [2]. Following publication of the guidance from this seminal meeting NHBD programmes were (re) introduced in many countries, and although they were initially focused on kidney retrieval, increasingly other organs were successfully procured and transplanted, such as livers, lungs and pancreas [3, 4].

Table 5.1 1995 Maastricht classification of non-heart beating donors

Category I	Dead on arrival	includes out of hospital victims who are not resuscitated, but are transported to the emergency department for donation purposes
Category II	Death with unsuccessful resuscitation	includes patients who are unsuccessfully resuscitated and declared dead in the hospital
Category III	Awaiting cardiac arrest	includes patients for whom circulatory death occurs after a planned withdrawal of life sustaining therapies, mainly cardiorespiratory support
Category IV	Cardiac arrest while brain dead	patients who after diagnosis of brain death and during donor management, but before the planned organ recovery suffer an unexpected CA.

5.3 Classification of DCD Donors

The terms 'non-heart beating' or 'cardiac death' were used interchangeably in cases of circulatory death, and the term of 'heart-beating' was used in cases of brain death. However, limitations of these terms arose, as they resulted in misunderstandings about the definition of death being based on a single organ (e.g. brain or heart) rather than a whole person. Thus, the Institute of Medicine—American National Academy of Sciences [5] proposed a clarification of the terms to specify that death could be declared or determined by a physician by the use of either neurologic criteria or by circulatory criteria. Donation after cardiac death was re-named Donation after Circulatory Death (DCD) and donation after brain death re-named Donation after Neurologic Determination of Death. This concept of Donation after Circulatory Death (DCD), to define organ donors after circulatory arrest (CA), has now been adopted by the World Health Organization (WHO) [6]. Following extensive discussion in the transplant community and during the DCD Conference in Paris in 2013 it was agreed to modify the original Maastricht Classification and update according to new developments but attempt to keep its relative simplicity intact. The result of this discussion is shown in following few paragraphs describing the various categories and summarised in Table 5.2.

5.3.1 Category I

Found 'dead on arrival' (by the emergency team) includes victims of out-of-hospital (OH) accidents who are not resuscitated for clear reasons such as death due to a broken neck or successful suicide. These deceased patients could be transported to the emergency department and become a donor if the organs are deemed appropriate for donation. One of the criteria for acceptance for donation is a warm ischaemia time (WIT; time between the circulatory arrest and the start of the

Table 5.2 Modified Maastricht classification of DCD in Paris 2013 [9]

Category I Uncontrolled	Found dead	Sudden unexpected circulatory arrest without any attempt of resuscitation by a medical team; WIT to be considered according to National life-recommendations in place; reference to in-or out of hospital life (IH-OH) setting
	1A. Out of hospital	
	1B. In hospital	
Category II Uncontrolled	Witnessed cardiac arrest	Sudden unexpected irreversible circulatory arrest with unsuccessful resuscitation – by a life-medical team; reference to in-or out-of-hospital (IH-OH) life setting
	IIA. Out of hospital	
	IIB In hospital	
Category III Controlled	Withdrawal of life-sustaining therapy	Planned withdrawal of life-sustaining therapy; expected circulatory arrest
Category IV Controlled	Cardiac arrest while life- brain death	Sudden circulatory arrest after brain death diagnosis during life-management but prior to planned organ recovery

cooling) of less than 45 min. To date, there are few examples of successful organ donation in this category, mainly because of the uncertainty about the duration of WIT.

5.3.2 Category II

'Unsuccessful resuscitation' includes patients brought to the emergency room while being resuscitated, but if cardiopulmonary resuscitation (CPR) is unsuccessful, the patient may be declared dead. At the Maastricht workshop, a 10-min period of "no-touch" after circulatory arrest to ensure a situation equivalent to brain death was proposed. In recent years, in most countries a period of 5 min has been adopted by medical societies and authorities, although depending on the jurisdiction a range from 2 min (USA) to 20 min (Italy) still exists. Countries with presumed consent (opting-out) can immediately proceed to the cooling preservation (detailed later), while countries with opting-in legislation might have to bridge the time until consent for organ donation has been given. Legislation in The Netherlands was introduced where 'preparatory handlings' could be allowed in order to preserve the organs for transplantation, before the person's or the family's wish was known. In some countries (Spain, France), two subcategories have been added due to different logistic conditions according to the site where CA occurs: IIa for out-of hospital (OH) and IIb for in-hospital (IH) [7, 8].

5.3.3 Category III

'Awaiting cardiac or circulatory death' includes those patients for whom circulatory death occurs after a planned withdrawal of life-sustaining therapies (WLST), mainly cardiorespiratory support. CA is expected and the medical decision of WLST is taken in a defined and multi-disciplinary approach, consistent with local/national legal requirements, by the clinical team together with the family, where further treatment is considered futile. In the initial description, the term "controlled" meant that the ischaemia time was short enough to consider recovery of liver, kidneys, pancreas and lungs. This category, which was defined in the 90s, does not include euthanasia or medical-assisted CA, an end-of-life practice authorized in some European countries (Belgium, Netherlands, Luxemburg).

5.3.4 Category IV

'Cardiac arrest in a brain-dead donor' includes patients who suffer an unexpected CA after diagnosis of brain death and during donor management but prior to the planned organ recovery. In this case, it is likely that health care professionals will try first to restore adequate circulation and perfusion of organs, but when unsuccessful, the patient can be considered for DCD donation (uncontrolled CA). In some countries, where the legislation does not accept brain death criteria (i.e. Japan) or when the patient will never meet the neurological criteria for the diagnosis of BD, the procedure for this potential DBD can be converted to a DCD (controlled CA).

5.4 DCD Utilization Rates

In Europe, there has been an increase in deceased donation as well as a rising contribution of DCD. In 2009, 9769 deceased donors were reported of which 661 (6%) were DCD, while in 2018 13,203 deceased donors were reported including 1856 DCDs (14%) [10]. In the Eurotransplant region the data [11] shows that the number of DCDs as well the percentage contribution of DCD of the total deceased donor pool has also grown considerably over the last 10 years. In 2009 144 of the 2074 (7%) of the deceased donor pool were DCDs, which increased to 269 of the 2159 (12%) in 2018. Out of the 8 countries however, only 3 countries (Austria, Belgium and Netherlands) have DCD programmes. The Netherlands has a very active and the longest existing programme. In 2018 65% of the deceased donors were DCDs, which was an increase from 40% in 2009. The UK [12] has the largest number of DCD donors, with 638 DCD's in 2018, which was equal to 40% of the total deceased donor pool.

The utilization rate of DCD is somewhat lower than DBDs. In the Netherlands, only 72% of DCDs that are registered for donation are eventually used. The main reason is that the retrieval does not proceed (non-proceeding DCD), this is because following the withdrawal of life sustaining treatment, the heart does not stop in the required period. The average number of organs used per donor is lower than in DBD donors. Within Eurotransplant the average number of organs per DCD donor stabilized around 2.4 organs per donor, while in the Netherlands there

has been an increase from 2.4 organs per donor in 2009 to 2.7 in 2018. This is lower than in DBDs from which 3.5 organs per donor were procured [13]. 36% of the donors are now multi-organ donors, compared with 18% in 2009. The 2018 UK data are comparable with a yield of 2.7 organs per DCD and 3.5 organs per DBD.

5.5 Donation After Circulatory Death Retrieval

The primary difference between controlled DCD (cDCD) and uncontrolled DCD (uDCD) is that cDCD occurs in hospital and is predictable and uDCD generally occurs out of hospital and is unpredictable. There are also distinct differences in the retrieval procedure between the two types which are described below.

5.6 Controlled Donors

In the UK, there are clear national guidelines on the process of DCD donation and once a suitable donor has been identified then an organ retrieval team is mobilised to the donor hospital. There is a national organ retrieval service (NORS) that comprises seven available abdominal teams and three available cardiothoracic teams. The process is coordinated by a locally based specialist nurse for organ donation (SN-OD) who liaises with the retrieval teams and the national hub, who oversee and help co-ordinate all the retrieval activity.

On arrival at the donor hospital the abdominal and thoracic (if present) retrieval team lead surgeons complete a final check to ensure there are no contra-indications to donation. Such details include a signed consent form, confirming blood group, review of medical history and virology test results. The retrieval team, local theatre staff, SN-OD and anaesthetist should confirm the withdrawal plan and logistics of transferring the patient into the operating theatre. As there are differences in priorities between the thoracic and abdominal retrieval teams this must be discussed and appreciated. The greatest urgency for the abdominal team is cannulation and cooling of the abdominal organs whereas the focus for the thoracic team is protection of the airway and inflation of the lungs or rapid procurement of the heart. Prior to treatment withdrawal the two teams need to discuss and agree the sequence of steps to ensure both thoracic and abdominal organs are optimally preserved and retrieved uninjured.

Treatment withdrawal usually occurs in the intensive care unit or in the anaesthetic room adjacent to theatre and the family may or may not be present. The retrieval team must be respectful of the presence of the family in the anaesthetic room and ensure noise from the operating theatre is not audible. The withdrawal of treatment is not standardised and is dependent upon the views of the local anaesthetic team and the type of life sustaining support of the patient. The endotracheal tube is removed and inotropic support is turned off although sedatives may continue as the patient should not be in distress. Once cardiac arrest occurs a 5 min 'hands-off' period must ensue before the patient can be certified dead. During this period the patient can be transferred into the operating theatre where the retrieval team will be set up, scrubbed and ready to proceed.

Once the patient has been certified dead and the identity confirmed by the lead surgeon the retrieval can commence. The patient is prepared and draped ensuring exposure is from the neck to the pubis. If the lungs are being retrieved the patient is re-intubated and the airway protected prior to manipulation of the abdominal organs and ideally prior to the abdominal incision.

A full thoraco-abdominal midline incision from the sternal notch to the pubis is made and rapid access into the thoracic and abdominal cavity is obtained, being careful not to damage the lungs and abdominal viscera, in particular the liver and small bowel.

5.6.1 Cardiac Retrieval

Since 2015 in the UK there has been a DCD heart program [14] that utilises perfusion technology to assess and preserve the heart. Hearts can be retrieved following Normothermic Regional Perfusion (NRP) or by direct procurement and perfusion (DPP) the details of which are described in the preservation section below. In DPP heart retrieval the heart is removed, flushed and placed on a perfusion device for assessment and transportation. If NRP is used then the cerebral circulation is occluded and the heart reanimated for assessment. This technique reduces the functional warm ischaemia time and allows in situ cardiac assessment.

5.6.2 Lung Retrieval

The lungs are recruited with a single breath and are flushed via the pulmonary artery with preservation solution (e.g. Perfadex®). Once they are removed the lungs are flushed via the pulmonary vein and can either be transported cold stored or using Ex Vivo Lung Perfusion (EVLP) which is described below.

5.6.3 Abdominal Retrieval

A large abdominal retractor is positioned and the assistant surgeon retracts the small bowel and right colon to the left side of the patient. The lead surgeon incises the peritoneum and isolates either the abdominal aorta just above the iliac bifurcation or the right common iliac artery, ensuring the ureter is not damaged in the process. The artery is controlled with ligatures and incised and either a double balloon or standard vascular cannula is secured in place. If a double balloon cannula is used, both balloons can be inflated and then perfusion can be commenced, however if a standard cannula is used the proximal aorta needs to be occluded to prevent reperfusion of the brain. This can be done by isolating the supracoeliac aorta or the descending aorta in the thorax. Once perfusion has commenced the venous system needs to be decompressed by incising or cannulating the right atrium/thoracic portion of the IVC or the IVC in the abdomen, see Fig. 5.1. The decision where to decompress the venous system depends on whether the cardiothoracic organs are being retrieved and whether there is straightforward

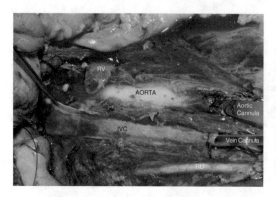

Fig. 5.1 Operative photograph showing part of the 'cold phase' dissection with aortic and venous cannulas in situ. Note the cut end of the left renal vein (RV), the inferior vena cava (IVC), aorta and right ureter (RU)

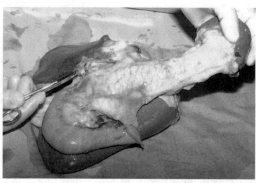

Fig. 5.3 Photograph of an en bloc retrieval of the liver and pancreas. The surgeon is holding the spleen which is connected to the tail of the pancreas and the stapled jejunum is also evident

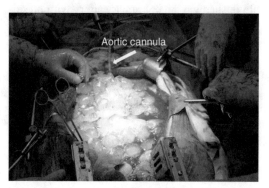

Fig. 5.2 Operative photograph showing an organ retrieval with an open abdomen and thorax filled with ice and the tubing with preservation fluid perfusing the donor via an aortic cannula

access into the thorax. The advantage of decompressing in the thorax is there is less effluent in the abdomen which makes the cold phase dissection easier. Once perfusion has commenced, the proximal aorta is occluded and the venous system has been decompressed, the abdomen is then filled with slushed ice to cool the organs, see Fig. 5.2. This step is crucial as it reduces the temperature, reduces metabolism and therefore reduces the warm ischaemic injury the organs sustain.

A volume of 4–5 litres of cooled preservation solution should be used to flush the organs *in situ,* unless otherwise indicated by the provider of the preservation solution. Once this step has been completed the cold phase dissection can begin. The specific technical details of the dissection of

the organs is beyond the scope of this chapter but the steps are noted sequentially in brief below (Fig. 5.3).

1. Liver and/or pancreas removal (see note below[1])
2. Removal of kidneys
3. Removal of common, external and internal iliac artery and vein bilaterally
4. Flushing, inspection and packaging of organs

Step 3 is carried out to aid vascular reconstruction of the liver and pancreas prior to transplantation. A healthy section of iliac vein and artery should be sent with each organ and if the iliac system is diseased they should be replaced with thoracic or neck vessels.

5.7 Uncontrolled Donors

Since the pioneering initiation of a uDCD programme in Madrid in 1995 protocols for uDCD retrieval have been implemented in Spain, France,

---

[1]The liver and pancreas can be removed *en bloc* or separately, Fig. 5.3. The advantages of *en bloc* removal are that it can be performed more quickly, and in the presence of abnormal vascular anatomy, in particular a replaced or accessory right hepatic artery, vascular damage can be minimised while working *in situ*. On the other hand, separation of liver and pancreas on the back-table in the donor hospital under less ideal conditions may be challenging.

Italy, the UK, and The Netherlands, and have been developed in Belgium, Switzerland, Austria, and in Saint Petersburg (Russia) and in New York City. Although the protocols differ slightly, there are defined stages that are consistent throughout. The list below details the common steps although there are procedural differences at each stage between the protocols. Step 7, organ retrieval follows the same procedure as in cDCD detailed above.

1. Cardiac arrest
2. Initiation of cardiopulmonary resuscitation
3. Cessation of cardiopulmonary resuscitation
4. Organ preservation during transport
5. Diagnosis of death
6. Cannulation and preservation
7. Organ retrieval

There are a number of ethical, legal and logistical issues that the protocols address, in particular what interventions can occur prior to family consent and confirmation of death. The key difference between the protocols is whether cannulation and organ preservation can occur during transport to the hospital. Normothermic-ECMO, following cannulation of the femoral vessels, is the most frequently used technique and this recirculates warmed, oxygenated blood to minimise warm ischaemic injury. On arrival at the hospital death must be confirmed following a defined period (5 min in the UK) without resuscitation or preservation. Consent must also be obtained prior to organ retrieval and the duration from time of cannulation to organ procurement varies from 120 to 360 min [15].

5.8 Preservation

The conventional storage method for all organs for transportation from the donor hospital to transplant centre used to be static cold storage (SCS) preservation. This involves immediate flush-out of blood at the time of retrieval, explantation, and submerging the organ in cold (5 °C) preservation solution within an organ bag or receptacle, which is then placed in an organ box surrounded by crushed melting ice to keep the temperature between 0–4 °C. Other preservation methods after retrieval when bridging between donor and recipient hospital have been developed to improve outcomes, prolong preservation time, assess viability and those specific to each organ are described below. Normothermic Regional Perfusion (NRP) is a technique applied *in situ* in the donor prior to explantation of donor organs and can be used as a method of preservation with, in the case of organs such as the heart and liver, the possibility to assess function. NRP involves using ECMO-based technology to recirculate autologous warmed, oxygenated blood to the abdominal organs and/or the heart. In brief, cannulas are secured in the abdominal aorta and the inferior vena cava and the cerebral circulation is excluded by clamping the thoracic aorta, or if the heart is included, the branches of the aortic arch, to avoid reperfusing the brain. Blood then drains from the venous system into the device where it is warmed and oxygenated and pumped back into the circulation via the aortic cannula. Cardiac and liver function can be assessed using physiological measurements and biochemical testing.

5.8.1 Kidney

Hypothermic machine perfusion (HMP) involves pumping the organ, via a cannula that connects to the aortic patch, with cooled preservation solution. There are a number of commercially available devices including Lifeport® (ORS, USA), KidneyAssist Transport® (Organ Assist, Groningen, NL), RM3® (Waters Medical System, USA). A seminal European multicentre trial in which paired kidneys (of both donor types DBD and DCD) were allocated to SCS or HMP showed that kidneys in the HMP group had less delayed graft function (DGF) and better 1 year. graft survival and eGFR [16]. In addition, in two separately powered studies in ECD and DCD donor kidneys significant benefit was observed for better graft survival in ECD and significant reduction of DGF in DCD [55, 56]. As a result, in The Netherlands, all kidneys nowadays undergo HMP from the donor hospital although the uptake in the rest of Europe is more variable and appears to be more focussed on the donor type. Two similar trials attempted in the UK were either stopped or failed to replicate the same findings due to different trial design and logistical problems resulting in realtively short perfusion times on HMP and therefore in the UK HMP use is centre and clinician specific [17, 18]. HMP can also be used once the organs arrive at the transplant centre for preservation and assessment and this is often for marginal organs. Oxygenated-HMP has been assessed in COMPARE and POMP, two of the COPE (Consortium for Organ Preservation in Europe) trials. The results for continuous prolonged oxygenated HMP in DCD donor kidneys while being transported to the recipient centre (7–8 h of HMP) (COMPARE) suggest that this is advantageous with lower graft failure, better eGFR at 12 months, and a significant reduction in rejection compared to standard HMP, while the combination of SCS with oxygenated HMP for a brief period (4–5 h) in the transplant centre of higher risk ECD kidneys (POMP) does not show any difference in outcomes [Abstract ESOT 2019 COMPARE; Abstract ATC 2020]. The latter POMP study outcome may affect current policy of many centres to either change to accepting higher risk donor kidneys on oxygenated HMP, or when initiating HMP only after the kidney has arrived in the recipient centre, letting it perfuse for a minimum of 7–8 h.

Ex vivo Normothermic Machine perfusion (EVNP or NMP) is a technique that involves pumping the kidney with a body temperature, blood-based, oxygenated solution. Early work by Hosgood and Nicholson suggested that DCD kidneys undergoing 1 h EVNP immediately prior to transplant had reduced rates of DGF compared with matched controls [19]. This question is currently being assessed in a multicentre RCT [20]. EVNP has also been used as a means of viability assessment, which has resulted in the successful transplantation of DCD kidneys declined for transplant, that would otherwise have not been utilised [21]. Prolonged periods of kidney perfusion may also be useful for regeneration, repair, viability assessment or, as with the liver, extending preservation without compromising out-

comes. A phase II clinical trial in deceased donor kidneys using the OrganOx kidney NMP device is due to commence in early 2020 and will assess preservation periods of up to 24 h of NMP.

5.8.2 Liver

NMP has recently been implemented in clinical practice in the UK and Europe following a seminal clinical trial that was part of COPE (Consortium for Organ Preservation in Europe) comparing SCS with NMP of deceased donor livers (although this was used in DCD and DBD organs). Livers accepted for transplant were allocated to SCS (n = 133) or NMP (n = 137) and those allocated to NMP were connected to the OrganOx metra device at the donor hospital. Early allograft dysfunction was reduced in NMP livers compared to SCS livers. In addition, utilisation was significantly higher in the NMP group and the median preservation duration was significantly increased in the NMP group without compromising outcome [22]. This has had a profound effect on the logistics of liver transplant and has allowed clinicians to safely extend preservation times and enabled elective cases, that would otherwise have been cancelled, to proceed. There is experimental evidence that HMP at the end of preservation may reduce ischaemic injury and therefore biliary complications [23, 24]. DHOPE-DCD is a European multicentre clinical trial of DCD livers comparing SCS with SCS plus 2 h HMP-O_2 immediately prior to transplant, on the incidence of non-anastomotic biliary strictures [25].

5.8.3 Pancreas

There are no clinical studies in pancreas perfusion and a limited number of preclinical studies which include both DBD and DCD organs. There is a case series using HMP in discarded human pancreas HMP which shows, on histological assessment, the technique is feasible and not injurious [26]. A similar study comparing HMP with SCS in both DBD and DCD pancreases showed no difference in perfusate flow, oedema and end-HMP ATP levels [27]. There is also a study of NMP assessment of discarded human pancreases that demonstrated perfusion was feasible although the viability of the organ appeared to be limited by the recirculation of proteolytic enzymes [28].

5.8.4 Lungs

Ex vivo lung perfusion (EVLP) is a technique where DCD and high risk DBD lungs are perfused with an acellular warmed solution to evaluate lung function prior to transplant. Following on from Steen et al. who pioneered the technique, the Toronto group showed in a non-randomised trial that physiologically stable lungs over 4 h had comparable outcomes with control lungs [29]. Their 10 year follow up of 230 patients who had undergone EVLP compared with 706 patients in the control group showed there was no significant difference in time to chronic lung allograft dysfunction (56% vs 56% at 5 years, and 53% vs 36% at 9 years, P = 0.68) or graft survival between the groups (62% vs 58% at 5 years, and 50% vs 44% at 9 years, P = 0.97) [30].

5.8.5 Heart

Perfusion technology is a central part of DCD cardiac retrieval and Transmedics OCS (Organ Conditioning System) is a transportable perfusion device that can be used for both heart preservation and assessment. At present, a combination of visual inspection, metabolic and flow parameters are used to determine organ viability. Remarkably this technique has, in an organ where early failure following transplant is often fatal, enabled clinicians to delay implantation time with no significant consequences [31]. There are two main protocols for DCD heart retrieval, the Sydney Direct Procurement Protocol (DPP) and the Papworth Normothermic Regional Perfusion (NRP). In brief, following circulatory death and thoracotomy, DPP involves rapid cooling and preservation of the heart, collection of 2 l donor blood, explantation of the heart and connection to the OCS NMP device. NRP is an adaptation of ECMO, where following death the aorta is cannulated, the arch vessels occluded and the heart is re-animated. Cardiac function can then be assessed and if appropriate the heart retrieved, cold stored (or placed on the OCS) and transplanted. So far, about 100 cases of DCD heart transplantation have been performed across six centres in Australia, United Kingdom and Belgium [32].

5.9 Outcomes

5.9.1 Kidney

Outcomes following DCD kidney transplant have remained fairly consistent in the UK over the past decade and NHSBT data from 13,310 patients in 2015 showed that there was no overall difference between DBD and DCD donors (Table 5.3). This is despite the age of donors and number of donor comorbidities increasing over that time period [33]. Data from The Netherlands Organ Transplant Registry (NOTR) has mirrored data from the UK showing equivalent long term outcomes from DCD and DBD kidney transplants but with higher rates of early graft loss and primary non-function (PNF) in DCD kidneys [34]. Compared with DBD donors, outcomes are also similar although rates of DGF are significantly higher in DCD donors. NOTR data (n = 6625) showed that the presence of DGF following transplant with a DCD kidney does not impact on the long-term outcome, although conversely the presence of DGF following DBD transplant equates to poorer long term graft survival [35].

Outcomes from uDCD donor kidneys (n = 499) transplanted in France from 2007–16 with 42% undergoing NRP showed PNF occurred in 37 cases (7.4%) and poor graft outcome, defined as eGFR at 1 year <30 ml/min or graft loss <1 year, occurred in an additional 66 patients (14.3%). These data were analysed to help improve protocols and outcomes in uDCD donors and showed that poor outcomes were associated with *in situ* cooling compared with NRP [36].

Table 5.3 Comparison of outcomes for DCD and DBD donor kidneys

	DCD $n = 3626$	DBD $n = 9684$	P-value	Risk-adjusted ratio (95% CI)	Risk ratio P-value
Primary non function	32% (115/3626)	2.6% (259/9684)	0.06[a]	OR 1.18 (0.9–15)	0.21[b]
Delayed graft function	48.5% (1417/2901)	24.9% (1745/5263)	<0.0001[a]	OR 2.81 (2.5–3.2)	<0.0001[b]
1-year eGFR	47.4 (35.6–61.2)	48.7 (37.3–61.1)	0.005[c]	RE −0.16 (−0.9–0.6)	0.69[d]
5-year eGFR	49.6 (35.1–64.7)	48.1 (35.8–62.2)	0.06[c]	RE 0.02 (−1.1–1.2)	0.97[d]
5-year death-censored graft survival	85.9%	84.5%	0.22[e]	HR 0.95 (0.8–1.1)	0.60[f]
5-year all-cause graft survival	76.8%	78.1%	0.15[e]	HR 0.97 (0.9–1.1)	0.55[f]
5-year patient survival	86.5%	89.4%	<0.0001[e]	HR 1.18 (0.8–1.1)	0.28[f]
10-year death-censored graft survival	74.9%	74.3%	0.20[e]	HR 0.95 (0.8–1.1)	0.42[f]
10-year all-cause graft survival	59.8%	60.7%	0.26[e]	HR 0.94 (0.9–1.0)	0.22[f]
10-year patient survival	71.7%	76.7%	<0.000[e]	HR 0.95 (0.8–1.1)	0.42[f]

Reproduced from NHSBT data [33]

Abbreviations: *CI* confidence interval, *DBD* donation after brain death, *DCD* donation after circulatory death, *eGFR* estimated glomerular filtration rate, *HR* hazard ratio, *OR* odds ratio, *RE* estimated difference in adjusted means

Data are for all deceased donors, kidney-only kidney transplants in first-time recipients performed between 2001 and 2012 inclusive. Data are median (interquartile range) or percentage (*n*). Risk adjustment for significant variables of donor age, cold ischemic time, recipient age, donor hypertension, donor premortem creatinine, transplant center, human leukocyte antigen (HLA) mismatch, machine perfusion, sensitization to HLA, donor cause of death, donor weight and cause of recipient primary renal disease. See our previous published work for more details of methodology, and the Supplementary Material online for models.[16] For the HR and OR, DBD is the reference group. For multiple linear regression for graft function, the coefficient of the variable that is 1 for DCD and 0 for DBD is the estimated mean difference in eGFR values between a recipient of a DCD donor kidney and a recipient of a DBD donor kidney, adjusted for the other terms in the model. For delayed graft function, patients who were pre-dialysis, or who had primary non-function, were excluded

[a]X^2

[b]Logistic regression

[c]Wilcoxon

[d]Multiple linear regression

[e]Log-rank

[f]Cox proportional hazards

Data from Madrid, the centre with one of the largest uDCD series showed uDCD outcomes were worse than SCD but superior to ECD kidneys. PNF rates were high at 12% although 5 and 10-year graft survival rates were 78% and 72% respectively [37]. Outcomes from Kidneys from uDCD donors having undergone NRP (n = 237) in Madrid were shown to have similar outcomes to a DBD population with (uncensored) graft survival between the uDCD and DBD groups at 5 years (80.9% vs 85.6%) and 10 years (71.1% vs 70.8%, respectively, P = 0.40) [38].

5.9.2 Liver

The early literature clearly shows outcomes from DCD liver transplant are inferior compared with DBD liver transplants. This includes lower transplant survival, higher rates or primary non-function (PNF) and higher rates of biliary complications, including ischaemic cholangiopathy [39–44]. A recently published study on behalf on the UK liver advisory group has replicated these findings showing that both 90 day (93.9% vs. 88.9%; p < 0.0001) and five-year post-

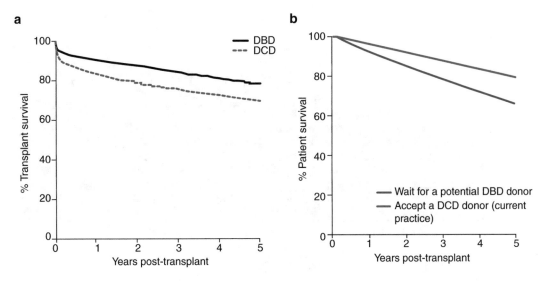

Fig. 5.4 Kaplan-Meier survival curves showing percentage survival of liver transplant recipients over time Graph A. Graph B shows survival rates of patients with a DCD liver transplant compared to those waiting for a suitable DBD liver

transplant survival were worse following DCD than DBD transplantation (69.1% vs. 78.3%; p < 0.0001). However, given 1325 (23%) patients either died or were removed from the waiting list without receiving a transplant if outcomes were modelled on DCD livers not being used at all then not only would overall survival on the waiting list be lower (Fig. 5.4) but the survival benefit of waiting for a DBD liver would also be lost. Thus, DCD liver transplant remains a valuable resource in the face of an expanding waiting list and fewer DBD donors. Clinicians attempt to mitigate the higher risks associated with DCD livers by being more selective about which DCD donors to accept for transplant, demonstrated by DCD donors having lower donor age, lower numbers with cerebrovascular cause of death, lower MELD and lower UKELD scores compared with DBD donors [45].

5.9.3 Lung

A recently published study of DCD lung outcomes from the International Society for Heart and Lung Transplantation (ISHLT) and Thoracic Transplant Registry showed that 5 yr.

DCD III outcomes were comparable with that of DBD (61% vs. 63%, p = 0.72) and donor type was not associated with survival (DCD-III vs DBD; hazard ratio 1.04; p = 0.61). This included 11,516 patients transplanted between January 2003 and June 2017 at 22 centres in North America, Europe, and Australia participating in the DCD Registry [46]. There have been two recent systematic reviews comparing outcomes in DBD and DCD lung transplant. Firstly, an analysis of 17 studies with 995 DCD recipients and 38,579 DBD recipients showed comparable 1-year overall survival between the groups (RR 0.89, 95% CI, 0.74–1.07, P = 0.54). The airway anastomotic complications rate in the DCD cohort was higher than that in DBD cohorts (RR 2.00; 95% CI, 1.29–3.11, P = 0.002) There was no significant difference between DCD and DBD in the occurrence of primary graft dysfunction, bronchiolis obliterans syndrome, acute transplantation rejection or length of stay [47]. The second SR combining 9 studies with 2973 patients (403 DCD, 2570 DBD) showed no difference in 1 year graft survival, chronic lung allograft dysfunction (CLAD) or primary graft dysfunction (PGD) between the groups [48].

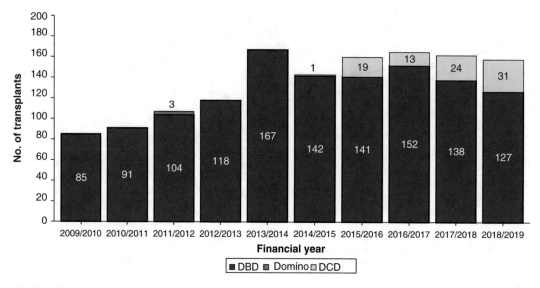

Fig. 5.5 Histogram showing the number of adult heart transplants by donor type in the UK over the past decade. Reproduced from NHSBT data [12]

5.9.4 Heart

Dhital et al. published the first series of DCD transplants in the modern era. 12 patients were transplanted from donors <40 years old and withdrawal times of <30 mins. All hearts were preserved using Transmedics OCS and in 2018 patient survival was 100% [48]. Papworth Hospital has the largest DCD heart transplant programme in the world with very encouraging early results. Recipient survival to discharge following DCD heart transplantation was 93%, with a post-operative ECMO requirement of 13%. Median stay was 5 days in intensive care and 20 days in hospital [49]. The group in Manchester, UK, have also published early results from their DCD programme, estimating an increase in transplant rates of about 25% with the use of DCD organs, although the numbers are small (n = 7). The overall 30-day survival rate was 100% and the 90-day survival rate was 86%. Postoperative extracorporeal membrane oxygenation was required in 43% [50]. A recent US study assessed the number and quality of hearts in one United Network for Organ Sharing (UNOS) Region and concluded that implementation of DCD heart transplantation in the United

States would improve overall donation rates [51]. To put survival following DCD heart transplant into context, 1 year survival following DBD heart transplant of 566 patients transplanted between 2014–18 was 82.4% [12]. Figure 5.5 shows the change in heart donor types in the UK over the past decade.

5.9.5 Pancreas

In comparison to DBD donors, there have been relatively small numbers of DCD pancreas transplants worldwide and the literature is quite thin. Concern about reperfusion pancreatitis and graft failure have meant that generally DCD donors are younger with lower risk scores than DBD donors. A 2017 meta-analysis of five studies, comparing DBD with DCD SPK recipients showed there was no difference in 1 yr. pancreas graft survival in SPK 87.2% vs. 86.5% or patient survival 95.3% vs. 96.5% respectively. However, there were higher rates of pancreas graft thrombosis in DCD pancreases of 9% vs 5.2% in DBD grafts [52]. A single centre study of 104 pancreas transplants from Leiden showed age was the only risk factor for pancreas graft failure [53].

5.10 Future Work

Many of the technologies being used for preservation, in particular in the context of DCD donors are slowly implemented into practice rather than tested in a clinical trial. Advances in practice utilising perfusion technology can be shown to be highly successful for individual patients, such as the paediatric patient who underwent a successful heart transplant following NRP then 2 h SCS [54]. However, to ensure the best use of technology clinicians and stakeholders should endeavour to work together to test them in multicentre clinical trials rather than highly selective series, as is often the case. In order for patients to benefit from organs that will provide excellent outcomes, deciding on the appropriate preservation and perfusion strategy and means of viability assessment for a particular organ is essential. This may include HMP, NMP, NRP or a combination of each and it may be different for individual organs from the same donor. There are many questions to answer and a plethora of trials ahead to reach the goal of negligible organ discard combined with excellent outcomes after transplant. The challenge for all of us involved is to design a sequence of strategies or combinations of methods of preservation that can be carried out in parallel across participating countries to demonstrate clinical evidence with benefit for patients and cost-effectiveness for our health care systems.

References

1. Organ Donation and Transplantation after cardiac death edited by David Talbot, Anthony D'Alessandro, Paolo Muiesan.
2. Kootstra G, Daemen J, Ommen A. Categories of non-heart beating donors. Transplant Poroc. 1995;27(5):2893–4.
3. Dubbeld J, Hoekstra H, Farid W, et al. Similar liver transplantation survival with selected cardiac death donors and brains death donors. Br J Surg. 2010;97:744–53.
4. Nijkamp DM, van der Bij W, Verschuuren EAM, Heemskerk MBA, de Bijuzer E, Erasmus ME. Non-heart-beating lung donation: how big is the pool? Heart Lung Transpl. 2008;9:1049–2.
5. National Academy Press. Institute of Medicine: Organ Donation: Opportunities for Action. Washington DC; 2006. http://www.nap.edu/catalog/11643/
6. Third WHO global consultation on organ donation and transplantation: striving to achieve self-sufficiency. WHO, The Transplantation Society and Organizacion Nacional de Trasplantes. Transplantation 2011;91(Suppl. 11):S27.
7. Donation after circulatory death in Spain: Current situation and recommendations. National Consensus Document. 2012. http://www.ont.es/infesp/Paginas/DocumentosdeConsenso.Aspx
8. Antoine C, Brun F, Tenaillon A, Loty B. Organ procurement and transplantation from non heart beating donors. Nephrol Therap. 2008;4:5.
9. Thuong M et al. New classification of donation afer circulatory death donor definitions and terminology. Transplant Int. 2016;29(7).
10. GODT Global Observatory on Donation & Transplantation 2009 and 2018.
11. Www.eurotransplant.org/statistics/report liberay/tabel1092P.
12. NHSBT Transplant activity report 2018–2019. https://www.odt.nhs.uk/statistics-and-reports/annual-activity-report/
13. Annual report DTF 2018.
14. Messer S, Page A, Axell R, Berman M, Hernández-Sánchez J, Colah S, Parizkova B, Valchanov K, Dunning J, Pavlushkov E, Balasubramanian SK, Parameshwar J, Omar YA, Goddard M, Pettit S, Lewis C, Kydd A, Jenkins D, Watson CJ, Sudarshan C, Catarino P, Findlay M, Ali A, Tsui S, Large SR. Outcome after heart transplantation from donation after circulatory-determined death donors. J Heart Lung Transplant. 2017 Dec;36(12):1311–8.
15. Ortega-Deballon I, Hornby L, Shemie SD. Protocols for uncontrolled donation after circulatory death: a systematic review of international guidelines, practices and transplant outcomes. Crit Care. 2015;19(1):268.
16. Moers C, Smits JM, Maathuis MH, Treckmann J, van Gelder F, Napieralski BP, van Kasterop-Kutz M, van der Heide JJ, Squifflet JP, van Heurn E, Kirste GR, Rahmel A, Leuvenink HG, Paul A, Pirenne J, Ploeg RJ. Machine perfusion or cold storage in deceased-donor kidney transplantation. N Engl J Med. 2009 Jan 1;360(1):7–19.
17. Summers DM, Ahmad N, Randle LV, O'Sullivan AM, Johnson RJ, Collett D, Attia M, Clancy M, Tavakoli A, Akyol M, Jamieson NV, Bradley JA, Watson CJ. Cold pulsatile machine perfusion versus static cold storage for kidneys donated after circulatory death: a multicenter randomized controlled trial. Transplantation 2019 Aug 8. https://doi.org/10.1097/TP.0000000000002907. [Epub ahead of print].
18. Watson CJ, Wells AC, Roberts RJ, Akoh JA, Friend PJ, Akyol M, Calder FR, Allen JE, Jones MN, Collett D, Bradley JA. Cold machine perfusion versus static cold storage of kidneys donated after cardiac death: a UK multicenter randomized controlled trial. Am J Transplant 2010 Sep;10(9):1991–9.
19. Nicholson ML, Hosgood SA. Renal transplantation after ex vivo normothermic perfusion: the first clinical study. Am J Transplant. 2013 May;13(5):1246–52.

20. Hosgood SA, Saeb-Parsy K, Wilson C, Callaghan C, Collett D, Nicholson ML. Protocol of a randomised controlled, open-label trial of ex vivo normothermic perfusion versus static cold storage in donation after circulatory death renal transplantation. BMJ Open. 2017 Jan 23;7(1):e012237.
21. Hosgood SA, Thompson E, Moore T, Wilson CH, Nicholson ML. Normothermic machine perfusion for the assessment and transplantation of declined human kidneys from donation after circulatory death donors. Br J Surg. 2018 Mar;105(4):388–94.
22. Nasralla D, Coussios CC, Mergental H, Akhtar MZ, Butler AJ, Ceresa CDL, Chiocchia V, Dutton SJ, García-Valdecasas JC, Heaton N, Imber C, Jassem W, Jochmans I, Karani J, Knight SR, Kocabayoglu P, Malagò M, Mirza D, Morris PJ, Pallan A, Paul A, Pavel M, Perera MTPR, Pirenne J, Ravikumar R, Russell L, Upponi S, CJE W, Weissenbacher A, Ploeg RJ, Friend PJ. Consortium for Organ Preservation in Europe. A randomized trial of normothermic preservation in liver transplantation. Nature. 2018 May;557(7703):50–6.
23. Schlegel A. Protective mechanisms of end-ischemic cold machine perfusion in DCD liver grafts. J Hepatol. 2013;58:278–86.
24. Dutkowski P. Rescue of the cold preserved rat liver by hypothermic oxygenated machine perfusion. Am J Transplant. 2006;6:903–12.
25. van Rijn R, van den Berg AP, Erdmann JI, Heaton N, van Hoek B, de Jonge J, Leuvenink HGD, Mahesh SVK, Mertens S, Monbaliu D, Muiesan P, Perera MTPR, Polak WG, Rogiers X, Troisi RI, de Vries Y, Porte RJ. Study protocol for a multicenter randomized controlled trial to compare the efficacy of end-ischemic dual hypothermic oxygenated machine perfusion with static cold storage in preventing non-anastomotic biliary strictures after transplantation of liver grafts donated after circulatory death: DHOPE-DCD trial. BMC Gastroenterol. 2019;19(1):40.
26. Branchereau J, Renaudin K, Kervella D, Bernadet S, Karam G, Blancho G, Cantarovich D. Hypothermic pulsatile perfusion of human pancreas: Preliminary technical feasibility study based on histology. Cryobiology. 2018.
27. Leemkuil M, Lier G, Engelse MA, Ploeg RJ, de Koning EJP, 't Hart NA, Krikke C, Leuvenink HGD. Hypothermic oxygenated machine perfusion of the human donor pancreas. Transplant Direct. 2018;4(10):e388.
28. Barlow AD, Hamed MO, Mallon DH, Brais RJ, Gribble FM, Scott MA, Howat WJ, Bradley JA, Bolton EM, Pettigrew GJ, Hosgood SA, Nicholson ML, Saeb-Parsy K. Use of ex vivo normothermic perfusion for quality assessment of discarded human donor pancreases. Am J Transplant. 2015 Sep;15(9):2475–82.
29. Cypel M, Yeung JC, Liu M, Anraku M, Chen F, Karolak W, Sato M, Laratta J, Azad S, Madonik M, Chow CW, Chaparro C, Hutcheon M, Singer LG, Slutsky AS, Yasufuku K, de Perrot M, Pierre AF, Waddell TK, Keshavjee S. Normothermic ex vivo lung perfusion in clinical lung transplantation. N Engl J Med. 2011;364(15):1431–40.
30. Divithotawela C, Cypel M, Martinu T, Singer LG, Binnie M, Chow CW, Chaparro C, Waddell TK, de Perrot M, Pierre A, Yasufuku K, Yeung JC, Donahoe L, Keshavjee S, Tikkanen JM. Long-term outcomes of lung transplant with ex vivo lung perfusion. JAMA Surg. 2019 Oct 9. https://doi.org/10.1001/jamasurg.2019.4079. [Epub ahead of print].
31. Ardehali A, Esmailian F, Deng M, et al. Ex-vivo perfusion of donor hearts for human heart transplantation (PROCEED II): a prospective, open-label, multicentre, randomised non-inferiority trial. Lancet. 2015;385:2577–84.
32. Chew HC, Macdonald PS, Dhital KK. The donor heart and organ perfusion technology. J Thorac Dis. 2019;11(Suppl 6):S938–45.
33. Summers DM, Watson CJ, Pettigrew GJ, Johnson RJ, Collett D, Neuberger JM, Bradley JA. Kidney donation after circulatory death (DCD): state of the art. Kidney Int. 2015;88(2):241–9.
34. Schaapherder A, Wijermars LGM, de Vries DK, de Vries APJ, Bemelman FJ, van de Wetering J, van Zuilen AD, Christiaans MHL, Hilbrands LH, Baas MC, Nurmohamed AS, Berger SP, Alwayn IP, Bastiaannet E, Lindeman JHN. Equivalent long-term transplantation outcomes for kidneys donated after brain death and cardiac death: conclusions from a nationwide evaluation. EClinicalMedicine. 2018;4–5:25–31.
35. de Kok MJ, McGuinness D, Shiels PG, de Vries DK, Nolthenius JBT, Wijermars LG, Rabelink TJ, Verschuren L, Stevenson KS, Kingsmore DB, McBride M, Ploeg RJ, Bastiaannet E, Schaapherder AF, Lindeman JH. The neglectable impact of delayed graft function on long-term graft survival in kidneys donated after circulatory death associates with superior organ resilience. Ann Surg. 2019;270(5):877–83.
36. Antoine C, Savoye E, Gaudez F, Cheisson G, Badet L, Videcoq M, Legeai C, Bastien O, Barrou B; National Steering Committee of Donation After Circulatory Death, Agence de la biomédecine, Saint Denis, France Kidney transplant from uncontrolled donation after circulatory death: contribution of normothermic regional perfusion. Transplantation. 2019 Apr 8. https://doi.org/10.1097/TP.0000000000002753. [Epub ahead of print].
37. Sánchez-Fructuoso AI, Pérez-Flores I, Del Río F, Blázquez J, Calvo N, Moreno de la Higuera MÁ, Gómez A, Alonso-Lera S, Soria A, González M, Corral E, Mateos A, Moreno-Sierra J, Fernández Pérez C. Uncontrolled donation after circulatory death: a cohort study of data from a long-standing deceased-donor kidney transplantation program. Am J Transplant. 2019;19(6):1693–707.
38. Molina M, Guerrero-Ramos F, Fernández-Ruiz M, González E, Cabrera J, Morales E, Gutierrez E, Hernández E, Polanco N, Hernández A, Praga M, Rodriguez-Antolín A, Pamplona M, de la Rosa F, Cavero T, Chico M, Villar A, Justo I, Andrés

A. Kidney transplant from uncontrolled donation after circulatory death donors maintained by nECMO has long-term outcomes comparable to standard criteria donation after brain death. Am J Transplant. 2019;19(2):434–47.

39. Laing RW, Scalera I, Isaac J, Mergental H, Mirza DF, Hodson J, et al. Liver transplantation using grafts from donors after circulatory death: a propensity score-matched study from a single center. Am J Transplant. 2016;16:1795–804.

40. Axelrod DA, Dzebisashvili N, Lentine KL, Xiao H, Schnitzler M, Tuttle-Newhall JE, et al. Variation in biliary complication rates following liver transplantation: implications for cost and outcome. Am J Transplant. 2015;15:170–9.

41. DeOliveira ML, Jassem W, Valente R, Khorsandi SE, Santori G, Prachalias A, et al. Biliary complications after liver transplantation using grafts from donors after cardiac death: results from a matched control study in a single large volume center. Ann Surg 2011;254:716–722, [discussion 722–713].

42. Foley DP, Fernandez LA, Leverson G, Anderson M, Mezrich J, Sollinger HW, et al. Biliary complications after liver transplantation from donation after cardiac death donors: an analysis of risk factors and long-term outcomes from a single center. Ann Surg. 2011;253:817–25.

43. Jay CL, Lyuksemburg V, Ladner DP, Wang E, Caicedo JC, Holl JL, et al. Ischemic cholangiopathy after controlled donation after cardiac death liver transplantation: a meta-analysis. Ann Surg. 2011;253:259–64.

44. O'Neill S, Roebuck A, Khoo E, Wigmore SJ, Harrison EM. A meta-analysis and meta-regression of outcomes including biliary complications in donation after cardiac death liver transplantation. Transpl Int. 2014;27:1159–74.

45. Taylor R, Allen E, Richards JA, Goh MA, Neuberger J, Collett D, Pettigrew GJ; Liver Advisory Group to NHS Blood and Transplant. Survival advantage for patients accepting the offer of a circulatory death liver transplant. J Hepatol. 2019 May;70(5):855–865. Jan 11.

46. Van Raemdonck D, Keshavjee S, Levvey B, Cherikh WS, Snell G, Erasmus M, Simon A, Glanville AR, Clark S, D'Ovidio F, Catarino P, McCurry K, Hertz MI, Venkateswaran R, Hopkins P, Inci I, Walia R, Kreisel D, Mascaro J, Dilling DF, Camp P, Mason D, Musk M, Burch M, Fisher A, Yusen RD, Stehlik J, Cypel M, International Society for Heart and Lung Transplantation. Donation after circulatory death in lung transplantation-five-year follow-up from ISHLT Registry. J Heart Lung Transplant. 2019 Dec;38(12):1235–45.

47. Zhou J, Chen B, Liao H, Wang Z, Lyu M, Man S, Pu Q, Liu L. The comparable efficacy of lung donation after circulatory death and brain death: a systematic review and meta-analysis. Transplantation. 2019 Dec;103(12):2624–33.

48. Palleschi A, Rosso L, Musso V, Rimessi A, Bonitta G, Nosotti M. Lung transplantation from donation after controlled cardiocirculatory death. Systematic review and meta-analysis. Transplant Rev (Orlando). 2020 Jan;34(1):100513.

49. Page A, Messer S, Large SR. Heart transplantation from donation after circulatory determined death. Ann Cardiothorac Surg. 2018 Jan;7(1):75–81.

50. Mehta V, Taylor M, Hasan J, Dimarakis I, Barnard J, Callan P, Shaw S, Venkateswaran RV. Establishing a heart transplant programme using donation after circulatory-determined death donors: a United Kingdom based single-centre experience. Interact Cardiovasc Thorac Surg. 2019 Sep 1;29(3):422–9.

51. Farr M, Truby LK, Lindower J, Jorde U, Taylor S, Chen L, Gass A, Stevens G, Reyentovich A, Mancini D, Arcasoy S, Delair S, Pinney S. Potential for donation after circulatory death heart transplantation in the United States: Retrospective analysis of a limited UNOS dataset. Am J Transplant 2019 Sep 17. https://doi.org/10.1111/ajt.15597. [Epub ahead of print].

52. van Loo ES, Krikke C, Hofker HS, Berger SP, Leuvenink HG, Pol RA. Outcome of pancreas transplantation from donation after circulatory death compared to donation after brain death. Pancreatology. 2017 Jan–Feb;17(1):13–8.

53. Kopp WH, Lam HD, Schaapherder AFM, Huurman VAL, van der Boog PJM, de Koning EJP, de Fijter JW, Baranski AG, Braat AE. Pancreas transplantation with grafts from donors deceased after circulatory death: 5 years single-center experience. Transplantation. 2018 Feb;102(2):333–9.

54. Tchana-Sato V, Ledoux D, Vandendriessche K, Van Cleemput J, Hans G, Ancion A, Cools B, Amabili P, Detry O, Massion PB, Monard J, Delbouille MH, Meyns B, Defraigne JO, Rega F. First report of a successful pediatric heart transplantation from donation after circulatory death with distant procurement using normothermic regional perfusion and cold storage. J Heart Lung Transplant. 2019 Oct;38(10):1112–5.

55. Treckmann J, Moers C, Smits JM, Gallinat A, Maathuis MH, van Kasterop-Kutz M, Jochmans I, Homan van der Heide JJ, Squifflet JP, van Heurn E, Kirste GR, Rahmel A, Leuvenink HG, Pirenne J, Ploeg RJ, Paul A. Machine perfusion versus cold storage for preservation of kidneys from expanded criteria donors after brain death. Transpl Int. 2011 Jun;24(6):548–54.

56. Jochmans I, Moers C, Smits JM, Leuvenink HG, Treckmann J, Paul A, Rahmel A, Squifflet JP, van Heurn E, Monbaliu D, Ploeg RJ, Pirenne J. Machine perfusion versus cold storage for the preservation of kidneys donated after cardiac death: a multicenter, randomized, controlled trial. Ann Surg. 2010 Nov;252(5):756–64.

Organ Preservation

6

Mahir Kirnap and Mehmet Haberal

6.1 Introduction

Organ transplantation has been one of the most significant advances in modern medicine in the second half of the twentieth century. It is regarded as the most effective treatment for end-stage organ failure. Progressin solid-organ transplantation from the level of experimental studies to becoming the criterion standard is undoubtedly due to advances in organ retrieval from deceased donors and their preservation. Organ preservation starts with making the diagnosis of brain death and continues until the time of the completion of vascular anastomoses and the return of proper organ function in the recipient. The objective of the preservation process is to preserve organ function and cellular integrity until the time of transplant [1, 2]. Because the number of patients on wait lists has increased and because of the limited organ and tissue pool, marginal grafts from deceased donors have become more frequently used. In this regard, organ and tissue preservation techniques are of even greater importance for outcomes attained with marginal grafts [3]. In this chapter, we will review and discuss injury mechanisms during the organ preservation process, the history of organ preservation techniques and solutions and currently used practices, and future perspectives.

6.2 History of Organ Preservation

First mentioned in the biography of Cesar Julien and Jean Le Gallois in 1812 and developed from the primitive concept of extracorporeal circulation, organ preservation has created a speculation that "if the heart's function can be mimicked via injection and if that injection can be regularly sustained, then life can be maintained infinitely" [4]. In 1938, Carrel and Lindbergh conducted a study that described the first isolated organ perfusion in which organs of cats, dogs, and chickens could be preserved under normothermic conditions [5]. Carrel perfused isolated cat thyroids in the Lindbergh apparatus with a thyroid solution composed of glucose, ions, and 40% to 50% homologous serum. He discovered that organs could survive for 3 to 21 days [6]. With the discovery of heparin, blood-containing substances necessary for continued survival of organs has been used as the perfusion fluid [7]. However, many studies conducted under normothermic conditions have shown that organs could only survive for an hour. This negative outcome has directed researchers from normothermic studies to hypothermic ones, making it clear that tissues may preserve their viability 10 times longer when

M. Kirnap · M. Haberal (✉)
Division of Transplantation, Department of General Surgery, Baskent University, Ankara, Turkey
e-mail: rectorate@baskent.edu.tr

© Springer Nature Switzerland AG 2021
N. Hakim et al. (eds.), *Transplantation Surgery*, Springer Specialist Surgery Series,
https://doi.org/10.1007/978-3-030-55244-2_6

their temperature is lowered to 4 °C compared with normothermic conditions [8, 9].

The discovery of hypothermic preservation methods led to a flood of organ preservation studies. Belzer et al. reported in 1967 that kidneys could be preserved for 72 h using a pulsatile perfusion device [10]. After it was understood how cell integrity and function are impaired in ischemia and that hypothermia augments ischemic injury by inducing cellular swelling, new irrigation and preservation liquids were developed. For this purpose, plasma, Perfadex, and Ringer lactate solutions were initially used. However, because kidney irrigation with these solutions did not yield superior outcomes versus embedding them in ice, researchers discovered that kidneys could be preserved for 30 h at 4 °C using solutions having intracellular properties and higher potassium and lower sodium content [11]. As greater understanding developed regarding the pathophysiology of ischemia-reperfusion injury and the differing resistances of organs to ischemia, focus on the importance of the contents of preservation solutions increased. Pharmacological agents added to preservation solutions can prolong organ preservation times. In 1988, Belzer and colleagues developed the University of Wisconsin (UW) solution [12]. Thanks to other subsequently developed solutions, the hypothermia-induced cellular dilemma was mitigated, allowing a longer preservation time for retrieved organs.

6.3 Pathophysiology of Ischemia-Reperfusion

There are three important points to remember for organ preservation: *hypothermia, cellular swelling, and reperfusion injury induced by free radicals*. With ischemia, structural alterations occur in the mitochondria, cell nucleus, endoplasmic reticulum, lysosomes, and cell membrane [1]. Although it is difficult to ascertain whether these alterations are reversible or irreversible, it is already known that injuries to mitochondria and cell membrane can cause permanent injury; that is, they can lead to irreversible impairments in

organ function. Ischemic changes begin at different times in each tissue of the human body, and each organ's ischemia endurance time is different. For example, ischemic changes start 5 min after ischemia in the heart and 30 min in the proximal tubules of the kidneys [13].

There are 2 main mechanisms of transplant tissue injury: ischemia/hypothermia and reperfusion.

6.3.1 Ischemia

Ischemia is the inability of the circulation to supply a tissue's need for oxygen and other metabolites and to remove waste products. Depending on ischemia time, reversible or irreversible changes can occur in the mitochondria, cell nucleus, endoplasmic reticulum, lysosomes, and cell membrane. During transplant, the two types of ischemia (cold and warm) follow each other [14].

Cold ischemia encompasses the cold preservation time after hypothermic perfusion has started with the cessation of the deceased donor's circulation. It ends when the organ is removed from the storage box.

Warm ischemia encompasses the time period between taking the organ out of the cold storage box and reperfusion. However, tissue injury caused by this process increases with increasing temperature. Hence, injury is reduced by taking measures such as shortening the warm ischemia time, reducing direct manual contact with the organ to limit an increase in temperature, and intermittent irrigation of the organ with isotonic saline [15].

6.3.2 Hypothermia-Induced Cellular Swelling

The main objective in organ preservation is to establish hypothermia, prevent cellular swelling, and minimize free radical-induced organ injury. Primary nonfunction of a transplanted organ is mainly due to preservation injury, where the death of the organ is inevitable [7, 16]. There are many complex physiological interactions during organ transplant. A thorough understanding of organ preservation, organ ischemia, and reperfusion pathophysiology is imperative [17].

The basic factor for slowing cellular metabolism is hypothermia. When an organ's temperature is kept at low levels, its metabolism is slowed, its need for oxygen and nutrients is reduced, the activity of hydratic enzymes is stopped, and the growth of microorganisms is arrested. With every 10 °C temperature decrease, organ metabolism reduces by 1.5 to 2.5 times, hence lowering approximately 10 times from 37 °C to 0 °C [1, 18]. In contrast to these favorable effects, hypothermia also has a detrimental effect, namely, cellular swelling. In this setting, ion pumps located at the cell membrane, particularly the sodium-potassium adenosine triphosphate (ATP) pump, are impaired. Normally, this mechanism pumps out intracellular sodium ions and pumps in extracellular potassium ions. Ischemia and hypothermia reduce the amount of ATP and hence impair the function of this pump. The most notable mechanism to preserve cellular integrity is the cell wall sodium-potassium pump, which maintains a cell's ionic composition.

When the activity of the sodium-potassium pump is impaired, sodium ions leak into the cell and potassium ions leak out. However, cells continue to function but at the expense of an anaerobic metabolic condition. This causes increased hydrogen ion and lactic acid production and hence acidosis. In addition, as a result of alterations in cell membrane permeability, calcium enters the cell and alters the intracellular acid buffering ability. Intracellular calcium triggers enzyme activation and induces cellular injury. At the same time, chlorine is transported outside the cell, intracellular oncotic pressure is increased, water is drawn into the cell, the cell swells, and cell death occurs (Fig. 6.1) [2, 19].

6.3.3 Reperfusion Injury

Another subject that is important for preservation, which has been recently intensely studied, is reperfusion injury caused by free oxygen radicals. Free oxygen radicals (FORs) and cytotoxins that are released when anastomoses are completed and organ reperfusion is established in the recipient are responsible for this type

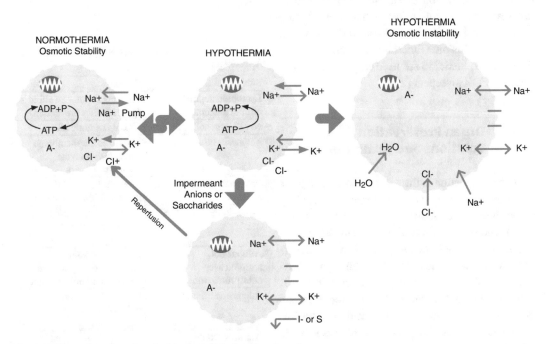

Fig. 6.1 Electrolyte alterations inside the cell during hypothermia

of injury. FORs are also responsible for augmented immunogenic properties of the graft. As ischemia time is prolonged, purine metabolites like xanthine and hypoxanthine, which are formed by ATP breakdown, are accumulated in the cell. An increase in calcium concentration causes the conversion of xanthine dehydrogenase into xanthine oxidase. A rapid and sudden oxygen supply to the tissue by reperfusion causes purine oxidation by xanthine oxidase and thus FOR formation. Lipid peroxidation, protein oxidative modification, and, by generating DNA chain breakdown, tissue injury form FORs. Cytokines are intercellular messenger molecules. Secretion of cytokines, including tumor necrosis factor-alpha, interferon-gamma, interleukin-1, and interleukin 8, is increased as a result of ischemia-reperfusion injury. Increased expression of these cytokines may cause leukocyte accumulation and formation of thrombocyte plugs, thus impairing graft function following revascularization.

With this understanding of the pathophysiology of reperfusion injury, some pharmacological agents that may prevent injury have been added to preservation solutions. Allopurinol is a xanthine oxidase inhibitor that has been shown to alleviate reperfusion injury when used before ischemia. Adenosine is used for ATP production during reperfusion. Glutathione, vitamin E, tryptophan, and histidine are used in perfusion solutions as FOR sweepers [20].

6.4   Organ Preservation Solutions and Techniques

Organ preservation is the most important step for all transplanted tissues and organs, including heart, lungs, liver, kidneys, cornea, pancreas, and small intestines. If metabolism can be slowed down during the ischemic process, which develops as a result of the cessation of an organ's vascular supply, then the resulting tissue injury will be proportionately reduced. Preservation solutions should protect organ viability and metabolism while the organ is transplanted to the recipient [1, 9]. An appropriate and effective preservation solution should consider the following:

- Reduce hypothermia-induced cellular swelling
- Prevent intracellular acidosis
- Not spread into the interstitial space during irrigation
- Protect the organ from cellular injury caused by FORs formed during reperfusion
- Provide necessary materials to reproduce ATP during reperfusion

6.4.1   Overview of Organ Preservation Solutions

Today, various solutions with different contents, but with a similar goal, are used for organ preservation. In general, preservation solutions contain electrolytes (sodium, potassium, chloride, gluconate, magnesium), acidity regulators (sulphate, bicarbonate, phosphate, lactobionate), sugars (glucose, trehalose, raffinose), colloids (HES, dextran), free oxygen radical scavengers (N-acetylcysteine, allopurinol, glutathione), and some other substances, albeit at variable proportions. The substances used in preservation solutions and their function are presented in Table 6.1 [21].

Table 6.1 Substances used in preservation solutions and their function

Substance	Function
Lactobionate, raffinose, citrate, gluconate	Prevents cellular swelling (permeability prevention)
Na, K, Mg, and Ca ions	Creates osmotic effects
Magnesium	Stabilizes the membrane and acts as enzyme cofactor
Phosphate, bicarbonate, histidine	Provides extracellular hydrogen ion balance
Colloid(albumin, HES)	Creates osmotic effect, preventing cellular swelling
Allopurinol, antiprotease, chlorpromazine	Suppresses cellular structural disruption via metabolic inhibitor effect
Adenosine, glutathione	Facilitates metabolic restoration during reperfusion
Amino steroids, glutathione, vitamin E, Desferal	Prevents free oxygen radical injury

6.4.2 Overview of Organ Preservation and Transplant

An organ must be preserved without being harmed during transport to the immunologically suitable recipient's hospital. With suitable preservation solutions and methods, a heart can currently be preserved for more than 6 h, a liver 24 h, a pancreas 48 h, and a kidney 100 h. The two basic techniques used for organ preservation are the continuous perfusion technique and the simple hypothermic preservation using preservative solutions [16, 22].

Organ preservation begins before donor surgery. Allowing a donor's hemodynamics to be maintained until organ retrieval allows healthier organs and longer graft survival to be achieved. Measures to be taken for this purpose include the following:

- Donor's blood pressure should be kept between 90 and 120 mmHg
- Donor should have a urinary output of 100 mL/h
- Hematocrit should be kept at 35%
- Arterial blood-gas Spo_2 value should exceed 95%
- Body temperature should be kept above 35 °C

All necessary information about the organ should be provided to the transplant team. In particular, information about the organ's anatomic structure and vascular anomalies should be provided. In addition, the exact time of harvest, how in situ perfusion was achieved, and the perfusion solution and its amount should be specified. *It should be remembered that transplantation is a race against time* [23].

6.5 The Simple Hypothermic Preservation Technique

6.5.1 Overview

Since the 1960s, static hypothermic preservation solutions have become the criterion standard for organ preservation. Static hypothermic preservation solutions include the irrigation of a retrieved organ with the preservation solution at 0 °C to 4 °C, with preservation in the solution at the same temperature until the time of transplant. The hypothermic medium is responsible for slowing cellular metabolism; a preservation solution reduces cellular metabolism and provides cytoprotection [1]. With the understanding of the cellular injury process during transplant, many preservation solutions have been developed to aid healing of injury. In 1969, Collins et al. developed a solution that could successfully protect kidneys for 30 h after organ retrieval until transplant, provided that the kidneys were perfused immediately after retrieval and preserved at 4 °C. Collins solution was the first preservation solution introduced to the commercial market [7]. It has been used to preserve kidney, heart, liver, and lung grafts. In 1980, the Collins solution was modified with an impermeant composition and an improved chemical stability. The renewed solution was called Euro-Collins solution, and it provided better preservation during prolonged cold ischemia [24]. In the mid-1980s. the University of Wisconsin (UW) solution was introduced. This solution is still used today for the preservation of intraabdominal organs [25].

In 1996, Haberal et al. were able to extend cold ischemia time to 111 h by using the simple hypothermic preservation technique. They reported that the organ functioned properly for 24 years [22]. The preservation solution is an intracellular-type solution characterized by a lower sodium ion concentration and a higher potassium ion concentration. Intracellular liquid-type solutions aim to prevent cellular edema by preserving intracellular ions over hypothermia-induced sodium/potassium ion pump dysfunction [26]. The simple hypothermic preservation technique is preferred by most transplant centers around the world due to its favorable properties, such as requiring no experienced team and complex devices, having low cost, allowing transport of organs to other centers, and having the advantage of not causing vascular damage seen in transplanted organs with the continuous perfusion technique [27].

During organ recovery with the simple hypothermic preservation method, organs are irrigated in situ with 2000 cm³ (4 °C) of preservation solution at a pressure of approximately 60 to 100 mmHg through a catheter placed inside the donor's aorta. The recovered organs are perfused separately with the same solution prepared in a sterile fashion at

4 °C. The solution volume varies by the type of organ recovered. Kidneys are irrigated with 200 to 400 cm^3, livers with 1000 to 1500 cm^3 (hepatic artery 150 cm^3, portal vein 1000 cm^3, common bile duct 100 cm^3), and pancreas with 200 to 500 cm^3. Recovered organs are then placed into bags containing the same solution at 4 °C. To prevent warming, crushing, and infection of the organ during transport, a second bag containing Ringer lactate and ice and a third bag as preservative are used. To maintain the temperature at 4 °C, the recovered organ is placed into a box filled with crushed ice, after which it is rapidly transported. During the period from placement of the organ into preservation solution to transplant, ice cubes inside the cold storage box are checked intermittently to ensure effective cooling is maintained [28].

6.5.2 Hypothermic Preservation Solutions Used Today

Over the past quarter century, 160 to 170 different solutions have been introduced. Among them are histidine-tryptophan-ketoglutarate (HTK), UW, Collins, Euro-Collins, UW-polyethylene glycol, polysol, Kyoto, and New Kyoto. However, HTK and UW solutions are the most widely used and studied solutions worldwide [29, 30].

6.5.2.1 Euro-Collins Solution
The aim of this solution is to reduce substance traffic between the intracellular and extracellular spaces during ischemia. For this purpose, high concentrations of potassium, magnesium, phosphate, and glucose and lower concentrations of sodium and bicarbonate are added to the solution prepared with intracellular properties. It has been shown to reduce delayed graft function when used for kidney preservation. This solution is used for both living-donor and deceased-donor transplant procedures [31, 32].

6.5.2.2 Ross-Marshall Citrate Solution
This solution has been developed as an alternative to Collins solution. Although its electrolyte content is similar to that of Collins solution, this solution uses citrate instead of phosphate and mannitol instead of glucose. Citrate forms a che-

late with magnesium and helps to stabilize the extracellular space [33].

6.5.2.3 Histidine-Tryptophan-Ketoglutarate Solution
Histidine-tryptophan-ketoglutarate solution (CUSTODİOL®, Odyssey Pharmaceutical, Hanover, Germany) was developed in the 1980s for cardioplegia. In this solution, mannitol and histidine create both an antioxidant and an osmotic effect. Ketoglutarate and tryptophan, on the other hand, have membrane-protective effects and act as a substrate of the Krebs cycle in an oxygen-deprived cell. Because potassium and sodium ion concentrations are low, it was first widely used for heart transplants. It offers a more rapid cooling effect and is characterized by a threetimes greater flow rate. Because its viscosity is lower (2.0 centipoise), it is used in high volumes and at a lower flow rate (approximately 10–12 lt and 100–175 mL/kg). Compared with UW solution, its cost is lower, and it forms no hyperpotassemia when used in flushing fashion [34]. In experimental studies, HTK was shown to be more effective than Euro-Collins and UW solutions at clearing blood cells in a microvascular bed. It was also as effective as UW solution in liver transplant [35]. In general, HTK solution lowers leukocyte adhesion rate, reduces capillary permeability, increases tissue oxygenation, reduces ATP consumption, and increases lactate dehydrogenase levels.

6.5.2.4 University of Wisconsin Solution
The UW solution (Via Span Belzer®, DuPont Pharmaceutical, Dublin, Ireland) is a solution developed by Belzer and colleagues at the University of Wisconsin. It is currently used in all organ transplant procedures. This solution was first formulated to reduce cellular swelling caused by hypothermia. Therefore, it has an intracellular character (contains low sodium and high potassium).

Glutathione and allopurinol as free-radical scavengers and xanthineoxidase as an inhibitor have been added to UW solution [36]. Both lactobionate and glutathione have been shown to be strong matrix metalloproteinase inhibitors. It also contains adenosine for ATP need, hydroxyethyl starch as an interstitial edema preventer, and phosphate as a pH stabilizer. Because it contains the same concentration of electrolytes as the intracellular space, it is cardiotoxic and its use in flushing fashion carries the risk of hyperkalemia [37]. Compared with HTK, UW has a higher viscosity; however, its endothelial protective effects are greater, and thus the incidence of ischemic biliary complications has been shown to be higher [38]. This solution also increases hepatic artery resistance and leukocyte aggregation [39].

6.5.2.5 Phosphate-Buffered Sucrose Solution

This solution contains 140 mmol/L sucrose, sodium hydrogen, and dihydrogen phosphate as a buffer. It is not widely used [40].

6.5.2.6 Celsior Solution

Celsior solution was originally introduced as a heart preservation solution in the 1990s and has been used as both a thoracic and abdominal organ preservation solution thereafter [28]. It has an extracellular character. Its content is very similar to that of UW solution. Because it does not con-

tain HES, its viscosity is lower. Similar to the HTK solution, it uses histidine buffer and a lower potassium ion concentration. However, its sodium ion concentration is much higher. It has equal properties as UW but with lower cost. Unlike UW solution, it contains glutamate as an antioxidant and an energy substrate. Other antioxidants like reduced glutathione, histidine, and mannitol have been added to the solution [41].

6.5.2.7 Kyoto Extracellular-Type Solution

Developed by Kyoto University, this solution contains higher concentrations of sodium, low concentrations of potassium, a disaccharide trehalose, and gluconate [41]. This extracellular-type solution is mostly used for experimental purposes.

Euro-Collins, HTK, and UW solutions have been in the commercial market since the 1980s; small modifications have been made to each of their compositions for marketing purposes. Table 6.2 provides a comparison of widely used preservation solutions [2].

Table 6.2 The most widely used preservation solutions and their pharmacological properties

Component	Euro-Collins	UW	HTK	Celsior
Cellular feature	Intracellular	Intracellular	Extracellular	Extracellular
pH	7.3	7.4	7.2	7.3
Sodium (mmol/L)	10	40	15	100
Potassium (mmol/L)	107	120	10	15
Magnesium (mmol/L)		5	4	13
Calcium (mmol/L)			0.015	0.25
Chloride (mmol/L)	15		50	
Sulfate (mmol/L)		5		
Lactobionate (mmol/L)		100		80
Phosphate (mmol/L)	57	25		
Raffinose (mmol/L)		30		
Adenosine (mmol/L)		5		
Glutathione (mmol/L)		3		3
Allopurinol (mmol/L)		1		
Ketoglutarate/glutamicacid (mmol/L)			1	20
Histidine (mmol/L)			198	30
Starch (g/L)		50		
Mannitol (mmol/L)			30	60
Glucose (mmol/L)	194			
Osmolarity (mOsm/L)	355	320	310	320
HES (g/L)		0.25		
Bicarbonate (mmol/L)	10	5		
Insulin		100		
Viscosity	Low	High	Low	Low

Abbreviations: HTK histidine-tryptophan-ketoglutarate, UW University of Wisconsin

6.6 The Continuous Hypothermic Perfusion Technique

The continuous perfusion technique was first used by Belzer et al. in 1967 [42]. Machine perfusion is a method that involves organ perfusion using a controlled perfusate flow. The main aims of this method is to provide oxygen and other nutrients through a perfusion device after organ retrieval, maintain the organ's temperature at between 8 °C and 12 °C, and remove metabolic products from the medium in a continuous manner. The cold ischemia time is the main bottleneck for transplanted organs, particularly those coming from marginal donors. Use of pumps to perfuse organs with an oxygenated fluid during cold ischemia time would allow cells to maintain their metabolic functions with less hypoxic injury [43, 44]. In a randomized study, kidneys from deceased donors stored with the machine perfusion method showed better graft survival than simple cooling [7].

The metabolic rate of cells is proportional to the medium's temperature. For example, at 0 °C to 4 °C, static cold preservation solutions reduce the metabolic rate by 5%. With hypothermic machine perfusion, the rate can be reduced by 10% at 0 °C to 8 °C. Normothermic machine perfusion can reduce at 35 °C to 38 °C by 70% to 80%, subnormothermic machine perfusion can reduce at 20 °C to 34 °C by 50%, and controlled oxygenated reheating can reduce at 8° to 20 °C by 20% to 25% (Fig. 6.2) [20].

6.6.1 Hypothermic Machine Perfusion

Hypothermic machine perfusion (HMP) (0–8 °C) is based on the concept of maintaining oxidative energy production at hypothermic temperatures via mitochondrial electron transport. Hypothermic machine perfusion constantly provides metabolic substrates for ATP production to replenish the graft tissue's energy. The first clinical HMP device was developed by Belzer in 1960; it was first used by Belzer et al. in 1968 to perform a preserved human kidney transplant. They performed kidney perfusion with hypothermic, diluted plasma or blood for 3 days [45, 46]. The newer HMP technology was shown to improve late graft function in marginal donors compared with simple cold preservation solu-

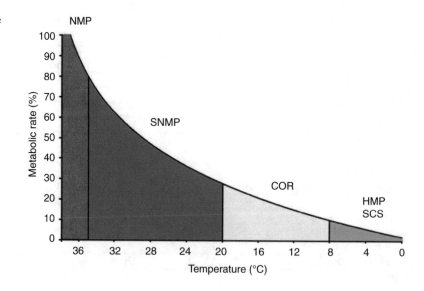

Fig. 6.2 Metabolic rate reduces with a decrease in temperature in humans. (SCS = static cold storage, HMP = hypothermic machine perfusion, COR = controlled oxygenated rewarming, SNMP = subnormothermic machine perfusion, and NMP = normothermic machine perfusion)

tions. In 2015, approximately 25% to 35% of all transplanted kidneys in the United States were preserved with HMP [47]. However, because the liver is perfused via both the portal vein and hepatic artery, use of HMP for liver transplant is challenging. Nevertheless, the first clinical study of liver grafts preserved with HMP showed shorter hospitalization times and reduced vascular and biliary complications. A few studies reported use of HMP for heart and lung transplants. Nakajima et al. reported that short-lived HMP (1–2 h) may increase energy levels in lung tissue and that it may improve ischemia-reperfusion injury by reducing the rate of reactive oxygen species production in rat lungs [48, 49]. Michel et al. showed that HMP protected the cellular structure of donor hearts better than simple cooling during prolonged ischemia times in pigs (Fig. 6.3) [50].

6.6.2 Normothermic Machine Perfusion

Normothermic machine perfusion (NMP) (35–38 °C) is a method that perfuses donor organs under physiological conditions to maintain activity and viability. Normothermic machine perfu-

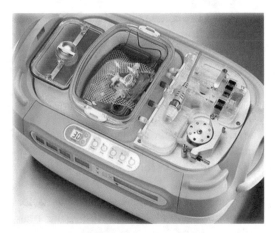

Fig. 6.3 Hypothermic machine perfusion device. The device shown here (Life Port Kidney Transporter by Organ Recovery Systems, Chicago, IL, USA) was used to preserve a kidney

sion provides oxygen and basic substrates and keeps donor organs at body temperature. In 2001, Steen et al. reintroduced the exvivo lung perfusion (EVLP) technique to assess lungs after cardiac death [51]. In 2007, the group performed the first human lung transplant using a donor lung rejected after being assessed by EVLP [52, 53]. The first clinical study on NMP in liver transplant was published in 2006; it assessed the outcomes of 16 transplant patients operated after NMP. The results suggested that 30-day graft survival was similar between the NMP and simple cooling techniques and that the median peak aspartate aminotransferase level was significantly lower in the NMP group compared with the simple cooling technique [54].

6.6.3 Subnormothermic Machine Perfusion

Subnormothermic machine perfusion (SNMP) (20–34 °C) is an intermediary approach between HMP and NMP. Although better preservation times have been provided with NMP compared with HMP, it has been considered that the cytoprotective benefits of reduced cellular metabolism under hypothermic temperatures would further improve organ preservation. In addition, adequate metabolism would be provided for viability assessment and organ repair/replenishment [55]. Although some studies have shown that livers and kidneys perfused with SNMP were superior to those preserved by the simple cooling technique, a recent study reported that swine kidneys preserved with SNMP had a higher rate of graft dysfunction than those preserved with the simple cooling technique [56, 57].

6.6.4 Controlled Oxygen Reheating

After cold ischemic protection, a sudden change of temperature from hypothermia to normothermia upon reperfusion may result in reperfusion-induced organ injury, affecting mitochondria and proapoptotic signal conduction. Hypothermic protection serves to help the ischemic organ by lowering metabolism. However, ischemic redox dyshomeostasis may disrupt mitochondrial membrane potential via mitochondrial passage opening. Mitochondrial injury may be worsened after reperfusion [58]. Controlled oxygen reheating (COR) (8–20 °C) is an alternative organ perfusion technique that involves a slow, gradual increase in perfusate temperature. Controlled oxygen reheating aims to minimize graft injury and prevent mitochondrial membrane potential disruption. Clinical studies have shown that COR could be used safely during liver transplant [59]. In 2016, COR was used effectively during 15 human liver transplant procedures [60].

6.6.5 Pulsatile Perfusion

Continuous perfusion can be accomplished by pulsatile or continuous techniques. Pulsatile flow can reduce capillary pressures, augment the expression of vasodilatory molecules, and provide a better solution flow, thereby improving organ function [44]. In addition, other agents like vasodilators and free oxygen radical scavengers can also be added to the solution. The use of a pump has dramatically improved organ use and its outcomes, particularly from marginal donors. In addition to improved graft function, it allows longer cold ischemia time. Several pumps are being developed for hepatic, cardiac, and pulmonary allografts. These pumps are portable and allow organ transport during pumping. The pump properties can also serve as a tool for diagnosis to decide whether a graft is suitable for use. Poor pump properties have been linked to a higher rate of graft dysfunction and thus higher rejection rates [1, 44]. In pulsatile perfusion, the solution used to perfuse the organ is usually given at a rate of 60 beats/min. The initial systolic pressure is 60 mmHg and diastolic pressure is 8 to 14 mmHg. Within hours after starting perfusion, the systolic pressure drops to 35 to 40 mmHg. The main superiority of pulsatile perfusion over continuous perfusion is that the former does not expose the organ's vascular structures to continuous pressure [40].

6.7 Summary of Continuous Perfusion Versus Simple Hypothermic Preservation and the Available Preservation Solutions

6.7.1 Advantages and Disadvantages of Continuous Perfusion Techniques Versus Simple Hypothermic Preservation Techniques

6.7.1.1 Advantages
The advantages of the continuous perfusion technique versus the simple hypothermic preservation technique are as follows:

- Preservation of organs with a long cold ischemia time
- Supporting organ metabolism with various factors (nutrient factors, osmotic and oncotic factors, oxygen, pH regulation, removal of metabolic wastes)
- Prevention of vasoconstriction
- Better removal of blood and its elements from the organ
- Ability to monitor the organ's physiological parameters
- Ability to determine levels of enzymes released from the organ, indicative of cellular injury
- Has been shown to have a reduced rate of primary graft organ dysfunction

6.7.1.2 Disadvantages
The advantages of the continuous perfusion technique versus the simple hypothermic preservation technique are as follows:

- Experienced personnel and perfusion devices may not be available in every center (thus, limiting transfer of organ to other centers)
- Organ injury may occur due to possible device malfunction
- May result in alterations induced by continuous pressure perfusion in the vascular system

6.7.1.3 Other Considerations

Ultrastructural examination of continuously perfused kidneys have shown that the vascular endothelium is affected [44]. Electron microscopic examination of biopsies taken 1 h after organ transplant detected endothelial cell and basal membrane injury. These injuries may be caused by high perfusion pressures and colloid concentrations found in perfusion solutions [2]. In kidneys treated with the simple hypothermic preservation technique, on the other hand, these injuries are far less common, which is the reason why the simple hypothermic preservation technique is widely utilized. Perfusion machines developed for organ preservation in clinical practice include the Belzer machine, GAmbro machine, and Waters machine. These machines are single-use devices that are similar in many aspects. Today, only the *Waters machine* is in active use [2].

Widely used perfusates, such as Steen solution and the Organ Care System perfusate, use glucose as the sole energy source. However, organs are perfused at body temperature during NMP. Glucose alone is not sufficient for organ metabolism. Adding more nutrients such as aminoacids, vitamins, lipids, and others should be considered to prolong NMP for organ repair. Aminoacids are the basic structural components of proteins and are essential for cell survival and proliferation. Vitamins may aid in utilizing chemical energy supplied for processing proteins, carbohydrates, and fats, which are necessary for cell metabolism [61].

In studies in liver and kidney transplants, aminoacids and extra glucose were added to the perfusate during NMP; this approach yielded promising results in dogs [62].

Although only a few prospective studies are available about continuous perfusion devices, several studies have indicated that it was effective for organ preservation. Nevertheless, the technique and its higher cost limit its use.

6.7.2 Which Is the Best Solution?

The answer is debatable, and there is no comprehensive study to answer this question. The UW solution and its derivatives are the most widely used solutions throughout the United States. There is some evidence that the HTK solution is less viscous than the UW solution, flows more smoothly through small vessels, and causes less vascular complications after transplant, especially in donors with prolonged cold ischemia time [1, 3, 43]. The Euro-Collins solution has been recently used mostly for kidney transplants. Haberal et al. reported that, with this solution, kidneys with a cold ischemia time of upto 111 h could be successfully transplanted [22]. In liver and pancreas transplants, the UW solution is widely used. With the use of this solution and the simple cooling technique, liver preservation can be successfully applied for 48 h under experimental conditions and for 36 h under clinical conditions, whereas pancreas preservation can extend to 48 to 72 h under experimental conditions and to 24 h in clinical practice [1, 2, 63].

6.7.3 Conclusions

Since the first speculations about organ preservation over 200 years ago, there has been enormous progress in this field. The introduction of the simple organ cooling technique in the 1960s caused a revolution. It has become a standard procedure for preserving organs in a static manner at hypothermic temperatures. With more demands to expand the organ donor pool, the current status of organ preservation has evolved from a simple cooling procedure to a continuous perfusion technique. These techniques have initiated in-depth studies about advanced graft preservation, viability assessment, and most importantly repair and regeneration. Studies on organ preservation continue intensively in many organ transplant centers worldwide, with the basic aim of prolonging preservation time without injuring the organ. Current techniques allow slowing, but not complete cessation, of organ metabolism. It is thought that complete, reversible cessation of metabolism and organ function is possible with the use of "cryopreservation." However, this technique has yet been developed for clinical practice.

References

1. Demirbaş A. Organ prezervasyonu. In: Haberal M, editor. Doku ve Organ Transplantasyonları. Ankara: Haberal Eğitim Vakfı; 1993. p. 69–75.
2. Haberal M, Emiroğlu R. Karaciğer transplantasyonu. In: Gulay H, editor. Temel ve Sistematik Cerrahi. İzmir: Güven Kitapevi; 2005. p. 711–38.
3. Brodie T. The perfusion of surviving organs. J Physiol. 1903;29:266–75.
4. Le Gallois M. Experiments on the principle of life, and particularly on the principle of the motions of the heart, and on the seat of this principle: including the report made to the first class of the Institute, upon the experiments relative to the motions of the heart. Philadelphia, PA: M. Thomas; 1813.
5. Carrel A, Lindbergh CA. The culture of whole organs. Science. 1935;81:621–3.
6. Carrel A. The culture of whole organs: I. technique of the culture of the thyroid gland. J Exp Med. 1937;65:515–26.
7. Collins GM, Bravo-Shugarman M, Terasaki PI. Kidney preservation for transportation. Initial perfusion and 30 hours' icestorage. Lancet. 1969;2:1219–22.
8. Ueda Y, Todo S, Imventarza O, Furukawa H, Oks A, Wu YM, et al. The UW solution for canine kidney preservation. Its specific effect on renal hemodynamics and microvasculature. Transplantation. 1989;48:913–8.
9. Taylor MJ, Baicu SC. Current state of hypothermic machine perfusion preservation of organs: the clinical perspective. Cryobiology. 2010;60(Suppl 1):20–35.
10. Belzer FO, Southard JH. Principles of solid-organ preservation by cold storage. Transplantation. 1988;45(4):673–6.
11. Calne RY, Pegg DE, Pryse-Davies J, Brown FL. Renal preservation by ice-cooling: an experimental study relating to kidney transplantation from cadavers. Br Med J. 1963;2:651–5.
12. Vreugdenhil PK, Belzer FO, Southard JH. Effect of cold storage on tissue and cellular glutathione. Cryobiology. 1991;28:143–9.
13. Mühlbacher F, Langer F, Mittermayer C. Preservation solutions for transplantation. Transplant Proc. 1999;31(5):2069–70.
14. Collins GM, Hartley LC, Clunie GJ. Kidney preservation for transportation. Experimental analysis of optimal perfusate composition. Br J Surg. 1972;59:187–9.
15. Starzl TE, Hakala TR, Shaw BW Jr, Hardesty RL, Rosenthal TJ, Griffith BP, et al. Flexible procedure for multiple cadaveric organ procurement. Surg Gynecol Obstet. 1984;158:223–30.
16. Arnault I, Bao YM, Dimicoli JL, et al. Combinedeffect of fasting and alanine on liver function recovery after cold ischemia. Transplant Int. 2002;15:89–95.
17. Pienaar BH, Lindell SL, Van Gulik T, Southard JH, Belzer FO. Seventy-two hour preservation of the canine liver by machine perfusion. Transplantation. 1990;49(2):258–60.
18. Guibert EE, Petrenko AY, Balaban CL, Somov AY, Rodriguez JV, Fuller BJ. Organ preservation: current concepts and new strategies for the next decade. Transfus Med Hemother. 2011;38(2):125–42.
19. Moray G, Sevmis S, Karakayali FY, Gorur SK, Haberal M. Comparison of histidine-tryptophan-ketoglutarate and University of Wisconsin in living-donor liver transplantation. Transplant Proc. 2006;38:3572–5.
20. Jing L, Yao L, Zhao M, Peng LP, Liu M. Organ preservation: from the past to the future. Acta Pharmacol Sin. 2018;39(5):845–57.
21. O'Callaghan JM, Morgan RD, Knight SR, Morris PJ. The effect of preservation solutions for storage of liver allografts on transplant outcomes. Ann Surg. 2014;260:46–55.
22. Haberal M, Moray G, Bilgin N, Karakayali H, Arslan G, Büyükpamukçu N. Ten-year survival after a cold-ischemia time of 111 hours in the transplanted kidney. Transplant Proc. 1996;28(4):2333.
23. ANZOD Registry. Australia and New Zealand Organ Donation Registry Report 2015. http://www.anzdata.org.au/anzod/v1/ar-2015.html. Accessed 4 Jun 2016.
24. Aydin G, Okiye SE, Zincke H. Successful 24-hour preservation of the ischemic canine kidney with Euro-Collins solution. J Urol. 1982;128:1401–3.
25. Jamieson RW, Friend PJ. Organ reperfusion and preservation. Front Biosci. 2008;13:221–35.
26. Okada Y, Kondo T. Preservation solution for lung transplantation. Gen Thorac Cardiovasc Surg. 2009;57:635–9.
27. Voigt MR, DeLario GT. Perspectives on abdominal organ preservation solutions: a comparative literature review. Prog Transplant. 2013;23:383–91.
28. Karam G, Compagnon P, Hourmant M, Despins P, Duveau D, Noury D, et al. A single solution for multiple organ procurement and preservation. Transpl Int. 2005;18:657–63.
29. Stewart ZA, Cameron AM, Singer AL, Montgomery RA, Segev DL. Histidine-tryptophan-ketoglutarate (HTK) is associated with reduced graft survival in deceased donor livers, especially those donated after cardiac death. Am J Transplant. 2009;9(2):286–93.
30. El-Wahsh M. Liver graft preservation: an overview. Hepatobiliary Pancreat Dis Int. 2007;6(1):12–6.
31. Groenewoud AF, Thorogood J. Current status of the Eurotransplant randomized multicenter study comparing kidney graft preservation with histidine tryptophan-ketogluterate, University of Wisconsin, and Euro-Collins solutions. The HTK Study Group. Transplant Proc. 1993;25:1582–5.
32. Latchana N, Peck JR, Whitson BA, Henry ML, Elkhammas EA, Black SM. Preservation solutions used during abdominal transplantation: current status and outcomes. World J Transplant. 2015;5(4):154–64.

33. Catena F, Coccolini F, Montori G, Vallicelli C, Amaduzzi A, Ercolani G, et al. Kidney preservation: review of present and future perspective. Transplant Proc. 2013;45:3170–7.

34. Feng L, Zhao N, Yao X, et al. Histidine-tryptophan-ketoglutarate solution vs. University of Wisconsin solution for liver transplantation: a systematic review. Liver Transpl. 2007;13(8):1125–36.

35. Ringe B, Braun F, Moritz M, et al. Safety and efficacy of living donor liver preservation with HTK solution. Transplant Proc. 2005;37(1):316–9.

36. Rentsch M, Post S, Palma P, Lang G, Menger MD, Messmer K. Anti-ICAM–1 blockade reduces postsinusoidal WBC adherence following cold ischemia and reperfusion, but does not improve early graft function in rat liver transplantation. J Hepatol. 2000;32:821–8.

37. Lynch RJ, Kubus J, Chenault RH, Pelletier SJ, Campbell DA, Englesbe MJ. Comparison of histidine-tryptophan-ketoglutarate and University of Wisconsin preservation in renal transplantation. Am J Transplant. 2008;8(3):567–73.

38. Mangus RS, Fridell JA, Vianna RM, Milgrom MA, Chestovich P, Chihara RK, Tector AJ. Comparison of histidine-tryptophan-ketoglutarate solution and University of Wisconsin solution in extended criteria liver donors. Liver Transpl. 2008;14(3):365–73.

39. Rayya F, Harms J, Martin AP, Bartels M, Hauss J, Fangmann J. Comparison of histidine-tryptophan-ketoglutarate solution and University of Wisconsin solution in adult liver transplantation. Transplant Proc. 2008;40(4):891–4.

40. Terasaki PI, McClelland JD, Yuge J, Cecka JM, Gjertson DW, Takemoto S, Cho YW.Advances in kidney transplantation: 1985–1995. Clin Transpl. 1995:487–501.

41. Montiel-Casado MC, Pérez-Daga JA, Blanco-Elena JA, Aranda-Narváez JM, Sánchez-Pérez B, Cabello-Díaz M, Ruiz-Esteban P, León-Díaz FJ, Gutiérrez-de la Fuente C, Santoyo-Santoyo J. Pancreas preservation with viaspan, celsior, and custodiol solutions: an initial experience. Transplant Proc. 2016;48(9):3040–2.

42. Belzer FO, May R, Berry M, Lee JC. Short term preservation of porcine livers. J Surg Res. 1970;10:55–61.

43. Fontes P, Lopez R, van der Plaats A, Vodovotz Y, Minervini M, Scott V, et al. Liver preservation with machine perfusion and a newly developed cell-free oxygen carrier solution under subnormothermic conditions. Am J Transplant. 2015;15:381–94.

44. Guarrera JV, Henry SD, Samstein B, Odeh-Ramadan R, Kinkhabwala M, Goldstein MJ, et al. Hypothermic machine preservation in human liver transplantation: the first clinical series. Am J Transplant. 2010;10:372–81.

45. Humphries AL, Russell R, Stoddard LD, Moretz WH. Successful five-day kidney preservation. Perfusion with hypothermic, diluted plasma. Investig Urol. 1968;5:609–18.

46. Belzer FO, Ashby BS, Dunphy JE. 24-hour and 72-hour preservation of canine kidneys. Lancet. 1967;2:536–8.

47. Henry SD, Guarrera JV. Protective effects of hypothermic ex vivo perfusion on ischemia/reperfusion injury and transplant outcomes. Transplant Rev. 2012;26:163–75.

48. Nakajima D, Chen F, Yamada T, Sakamoto J, Osumi A, Fujinaga T, et al. Hypothermic machine perfusion ameliorates ischemia-reperfusion injury in rat lungs from non-heart-beating donors. Transplantation. 2011;92:858–63.

49. Nakajima D, Chen F, Okita K, Motoyama H, Hijiya K, Ohsumi A, et al. Reconditioning lungs donated after cardiac death using short-term hypothermic machine perfusion. Transp J. 2012;94:999–1004.

50. Michel SG, LaMuraglia GM II, Madariaga MLL, Titus JS, Selig MK, Farkash EA, et al. Twelve-hour hypothermic machine perfusion for donor heart preservation leads to improved ultrastructural characteristics compared to conventional cold storage. Ann Transplant. 2015;20:461–8.

51. Steen S, Liao Q, Wierup PN, Bolys R, Pierre L, Sjöberg T. Transplantation of lungs from non-heart-beating donors after functional assessment ex vivo. Ann Thorac Surg 2003;76:244–52; discussion 252.

52. Erasmus ME, Fernhout MH, Elstrodt JM, Rakhorst G. Normothermic ex vivo lung perfusion of non-heart-beating donor lungs in pigs: from pretransplant function analysis towards a 6-h machine preservation. Transpl Int. 2006;19:589–93.

53. Cypel M, Yeung JC, Hirayama S, Rubacha M, Fischer S, Anraku M, et al. Technique for prolonged normothermic ex vivo lung perfusion. J Hear Lung Transpl. 2008;27:1319–25.

54. Ravikumar R, Jassem W, Mergental H, Heaton N, Mirza D, Perera MTPR, et al. Liver transplantation after ex vivo normothermic machine preservation: a phase 1 (first-in-man) clinical trial. Am J Transplant. 2016;16:1779–87.

55. Bejaoui M, Pantazi E, Folch-Puy E, Baptista PM, García-Gil A, Adam R, et al. Emerging concepts in liver graft preservation. World J Gastroenterol. 2015;21:396–407.

56. Hoyer DP, Gallinat A, Swoboda S, Wohlschläger J, Rauen U, Paul A, et al. Subnormothermic machine perfusion for preservation of porcine kidneys in a donation after circulatory death model. Transpl Int. 2014;27:1097–106.

57. Adams TD, Patel M, Hosgood SA, Nicholson ML. Lowering perfusate temperature from 37 °C to 32 °C diminishes function in a porcine model of ex vivo kidney perfusion. Transplant Direct. 2017;3:e140.

58. Schopp I, Reissberg E, Lüer B, Efferz P, Minor T. Controlled rewarming after hypothermia: adding a new principle to renal preservation. Clin Transl Sci. 2015;8:475–8.

59. Hoyer DP, Mathé Z, Gallinat A, Canbay AC, Treckmann JW, Rauen U, et al. Controlled oxygenated rewarming of cold stored livers prior to transplantation. Transplantation. 2016;100:147–52.
60. Hoyer DP, Paul A, Minor T. Prediction of hepatocellular preservation injury immediately before human liver transplantation by controlled oxygenated rewarming. Transplant Direct. 2017;3:e122.
61. Bender DA. Nutritional biochemistry of the vitamins. Cambridge: Cambridge University Press; 2003.
62. Kaths JM, Echeverri J, Goldaracena N, Louis KS, Chun YM, Linares I, et al. Eight-hour continuous normothermic ex vivo kidney perfusion is a safe preservation technique for kidney transplantation: a new opportunity for the storage, assessment, and repair of kidney grafts. Transplantation. 2016;100:1862–70.
63. Jing L, Yao L, Zhao M, Peng L-p, Liu M. Organ preservation: from the past to the future. Acta Pharmacol Sin. 2018;39:845–57.

Cardiac Replacement, Assistance, Repair or Regeneration for Heart Failure

7

Daniel G. Tang, Jenna E. Aziz, Katherine Klein, and Salim Aziz

7.1 Introduction

The number of patients with end-stage heart failure is increasing and they are more complex. As management of acute coronary syndromes has improved acute mortalities have decreased but this has increased the percentage of patients developing chronic heart failure. In the USA, approximate six million patients have CHF and of these 5–10% [1] have advanced heart failure or stage D disease.

The 1-year mortality for these patients is worse than most forms of cancer with over 50% dying within a year [2]. The management of end stage severe chronic heart failure remains a challenge.

We have come a long way since the first successful human heart transplant by Christian

Barnard in 1967 [3]. Heart transplantation is now an established form of therapy for end stage heart failure. Over 140,000 heart transplants have been performed worldwide with current 1 year survival approaching 90%, and 50% of patients surviving 15 years [4] (Fig. 7.1). In those early days, limited immunosuppressive regimens together with inability to treat opportunistic infections and rejection were associated with poor short and long- term survivals. The introduction of cyclosporine by Calne et al. [5] allowed for an exponential increase in organ transplantation, globally.

A major stumbling block to more widespread use of cardiac transplantation is the lack of suitable donors, approximately 2000 heart transplants are performed per year in the US. Despite the growing number of patients being listed for transplantation, the number of transplants performed worldwide has remained stagnant with <5000 being done annually [4]. In the last few years, this has increased approximately 20% primarily because of increase in North American transplants (now ~3000/year) and it is speculated that the opioid epidemic has played a role. A change in allocation systems has also recently been introduced so as to ensure best use of donor organs for the sickest patients.

Lack of suitable and adequate donors has led to the increasing use of mechanical devices ranging from ventricular assist devices (VADs) that support either ventricle to use of the total artificial

D. G. Tang
Inova Heart and Vascular Institute,
Falls Church, VA, USA
e-mail: Daniel.Tang@inova.org

J. E. Aziz
Howard University Hospital, Washington, DC, USA
e-mail: jenna.aziz@bison.howard.edu

K. Klein
Division of Cardiac Surgery at Virginia
Commonwealth University, Richmond, VA, USA
e-mail: Katherine.Klein@vcuhealth.org

S. Aziz (✉)
George Washington University,
Washington, DC, USA
e-mail: salimaziz@gwu.edu

© Springer Nature Switzerland AG 2021
N. Hakim et al. (eds.), *Transplantation Surgery*, Springer Specialist Surgery Series,
https://doi.org/10.1007/978-3-030-55244-2_7

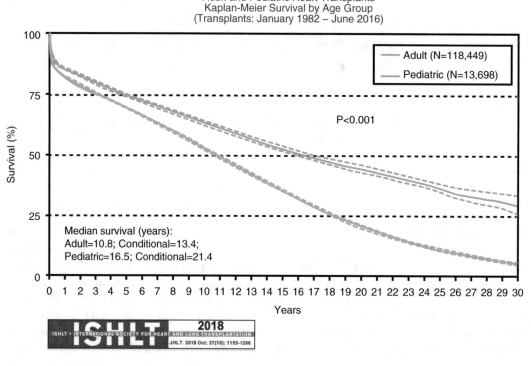

Fig. 7.1 ISHLT survival

heart [6]. These have been used both as a bridge to transplantation (BTT) as well as destination (BTD) therapy. However, VADs are associated with a number of ongoing problems including thromboembolic events, strokes, gastrointestinal bleeding, driveline infections etc., [7].

Advances in the detection of early rejection, improved organ preservation procedures, and the introduction of new immunosuppressive therapy protocols have improved survival results in heart transplantation [4]. Late graft atherosclerosis remains a serious threat despite retransplantation and, in some cases, mechanical cardiac support [8, 9].

7.2   Indications for Heart Transplantation

Figure 7.2 outlines the types of patients receiving heart transplantation (ISHLT 2018). In Western countries, the main indications for cardiac transplantation remain ischemic heart disease and idiopathic cardiomyopathies. In the current era, heart transplant recipients are more complex, are older,

may be on mechanical circulatory systems (MCS), have pre-formed antibodies and tend to have other system involvement. In rare conditions such as post-partum cardiomyopathy the failing heart can recover if allowed a period of "rest" using MCS or appropriate medical therapy [10].

7.2.1   Recipient Selection for Heart Transplantation

A thorough work up must be done before listing a patient for heart transplantation including a full psychosocial assessment. Table 7.1 outlines standard and extended recipient selection crtieria and work-up need before a patient can be listed for heart transplantation. Generally speaking, most centers limit the upper age limit to 65 years. Although reports do suggest that suitable outcomes can also be achieved in patients older than 70 years of age [11]. As always, a multidisciplinary team approach must be used in establishing each center's willingness to expand from standard criteria. Also, the presence of other co-morbid conditions in the recipient can pre-

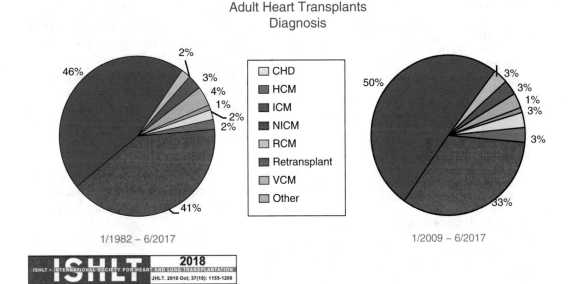

Fig. 7.2 ISHLT 2018 types of patients getting Heart Transplants

Table 7.1 Work of patient before being listed for heart transplantation

Recipient evaluation for cardiac transplantation:
Right and left heart catheterization
Cardiopulmonary testing.
Labs: CNBC, CMP, coagulation studies, thyroid function tests,
HIV, hepatitis screen, PPD, CMV IgG, RPR, VDRLK, PRA
Blood group, lipids
CXR, PFTs including DLCO, EKG
Substance abuse history, screening, abstinence for at least 6 months
Mental health evaluation, social support
Financial support
Weight not more than 140% of ideal body weight
Extended recipient criteria:
Re-transplantation for acute graft failure.
Re-do heart-lung transplantation
Age > 70 year.
Combined organ transplantation: (heart-liver, heart-kidney)

clude selection of the recipient for transplantation. Some disease can recur in the donor heart e.g. sarcoidosis, amyloidosis etc. leading to different centers have varying selection criteria. Standard and extended donor selection criteria are outlined in Table 7.2. The subject of using marginal donors for marginal recipients has been considered and used by some centers [12]. Finally, the donor must be "matched" to the recipient Table 7.3.

7.3 Pre-sensitized Recipients

Presensitized patients are at risk for antibody mediated rejection [13]. It is important to detect the identity and intensity of anti-HLA antibodies that are present. This helps in finding a safe donor organ for the recipient and also in evaluating which sensitized patients require treatment prior to transplantation. A threshold of the calculated PRA (cPRA), which is the frequency of unacceptable HLA in the donor, is used to decide on treatment of the sensitized patient [14].

A number of approaches are used either in isolation or in combination in the management of the sensitized patients. These involve protocols that target antibodies by inactivation (intravenous immune globulin), removal (plasmapheresis), and decreased production (rituximab and bortezomib) [13, 15, 16].

With increasing use of assist devices, patients who have received blood and blood products is likely to increase. In patients with a history of elevated PRAs and/or pre-sensitization flow cross-matching should be used prior to performing the implant. Post-operative flow cross matching may be useful in monitoring an increase in donor reactive antibodies so that measures can be taken to decrease the development of full blown humoral medicated rejection by adjusting immunosuppression [17].

Table 7.2 Donor selection criteria

Standard cardiac donor criteria and evaluation:
Age < 50–60
Absence of the following:
Prolonged cardiac arrest
Prolonged severe hypotension
Pre-existing cardiac disease
Intra-cardiac drug injection
Severe chest trauma with evidence of cardiac injury
Septicemia
Extra-cerebral malignancy and glioblastoma
Positive serologies for human immunodeficiency virus, hepatitis B (active), or hepatitis C.
Hemodynamic stability without high-dose inotopic support (<20 ug/kg/min dopamine)
Evaluation/tests:
Past medical history and physical examination
EKG
Arterial blood gases
Laboratory tests: (blood group, HIV, HBV, HCV)
ECHO
Pulmonary artery catheter.
If indicated a cardiac catheterization (? Role for cardiac CT angiogram)
Extended donor criteria
Age > 60
Long ischemic times likely
Size mismatch
LVH
Positive serology (Hep B inactive)
Presence of CAD
Valve abnormality present
Cardiac death donor (DCD)

Table 7.3 Factors involved in matching donor to recipient

Matching donor and recipient:
Severity of illness
ABO blood group (match or compatible)
Donor weight to recipient ratio (must be 75–125%)
PRA issues: Is prospective flow cross-matching required?
Location of donor/ischemic time issues (may be less so with use of OCS)
In recipients with elevated pulmonary pressure more attention may need to be paid to D/R size, ischemic times etc.

7.4 Cardiac Re-transplantation

Another topic that has differing opinions is how to handle recipients with a failed heart transplant (a) acute primary graft failure, hyperacute rejection, acute rejection and (b) chronic rejection,

AGA. In the climate of limited donors, many centers do not offer re-transplantation. Analysis of UNOS data clearly shows that re-transplantation for early acute allograft failure has decreased survival and should generally not be done [18]. For these patients, the TAH and or other MCS should be considered. However, survival results for second or third-time re-transplantation for AGA are not inferior to first time transplantation.

7.5 Limitations for Widespread Use of Heart Transplantation

The major limitation has been the shortage of suitable donors for the increasing number of recipients. A chronic shortage of donor organs has led to innovative approaches to enhance donor supply have included, use of marginal donors, use of cardiac death donors and use of extracorporeal systems to resuscitate/evaluate cardiac allografts [19, 20]. Efforts to redress this imbalance have included the use of marginal donors. This has increased the number of donors especially if these are used for marginal recipients e.g. older patients. Another recent innovation is to use cardiac death (DCD) donors [20].

7.5.1 Donor Selection Criteria

Suitable criteria and extended for donor evaluation are outlined in Table 7.2 and are from usually harvested from brain dead donors. However, with increasing waiting lists experienced centers have liberalized their donor selection criteria. Organ Care System (OCS) can be used in situations where there is an adverse donor-recipient profile. Some of these like the TransMedics system allow allograft perfusion after explant and until implantation (Fig. 7.3). They can be particularly useful in evaluating marginal donors or extended criteria donors e.g. reduced EF, presence of LVH, cardiac arrest, long ischemic times, on high dose inotropes, donors where status of coronary arteries is unknown etc. In addition, in cases where recipient implantation is likely to be problematic e.g. hostile mediastinum, presence

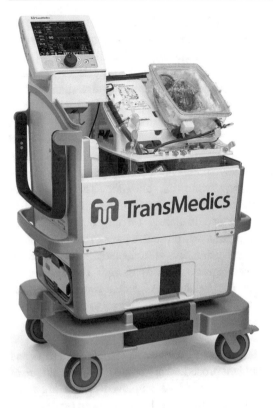

Fig. 7.3 Tansmedics Organ Care System (OCS™) image courtesy of TansMedics, Inc

of LVAD etc. the OCS allows the recipient team to work carefully without increasing the "ischemic times" [21].

Efforts are made to "match" donors to recipients. Although height and weight have been used extensively, a better option is to "match the donor recipient cardiac mass [22]. Most centers limit cold ischemic times to less than 4 hours as this has been shown to have a bearing on outcomes [23].

The concept of using organs from donors death after cardiac (DCD) is not new. Using these donors as a source of cardiac allografts is receiving increasing attention [20]. Investigators in Cambridge, UK and Australia have shown that, properly managed, procured and preserved, these donors can increase donor supply. Recipients so implanted have comparable outcomes to those implanted with brain death donors [20, 24].

7.6 The Donor Explant Procedure

The techniques for allograft procurement are straight forward and not complex. Although this is often delegated to trainees or junior surgeons, procurement is nonetheless key to a functioning and successful transplant. The increased availability of diagnostic angiography and echocardiography helps with allograft prescreening and avoiding unnecessary travel. However, all tests are subject to interpretation and the procuring surgeon should personally review the available diagnostic imaging. On arrival, appropriate verification of the declaration of brain death, consent for organ donation, and final review of the donor's evaluation including serology and blood type match with the recipient is performed. With emphasis on maximizing available donor organs, coordination with other potential procuring surgeons (such as the lung and abdominal team) is necessary. Development of vascularized composite allotransplantation (such as the face and hand) has seen remarkable success and these donors require significant coordination for the extra dissection time required.

A median sternotomy connected to an extended laparotomy is made. Inspection of the donor heart is important before making the final decision to proceed with transplant. The coronary arteries and atria are inspected and palpated for unexpected stenosis or thrills. The left and right ventricular function is assessed. As noted above, angiography and echocardiography are widespread and unexpected findings are less common. Assessment of the right ventricular function prior to final acceptance is perhaps the most important part of procurement. Dynamically sensitive to preload and afterload, RV function can readily deteriorate in the interim between initial testing and the time of procurement. Large volume resuscitation, evolution of cardiac contusion, pulmonary embolism, arrhythmia, or other hemodynamic deterioration can present the procuring surgeon with an unexpected distended struggling right heart. Intraoperative maneuvers (such as diuresis, inotropes, etc.) are reasonable but if there is not demonstrable improvement, the risk/benefit ratio to the recipient and allograft declination should be considered. Once accepted, limited dissection is necessary prior to procurement. Mobilization of the great vessels is helpful. The pulmonary artery, left atrium, and IVC are shared between their respective organs and good communication is important such that each team has adequate lengths for implantation. Separation of the aorta from the pulmonary artery facilitates subsequent aortic cross clamp and separate cardio/pulmonoplegia. Mobilization of the IVC from the diaphragm and opening oblique sinus facilitates division of the IVC. Ligation of the azygous vein allows for maximal harvest of the SVC (particularly for congenital heart transplants. Mobilization of the interatrial (Waterston's) groove can facilitate safe separation of the right sided pulmonary veins from the right atrium / cava. Once all the procuring teams are ready, heparin 30,000 U IV is given. A cardioplegia catheter is placed in the ascending aorta. If lungs are being procured the mid pulmonary artery is cannulated. Also, during the time of donor procurement, care must be taken to prevent pulmonoplegia solution from entering the coronary arteries and damaging the myocardium.

The SVC is ligated and the right atrium/IVC junction is incised. A pool tip suction catheter is passed down the IVC to exsanguinate all returning warm blood. The heart is allowed to empty for 1–2 beats. The aorta is cross clamped and cardioplegia is given. There is wide heterogeneity in solutions used for cardioplegia although University of Wisconsin and HTK are common. Distention of the aortic root for adequate delivery of cardioplegia and flaccid decompression of the left ventricle are verified by amputating the tip of the left atrial appendage or incising the left atrium above the pulmonary veins to vent the left ventricle. If the lungs are not being procured, the left inferior pulmonary vein can be divided. The field is then flooded with iced saline. Once completed, the heart is excised confirming the various cuffs with the lung and abdominal team. The IVC division is completed. The left atrium is transected just anterior to the pulmonary veins. Use of a bicaval anastomosis for implantation requires suitable length of SVC and IVC be taken. If lungs are not procured the pulmonary veins can be divided and the left atrium opened later.

The main pulmonary artery is divided half way between the pulmonary valve sinus and the PA bifurcation. The aorta is divided at the takeoff of the innominate artery. The previously ligated azygous is divided and the SVC is divided just below the innominate vein. Care must be taken that any central lines present in the SVC do not embolize into the allograft. They are either retracted or divided and removed. The allograft is rinsed and inspected for any potential missed abnormality. If present, a patent foramen ovale is closed primarily. If amputated, the left atrial appendage is similarly closed. The allograft is then packaged in the ice cold cardioplegia solution and transported back to the recipient hospital.

Recipient Procedure Both the explant and implant procedure are related to the technique of implantation to be employed. There are three techniques that have been described (a) The standard bi-atrial Shumway and Lower technique (b) bicaval (with left atrial), and (c) bicaval with separate pulmonary venous anastomosis [25–27].

Irrespective of the technique being used, assiduous attention must be paid to myocardial protection during the implantation period [28]. In the early days at Stanford, a "cold line" was used to infuse cold saline into the recipient heart via the left atrial appendage during the implantation period.

The standard bi-atrial technique was developed by Lower and Shumway [25] in the 1960s. Efficient and reproducible, the technique was associated with distortion of the atrial geometry which lead to subsequent tricuspid regurgitation and dysrhythmias. In the early 1990s, several centers developed a technique with complete excision of the left and right atria with separate pulmonary venous and caval anastomoses. The benefits of a more anatomic implant over the increased complexity of four additional anastomoses were indeterminate. Bi-caval and left atrial implantation was developed as a hybrid of the two techniques and is the most commonly utilized technique today. The bi-caval technique [26] has been shown to decrease the incidence of atrial arrhythmias, need for permanent pacemaker implantation and significant tricuspid regurgitation because of the preservation of sinus function and atrial geometry. The group at Cedar Sinai have reported excellent results using total excision of recipient's atria with bi-caval and pulmonary venous anastomoses [27]. UNOS registry analysis of bi-caval versus bi-atrial implants demonstrated a lower incidence of dysrhythmias requiring pacemaker implant and a small survival benefit [29]. Here we describe the bi-caval and left atrial anastomosis technique.

(a) **Recipient Explant**. Close coordination must take place between the donor harvesting team and the recipient site so that ischemic times are minimized for the allograft. In patients with no prior sternal entry a standard median sternotomy approach is used. Once the sternum is opened the ascending aorta and SVC are exposed for cannulation. Bi-caval (SVC and IVC) cannulae are used. The ascending aorta is clamped, and the ascending aorta and main pulmonary arteries transected above their valves by using the transverse sinus as a plane. We tend to mark the 3 and 9 'o'clock positions on the PA so as to allow best orientation during implantation of this floppy structure.

Heart failure patients are often at risk for thromboembolism and early (cross clamp) aortic control is recommended. Once the aorta is clamped, the proximal aorta should be incised (or transected) to vent the left side. The left atrial excision plane is just posterior to the coronary sinus. The right atrium is divided at the SA node and the coronary sinus. This maintains the entire length of the SVC and IVC to be later trimmed and tailored to the allograft. A common modification to the bi-caval technique is to leave the posterior wall of the right atrium connecting the SVC and IVC. This prevents retractions of the vessels and facilitates large spatulated anastomoses to prevent stenosis but still maintain atrial geometry.

(b) **The implant procedure** (Fig. 7.4): Explant of the native heart is done in coordination with the arrival of the donor allograft to minimize ischemia. On arrival, the allograft is unpackaged and re-inspected. There is wide variation on whether to give another dose of cardioplegia to the allograft and whether to repeat if at all. If not previously done, closure of patent foramen ovale and repair of an amputated left atrial appendage are performed. Size matching of the donor cuffs to the recipient is assessed. Implanting surgeons must be prepared to use innovative techniques should improper length/cuff of tissue be left for implantation. The donor and recipient left atria are first anastomosed using long 3/0 Prolene. Care must be taken to have endocardium opposed to endocardium. Next, we sew in the IVC and SVC, followed by the PA and the aorta. Care must be taken to trim the PA. Due to the posterior course of the pulmonary artery, an overly long length to the PA can be associated with kinking and inadvertent RV outflow obstruction. The usual de-airing maneuvers are made before unclamping the aorta. Prior to weaning off CPB careful inspection is made of all anastomoses. In special circumstances of unanticipated long ischemic times, the aortic anastomosis can be completed immediately following the left atrial anastomosis. The allograft is then reperfused while the remaining anastomoses are completed.

Weaning off CPB Is done with particular attention to de-airing and evaluation of the right heart function. In some cases, a gradual wean may be needed. Intra-op TEE is useful for evaluating de-airing and overall cardiac function. In patients with prior elevated pulmonary pressures nitric oxide or pulmonary vasodilators may be needed. Any evidence of right and or left heart dysfunction that does not respond to the usual measures and inotropes etc., should be supported by an IABA, ECMO or temporary VAD. In most centers, the incidence of PGF is fortunately less than

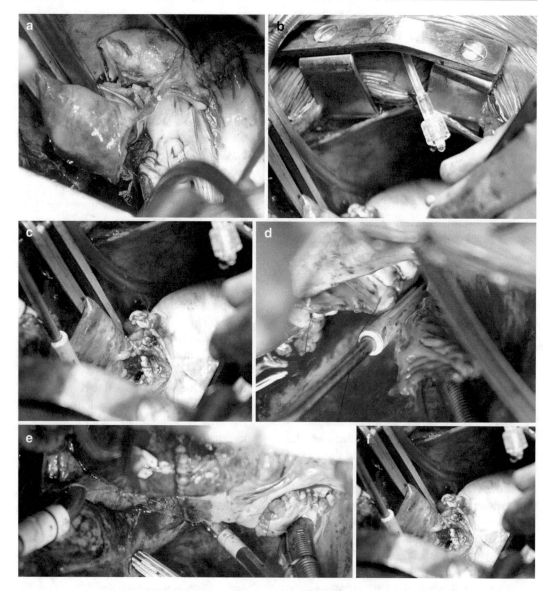

Fig. 7.4 Recipient implant technique. (**a**) Left atrial anastromosis. (**b**) Use of topical cooling during implantation. (**c**) Pulmonary artery anastomosis. (**d**) and (**e**) Bicaval (IVC and SVC anastomosis), (**f**) Aortic anastomosis

5% [30]. A period of MCS can help the dysfunctional transplant heart recover.

Special Circumstances: Heart Transplantation in Patients Already on MCS The use of mechanical circulatory support as a bridge to transplantation continues to grow [4]. In 2018, 55% of adult heart transplants were performed in patients supported with a VAD, TAH, or ECMO. Ideally, efforts to make re-entry "safer"

at the time of transplantation should be considered at the time of device implantation. Liberal coverage of the heart and device with thin sheets of PTFE minimizes adhesions and significantly reduces the bleeding associated with mobilization for explant of the device and native heart. A substernal strip of silastic can be an effective buffer to the oscillating saw. With appropriate planning, sternal re-entry, explant and transplant with minimal to no blood transfusion is possible.

Planning for sternal re-entry at the time of listing is important. CT scan imaging to assess the proximity/fixation of structures (e.g. coronary bypass grafts, right ventricle, LVAD outflow graft lie and attachment) underneath the sternum and assessment of the peripheral arterial access is important. Pre-operatively the anticoagulation on Coumadin needs correction with fresh frozen plasma or PCC to decrease bleeding related issues. Some centers use PCC after completion of the implant and when off CPB.

Unique Considerations in LVAD Patients The vast majority of MCS patients are supported with a continuous flow LVAD. The introduction of intra-pericardial placed centrifugal flow devices has made the explant procedure easier, but there are still many patients supported with devices placed in the pre-peritoneal space. While much easier to explant than the large first generation pneumatic pre-peritoneal devices, careful mobilization is still important to avoid intra-abdominal injury. As current continuous flow devices do not have valves, regurgitant flow will occur if turned off. Once on bypass, LVAD flow is continued to prevent retrograde flow but turned down to prevent blood trauma.

There seem to be two schools of thought on how best to approach LVAD patients. In patients at high risk for re-entry, peripheral cannulation (via the axillary and/or femoral vessels) facilitates safe and expeditious re-entry. When cannulated peripherally, the femoral venous cannula is placed at the IVC/RA junction and the SVC is then directly cannulated once exposed.

1. Some centers expose the right axillary/subclavian artery and sew an 8 mm graft in an end to side fashion to use at the arterial site for CPB [31] and use either open or percutaneous placed long femoral venous cannula (Size 25 F) that is parked at the IVC RA junction and go on partial CPB prior to opening the chest using an oscillating saw. During this time, the LVAD flows are reduced but not stopped. In most cases a prior sheet of PTFE is usually placed to cover the heart/LVAD and the outflow limb of the LVAD is usually curved laterally away from the midline to avoid injury during re-entry.

2. Another approach in patients with an LVAD is to use the re-do median sternotomy approach using an oscillating saw. Some surgeons place femoral artery and vein cannulae and start partial bypass prior to starting the sternal entry. It is imperative that pre-operative evaluation has shown that the outflow graft to the ascending aorta is well away from the midline.

The aortic cannula needs to be placed at a point on the ascending aorta or arch so that the ascending aorta can be transected at a higher level to include the graft/aorta anastomosis. Also, the donor harvesting team should get as long a segment of ascending aorta and arch as possible. Once the device is exposed and on full flow support bypass, the outflow graft is clamped and the device turned off.

Heart Transplant in a Patient with a TAH Although there are a few trials using recently developed TAH devices, the majority of patients with a TAH have the Syncardia device [32]. Many centers tend to place a PTFE patch to separate the TAH from the sternum and other surrounding structures. This makes the chance of inadvertent surgical mishaps during re-entry less likely.

Transition from TAH to CPB and Explant of the TAH Once the chest is suitably entered, the ascending aorta, SVC and IVC are dissected and sutures placed for cannulation. The patients are placed on CPB, the TAH is switched off and the aortic cross-clamp applied high on the ascending aorta. The TAH is removed using the same plane of explant (beneath the coronary sinus level/ atrioventricular junctions) as for a regular recipient "heart" explant. This can be further adjusted depending on the technique of implantation to be used for the allograft.

7.7 Patients on ECMO

If the recipient is on central VA ECMO the right atrial cannula is converted to SVC/IVC bi-caval cannulation. In patients on peripheral VA ECMO, the femoral venous cannula maybe left in place and an additional SVC cannula added and "Yed" to this.

7.7.1 ICU Care

The transplanted heart is denervated although the atrial remnant of the recipient remains innervated, these impulses do not cross the suture line. It is the donor atrium that is responsible for heart rate generation. The transplanted heart has a higher resting rate (90–110/min) and demonstrates reduced rate variability. In the denervated heart the initial response via the Frank-Starling mechanism is an increase in stroke volume dependent on an adequate left ventricular end diastolic volume. The increased contractility secondary to heart rate is a secondary effect and is dependent on circulating catecholamine. The transplanted heart is sensitive to preload [33]. The higher rate in the denervated heart is fortuitous as the decreased filling time minimizes stress to the allograft RV while maintaining cardiac output. Temporary atrial pacing and chronotropic agents such as isoproterenol, epinephrine, dopamine, and dobutamine are useful adjuncts in maintaining a higher rate.

Other features that may impact early allograft function include presence of tricuspid and mitral regurgitation. With increasing use bi-caval anastomosis, the former is less likely. The pulmonary artery catheter helps monitor the pulmonary pressures and need for pulmonary dilators etc. Chest drains and temporary RA and RV pacing wires are placed. Patients are kept intubated usually until the next day.

Vasoconstrictors When vasoconstrictors are required, especially on patients who were on angiotensin receptor blockers, Vasopressin, which produces less pulmonary vasoconstriction as compared to systemic vasoconstriction, should be considered over standard alpha-agonists.

7.7.2 Renal Dysfunction

A long period of chronic low cardiac output in itself can result in renal dysfunction in many patients awaiting heart transplantation [34]. Further insult with prolonged non-pulsatile CPB, CNI, hypotension and hypertension etc. can compound an already precarious situation. At times an early and short course of renal replacement therapy (RRT) may be required with judicious use of CNI. Some centers resort to using induction therapy to allow a delayed introduction of potential nephrotoxic immunosuppressive agents.

7.7.3 Bleeding

The recipient has a number of factors before going to the operation that predispose to bleeding. These include, being on oral anticoagulation until the time of transplantation, liver congestion and associated coagulation factors produced by the liver abnormality. These will be compounded by heparinization and hypothermia during CPB. In patients with re-sternotomies, added dissection, adhesions can increase areas of bleeding. The presence of LAVDS or being on ECMO can also affect von Willebrand factor (vWF) form and function [35].

The use of TEG (thromboelastography) to help guide blood product replacement therapy is useful. Although a variety of "agents" have been used to correct the coagulopathy such as platelets, fresh frozen plasma or plasma protein concentrate (PCC) and recombinant factor VII we tend to use PCC. In cases where the coagulopathy cannot easily be corrected, we resort to a delayed sternal closure technique, using either negative pressure suction or Esmark sternal coverage. It must be remembered that patients with a coagulopathy may develop hemodynamic compromise and may need early re-exploration for tamponade.

7.7.4 Hypertension

Is not uncommon in the early postoperative period. The etiology of this is probably multifactorial and includes use of calcineurin inhibitors, steroids, baroreflex related hypertension, catecholamine dysregulation etc. [36]. These patients may also have cardio renal-neuroendocrine aberrations with a denervated allograft. The hypertension should be appropriately managed using vasodilators and calcium channel blockers. In the setting of renal dysfunction, angiotensin receptor blockers and/or inhibitors should be avoided.

7.8 Postoperative Complications

These are outlined in Table 7.4. They include early graft failure (RV, LV, biventricular), low cardiac output requiring MCS (ECMO, VADs), neurological (cerebrovascular accident (CVA), TIAs, seizures), bleeding requiring blood and products and need for re-exploration, renal failure requiring renal replacement therapy, pericardial effusion, arrhythmias and node dysfunction. Once the patient arrives in ICU after surgery with some differences, the postoperative care is similar to other open-heart surgery cases. After the patient has stabilized with no evidence of mediastinal bleeding, neurologic or respiratory dysfunction, weaning off mechanical ventilation is done. This is usually within 24 hours. In patients who have been on preoperative ACE inhibitors, vasoconstrictors may be needed to maintain adequate systolic pressures (90-110 mm Hg). We try to maintain adequate vital signs: As the transplanted heart is denervated, we tend to use dobutamine and/or isoproterenol to keep the heart rate 90–110 beats/min. Pulmonary vasodilators may be needed if the systolic PA is >40 mm Hg. We tend to use PGE1 or inhaled Flolan or iloprost. Particular attention in this regard must be paid in cases with a pre-operative history of elevated pulmonary pressures.

(A) Patients with explanted LVAD prior to transplantation: With the increasing use of LVADS as BTTx, up to 55% of cases coming to transplantation have a chronically implanted LVAD [4]. These patients tend to have a more complicated post-operative management because (a) pre-operatively they are on anticoagulants (b) have undergone a redo-sternotomy (c) longer bypass times and (d) more prone to requiring blood products.

(B) Patients with explanted TAH prior to transplantation: As these patients also have been on pre-operative anticoagulation they can be prone to requiring blood and blood products.

(C) On pre-transplant ECMO. Again, the majority of these patients have been on anticoagulation, have associated coagulation abnormalities pre-operatively and hence may be more prone to bleeding problems.

Table 7.4 Post-Op complications

Postoperative complication:
Surgical: Bleeding, tamponade, aortic pseudoaneurysm (cannulation sites) sternal complications.
Medical: Tricuspid regurgitation
RV failure: Pulmonary artery compression Stenosis, pulmonary hypertension
LV failure: Ischemia, poor protection, operative injury, rejection (acute, hyperacute)
Rejection:
Acute. (a) Cellular (b) antibody mediated (humoral)
Rhythm issues: Sinus node dysfunction, bradyarrhythmias, atrial fibrillation, ventricular arrhythmias, may need permanent pacemaker.
Respiratory failure: Cardiogenic and non-cardiogenic pulmonary edema Infection, prolonged intubation
Renal and hepatic dysfunction: Exacerbation of previous dysfunction, new dysfunction. Need for RRT (CVVH, HD)
Infection: Early, late. Bacterial, viral, fungal, "opportunistic"
Complications related to immunosuppression:
Early: Related to need for increased immunosuppression in the peri-operative period e.g. use of induction therapy, steroids, etc)
Late: Hypertension, steroid related, renal dysfunction, PTLD
Hypertension.
Elevated pulmonary pressures.

7.9   Immunosuppression

Although protocols may vary from center to center [37, 38], in essence four classes of drugs [39] are used they consist of a calcineurin inhibitors (Cyclosporine and Tacrolimus), anti-proliferative agents (Azathioprine and Mycophenolate Mofetil: MMF/Cellcept), m-TOR inhibitors (Sirolimus and Everolimus) and steroids. Corticosteroids have been used as part of induction therapy, treatment of rejection and for maintenance therapy. They provide non-specific immunosuppression. They are started at the time of surgery in higher doses and then rapidly tapered to maintenance dose. An immunosuppressive protocol is outlined in Table 7.5.

7.9.1   Induction Therapy

Induction therapy is traditionally given in the peri-operative period to decrease the risk of early rejection [40, 41]. Many centers now used it to delay introduction of CNI and steroid use. Agents used for induction therapy have included polyclonal anti-thymocyte globulin such as rabbit derived Thymoglobulin (rATG, Genzyme Corporation, Cambridge, MA) or equine derived ATGAM (Pharmacia Upjohn, Pfizer, NY) can induce rapid depletion of T lymphocytes by complement mediated cytolysis or cell mediated

Table 7.5 Immunosuppression protocols. (Inova)

Immunosuppressive protocol:
Induction plan decided by team at time of listing
Non-sensitized, renal dysfunction: Basiliximab
Sensitized: rATG
Preop
MMF 1000 mg PO × 1
Intraop
Methylprednisolone 1 gm IV
Postop
MMF 1500 IV/PO q12
Methyprednisolone 125 mg IV q8 × 3 then taper to prednisone 15–20 mg qd by 2 weeks
Tacrolimus 2 mg Q12 starting 24–48 h post surgery (target trough 10–12 for first 3 mo

Augmented immunosuppression during rejection episodes (mild, moderate, severe

opsonization. Newer agents include interleukin 2 receptor IL-2R antagonists [42] such as basiliximab (Simulect) which blocks IL-2 mediated T cell proliferation. However, as maintenance immunosuppression has improved, the benefits of either induction therapy in heart transplantation is questionable. Similar to studies in other organs, the use of induction therapy has not been shown to have a significant impact on long term graft function or survival. Studies suggest it may result in a small decrease in the incidence of early rejection but an increase in viral and fungal infections and malignancy. Reflecting the lack of consensus, ISHLT registry demonstrates that currently one half of heart transplant patients receive no induction therapy. Of the remaining half, ~30% receive ILR antagonist, and ~ 20% receive polyclonal ATG.

Many programs have taken a graduated approach to the use of induction therapy. Patients at the highest risk for rejection (such as known HLA sensitizatioin, younger recipients, African American recipients, MCS recipients) are considered. Also, patients with renal dysfunction, who may benefit from delaying the start of calcineurin inhibitors are considered.

7.10   Rejection

Hyperacute Rejection Luckily with preoperative evaluation of PRAs, cross-matching techniques, hyperacute rejection is very uncommon [43]. A scientific statement from the American Heart Association on this subject is all encompassing regarding diagnosis and treatment [44]. Should it occur or be suspected plasmapheresis, agents targeting humoral mediation should be employed [17, 44]. In addition, early use of MCS can be used should there be serious hemodynamic instability.

Acute Rejection Histological criteria have been established for diagnosing acute rejection [45].

Cellular The gold standard for diagnosis remains the endomyocardial biopsy (EMBx). The grading criteria is outlined in Table 7.6. With current immunosuppressive regimens, severe acute rejection is unusual. Should it occur steroid bolus therapy, intravenously is used. Also, with milder forms of rejection, augmented immunosuppression using lower dose steroids can be used.

Humoral (antibody mediated) rejection. Again, special staining techniques on the EMBx should be performed to make this diagnosis. Agents to treat this type of rejection include plasmapheresis, IVIG, Rituximab, Alemtuzumab, Bortezomib, Eculizumab, Cyclophosphamide, Mycophenolate and total lymphoid irradiation [44].

Treatment of Rejection   Rejection is treated by augmented immunosuppression and agents used depend on whether it is cellular and the grade on histology or if it is humoral, antibody mediated. With any rejection episode if severe hemodynamic compromise results that is not response to inotropic agents and anti-rejection therapy, consideration to using MCS including ECMO should be given, early.

Monitoring Rejection   An early EMBx is done on the seventh postoperative day and thereafter

based on protocol at a particular institution. Suggested frequency can include weekly biopsies for the first month, then every month for the first 3 months, then every third month for the first year, and every fourth month in the second year, then annually depending on the presence or absence of rejection. We and other use molecular systems to increase the accuracy of making a diagnosis of rejection and also to reduce the frequency of doing EMBx [46, 47].

Infection   Antibiotics: Perioperative antibiotics include gram positive and negative coverage. In addition, as with other organ transplants, immunosuppressant predisposes to increased infection risk. Attention must be paid to decreasing risk of viral, fungal and P. carnii infections. This is particularly important when there is donor recipient "mismatching" e.g. of CMV status.

Mortality After Heart Transplantation   The cause of death after heart transplantation is time dependent. Early postoperative period: graft failure, multi-organ failure and infections, Fig. 7.5. In most centers, overall 1-year mortality is 88%.

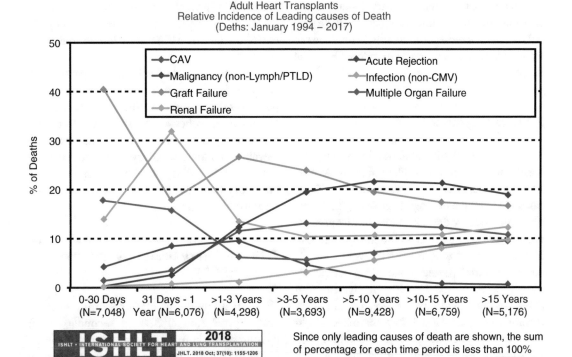

Fig. 7.5 ISHLT graph of Mortality

Factors that increase mortality include, age, long donor ischemic times, rejection episodes, infections, re-do sternotomy, pulmonary hypertension, presence of MCS etc.

7.11 Effects of Donor/Recipient Sizing

Donor/recipient size mismatching can impact the post-operative course. The term "Big heart syndrome" is used when the D/R size ratio is >2. This can result in systemic hypertension syndrome with resultant effects on the central nervous system symptoms e.g. seizure, coma etc. The hypertension must be carefully controlled. On the other end a D/R ratio < 1 has been reported to cause post-operative heart failure [48, 49].

7.11.1 Post-Operative Pericardial Effusions

Occur in 9–21% of adult recipients [50]. This may in part be due to the increased pericardial volume that results when regular sized heart replaces a dilated removed heart. Usually these effusions do not require surgical drainage and only require intervention should hemodynamic instability occur. They can be monitored by serial ECHOs.

7.11.2 Arrhythmias

The commonest rhythm abnormality is bradycardia. In the early post-transplant sinus node dysfunction is reported to occur in up to 44% of cases [51] and the etiology is probably multifactorial. In the early days, a continuous isoproterenol infusion was used as a chronotrope agent to increase the heart rate. Other options include AV pacing or atrial pacing alone using temporary pacing wires placed intraoperatively. In most cases the sinus node dysfunction is temporary. Approximately 2–5% will have permanent dysfunction requiring pacemaker implantation [52]. As some of the calcium channel blockers can interfere with immunosuppression their use should be avoided.

7.12 Pulmonary Vascular Resistance and RV Failure

Since the early days if transplantation the deleterious effects of recipient elevated PVR on allograft RV dysfunction/failure was quickly realized [53]. Pulmonary artery pressures greater than 50 mm Hg, transpulmonary gradient (TPG) greater than 15 mm Hg and PVR greater than 6 Woods units that are not responsive to vasodilators, are contraindications to orthotopic heart transplantation. Several studies have shown that elevated fixed PVR > wood units are associated with a high risk of RV failure and death [54]. In the immediate post-implant period of heart transplantation, the etiology of RV failure is multifactorial and can be compounded by the presence of elevated pulmonary hypertension. Factors include poor donor heart preservation during procurement and implantation, ischemia/reperfusion injury, prolonged ischemic times, SIRS associated with CPB and pulmonary vascular hyperreactivity [55] which increases and further strains the RV. If this RV failure is not managed properly (chemical and or MCS) graft failure and death can result.

The management of pulmonary hypertension and RV failure must continue into the early post-operative period. An indwelling PA catheter and use of echocardiography can be complimentary in this regard. Agents that decrease elevated pulmonary artery pressures include iNO, prostaglandins, phosphodiesterase type-5 inhibitor such as Sildenafil and endothelin receptor blockers [56].

7.13 Primary Graft Dysfunction (PGD)

Graft dysfunction is classified into primary graft dysfunction (PGD) or secondary graft dysfunction where a discernible cause can be identified e.g. hyperacute rejection, pulmonary hypertension, or surgical complications. PGD must be diagnosed within 24 hours of transplantation. It is said to occur in up to 20–30% of patients in the first 30 days post-transplantation and is said to be the etiology of up to 20% of deaths in the first 30 days [57, 58]. PGD is divided into PGD of the left or right ventricle and categorized into mild, moderate, or severe grades depending on the level of cardiac function and need/extent of supportive therapy (inotropes and MCS such as VADs, ECMO or TAH).

7.13.1 Renal Dysfunction

Recipients with long-standing heart failure may either heart failure related or unrelated renal dysfunction. This may be compounded by CPB, immunosuppressive agents, need for vasoconstrictors in the post-operative period etc. Fluid overload due to volume resuscitation in the face of renal dysfunction and diuretic resistance may necessitate renal replacement therapy or simple ultra-filtration. Acute renal failure occurs post-operatively in approximately 3–10% of heart transplant recipients [59].

7.13.2 After Hospital Discharge

Close follow-up by the transplant cardiologist team is essential. These visits decrease in frequency as after the first few months. The goals being to monitor cardiac allograft function, detect rejection, infection, adjust immunosuppression. Patients are also monitored for development of PTLD and other tumors. Transplant patients have a 100-fold increase in the prevalence of malignant tumors as compared with age-matched controls. The most common is PTLD (post-transplantation lymphoproliferative disorder), a type of non-Hodgkin's lymphoma believed to be related to EBV (Epstein Barr Virus). The incidence can be as high as 50% in EBV-negative recipients of EBV positive hearts. Treatment involves reduction of immunosuppressive agents, use of acyclovir and chemotherapy for widespread disease.

7.13.3 Allograft Vasculopathy

Ever since this entity was recognized after cardiac transplantation was started in South Africa, we have made little progress in its overall prevention [60]. Even though acute and severe rejection frequency has decreased with immunosuppressive regimens AGA still remains an important cause of late allograft failure and need for re-transplantation. It is best evaluated by coronary angiography imaging which is also notorious for under estimating its severity. The role of CT angiography is also being evaluated. Use of IVUS and other intravascular techniques has highlighted its severity. In severe cases cardiac re-transplantation is the only recourse.

7.13.4 Role of MCS (TAH, LVAD, RVAD, bi-VAD, ECMO) in Chronic Heart Failure

The concept of using MCS (mechanical circulatory systems) to support patients with heart failure is not new. As technology has improved these devices have also been miniaturized and designs have moved away from the first-generation devices that were pusher plate systems to continuous flow (CF) systems either axial flow or centrifugal flow based. The CF devices are smaller and easier to implant. We are beginning to better understand the long-term effects of CF systems.

MCS can be used as a bridge to transplantation for suitable patients. They are a variety of systems, devices temporary/ short term and long-term devices. The frequency and type of configuration used is outlined in Fig. 7.6 (ISHLT). The

Table 7.6 LVAD complications

1.	Stroke (etiology multifactorial. Hemorrhagic, ischemic).
2.	Aortic insufficiency. Approximately 30% by two years. Etiology multifactorial.
3.	Right heart failure. May be early or delayed.
4.	Pump thrombosis. Inadequate anticoagulation, mechanical, low-flow.
5.	Driveline infection. Occurrence, variable timeline.
6.	Gastrointestinal bleeding. 15–30% incidence.
7.	Bleeding: Early: Usually surgery related.
8.	Device malfunction.
9.	Hemolysis
10.	Arrhythmias

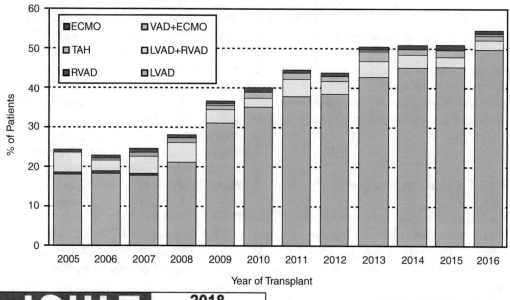

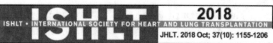

Fig. 7.6 Types of MCS used as BTTx

REMATCH trial using first generation systems was the first randomized trial that showed LVADS had an advantage of maximal medical therapy in chronic heart failure patients [61]. Another approach has been use of MCS as "destination therapy". These are patients who are not transplant candidates. For the majority of these patients LVADS are used [62]. However, the great disparity between donor supply and recipient need has not improved with use of MCS. The use of MCS as a bridge to transplant therapy has increased the list of patients awaiting transplantation.

Types of Commonly Implanted Long-term LVADS The two commonly implanted LVADS [63] are: (a) Heartware (HVAD, Medtronic). This is a centrifugal pump (Fig. 7.7) and (b) the Heartmate (HM, Abbott). The axial flow pump version HM2 has now been superseded by the centrifugal design HM3 (Fig. 7.8) which in recent reports is associated with less complications [64]. These devices are mainly implanted on CPB and

via a median sternotomy. However alternate approaches avoiding a median sternotomy have been described, e.g. via a left thoracotomy for accessing the LV apex and use of the subclavian artery for the outflow anastomoses in cases of a hostile mediastinum and/or in an effort to prevent sternal re-entry issues [65].

Complications associated with LVADS: These are listed in Table 7.6 and include, RV failure, infection, stroke, TIAs, gastrointestinal bleeding, VW factor abnormalities, pump thrombosis and embolism and death [66]. Early results suggest that with better designs, some of these complications may be reduced [66]. The role of lack of pulsatility and attempts to create pulsatility continue to be evaluated.

Temporary MCS In cases where a heart failure patient deteriorates rapidly and time is required to plan overall care, temporary or short-term support devices may be used to support the left and/or right ventricle [67]. These devices include IABA, ECMO, Impella, Tandem Heart, ProTek

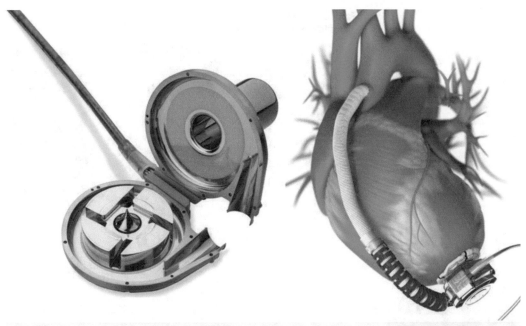

HeartWare HVAD. A continuous flow device designed to draw blood from the LV & propel it through an outflc graft connected to the patient's ascending aorta. The inflow cannula is surgically implanted into the left ventric blood is conveyed through the pump via an impeller at operating speeds of 2400-3200 rpm (resulting in up t 10L/min of blood flow)(Courtesy of HeartWare International Inc, Framingham, Massachusetts, USA.)

Fig. 7.7 Heartware

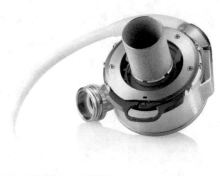

Thoratec HeartMate 3 (picture reprinted with friendly permission of Thoratec).

Fig. 7.8 HM3

Duo etc. (Fig. 7.9). These devices can play a useful role as a "bridge to further decision", be that as a "bridge to a bridge", bridge to implantable MCS, or transplantation, etc.

Use of the Total Artificial Heart (TAH) This should be considered as replacement therapy where there is severe biventricular heart failure, in restrictive and infiltrative cardiomyopathies, in severe structural heart disease and in

patients on ECMO with biventricular failure. Presently the largest experience is with the Syncardia TAH with over 1800 being implanted. They are used as a bridge to transplant. The implantation technique is depicted in Fig. 7.10a, b, c. The explantation technique at the time of transplantation is similar to a "native heart" explant. With improvement in patient selection, implantation techniques and postoperative care and targeted anticoagulation therapy excellent immediate and longer-term results are reported. Complications include, infection, stroke, device malfunction and bleeding.

7.14 Cardiac Procedures on the Native Heart

In some patient surgical procedures may help manage/correct the etiology of the heart failure. These include: (a) revascularization (coronary artery bypass grafting) especially in

**Temporary (Short to Mid-term)
Circulatory Support Devices)**

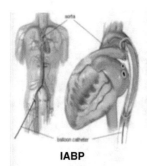

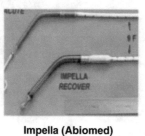

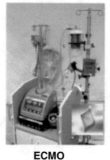

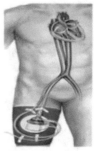

IABP

Impella (Abiomed)

ECMO

TandemHeart

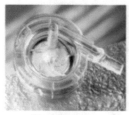

Centrimag

Fig. 7.9 Percutaneous temporary MCS. Permission from Michael A Acker MD, Chief CV Surgery, University of Pennsylvania

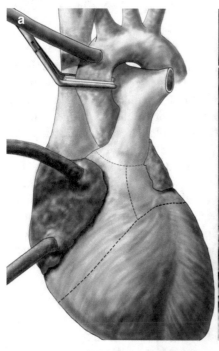

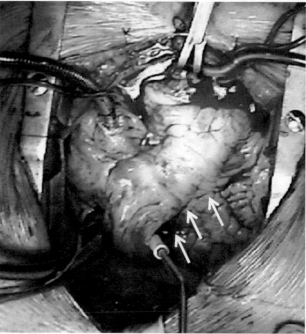

Fig. 7.10 (**a**) Excision of the right and left ventricle. The RV and LV are excised leaving a 1 cm ventricular cuff beyond the mitral and tricuspid annulus. Arrows point to the incision along the anterior wall of the RV. The incisions are extended through the left and right ventricular outflow tracts and through the aortic and pulmonic valves. (**b**) Quick connects and Gortex Prelude implanted. The atrial quick connects and vascular grafts are sewn to their respective orifices. The pericardium is lined with a Gortex membrane to facilitate subse-quent reentry for transplantation. (**c**) A saline implant is used to maintain the pericardial apical space for transplantation. (**d**) Device implanted. The device implanted just prior to chest closure. TAH: Recipient heart explant and Syncardia IMPLANT (Citation for TAH implant figure. Tang, D. G., Shah, K. B., Hess, M. L., Kasirajan, V. Implantation of the Syncardia Total Artificial Heart. *J. Vis. Exp.* (89), e50377, https://doi.org/10.3791/50377 (2014)

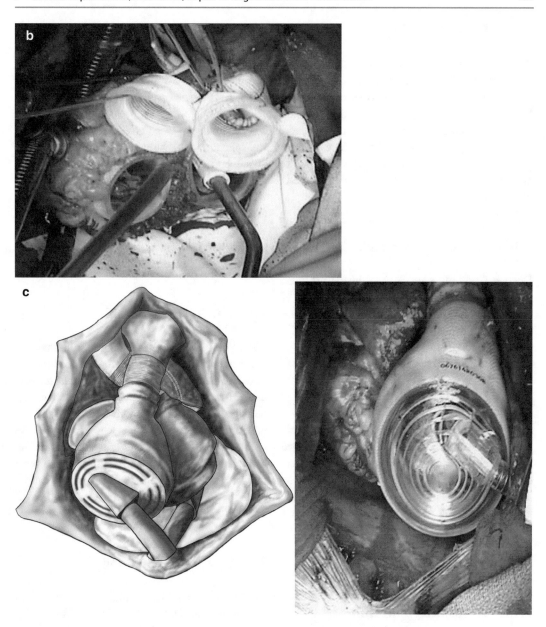

Fig. 7.10   (continued)

segments of the heart that are viable or hibernating (b) repair/replace valvular defect causing/contributing to the failure e.g. aortic, mitral, tricuspid valve disorders (c) treat the "electrical issues" arrhythmias contributing to cardiac dysfunction (d) repair myocardial structural abnormalities such as ventricular aneurysms e.g. Dor procedure (e) "reverse/reduce severe pulmonary hypertension contributing to right heart failure e.g. pulmonary thrombo-endartectomy for severe pulmonary hypertension due to thromboembolic disease. (f) correction of congenital heart defects contributing to heart failure.

7.14.1 Future Direction

A better understanding of molecular mechanisms of heart failure should allow introduction of further medical therapies to stop worsening heart failure. Use of genomics and cell-based therapies could assist in recovery of the damaged heart before severe heart failure ensues. Also, the concept or depopulating donor hearts and repopulating them with recipient stem cells hold some promise.

7.14.2 "Re-furbished hearts"

Donors: Currently only 34% of hearts are used from potential donors annually in the US.Use of ex-vivo systems [68] where the donor heart can be placed after explantation to replenish metabolic derangements should increase donor supply.

7.14.3 Recent Developments in TAH

Although the majority of current TAH implants involve Syncardia, other TAH devices that have been developed. Some have been implanted clinically such as CARMAT and the Abiomed TAH. Others are in various stages of development. An exciting device design is the Bivacor heart which can be used as a VAD or TAH [69]. Isolated reports describe using two CF pumps placed in series in lieu of implanting a TAH.

7.15   Xenotransplantation

As a source of donor organs, xenografts holds promise to address the critical shortage of organs. Much progress has been made in the ability to control the initial hyperacute rejection which is driven primarily by innate immune and inflammatory responses. The results of orthotopically transplanted transgenic pigs hearts into baboons are encouraging [70, 71].

A fear of xenotransplantation has been transmission of pig retroviruses. The availability of CRISPR molecular tools to remove pig retroviruses should hopefully speed up their use in clinical transplantation [72, 73].

7.15.1 Tolerance

The encouraging results of Treg cells in renal transplantation to help create "chemical tolerance" bodes well for extending to other solid organs including cardiac transplantation. This would decrease the unfortunate complications associated with long term immunosuppression. It will be interesting to see if this also impacts the severity and incidence of AGA, a major cause for cardiac re-transplantation [74, 75].

7.15.2 Cell Based Therapies

The role of using cells to "support" the myocardium is continuing to be evaluated. In the early days the patient's own skeletal myoblasts were used. However, these were associated with development of ventricular arrhythmias [76] and are no longer used.

The role of stem cells to repopulate the failing heart are current being actively evaluated. Now that induced pluripotent stem (ips) cells can be used instead of using an embryonic source of stem cells, the field has expanded [77].

7.15.3 Tissue Engineering

The concept of depopulating donor organs and then repopulating the "acellular scaffold" with recipient cells is receiving increasing attention [78]. There have been some encouraging experimental results [79] using this approach.

7.16   Conclusion

We owe much to the early intrepid investigators. The field of managing heart failure is set for rapid expansion. Advances in bioengineering, regenerative medicine, immunology, molecular biology and xenotransplantation will all play a vital role in selecting a patient/disease centered approach to managing heart failure.

References

1. American Heart Association. Heart diseases and stroke statistics: 2008 update. Dallas, Tex: American Heart Association; 2008.
2. Mozzafarian D, Benjamin EJ, Go AS, et al. On behalf of the American heart association statistics committee and stroke statistics subcommittee. Heart disease and stroke statistics—2016 update: a report from the American heart association. Circulation. 2016;133:e38–e360.
3. Barnard CN. The operation. A human cardiac transplant: an interim report of a successful operation performed at Groote Schuur hospital, Cape Town. S Afr Med J. 1967;41:1271–4.
4. ISHLT 2018 Registry data.
5. Calne R, Rolles K, Thiru S, McMaster P, Craddock G, Aziz S, White D, Evans D, Dunn D, Henderson R, Lewis P. Cyclosporin-a as the only immunosuppressant in 34 recipients of cadaveric organs: 32 kidneys, 2 pancreases and 2 livers. Lancet. 1979;2:1033–6.
6. James KK, Francis PD, Robert KL, Lynne SW, Elizabeth BD, Susan ML, Marissa MA, John BT, James YB, David NC. Eighth annual INTERMACS report: special focus on framing the impact of adverse events. J Heart Lung Transplant. 2017 July;36(10):1080–6.
7. Han JJ, Acker MA, Atluri P. Left ventricular assist devices. Synergistic model between technology and medicine. Circulation. 2018;138:2841–51.
8. Thompson JG. Atheroma in a transplanted heart. Lancet. 1969;2:1088–92.
9. Sharon A. Hunt. Cardiac allograft vasculopathy. It really has changed over time. JACC: Heart Failure. 2017 Dec;5(12):902–3.
10. Dandel M, Hetzer R. Myocardial recovery during mechanical circulatory support: long-term outcome and elective ventricular assist device implantation to promote recovery as a treatment goal. Heart Lung Vessel. 2015;7(4):289–96.
11. Cooper LB, Lu D, Mentz RJ, Rogers JG, Milano CA, Felker GM, Hernandez AF, Patel CB. Cardiac transplantation for older patients: characteristics and outcomes in the septuagenarian population. J Heart Lung Transplant. 2016 Mar;35(3):362–9.
12. Russo MJ, Davies RR, Hong KN, Chen JM, Argenziano M, Moskowitz A, Ascheim DD, George I, Stewart AS, Williams M, Gelijns A, Naka Y. Matching high-risk recipients with marginal donor hearts is a clinically effective strategy. Ann Thorac Surg 2009 Apr;87(4):1066–1070. discussion 1071.
13. Michelle Maya Kittleson, Jon A Kobashigawa. Management of the highly sensitized patient awaiting heart transplant. ACC Jan 08, 2015.
14. Kittleson MM, Kobashigawa A. Management of pre-sensitized recipient. Curr Opin Organ Transplant. 2012;17:551–7.
15. Vo AA, Lukovsky M, Toyoda M, et al. Rituximab and intravenous immune globulin for desensitization during renal transplantation. N Engl J Med. 2008;359:242–51.
16. Patel J, Everly M, Chang D, et al. Reduction of alloantibodies via proteasome inhibition in cardiac transplantation. J Heart Lung Transplant. 2011;30:1320–6.
17. Aziz S, Hassantash S, Nelson K, Levy W, Kruse A, Reichenbach D, Himes V, Fishbein D, Allen M. The clinical significance of flow cytometry crossmatching in cardiac transplantation. J Heart Lung Transplant. 1998;17:686–92.
18. Rizvi SS, Luc JG, Choi JH, Phan K, Moncho Escriva E, Patel S, Massey HT, Tchantchaleishvili V. Outcomes and survival following heart transplantation for cardiac allograft failure: a systematic review and meta-analysis. Ann Cardiothorac Surg. 2018;7(1):12–8.
19. Laks H, Marelli D, Fonarow G, Hamilton M, Ardehali A, Moriguchi J, Bresson J, Gjerton D, Kobashigawa J. Use of two recipient lists for adults requiring heart transplantation. J Thorac Cardiovasc Surg. 2003;125:49–59.
20. Berman M, Pavlushkov E, Doshi H, Balasubramanian S, White D, Claydon S, Ballantyne H, Ellis C, Tsui S. Transition of DCD heart transplantation from research to a clinical programme – challenges and lessons learned. J Heart Lung Transplant. 2017;36(4, Supplement):S46.
21. Popov A-F, Sáez DG, Sabashnikov A, Patil NP, Zeriouh M, Mohite PN, Zych B, Schmack B, Ruhparwar A, Kallenbach K, Dohmen PM, Karck M, Simon AR, Weymann A. Utilization of the organ care system – a game-changer in combating donor organ shortage. Med Sci Monit Basic Res. 2015;21:29–32.
22. Mitchell BD, Rajagopal K, Scharf S, Eberlein M. Cardiac size and sex-matching in heart transplantation: size matters in matters of sex and the heart. JACC Heart Failure. 2014 Feb;2(1):73–83.
23. Hong KN, Iribarne A, Worku B, et al. Who is the high-risk recipient? Predicting mortality after heart transplant using pretransplant donor and recipient risk factors. Ann Thorac Surg. 2011;92:520–7.
24. Dhital KK, Iyer A, Connellan M, et al. Adult heart transplantation with distant procurement and ex-vivo preservation of donor hearts after circulatory death: a case series. Lancet. 2015;385:2585–91.
25. Lower RR, Stofer RC, Shumway NE. Homovital transplantation of the heart. J Thorac Cardiovasc Surg. 1961;41:196–204.
26. Sievers HH, Weyand M, Kraatz EG, Bernhard A. An alternative technique for orthotopic cardiac transplantation, with preservation of the normal anatomy of the right atrium. Thorac Cardiovasc Surg. 1991;39:70–2.
27. Blanche C, Valenza M, Aleksic I, Czer LSC, Trento A. Technical considerations of a new technique for orthotopic heart transplantation. Total excision of

recipient's atria with bicaval and pulmonary venous anastomoses. J Cardiovasc Surg. 1994;35(4):283–7.

28. Aziz S, Panos A. Current techniques of myocardial protection for cardiac transplantation. In: Cooper DKC, Miller LW, Patterson GA, editors. The transplantation and replacement of thoracic organs. 2nd ed. Hingham, MA: Kluwer Academic Publishers; 1996.

29. Ryan RD, Mark JR, Jeffrey AM, Robert AS, Yoshifumi N, Jonathan MC. Standard versus bicaval techniques for orthotopic heart transplantation: an analysis of the united network for organ sharing database.

30. Kobashigawa J, Zuckermann A, Macdonald P, Leprince P, Esmailian F, Luu M, Mancini D, Patel J, Razi R, Reichenspurner H, Russell S, Segovia J, Smedira N, Stehlik J, Wagner F. Consensus conference participants. Report from a consensus conference on primary graft dysfunction after cardiac transplantation. J Heart Lung Transplant. 2014 Apr;33(4):327–40.

31. Cheng A, Slaughter MS, Technique S. Heart transplantation. J Thorac Dis. 2014 Aug;6(8):1105–9.

32. Torregrossa G, Gerosa G, Tarzia V, Morshuis M, Copeland J. Long term results with total artificial heart: is it prime time for destination therapy? JHLT 2013 1 April;32(4):Supplement S118.

33. Cotts WG, Oren RM. Function of the transplanted heart: unique physiology and therapeutic implications. Am J Med Sci (Heart Transplantation Symposium). September 1997;314(3):164–72.

34. Cole RT, Masoumi A, Triposkiadis F, Giamouzis G, Georgiopoulou V, Kalogeropoulos A, Butler J. Renal dysfunction in heart failure. Med Clin North Am. 2012 Sep;96(5):955–74.

35. Nascimbene A, Neelamegham S, Frazier OH, Moake JL, Dong JF. Acquired von Willebrand syndrome associated with left ventricular assist device. Blood. 2016 Jun 23;127(25):3133–41.

36. Bennett AL, Ventura HO. Hypertension in patients with cardiac transplantation. Med Clin North Am. 2017 Jan;101(1):53–64.

37. Koomalsingh K, Kobashigawa JA. The future of cardiac transplantation. Ann Cardiothorac Surg, 2018 Jan. 7(1):135–42.

38. Valantine H, Khush K, Stadnick E. Drugs used for immunosuppression post transplant. Cardiology Advisor.

39. Kobashigawa J, Zuckermann A, Macdonald P, Leprince P, Esmailian F, Luu M, Mancini D, Patel J, Razi R, Reichenspurner H, Russell S, Segovia J, Smedira N, Stehlik J, Wagner F. Consensus conference participants. Report from a consensus conference on primary graft dysfunction after cardiac transplantation. J Heart Lung Transplant. 2014 April;33(4):327–034.

40. Aliabai A, Grommer M, Cochrane A, Salamch O, Zuckermann A. Induction therapy in heart transplantation: where are we now? Transpl Int. 2013;26:684–95.

41. Barten MJ, Schulz U, Beiras-Fernandez A, Berchtold-Herz M, Bocken U, et al. A proposal for early dosing regimens in heart transplant patients receiving thymo-globulin and calcineurin inhibition. Transplant Direct. 2016;2:e81.

42. Furiasse N, Kobashigawa JA. Immunosuppression and adult heart transplantation: emerging therapies and opportunities. J Exp Rev Cardiovasc Ther. 2017;15(1):59–69.

43. Weil R III, Clarke DR, Iwaki Y, Porter KA, Koep LJ, Paton BC, Terasaki PI, Starzl TE. Hyperacute rejection of a transplanted human heart. Transplantation. 1981 Jul;32(1):71–2.

44. Colvin MM, Cook JL, Chang P, Francis G, Hsu DT, Kiernan MS, Kobashigawa JA, Lindenfeld J, Masri SC, Miller D, O'Connell J, Rodriguez ER, Rosengard B, Self S, White-Williams C, Zeevi A. American heart association heart failure and transplantation committee of the council on clinical cardiology, council on cardiopulmonary, critical care, perioperative and resuscitation, council on cardiovascular disease in the young, council on cardiovascular and stroke nursing, council on cardiovascular radiology and intervention, and council on cardiovascular surgery and anesthesia. Antibody-mediated rejection in cardiac transplantation: emerging knowledge in diagnosis and management: a scientific statement from the American heart association. Circulation. 2015;131: 1608–39.

45. Stewart S, Winters GL, Fishbein MC, Tazelaar HD, Kobashigawa J, Abrams J, Andersen CB, Angelini A, Berry GJ, Burke MM, Demetris AJ, Hammond E, Itescu S, Marboe CC, McManus B, Reed EF, Reinsmoen NL, Rodriguez ER, Rose AG, Rose M, Suciu-Focia N, Zeevi A, Billingham ME. Revision of the 1990 working formulation for the standardization of nomenclature in the diagnosis of heart rejection. J Heart Lung Transplant. 2005, Nov;24(11):1710–20.

46. Hermida-Prieto M, Crespo-Leiro MG, Paniagua MJ, Castro-Beiras A. Identification of a cardiac allograft rejection marker using microarray gene expression analysis in lymphocytes from heart transplant patients. Rev Esp Cardiol. 2007;60(2):217–8.

47. Halloran PF, Potena L, Van Huyen JD, Bruneval P, Leone O, Kim DH, Jouven X, Reeve J, Loupy A. Building a tissue-based molecular diagnostic system in heart transplant rejection: the heart molecular microscope diagnostic (MMDx) system. J Heart Lung Transplant. 2017 Nov;36(11):1192–200.

48. Reichart B. Size matching in heart transplantation. J Heart Lung Transplant. 1992;11(4 Pt 2):S199–202.

49. Tamisier D, Vouhé P, Le Bidois J, Mauriat P, Khoury W, Leca F. Donor-recipient size matching in pediatric heart transplantation: a word of caution about small grafts. J Heart Lung Transplant. 1996;15(2):190–5.

50. Quin JA, Tauriainen MP, Huber LM, et al. Predictors of pericardial effusion after orthotopic heart transplantation. J Thorac Cardiovasc Surg. 2002;124(5):979–83.

51. Thajudeen A, Stecker EC, Shehata M, Patel J, Wang X, McAnulty JH Jr, Kobashigawa J, Chugh SS. Arrhythmias after heart transplantation: mechanisms and management. J Am Heart Assoc. 2012 Apr;1(2):e001461.

52. Mallidi HR, Bates M. Pacemaker use following heart transplantation. Ochsner J. 2017 Spring;17(1):20–4.
53. Kirklin JK, Naftel DC, McGiffin DC, et al. Analysis of morbid events and risk factors for death after cardiac transplantation. JAMA. 1988;11:917–24.
54. Natale ME, Pina IL. Evaluation of pulmonary hypertension in heart transplant candidates. Curr Opin Cardiol. 2003;18:136–40.
55. Cimato TR, Jessup M. Recipient selection in cardiac transplantation contraindications and risk factors for mortality. J Heart Lung Transplant. 2002;21:1161–73.
56. Perez-Villa F, Farrero M, Sionis A, Castel A, Roig E. Therapy with sildenafil or bosentan decreases pulmonary vascular resistance in patients ineligible for heart transplantation because of severe pulmonary hypertension. J Heart Lung Transplant. 2010;29:817–8.
57. Chew HC, Kumarasinghe G, Iyer A, Hicks M, Gao L, Doyle A, Jabbour A, Dhital K, Granger E, Jansz P, Hayward C, Keogh A, Kotlyar E, Spratt P, Macdonald P. Primary graft dysfunction after heart transplantation. Current Transplant Rep. 2014 Dec;1(4):257–65.
58. Isaac D. Primary cardiac graft failure-defining, predicting, preventing. J Heart Lung Transplant. 2013 Dec;32(12):1168–9.
59. De Santo LS, Romano G, Amarelli C, Maiello C, Baldascino F, Bancone C, Grimaldi F, Nappi G. Implications of acute kidney injury after heart transplantation: what a surgeon should know. Eur J Cardiothorac Surg. 2011 Dec;40(6):1355–61.
60. Chih S, Ching Y, Mielniczuk LM, Bhatt DL, Beanlands RSB. Cardiac allograft vasculopathy. The achilles' heel of heart transplantation. JACC. 2016 July 5;68(1):80–91.
61. Rose E, et al. Long-term use of a left ventricular assist device for end-stage heart failure. N Engl J Med. 2001;345:1435–43.
62. Fukunaga N, Rao V. Left ventricular assist device as destination therapy for end stage heart failure: the right time for the right patients. Curr Opin Cardiol. 2018 Mar;33(2):196–201.
63. Schroder JN, Milano CA. A tale of two centrifugal left ventricular assist devices. JTCVS. 2017 Sept;154(3):850–2.
64. Mehra MR, Uriel N, Naka Y, Cleveland JC Jr, Yuzefpolskaya M, Salerno CT, Walsh MN, Milano CA, Patel CB, Hutchins SW, Ransom J, Ewald GA, et al. MOMENTUM 3 investigators. A fully magnetically levitated left ventricular assist device — final report. NEJM March. 2019;17:1618–27. https://doi.org/10.1056/NEJMoa1900486.
65. Pantino DW, Khalpey Z. Off pump robotic-assisted LVAD (HeartWare, HVAD) placement via left mini thoracotomy. Oper Tech Thorac Cardiovasc Surg. 2017;22:68–77.
66. Han JJ, Acker MA, Atluri P. Left ventricular assist devices. Synergistic model between technology and medicine. Circulation. 2018 Dec 11;138(24):2841–51.
67. Federica Jiritino, Valeria Lo Coco, Matteo Matteucci, Dario Fina, Roberto Lorusso. Temporary Mechanical Circulatory Support in Acute Heart failure. Cardiac Failure reviews 2020:6:e01. DOL https://doi.org/10.15420/cfr.2019.02.
68. Stamp NL, Shah A, Vincent V, Wright B, Wood C, Pavey W, Cokis C, Chih S, Dembo L, Larbalestier R. Sucessful heart transplant after ten hours out-of-body time using the TransMedics organ care system. Heart Lung Circ. June 2015;24(6):611–3.
69. Sotirios S, Vera H, Andrae W, Otto D. Current state of total artificial heart therapy and introduction of the most important total artificial heart systems. De Gruyter. Published Online: 2018-06-14.
70. Murthy R, Bajona P, Bhama JK, Cooper DKC. Heart xenotransplantation: historical background, experimental Progress, and clinical prospects. Ann Thorac Surg. April 2016;101(4):1605–13.
71. Cooper DKC, Pierson RN III, Hering BJ, Mohiuddin MM, Fishman JA, Denner J, Ahn C, Azimzadeh AM, Buhler LH, Cowan PJ, Hawthorne WJ, Kobayashi T, Sachs DH. Regulation of clinical xenotransplantation—time for a reappraisal. Transplantation. 2017 Aug;101(8):1766–9.
72. Michael J. Ross and P toby Coates. Using CRISPR to inactivate endogenous retroviruses in pigs: an important step toward safe xenotransplantation? Kidney Int. 2018;93:4–6.
73. Dong N, Wei H-J, Lin L, George H, Wang T, Lee I-H, Zhao H-Y, Wang Y, Kan Y, Shrock E, Lesha E, Wang G, Luo Y, Qing Y, Jiao D, Zhao H, Zhou X, Wang S, Wei H, Güell M, Church GM, Yang L. Inactivation of porcine endogenous retrovirus in pigs using CRISPR-Cas9. Science. 2017 Sep 22;357(6357):1303–7.
74. Jeroen B. van der Net, Bushell A, Wood KJ, Harden PN. Regulatory T cells: first steps of clinical application in solid organ transplantation. Transplant Int. First published: 2015 15 May https://doi.org/10.1111/tri.12608.
75. Kawai K, Uchiyama M, Hester J, Wood K, Issa F. Regulatory T cells for tolerance. Hum Immunol. 2018 May;79(5):294–303.
76. Fernandes S, Amirault J-C, Lande G, Nguyen J-M, Forest V, Bignolais O, Lamirault G, Heudes D, Orsonneau J-L, Heymann M-F, Charpentier F. Patricia Lemarchand. Autologous myoblast transplantation after myocardial infarction increases the inducibility of ventricular arrhythmias. Cardiovasc Res. 2006, 1 Feb;69(2):348–58.
77. Haider KH, Aziz S. Second volume "Stem Cells: From Hype to Real Hope". De Gruyter (2018).
78. Iop L, Sasso ED, Menabò R, Di Lisa F, Gerosa G. The rapidly evolving concept of whole heart engineering. Stem Cells Int. 2017;2017:8920940.
79. Ott HC, Matthiesen TS, Goh SK, et al. Perfusion-decellularized matrix: using nature's platform to engineer a bioartificial heart. Nat Med. 2008;14(2):213–21.

Lung and Heart-Lung Transplantation and Other Therapies for Lung Failure

8

Salim Aziz, Lambros Tsonis, Jenna E. Aziz,
Jai Shankar Raman, and Wickii T. Vigneswaran

8.1 Introduction

We have come a long way since the first lung transplantation was performed by James Hardy in 1964 [1]. With the advent of calcineurin inhibitors [2], the issues related to bronchial/tracheal healing have been minimized. Surgical techniques have largely been standardized. "Lung supportive therapy", extracorporeal membrane oxygenation (EC MO) before, during, and after transplantation has enhanced management of complex patients [3]. ISHLT (International Society of Heart and Lung Transplantation) reports that over 50,000 transplants have been performed worldwide with approximately 4600 performed in 2017 (Fig. 8.1), with 1 and 5 year survivals of 80% and 54% respectively [4]. The Achilles heel of long-term survival after trans-

plantation remains bronchiolitis obliterans [5]. A continued shortage of donors limits wider use of lung transplantation.

Lung transplantation is a potential treatment option for carefully selected patients with very advanced chronic lung disease who continue to deteriorate despite best medical therapy. However, it must be remembered that pulmonary transplantation in itself is not a cure, but rather another form of treatment. The post-transplant care requires close management of the patient and the long-term use of immunosuppressive therapy and monitoring for rejection, infection etc.

Numerous studies have shown that after successful lung transplant there is a marked improvement in quality of life and survival advantage in patients with cystic fibrosis (CF), idiopathic pulmonary fibrosis and pulmonary hypertension. However, for other conditions such as chronic obstructive pulmonary disease (COPD), improved quality of life may not be associated with an overall increase in survival. In the climate of limited donor supply these factors must be taken into account (Fig. 8.2). Patients with end-stage lung disease who may be candidates for lung transplantation must be referred to centers of excellence early, so that appropriate evaluation and bridge to transplantation options are considered. On the horizon are other mechanical and biological therapies that can support the failing lung and will also be addressed in this chapter.

S. Aziz
George Washington University,
Washington, DC, USA

L. Tsonis · W. T. Vigneswaran (✉)
Loyola University Health System,
Maywood, IL, USA
e-mail: LTSONIS@lumc.edu;
Wickii.vigneswaran@lumc.edu

J. E. Aziz
Howard University College of Medicine,
Washington, DC, USA
e-mail: Jenna.aziz@bison.howard.edu

J. S. Raman
University of Melbourne, Melbourne, Australia

© Springer Nature Switzerland AG 2021
N. Hakim et al. (eds.), *Transplantation Surgery*, Springer Specialist Surgery Series,
https://doi.org/10.1007/978-3-030-55244-2_8

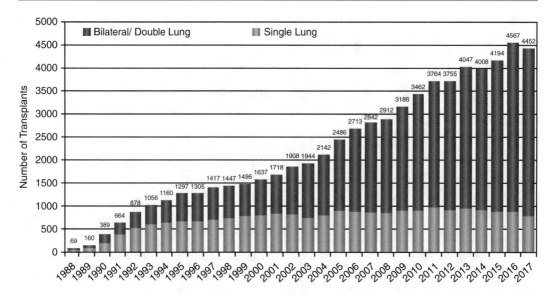

Fig. 8.1 Number of adult lung transplants by year and procedure type (transplants: 1988–2017). Ref: J Heart Lung Transplant. 2019 Oct; 38(10):1042–1055. Published online 2019 Aug 8

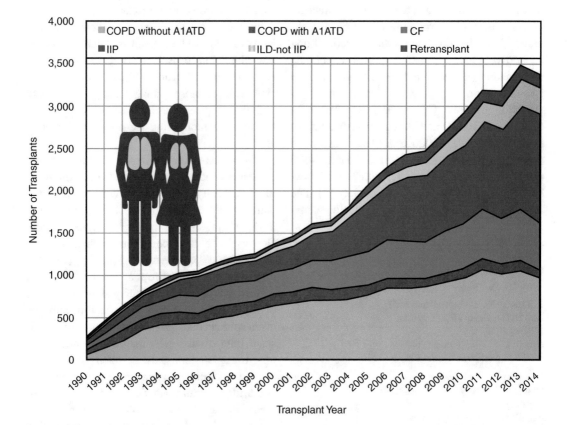

Fig. 8.2 Major indications for adult lung transplantation by year (absolute number; transplants: 1990–2017). *A1ATD* alpha-1-antitrypsin deficiency, *CF* cystic fibrosis, *COPD* chronic obstructive pulmonary disease, *IIP* idio- pathic interstitial pneumonia, *ILD-not IIP* interstitial lung disease-not idiopathic interstitial pneumonia. Ref: J Heart Lung Transplant. 2019 Oct; 38(10): 1042–1055. Published online 2019 Aug 8

8.1.1 Recipient Selection

Patients should be considered for lung transplantation when the risk of mortality from their lung disease is greater than 50% within the next 2 years. If transplantation is performed before this point, the peri-operative mortality risks may outweigh the potential benefits. Selecting this "tipping point" in risk requires experience and judgement. Guidelines are provided by ISHLT, Table 8.1.

Disease-specific indications are shown in Table 8.1. Recipient evaluation and contraindications are outlined in Table 8.2. The type of operation is considered, single, double, lobar or heart-lung block Lung transplantation. This is determined when the patient is listed for transplantation.

Currently the upper limit of recipient age in most centers is 65 years, although older patients without added comorbidities are transplanted in centers with a large experience. Indications for lung transplantation are outlined in Table 8.1.

The timing of listing a patient for lung transplantation is also important. General contraindications are outlined in Table 8.2. We know that certain subsects of patients requiring lung transplantation are at higher risk of dying while waiting for transplant, e.g. patients with pulmonary arterial hypertension and pulmonary fibrosis. These patients get extra "points" added and are placed higher on the waiting list. The latest UNOS listing scheme for recipients is outlined in Table 8.3, which take into account these recipient factors for lung allocation.

The role of re-transplantation for acute and or chronic graft failure (largely due to bronchiolitis obliterans) remains a topic of debate, especially in the current climate of donor shortage [8, 9].

Now with ECMO therapy being widely available, patients who are deteriorating can be supported (and allowed mobility) without recourse to intubation [3]. Emerging data suggest limiting anticoagulation therapy is safe during protracted ECMO and hopefully this will decrease the need for transfusions and the added risk thereby of increasing antibody formation [10].

Table 8.1 Disease-specific indication for transplant [6]

Guidelines for lung transplantation for common disease indications	
Idiopathic pulmonary fibrosis	COPD
Timing of Referral: At the time of clinical diagnosis Timing of Listing FYC<65% predicted · DLCO<40% predicted 6 MWD <250 m ≥10% decline in FVC over 6 months ≥15% decline in DLCO over 6 months >50 m decline in 6 MWD over 6 m Desaturation to <88% during 6 MW Extensive and or worsening fibrosis on HRCT Presence of significant pulmonary hypertension Moderate to severe and or worsening dyspnea · History of respiratory hospitalization	Timing of Referral (presence of 1 or more): · BODE index (composite score of body mass index, FEV_1, degree of dyspnea and 6 minute walk distance) ≥5 Hypoxemia (PaO_2 < 60 mmHg) and or hypercapnia ($PaCO_2$ >50 mmHg) FEV_1 < 25% of predicted Progressive disease despite optimal medical therapy, including pulmonary rehabilitation Timing of listing (presence of 1 or more) BODE index ≥ 7. FEV_1 < 15% to 20% predicted. Frequent exacerbations · Episode of acute hypercapnic respiratory failure · Moderate to severe pulmonary hypertension
Cystic fibrosis	Pulmonary Arterial Hypertension (PAH)
Timing of Referral: · FEV_1 < 30% of predicted, or a rapid decline in FEV_1, particularly in females · Increasing frequency of exacerbations · Exacerbation requiring non-invasive ventilation · Recurrent or refractory pneumothorax or massive hemoptysis · Worsening nutritional status despite supplementation · Increasing antibiotic resistance · 6 min walk <400 m Timing of Transplant Hypercapnia ($PaCO_2$ > 50 mmHg) Hypoxemia (PaO_2 < 60 mmHg) Advanced functional limitation · Pulmonary hypertension	Timing of Referral · NYHA functional class III–IV with escalating therapy · Rapidly progressive disease · Known or suspected pulmonary venoocclusive disease or pulmonary capillary hemangiomatosis · Timing of Transplant · Persistent NYHA class HI–IV despite maximal medical therapy · Cardiac index <2 L/min/m² · Right atrial pressure>15 mmHg · Other clinical and/or imaging evidence of RV failure · Massive hemoptysis

Table 8.2 Absolute and relative contraindications for transplant [6]

Absolute contraindications	Relative contraindications
Active smoking or substance abuse	Age > 65
Current malignancy (excluding some skin cancers)	Bilateral pulmonary sepsis or infection with multi-drug resistant organisms (for single lungs)
Co-existing organ failure, other than pulmonary failure	Ventilator or ECMO dependence
Active *Mycobacterium Tuburculosis* infection	Severe malnutrition or obesity
Irreversible left heart failure or uncorrectable severe coronary artery disease	Dependence on high dose steroids
Medical instability, including, but not limited to, sepsis, myocardial infarction, or liver failure, or uncontrollable bleeding diathesis	Active hepatitis B or C with signs of liver damage
Severe connective tissue disorders with significant extra-thoracic manifestations	Severe, symptomatic osteoporosis
Severe untreated psychiatric disorders or significant medical non-compliance	Extensive prior thoracic surgery, lung resection, or pleurodesis
Infection with highly virulent or multi-drug resistant organisms including bacteria, mycobacteria, or fungi in extrapulmonary locations or with poor control pre-transplant	Recent history of malignancy (within 2 years for most malignancies and within 5 years for breast cancer or melanoma)
Inability to walk with poor rehabilitation potential	Presence of significant esophageal dysfunction
Lack of health insurance or financial means to pay for medical care	HIV infection (transplant can be considered if undetectable HIV-RNA and compliance with good anti-retroviral regimen)
	Spinal deformity that would cause pulmonary restriction
	Infection with *Burkholderia cenocepacia, Burkholderia gladioli,* or *Mycobacterium abscessus*
	Lack of social or family support
	Availability of an alternative treatment plan

8.2 Effect of Elevated Panel Reactive Antibodies (PRA)

In lung transplantation it has been reported that PRA-positive patients have higher rates of cellular rejection and BOS rates [11]. Ashish et al. [12] in examination of UNOS data set looking at over 10,000 patients (1987–2005), reported that PRA exceeding 25% is associated with increased death. Their study also suggested that from 1998 through 2005, highly sensitized patients no longer have the same mortality risk. However, the risk of rejection and chronic allograft failure was not reported.

8.2.1 The Donor

There remains a major imbalance between donor supply and recipient demand in lung transplanta-

tion. Presently less than 30% of multi-organ donors are suitable for lung transplantation. Characteristics of the ideal donor are outlined in Table 8.4. Unfortunately, few donors meet the ideal criteria and extended criteria and marginal donors are often considered. At times a marginal donor can be improved prior to explantation by assiduous attention to donor management. Careful fluid balance should be maintained and requires close cooperation between the various harvesting teams and the local organ procuring organization (OPO). Fluid overload resulting in pulmonary edema must be avoided. Pulmonary toilet including use of frequent bronchoscopy and early involvement of the pulmonary team is helpful. Sometimes only one lung may be able to be procured.

In addition to size measurement on CXR and comparisons of estimated total lung capacity (TLC) between donor and recipient there must be blood group compatibility.

Table 8.3 The lung allocation score [7]

Clinical variables used for lung allocation score calculation	
Characteristics for waiting list model	Characteristics tor post-transplant model
Age (years)	Age at transplant (years)
Body mass index (kg/m²)	Creatinine at transplant (mg/dL)
Diabetes	New York Heart Association functional class
New York Heart Association functional class	Forced vital capacity for groups B and D (% predicted)
Forced vital capacity (% predicted)	Pulmonary capillary wedge pressure mean ≥20 mm Hg for group D
Pulmonary arterial systolic pressure for diagnosis groups A, C, and D	Mechanical ventilation
Oxygen requirements at rest (L/mm)	Diagnosis groups[a]
Six-minute walk distance (feet)	Diagnosis detailed[b]
Continuous mechanical ventilation	
Diagnosis groups[a]	
Diagnosis detailed[b]	

[a]Diagnosis groups
A = Obstructive lung disease
B = Pulmonary vascular disease
C = Cystic fibrosis or immunodeficiency disorder
D = Restrictive lung disease
[b]Diagnosis detailed
Bronchiectasis
Eisenmenger syndrome
Lymphangioleiomyomatosis
Obliterative bronchiolitis
Pulmonary fibrosis, other
Sarcoidosis and pulmonary arterial pressure mean >30 mm Hg
Sarcoidosis and pulmonary arterial pressure mean ≤30 mm Hg
- The waitlist urgency measure (WLi), which predicts the number of days an individual with a specific set of characteristics is expected to live during the next year on the waiting list (range 0–365).
- The post–transplant survival measure (PTi), which predicts the number of days an individual is expected to live during the first year after the lung transplantation (range 0–365).
The raw allocation score is calculated using the following equation:
Raw Score = PTi − 2WLi
The raw score can range from −730 to 365. A final lung allocation score (0–100) is obtained by normalization of the raw score

$$\text{Lung Allocation Score} = 100\left[\text{Raw Score} - \text{minimum}\right]/\text{Range}$$
$$= 100\left[\text{Raw Score} - (-730)\right]/1095$$
$$= 100\left[\text{Raw Score} = 730\right]/1095$$

8.2.2 Recent Developments to Enhance Donor Use

Two recent developments increase the availability of donors for transplantation. (1) Use of ex vivo perfusion techniques as a means to assess and "optimize" marginal or unsuitable donor lungs [13]. (2) Use of donors of cardiac death (DCD) [14]. Evidence suggest that outcomes in recipients of DCD are comparable to brain death (BD) donors [15] without an increase in primary graft dysfunction (PGD).

Steen et al. [13] were the first to use ex vivo lung perfusion (EVLP) prior to transplant, and experience has been steadily growing with the use of EVLP to optimize marginal lungs. EVLP involves controlled ventilation and perfusion of the lungs, with a number of different perfusates being available [15, 16]. This has allowed lungs to be optimized in controlled environment and rule in or out a suboptimal lung such as allowing us to screen out lungs with early pneumonia, which typically do not improve on EVLP and can then be discarded [17].

In special circumstances living (related and non-related) donors have been used for lobar transplantation particularly in cystic fibrosis, or where in circumstances where cadaveric lung donation is limited [18]. This type of operation however is limited due to donor associated risks. The rate of heart-lung en-block transplantation worldwide has declined over the past few years (Fig. 8.3).

8.3 The Operation

8.3.1 Donor Procurement

Prior to starting the explant procedure, flexible bronchoscopy is repeated. This is done both to

Table 8.4 Ideal lung donor criteria

Age	20–45
PaO$_2$:FiO$_2$	>350
Smoking history	None
Chest X-ray	Clear
Ventilation days	<5
Microbiology	Grain stain negative
Bronchoscopy	Clear
Ischemic time	<4 h

clear any secretions that may be present and to assess bronchial anatomy. Secretions that clear easily and reveal normal, non-erythematous mucosa are not significant [19]. Secretions that re-accumulate after appropriate suctioning indicate the presence of pneumonia and generally indicate unsuitability of the donor's lungs for transplantation, but if this is confined to one lung the other lung may be used. If bronchial abnormalities, such as takeoff of the right upper lobe bronchus from the trachea, are found, this does not preclude the use of the donor's lungs but this needs to be communicated to the implanting team.

A median sternotomy incision is made, followed by creating a pericardial well after both pleura are widely opened and lungs are inspected. Initially, the lungs are palpated to evaluate for masses or adhesions, and visually inspected to look for consolidation or contusion. The lungs are then gently expanded to 25 cm H$_2$O pressure, and any areas of atelectasis are examined to ensure they are recruitable. The anesthesiologist is then instructed to break the ventilator circuit and the lungs are observed as they deflate. Palpation of the deflated lungs is performed to look for occult masses. Ventilation is then

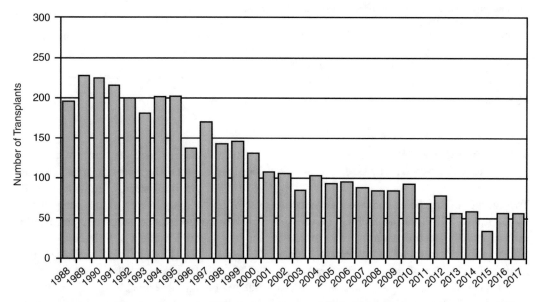

Fig. 8.3 Number of adult heart-lung transplants by transplant year. Ref: J Heart Lung Transplant. 2019 Oct; 38(10):1042–1055. Published online 2019 Aug 8

resumed, typically at tidal volumes of 6–8 cc/kg of tidal volume, FiO_2 of 1.00, and PEEP of 5 to minimize barotrauma. [20]. Arterial blood gases are generally checked about 15–20 min after the bronchoscopy, and PO_2 should be >300 on the above settings. Selective pulmonary venous gases may be drawn during procurement if needed. During procurement, every effort is made to minimize fluid administration during the case, and, in some cases, diuretics may be necessary to treat pulmonary edema. Recruitment maneuvers with gentle "hand-bagging" and the administration of bronchodilators may also be used. Contusions, areas of consolidation, masses, significant bullae, or areas of infarction are generally contraindications to the use of a set of lungs.

Once the lungs are deemed to be appropriate for transplantation, this is communicated to the recipient team so that the recipient operation can be scheduled to keep ischemia time less than 8 h [21, 22].

Dissection is carried out to separate the pulmonary artery from the aorta. The aorta is circumferentially controlled and separated not only from the main pulmonary artery, but also from the right pulmonary artery as it courses under the ascending aorta. The superior vena cava (SVC) is also separated from the right pulmonary artery. The trachea is usually exposed above the innominate vein and is circumferentially controlled. The SVC is controlled above the attachment of the azygos vein, and the azygos is ligated and divided. During this time, there is an ongoing discussion with the cardiac procurement team regarding sites of pulmonary arterial cannulation, strategy for venting the left side of the heart, and cuff length of the left atrium. Venting the left side of the heart can be accomplished either by dividing the left atrial appendage or by direct entry into the left atrium via Sondergaard's grove. Developing Sondergaard's groove adequately is essential to ensuring adequate left atrial cuff length (Fig. 8.4). Since this can cause bleeding or atrial fibrillation, this step can be done after heparin administration just prior to crossclamp. If the heart is not going to be transplanted, this mobilization should be done by the lung team to

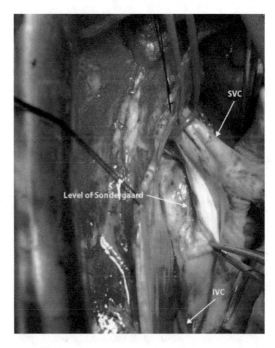

Fig. 8.4 Incision in the Atrium along the Sodergaard grove

ensure all the left atrium is left attached to the pulmonary veins during procurement [23].

When the time is ready to procure, the lung and heart team must work in concert. The donor is heparinized with 30,000 units of heparin, and given 3 min to circulate. A purse-string suture with 4–0 Prolene is placed at the bifurcation of the pulmonary artery and the pulmonary artery is cannulated. This cannula is directed towards the pulmonic valve to ensure equal perfusion of both lungs. Once all teams are ready, 500 ucg of PGE1 is given directly into the pulmonary artery [24]. This serves as a potent pulmonary vasodilator, and will often cause significant systemic hypotension. Once this is given, the SVC is ligated, the left atrium is opened (either through the left atrial appendage or via Sondergaard's groove), the anterior part of the IVC is divided, and the aortic crossclamp is applied. The early studies by Haverich et al. showed the benefit of using flush techniques using Euro-Collins solution [25]. Presently many centers use Perfadex [26] and 60 ml/kg is given. The antegrade pulmonoplegia is then started, taking care to keep the infusion pressure 10–15 mmHg. This is best accomplished by hanging the bag about 30 cm above the donor and allowing the infusion to run in by gravity. Care is taken to keep pulmonoplegia away from the coronary tree. As the lungs are being perfused, the heart and lungs are covered in cold saline and icy slush. Every effort is made to avoid lifting the heart (as this can cause incompetence of the pulmonic valve), and the effluent from the left atrium is examined to ensure it adequately clears. The atriotomy on the left atrium needs to be adequate to ensure the left atrium is completely decompressed. The lungs are also examined to make sure they blanche appropriately. The lungs continue to be ventilated, but the FiO_2 is reduced to 50%.

Once the pulmonoplegia has been given, the heart explant is performed. The SVC is divided, and any remaining attachments to the right pulmonary artery are divided. The IVC is transected, and the pericardium up to the right inferior pulmonary vein is divided. The left atrium is then divided, leaving an adequate cuff of left atrium attached to the pulmonary veins. On the left side, the midpoint between the base of the left atrial appendage and the takeoff of the left superior pulmonary vein is incised (Fig. 8.5). On the right side, adequate development of Sondergaard's AV

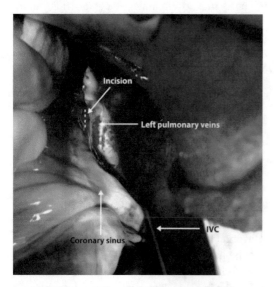

Fig. 8.5 Incision on the left side of the left atrium, showing the relative locations of the left pulmonary veins and the coronary sinus

groove will facilitate this division. Care must be taken as one cuts under the IVC to leave some left atrium attached to the heart and also some attached to the right inferior pulmonary vein. It is essential to visualize each pulmonary vein to avoid injuries as the atrium is divided. Superiorly, the coronary sinus should be avoided, and the adventitial attachments to the right pulmonary artery will need to be divided. The aorta is then divided, and the pulmonoplegia cannula is removed and the cannulation site is incised. The pulmonary artery is then divided at its bifurcation; this is often best visualized from the left side of the operating table. The heart is then able to be removed [27].

The pulmonary explant is begun by dividing the pericardium at the level of the diaphragm down to the inferior pulmonary ligaments bilaterally. These incisions are then connected in front of the esophagus, taking care to avoid the cut end of the IVC. The inferior pulmonary ligaments are then divided, down to the inferior pulmonary veins. The lungs are then each medially rotated, and the posterior mediastinal pleura is divided up to the lung apices. On the right, this means dividing the azygos vein. Above the carina, the esophagus will need to be carefully separated from the trachea to avoid injury to the membranous portion. On the left, the aorta will be encountered and should be divided. The innominate vein is then divided, and the tissues anterior to the trachea are incised. The soft tissues on the right of the trachea are divided down to the level of the esophagus. The soft tissues on the left are divided down to the level of the transected aorta. The trachea is then palpated, and the endotracheal tube is pulled back by the anesthesiologist if needed. Two firings of a TA-30 stapler with 4.8 mm staples are used to staple the trachea with the lungs inflated to 25 cm H_2O pressure. The trachea is incised with a scalpel between the staple lines, and any remaining soft tissue is divided. The lungs are then brought out to the back table. If the retrograde flush was not done in the field, it can be done at this time. The lungs are then separated on the back table. This is done by first dividing the left atrium into left and right halves. The pulmonary arteries are

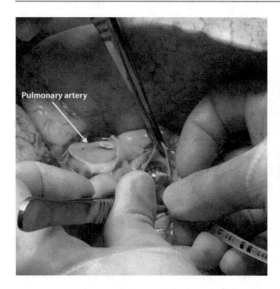

Fig. 8.6 Retrograde flush through individual pulmonary veins

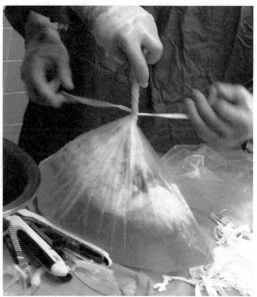

Fig. 8.7 Each of the lungs is then triple bagged, with 1 L of Perfadex solution placed in the innermost bag and 1 L of cold saline and ice in each of the other bags

then divided along the bifurcation ridge into left and right halves. The pericardium is then divided up to the carina. Finally, the left bronchus is separated from the trachea and the right bronchus with a single firing of a GIA 60 stapler with 4.8 mm staples.

A retrograde flush through individual pulmonary veins are performed of the lungs typically using 500 ml of cold Perfadex solution, following the antegrade flush. This can be done either in the field at this time, or on the back table after the lungs are taken out (Fig. 8.6). As this is being done, the effluent from the pulmonary arteries is examined to ensure that the effluent becomes clear. It is often than not there may be clots or debris in the effluent.

Each of the lungs is then triple bagged, with 1 L of Perfadex solution placed in the innermost bag and 1 L of cold saline and ice in each of the other bags. Each bag is securely tied after all the air is evacuated, and the bags are labelled for laterality and placed on ice for transport to the recipient hospital (Fig. 8.7).

In cases where EVLP systems are being used, the system and protocols should be used as described by the individual center. In general, the lungs are not separated during an EVLP procurement.

Injuries during procurement are relatively uncommon. Tracheal injuries usually affect the membranous trachea and can cause rapid deflation of the lungs. If this occur, an endotracheal tube can be inserted into the cut end of the trachea, and the lungs can be hand-bagged to appropriate expansion. Once the level of the tracheal injury has been identified, the trachea can be clamped below this level and stapled to allow the lungs to remain inflated.

The most common arterial injury is division of the right pulmonary artery instead of the main pulmonary artery. If the right or left pulmonary artery is injured, a segment of descending aorta can be harvested to use as an interposition graft. Pulmonary venous injuries can be much more difficult to manage, as the cut pulmonary vein may retract into the lung parenchyma if it is completely transected. This is most often caused by inadequate visualization of the pulmonary veins during division of the left atrium, or during the division of the inferior pulmonary ligament. In those cases, donor pericardium can be used to help reconstruct the pulmonary vein. As always, communication with the recipient team when an injury is discovered is essential.

8.4   Recipient Operation

8.4.1   Explantation Procedure

For all lung transplants, we typically place a double-lumen endotracheal tube and a Swan-Ganz catheter. For a single lung transplant, the patient is usually positioned in a lateral or semi-lateral position and a left or right thoracotomy incision is made in the fifth intercostal space. Whenever possible, muscle-sparing incisions should be used. For a double lung transplant, the patient is placed supine on the operating table, and the arms are extended above the patient's head and appropriately supported in a neutral position. Either bilateral thoracotomies or a clam-shell incision are made (Fig. 8.8). The clam-shell provides excellent exposure to the whole thorax, and makes central cannulation easier if cardiopulmonary bypass is needed, but requires division of both internal mammary arteries and there are reports of poor sternal healing. Alternatively, some centers perform a median sternotomy for double lung transplant. This only requires a single lumen endotracheal tube, but does require cardiopulmonary bypass. Also, exposure to the pulmonary hila can be difficult from this approach, especially with any degree of cardiac hypertrophy or mediastinal lymphadenopathy.

Regardless of the approach used, all adhesions must be carefully taken down and meticulous attention to hemostasis is essential. With a sternotomy, this is especially important as the posterior mediastinum cannot be easily visualized once the lungs have been implanted. Depending on the patient's diagnosis, abscesses or significant mediastinal lymphadenopathy may complicate the pneumonectomy. While exposure and control of the pulmonary vessels can be obtained at any time, division of the vessels is not done until the donor lung is in the operating room. The pulmonary veins are either ligated and divided or stapled as distal as possible. The pulmonary artery is also kept as long as possible and divided with staplers. Care is taken to pull back the Swan-Ganz catheter before division of the pulmonary artery. The bronchus is divided after the takeoff of the lobar bronchi using electrocautery. Mediastinal lymph nodes other than those around the bronchus or pulmonary artery are generally left undisturbed if possible, to minimize bleeding. Bleeding from bronchial arteries is controlled with clips or electrocautery. Dissection around the bronchus is minimized to avoid disrupting the bronchial circulation, but the bronchus is separated from the pulmonary artery and prepared with the knife before anastomosis. Next, the pericardial reflection around the pulmonary artery and vein is divided. This helps facilitate clamp placement.

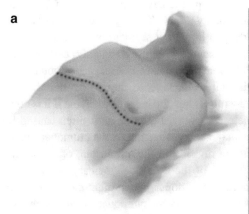
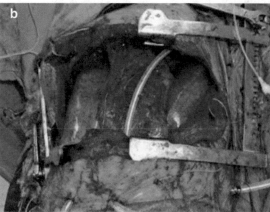

Fig. 8.8 (**a**) Bilateral thoracotomies or (**b**) a clam-shell incision

8.4.2 Implant Procedure [24, 27, 28]

Once the donor lung arrives in the operating room, it is carefully examined for surgical damage and for atrial cuff size, PA size, and bronchial size. The PA, atrial cuff and bronchus are mobilized from each other. We perform a retrograde flush with cold Perfadex solution in the back bench prior to starting implantation. On the back table, the bronchus is divided, deflating the lung and obtaining a specimen for bronchial culture. The bronchus is then divided, leaving no more than 2 rings between the cut end of the bronchus and the takeoff of the first lobe. The order of sewing structures can be variable depending on surgeon preference. We prefer to perform the PA anastomosis last. Most surgeons will sew the bronchus or left atrial anastomosis first. If you are performing the atrial anastomosis the recipient bronchus is not cut until the donor lung is seated in the chest. We typically use a running 4–0 PDS suture for the membranous portion of the bronchus, and interrupted 4–0 PDS figure-of-eight sutures for the cartilaginous portion of the bronchus. We tend to use 4–0 Prolene for atrial and 5–0 Prolene for PA anastomoses. Care must be taken to avoid kinking of the pulmonary artery particularly on the right side and excess tissue needs to be removed before anastomosis. For LA anastomosis, care must be taken to approximate intima to intima to avoid a nidus for thrombus formation. This anastomosis should be performed widely to avoid obstruction of venous outflow. Suitable measures to de-air the pulmonary circulation must be used before the LA clamp is finally removed. Gradual reperfusion must be established to minimize injury from ischemia–reperfusion. When performing sequential double lung transplant, adequate time for reperfusion of the newly transplanted lung is given before the second pneumonectomy is performed. Once the transplant is completed, the Swan-Ganz is re-advanced into the pulmonary artery while the chest is open. Meticulous hemostasis is achieved before closing the chest. Bronchoscopy is performed at the end of the case, both to assess the bronchial anastomoses and to clear any secretions, blood clots and debris present.

It is unusual to have technical complication with this technique of allograft implantation. However, one must keep in mind possibilities of pulmonary vein stenosis, gradients across pulmonary artery anastomosis, bronchial stenosis, stricture and dehiscence. TEE and flexible bronchoscopy are useful in evaluating such concerns. When detected early, appropriate intervention must be considered (endovascular, stents or open repair) [24].

8.4.3 Lobar Lung Transplantation

Living donor lobar lung transplantation is a rare procedure performed in some centers in the US. It was championed by Starnes [18] and colleagues, but has also been used in Japan, England, Brazil, and China. The most common indication is cystic fibrosis, although other indications has been treated with lobar transplantation. It is most often performed in children or young adults. It is typically performed by harvesting lower lobes from two living donors and then transplanting the lobes into a single recipient. Usually, the larger donor has their right lower lobe harvested, and the smaller donor has their left lower lobe harvested. Size matching of both donor lobes and the recipient are essential for good outcomes, both in terms of anatomic size and function. The recipient operation is usually performed via a clamshell incision and with the use of cardiopulmonary bypass. The technical aspects of the implant are similar to the technique described above.

8.4.4 General Anesthesia Issues

In our practice, all patients have a double-lumen endotracheal tube and a Swan-Ganz catheter placed preoperatively. Single lung transplants are not performed on patients with significant pulmonary hypertension; those patients either receive double lung transplants or have their transplant deferred if discovered intraoperatively. Nitric oxide or inhaled prostaglandins (Velitri) are useful adjuncts in this setting. In some patients with advanced lung disease, ECMO may be started preoperatively; this is typically contin- ued postoperatively as needed. If cardiopulmo- nary bypass (CPB) is needed during the transplant, either central cannulation or femoral cannulation can be used and partial or full flow may be used depending on the circumstance. In centers that do double lung transplant using a median sternotomy with full CPB, single lumen alone may be adequate but having double lumen intubation help to independently ventilate lung if necessary.

Fluid management is essential to avoid signifi- cant pulmonary edema. In single lung transplant, acute increases in pulmonary airway pressures or hemodynamic instability may indicate tension pneumothorax of the contralateral side or signifi- cant auto-PEEP. This must be rapidly recognized and corrected.

8.4.5 Role of ECMO in Lung Transplantation

With better circuitry (cannula, pumps, heparin bonded tubing, miniaturization) and the ability to minimize heparin doses or use alternate anti- coagulants, there has been increasing consider- ation to use ECMO at various stages of lung transplantation process. *Donor*: Experience sug- gests it can be used to better manage the donor prior to organ harvesting, to manage the explanted allograft to "recover" marginal donors and "test them" for suitability for implantation (EVLP) and to extend the "safe" period of lon- ger ischemic times (Fig. 8.9). *Recipients*: ECMO can also be used to manage the deterio- rating recipient prior to lung transplantation and thereby avoid use of conventional mechanical ventilation. In these patients, it is usually used in the VV (veno-venous ECMO) format and often as a single cannula with double lumen configuration via the internal jugular vein which allows for ambulation and rehabilitation. It can also be used intra-operatively in lieu of using classical CPB circuits. Postoperatively ECMO can be used to support the allograft and or the recipient in a VV or VA (Veno-arterial format) configuration for primary graft failure (PGF), severe rejection, infectious or technical complications.

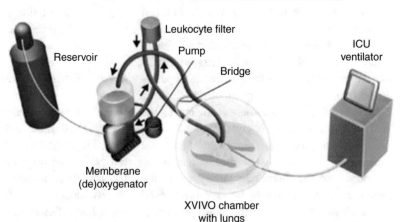

Fig. 8.9 Toronto Ex Vivo Lung Perfusion (EVLP) system

8.4.6 Post-Transplant Issues

These maybe considered at different time periods (a) early post operatively within days to weeks after transplantation (b) weeks to months and then finally long-term complications (months to years).

8.4.7 Intra-Operative Management

Prior to allowing reperfusion of the transplanted lung, 500–1000 mg of Solumedrol are given. It is key to prevent hyper-perfusion of the newly implanted lung and also to prevent excessive airway pressure during re-establishment of ventilation of the implanted lung. Gentle "hand bagging" efforts to open areas of atelectasis /collapse are employed.

8.4.8 Immediate Post-Operative Management

The double lumen tube is changed to a single lumen tube at the end of surgery. Patients are ventilated with pressure control ventilation, aiming to use a lung protective strategy. The usual parameters of ventilator weaning are used. Most patients are extubated within hours of the completion of the transplant assuming there are no issues related to the transplanted lung (severe reperfusion injury, bleeding, pulmonary edema, evidence of PGF etc.). Evidence of lung injury (ischemia-reperfusion, preservation, immune mediated etc.) may necessitate a more prolonged period of intubation. Careful attention to fluid management in the early post-operative period is essential. The transplanted lung is devoid of functioning lymphatics and is especially sensitive to volume loading. Early use of diuretics helps optimize lung function, and will help with minimizing chest tube output. Nitric oxide, intravenous or inhaled prostaglandins (Flolan, Veletri), or intravenous vasodilators are helpful in managing early pulmonary hypertension. In cases with early primary graft dysfunction, ECMO is a useful adjunct and should be used early.

8.4.9 Primary Graft Dysfunction (PGD) After Lung Transplantation

The term really includes a spectrum from mild to severe lung injury seen within the first 72 h after lung transplantation. The etiology is probably multifactorial (Table 8.5). The incidence is between 11 and 57% and is said to account for approximately 25% of the deaths within 30 days [29, 30]. In 2005, the ISHLT published their standardized definition that was updated in 2016 (Table—ISHLT PGD definition). Approximately 10–15% of recipients develop the severe form of PGD (Table 8.6).

Table 8.5 Key factors that may confound and/or amplify a diagnosis of primary graft dysfunction

Key post-lung transplant factors that may confound and/or amplify a diagnosis of primary graft dysfunction[a]
Airway
Blocked endotracheal lube/poor positioning
Blocked bronchus/distal airways with sputum or blood
Vascular
Arterial anastomotic obstruction
Venous anastomotic obstruction
Cardiac
Acute Left ventricular cardiac dysfunction
Right and left ventricular dys-synchrony in patients with
Significant pre-operative pulmonary hypertension
Parenchymal
Infection
Rejection
Aspiration
Hemorrhage
Transfusion-related acute Lung injury
Systemic inflammatory response syndrome
Pleural
Hemorrhage
Effusion
Pneumothorax
Open chest

[a]Not exhaustive and not listed, in order of frequency

8.4.10 Infection

All patients treated with immunosuppressants are prone to opportunistic infections. In addition, at times of augmented immunosuppression e.g. to treat rejection or in the early phase when induction therapy is being used, there is also an increased incidence of infections.

Infection related to the allograft. The source of allograft infections can be from the donor lung, such as occult pneumonia, or from organisms already present in the recipient at the time of transplantation, especially in cystic fibrosis. Also, patient transplanted across CMV mismatch status can get CMV infections.

8.4.11 Immunosuppression

Although these may vary from center to center, Table 8.7 [31] outlines a commonly used approach. In the meantime, challenges remain of managing the long-term complications of chronic immunosuppression. Ideally regimens that allow development of tolerance will be the key to successful long-term allograft implantation. Such approaches utilizing a combination of Treg and minimal immunosuppression are being evaluated in renal transplantation [32].

Other long-term complications associated with lung transplantation are outlined in Table 8.8.

Table 8.6 International society for heart and lung transplant primary graft dysfunction definition

The 2016 international society for heart and lung transplantation primary graft dysfunction definition		
Grade	Pulmonary edema on chest X-ray	Pao_2/Fio_2 ratio
PGD grade 0	No	Any
PGD grade 1	Yes	>300
PGD grade 2	Yes	200–300
PGD grade 3	Yes	<200

Table 8.7 Immunosuppression strategies for lung transplant

Basiliximab (standard Induction therapy): 20 mg IVPB intra-operatively and on post-operative day 4
Corticosteroids (standard maintenance therapy): Methylprednisolone 1,000 mg IV Intra-operatively than 125 mg IV every 12 h X 2 doses on post-operative day 1 than 20 mg IV every 12 h X 6 doses on post-operative day 2–4 then prednisone 0.5 mg/kg/day for 7 doses on post-operative day 5–11 with further taper by 5 mg every 7 days down to 20 mg dally through month 1. If no refection at 1 month bronchoscopy, taper by 2.5 mg per month to 5 mg daily by month 6 post-transplant
Calcineurin inhibitor (standard maintenance therapy)
Tacrollmus (first-line): 1mg sublingual every 12 h beginning post-operative day 1 (may delay start If shock or acute kidney injury), titrate every 2–3 days to goal 12-h trough level; convert to oral route (2X sublingual dose) when able except continue sublingual route in cystic fibrosis patients due lo absorption concerns
Goal 12-h trough levels (ng/ml):
Months 1–6:10–12
Months 7–12: 8–10
Year 1–2: 6–10
>2 years: 6–8
If on mTOR inhibitor for rental Insufficiency: <1 year: 4–6 or >1 year 3–5
Cyclosporine, modified (second-line If Intolerant to tacrollmus): 100 mg by mouth or via feeding tube every 12 h; titrate every 2–4 days to goal li-h trough level
Goal 12-h trough levels (ng/ml):
Months 1–6: 250–300
Months 7–12: 200–250
Year 1–2: 150–200
>2 years: 100–150
If on mTOR inhibitor for renal insufficiency: <1 year 100–150 or a 1 year 50–100
Anti-metabolite/Cell Cycle Inhibitor (standard maintenance therapy):

Table 8.7 (continued)

Mycophenolate mofetil (first-line): 1000 mg by mouth pre-operatively then 1000 mg IVPB every 12 h post-operatively converted to by mouth/feeding tube route when able
– Mycophenolate mofetil dose can be Increased to 1500 mg every 12 h to control severe rejection
– Consider reduction in mycophenolate mofetil dose to 500 mg every 12 h or holding during severe infections
Azathioprine (second-line If Intolerant to mycophenolate): 2 mg/kg/day (round to nearest 25 mg)
Adjustments to mycophenolate mofetill or azathioprine dose for neutropenia:
– Reduce dose by one half for absolute neutrophil count (ANC) <2000 cell/mm^3 and hold for ANC <1000 cell/mm^3
– Resume poor dosing once ANC >2000 cell/mm^3 for 2 consecutive weeks
– For patients on azathioprine that develop mycophenolate consider checking thiopurine methyltransferase (TPMT) enzyme level
mTOR Inhibitor/Proliferation Signal inhibitor (alternate maintenance therapy):
Everolimus or Sirolimus: Used as a third-line agent if >30 days post-transplant, no open wounds, and no significant proteinuria at discretion of transplant physician for the following indications:
– Renal dysfunction: used in combination with low dose CNI, cell cycle inhibitor, and prednisone
– Cell cycle inhibitor intolerance: used in place of cell cycle inhibitor with standard dose CNI and prednisone
– Malignancy: used in place of cell cycle inhibitor with reduced dose or suspension of CNI and prednisone
– Chronic/persistent rejection: used in combination with standard-dose CNI, cell cycle inhibitor, and prednisone
Everollmus usual starting dose in absence of significant CYP 3A4 Inhibitors/Inducers: 0.75–1 mg by mouth every 12 h; titrate dose every 5 days to goal 12-h trough level 4–6 ng/ml (if in combination with CNI)
Strollamus usual starting dose in absence of significant CYP 3A4 Inhibitors/Inducers: 4 mg by mouth daily for 2 days then 2 mg by mouth daily; titrate dose every 7 days to goal 12-h trough level 4–7 ng/ml (if In combination with CNI)

Table 8.8 Chronic Complications of lung transplantation

Organ system or type of complication	Specific disorders
Cardiovascular	Systemic hypertension
	Cardiac rhythm disturbances
	Thromboembolism
	Atherosclerotic heart disease
Renal	Chronic renal insufficiency
	Renal failure
Gastrointestinal	Gastroesophageal reflux
	Biliary tract disease
	Bowel disorders (motility disorders, diverticulitis, etc.)
Metabolic/endocrine	Dyslipidemia
	Diabetes
	Excessive weight gain, obesity
	Electrolyte abnormalities
Musculoskeletal	Osteoporosis
	Myopathy
Hematologic	Anemia
	Cytopenia (leukocytes, platelets)
Neurologic	Tremor
	Secure
	Memory loss
	Neuropathy
Drug toxicity and side effects	Immunosuppressants
	Drug-drug interactions
Malignancy	Post-transplant lymphoproliferative disease
	Primary lung cancer
	Other malignancy

(continued)

Table 8.8 (continued)

Organ system or type of complication	Specific disorders
Lung allograft	Acute cellular rejection
	Infection
	Chronic lung allograft dysfunction
	Diaphragmatic dysfunction
	Disease recurrence
Native lung complications	Hyperinflation (emphysema as transplant indication)
	Infection
	Pneumothorax
Pleural disease	Effusion
	Pleural space infection
Chronic infection	Paranasal sinus disease
	Bronchiectatic lung (native or allograft)
Psychosocial problems	Disrupted support system
	Depression
	Medical noncompliance
	Multiple hospitalizations
	Resumption of addictive behaviors
Socioeconomic problems	Inadequate funds to cover medical costs
	Pressure on relationships
	Loss of insurance
	Disability, inability to find gainful employment

8.4.12 Rejection

Acute rejection: This may be cellular and or humoral. In this day and age, with current immunosuppressive regimens the incidence of acute rejection is between 50 and 60% [33, 34]. Clinical and radiological features may be suspicious for rejection. The diagnosis is confirmed by transbronchial biopsy and is made on H&E stains. The role of C4d immunostaining for antibody-mediated rejection in the lung is still evolving [35]. Immunostaining for lymphocyte markers (B- and T-cells) and in situ hybridization for EBV mRNA (EBER) and CMV can also e used as required. Treatment is usually with augmented immunosuppression.

8.4.12.1 Chronic Lung Allograft Dysfunction (CLAD)

It now appears that CLAD represents a range of disorders including BO [36] and restrictive allograft syndrome (RAS) [37]. RAS as a more aggressive clinical course with the lungs becoming smaller and smaller causing difficulty in lung expansion. BO is associated with clinical and histological features (Table 8.9 and Fig. 8.10). The etiology is probably multifactorial and is the main cause long term allograft dysfunction and re-transplantation.

These may be considered as general issues related to (a) effects of chronic Immunosuppression, and (b) those related to the transplanted lung itself. The transplanted lung itself eventually succumbs to BO, a phenomena whose clinical course and pathology is well described but whose therapy is far from effective.

8.4.13 Treatment of BO

The long-term impairment to successful lung transplantation remains bronchiolitis obliterans (BO). The etiology is probably multifactorial and includes ischemia-reperfusion injury, preservation, infection ongoing rejection etc. Some evidence suggests a role for injury-induced exhaustion of airway epithelial stem cells [39]. In its advanced stages, lung re-transplantation remains the only option. Results for re-transplantation are not as good as for primary transplantation and in these days of limited donor supply, careful consideration must be given to this therapy.

Table 8.9 Algorithm for clinical evaluation of suspected bronchiolitis obliterans syndrome [38]

```
            ┌─────────────────────────────────┐
            │ Suspected decline in lung function │
            └─────────────────────────────────┘
                             │
                             ▼
       ┌───────────────────────────────────────────┐
       │ Clinical evaluation                        │
       │   History and physical examination         │
       │   Spirometry (in PFT laboratory)           │
       │   Routine thoratic imaging (chest radiography) │
       │   Other testing based upon clinical presentation │
       └───────────────────────────────────────────┘
```

No significant abnormality
or
spirometric decline identified

FEV1 <90% of baseline
and/or FEF25-75% ≤75 of baseline
Non-BOS cause not identified

Observe

Consider HRCT if not recently performed[#]
Bronchoscopy
   Transbronchial biopsy
   Bronchoalveolar lavage
Evaluate for GOR

BOS is likely cause[¶]
Sustained and persistent FEV1
decline (FEV1 <80% baseline)

Other cause identified

Clinical diagnosis of BOS

Treat cause

Re-evaluate

Algorithm for clinical evaluation of suspected bronchiolitis obliterans syndrome (BOS). This algorithm is a description of the collective clinical practices of the committe members. It is not based upon systematically developed evidence-based diagnostic recommendation. PFT: pulmonary function test; FEV1: forced expiratory volume in 1 s: FEF25-75%: forced expiratory flow at 25–75% of the forced vital capacity; HRCT: high-resolution computed tomography GOR: gastro-oesophageal reflux. [#]: obtain both inspiratory and expiratory views to evaluate for air trapping; [¶]: the presence of bronchiolitis obliterans lessions on lung biopsy (if obtained) is considered diagnostic and HRCT findings consistent with bronchiolitis (*e.g.* air-trapping) are supportive, restrictive allograft syndrome is an alternative diagnostic consideration if a restrictive pattern is found on pulmonary function testing.

8.4.14 Survival

Survival after lung transplantation is significantly greater in the most recent era (2010–June 2017) compared to previous eras, however the difference has not been as profound as previously noted in the recent past (Fig. 8.11). For adults who underwent primary lung transplantation in the most recent era, the median survival was 6.7 years (Fig. 8.12). For adult recipients who survived to 1 year after primary transplant, the median survival in the most recent cohort was 8.9 years. Female recipients, recipients with CF as the indication for transplantation and recipi-

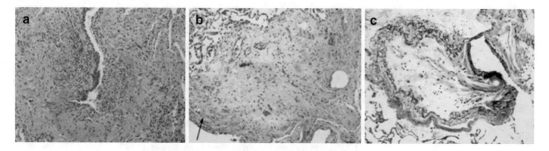

Fig. 8.10 Histological features of bronchiolitis obliterans on lung biopsy. (**a**) Bronchiolitis obliterans in a surgical lung biopsy with partial luminal compromise accompanied by mild chronic inflammation in the wall and focal ulceration of the mucosa. (**b**) Bronchiolitis obliterans on a transbroncheal biopsy with complete luminal obliteration. Scant bronchiolar muscle (arrow) helps to identify the scarred structure as residual airway (haematoxylin and eosin stain). (**c**) An elastic tissue stain from a slightly deeper section of the same bronchiole (shown in **b**) highlights the residual elastica present. In contrast to the accompanying artery on the right, there is only one elastic lamella in the bronchiolar wall. Original magnification: 100×

Fig. 8.11 Kaplan-Meier survival for adult lung transplant recipients by transplant era (transplants: 1992–June 2017)

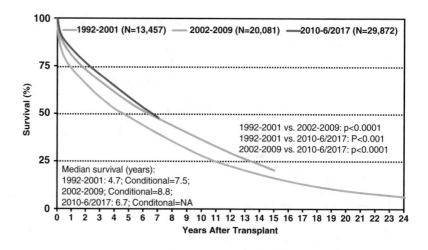

Fig. 8.12 Adult and Pediatric Lung Transplants Kaplan Meier Survival by Age Groups (transplants January 1990–2016). Ref: J Heart Lung Transplant. 2019 Oct; 38(10): 1042–1055

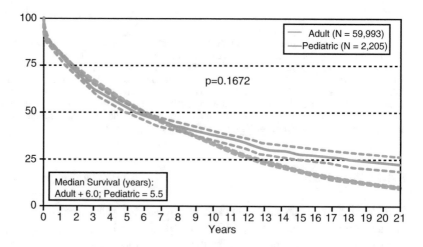

ents of bilateral lung transplants continue to experience longer survival [4, 40].

8.5 Heart and Lung Transplantation (HLTX)

In the early days of HLTX, indications included idiopathic pulmonary hypertension (iPAH) and congenital heart disease [41]. As increasing evidence showed resolution of right ventricular after double lung transplantation (DLTx), this latter procedure became the operation of choice for iPAH patients. Presently HLTX is reserved for congenital heart disease (CHD) [42] and those patients with acquired heart disease combined with pulmonary hypertension and/or lung parenchymal disease. As compared with lung transplantation, early survival with HLTx is decreased [43]. Indications for listing patients for HLTx are less uniform.

Kaplan-Meier survival curve for adult HLTx recipients transplanted in 1982–1993, 1994–2003, and 2004–2015. Conditional median survival is defined as the time to 50% survival in 1-year survivors [from Lund et al. [43], with permission]. HLTx, heart-lung transplantation.

8.5.1 Postoperative Care

Postoperative care after HLTx is similar to that of DLTx or single-lung transplantation. Indeed, it is lungs not the heart related issues that are the source of most postoperative complications and include infections and both acute and chronic rejection [44].

Rejection: Acute cellular rejection in either the lungs or heart after HLTx is less common than after isolated heart or lung transplantation. Acute cellular rejection tends to involve the lungs more often than the heart [44]. Also, rejection of the heart may occur independently of lung rejection [45].

8.5.2 Further Developments

8.5.2.1 Biological Solutions
(a) The role of gene based therapies to treat genetic disorders such as alpha 1 anti-trypsin [46] and cystic fibrosis [47] is increasing.
(b) Lung Regeneration [48]. Regenerative medicine has the potential to play an important role in new therapies for a variety of lung diseases. Lung re-cellularization with induced pluripotent stem cells after decellularization could lead to "on-demand", patient specific allografts for transplantation. Another approach is direct transplant of stem cell lines that are capable of developing into lung tissue [49].
(c) Xenotransplantation: Developments in transgenic animals such as the pig as a source of lung xenografts are ongoing [50]. Using lungs from transgenic pigs together with drugs that target complement activation, coagulation and inflammation plus immunosuppression has yielded encouraging results [51].

8.5.3 Mechanical Solutions

The concept of an implanted membrane based lung assist device (LAD) is not new. Much work is in progress and clinical trials are on the horizon. Early concepts include paracorporeal devices attached either in series or parallel [52, 53].

8.6 Summary

Lung transplantation, presently is therapy for end stage lung failure in select patient populations. There remains a disparity between donor supply and recipient needs. The use of EVLP techniques and DCD donors increase the donor supply. Xenotransplantation should enhance donor supply but still not realized. Temporary "mechanical" (ECMO) approaches have become widespread. Implantable lung devices that would permit longer term use are under current investigation.

References

1. Hardy JD, Webb WR, Dalton ML, Walker GR. Lung homotransplantation man. JAMA. 1963;186:1065–74.
2. Calne R, Rolles K, Thiru S, McMaster P, Craddock G, Aziz S, White D, Evans D, Dunn D, Henderson R, Lewis P. Cyclosporin-a as the only immunosuppressant in 34 recipients of cadaveric organs: 32 kidneys, 2 pancreases and 2 livers. Lancet. 1979;2:1033–6.
3. Bazan VM, Zwischenberger JB. ECMO in lung transplantation: a review. Clin Surg. 2018;3:2016.
4. Chambers, DC, Cherikh, WS, Harhay, MO et al. The international thoracic organ transplant registry of the international society for heart and lung transplantation: thirty-sixth adult lung and heart–lung transplantation report—2019; Focus theme: Donor and recipient size match. J Heart Lung Transplant. 2019 Oct; 38(10): 1042–1055. https://doi.org/10.1016/j.healun.2019.08.001. Published online 2019 Aug 8.
5. Estenns M, Hertz MI. Bronchiolitis obliterans after human lung transplantation. AJRCCM. 2002 15 Aug;166(4):440–4.
6. Weill D, Benden C, Corris PA, et al. A consensus document for the selection of lung transplant candidates: 2014-an update from the pulmonary transplantation council of the international society for heart and lung transplantation. J Heart Lung Transplant. 2015;34(1):1–15.
7. Gries CJ, et al. Lung allocation score for lung transplantation. Chest. 2007;132(6):1954–61.
8. Otani S, Oto T, Miyoshi S. Living-donor lobar lung retransplantation for an adult patient with bronchiolitis obliterans syndrome: an option for retransplantation. JHLT. 2013 April;32(4):469–70.
9. Neujahr DC. Lung retransplantation: practical and ethical considerations raised by the hannover protocol. Transplantation. 2018 March;102(3):355–6.
10. Jai Raman, Mazahir Alimohamed, Nikola Dobrilovic, Omar Lateef, Salim Aziz. A comparison of low and standard anticoagulation regimens in extracorporeal membrane oxygenation. JHLT. 2019 Jan. (In press).
11. Grinita AL, McCurry KR, Iacono AT et al. HLA-specific antibodies are associated with high grade and persistent recurrent lung allograft acute rejection. J Heart Lung Transplant. 2004;23:1135–1141. Showed that patients who have elevated preoperative PRA and also patients in whom antibodies develop after transplantation have higher increased rates of cellular rejection and BOS.
12. Ashish SS, Nwakanma L, Simpkins C, Williams J, Chang DC, Conte JV. Pretransplant panel reactive antibodies in human lung transplantation: an analysis of over 10,000 patients. Ann Thorac Surg. 2008 June;85(6):1919–24.
13. Steen S, Ingemansson R, Eriksson L, et al. First human transplantation of a nonacceptable donor lung after reconditioning ex vivo. Ann Thorac Surg. 2007;83:2191–4.
14. Steen S, Sjoberg T, Pierre L, et al. Transplantation of lungs from a non-beating donor. Lancet. 2001;357:825–9.
15. Machuca TN, Cypel M, Keshavjee S. Advances in lung preservation. Surg Clin North Am. 2013;93:1373–94.
16. Cypel M, Yeung JC, Machuca T, et al. Experience with the first 50 ex vivo lung perfusions in clinical transplantation. J Thorac Cardiovasc Surg. 2012;144:1200–6.
17. Botha P, Rostron AJ, Fisher AJ, Dark JH. Current strategies in donor selection and management. Semin Thorac Cardiovasc Surg. 2008;20:143–51.
18. Starnes VA, Bowdish ME, et al. A decade of living lobar lung transplantation: recipient outcomes. J Thoracic and CV Surgery. 2004 Jan;127(1):114–22.
19. Puri V, Patterson GA. Adult lung transplantation: technical considerations. Semin Thorac Cardiovasc Surg. 2008;20:152–64.
20. Ventilation with lower tidal volumes as compared with traditional tidal volumes for acute lung injury and the acute respiratory distress syndrome. The acute respiratory distress syndrome network. N Engl J Med. 2000;342:1301–8.
21. Tuttle-Newhall JE, Collins BH, Kuo PC, Schoeder R. Organ donation and treatment of the multi-organ donor. Curr Probl Surg. 2003;40:266–310.
22. Mayer E, Puskas JD, Cardoso PFG, Shi S, Slutsky AS, Patterson GA. Reliable eighteen-hour lung preservation at 4 degree and 10 degree Celsius by pulmonary artery flush after high-dose prostaglandin E1 administration. J Thorac Cardiovasc Surg. 1992;103:1136–42.
23. Sundaresan S, Trachiotis GD, Aoe M, et al. Donor lung procurement: assessment and operative technique. Ann Thorac Surg. 1993;56:1409–13.
24. Vigneswaran W, et al. Single-lung transplantation: technical aspects. Lung transplantation principles and practice, pp. 145–158.
25. Haverich A, Aziz S, Scott W, Jamieson S, Shumway N. Improved lung preservation using euro-Collins solution for flush perfusion. Thorac Cardiovasc Surg. 1986;34:368–76.
26. Gohrbandt B, Simon A, Warnecke G, et al. Lung preservation with Perfadex or Celsior in clinical transplantation: a retrospective single-center analysis of outcomes. Transplantation. 2015;99(9):1933–9.
27. Todd TR, Goldberg M, Koshal A, et al. Separate extraction of cardiac and pulmonary grafts from a single organ donor. Ann Thorac Surg. 1988;46:356–9.
28. Hartwig MG, Davis RD. Surgical considerations in lung transplantation: transplant operation and early postoperative management. Respir Care Clin N Am. 2004;10:473–504.
29. Lee JC, Christie JD, Keshavjee S. Primary graft dysfunction: definition, risk factors, short- and

long-term outcomes. Semin Respir Crit Care Med. 2010;31(2):161–71.

30. Snell GI, Yusen RD, Weill D, et al. Report of the ISHLT working group on primary lung graft dysfunction, part i: definition and grading—a 2016 consensus group statement of the international society of heart and lung transplantation. J Heart Lung Transplant. 2017;36(10):1097–103.

31. McDermott JK, Girgis RE. Individualizing immunosuppression in lung transplantation. Glob Cardiol Sci Pract. 2018;2018(1):5.

32. Jeroen B. van der Net, Andrew Bushell, Kathryn J. Wood, Paul N. Harden regulatory T cells: first steps of clinical application in solid organ transplantation. Transplant International First published: 15 May 2015 https://doi.org/10.1111/tri.12608

33. Knoop C, et al. Acute and chronic rejection after lung transplantation. Semin Respir Crit Care Med. 2006;27(5):521–33.

34. Stewart S, Fishbein MC, Snell GI, et al. Revision of the 1996 working formulation for the standardization of nomenclature in the diagnosis of lung rejection. J Heart Lung Transplant. 2007;26(12):1229–42.

35. Roden AC, Aisner DL, et al. Diagnosis of acute cellular rejection and antibody- mediated rejection on lung transplant biopsies. A perspective from members of the pulmonary pathology society. Arch Pathol Lab Med. 2017;141:437–44.

36. Christie JD, Edwards LB, Kucheryavaya AY, et al. The registry of the International Society for Heart and lung transplantation: twenty-eighth adult lung and heart-lung transplant report-2011. J Heart Lung Transplant. 2011;30:1104–22.

37. Ofek E, Sato M, Saito T, Wagnetz U, Roberts HC, Chaparro C, Waddell TK, Singer LG, Hutcheon MA, Keshavjee S, Hwang DM. Restrictive allograft syndrome post lung transplantation is characterized by pleuroparenchymal fibroelastosis. Mod Pathol. 2013;26:350–6.

38. Meyer KC, et al. An international ISHLT/ATS/ERS clinical practice guideline: diagnosis and management of bronchiolitis obliterans syndrome. Eur Respir J. 2014;44:1479–503.

39. Swatek AM, Lynch TJ, Crooke AK, et al. Depletion of airway submucosal glands and TP63(+)KRT5(+) basal cells in Obliterative bronchiolitis. Am J Respir Crit Care Med. 2018;197:1045–57.

40. Long term survival after lung Tx ISHLT data set 2018.

41. Reitz BA, Wallwork JL, Hunt SA, et al. Heart-lung transplantation: successful therapy for patients with pulmonary vascular disease. N Engl J Med. 1982;306:557–64.

42. Goerler H, Simon A, Gohrbandt B, et al. Heart-lung and lung transplantation in grown-up congenital heart disease: long-term single Centre experience. Eur J Cardiothorac Surg. 2007;32:926–31.

43. Lund LH, Khush KK, Cherikh WS, et al. The registry of the International Society for Heart and Lung Transplantation: thirty-fourth adult heart transplantation Report-2017; focus theme: allograft ischemic time. J Heart Lung Transplant. 2017;36:1037–46.

44. Idrees JJ, Pettersson GB. State of the art of combined heart-lung transplantation for advanced cardiac and pulmonary dysfunction. Curr Cardiol Rep. 2016;18:36.

45. Pinderski LJ, Kirklin JK, McGiffin D, et al. Multiorgan transplantation: is there a protective effect against acute and chronic rejection? J Heart Lung Transplant. 2005;24:1828–33.

46. Chluchiolo MJ, Crystal RG. Gene therapy for alpha −1 antitrypsin deficiency lung disease. Ann Am Thorac Soc. 2016 Aug;13(Suppl 4):s352–69 and cystic fibrosis.

47. Burney TJ, Davies JC. Gene therapy for the treatment of cystic fibrosis. Appl Clin Genet. 2012;5:29–36.

48. Nichols JE, La Francesca S, Niles JA, Vega SP, Argueta LB, Frank L, Christiani DC, Pyles RB, Himes BE, Zhang R, Li S, Sakamoto J, Rhudy J, Hendricks G, Begarani F, Liu X, Patrikeev I, Pal R, Usheva E, Vargas G, Miller A, Woodson L, Wacher A, Grimaldo M, Weaver D, Mlcak R, Cortiella J. Production and transplantation of bioengineered lung into a large-animal model. Sci Transl Med. 2018 1 Aug;10(452):aao3926.

49. Ma Q, Ma Y, Dai X, Ren T, Fu Y, Liu W, Han Y, Wu Y, Cheng Y, Zhang T, Zuo W. Regeneration of functional alveoli by adult human SOX9+ airway basal cell transplantation. Protein Cell. 2018 Mar;9(3):267–82.

Management of Primary Graft Dysfunction: Lung Transplantation Surgery

Yoshikazu Suzuki and Christian A. Bermudez

9.1 Introduction

Lung transplantation is an effective treatment option for selected patients with end-stage lung disease. However, the effectiveness of this therapy is hampered by the limited number of suitable organs for transplant, the development of primary graft dysfunction (PGD), adverse effects of life-long immunosuppressive therapy, and chronic lung allograft dysfunction. Among these challenges, PGD influences each of the others and has been demonstrated to have significant impact on short and long-term outcomes [1].

There are no effective treatments available for recipients who develop PGD and successful outcome depend on supportive care [2]. Therefore, risk reduction strategies and advanced support adjuncts are necessary to salvage recipients who develop a severe form of PGD; otherwise early mortality with severe PGD has been reported to be between 23 and 42% [1]. Because "standard criteria" lungs only comprise about 5–15% of donors, no definitive predictive criteria are yet available, and decisions on organ suitability are complex, transplant teams must consider pre-, intra- and postoperative strategies to optimize organ recovery and patient outcome [3] (Table 9.1).

Systematic prevention of PGD can be achieved by decision on donor-recipient matching and surgical planning, by decision on marginal donor lung suitability at procurement, by preventive measures at procurement, and by preventive measures at implantation. Although decision factors principally rely on art and science of surgeon's experience and expertise, Lung Allocation Score (LAS) and ex-vivo lung perfusion are innovative advances [4–6]. Many advances in measures to prevent PGD at procurement, evaluation, protection, preservation, and implantation have been made. With all considerable endeavors in the field, safe expansional use of donor lungs with certain marginality has been successfully achieved, which increased number of lung transplantation with improved outcomes [5, 7–14] (Figs. 9.1, 9.2, 9.3, 9.4 and 9.5).

From surgeon's perspective, we describe our current approach in the management of PGD emphasizing an: (1) cautious clinical decision making on donor-recipient matching and surgical planning; (2) cautious clinical decision making on marginal donor lung suitability for transplantation; (3) simple implementation of preventive measures at procurement with more attention to protection from alveolar side ("Open

Y. Suzuki (✉) · C. A. Bermudez
Division of Cardiovascular Surgery, Department of Surgery, Perelman School of Medicine, University of Pennsylvania, Hospital of the University of Pennsylvania, Philadelphia, PA, USA
e-mail: Yoshikazu.Suzuki@pennmedicine.upenn.edu; Christian.Bermudez@pennmedicine.upenn.edu

© Springer Nature Switzerland AG 2021
N. Hakim et al. (eds.), *Transplantation Surgery*, Springer Specialist Surgery Series,
https://doi.org/10.1007/978-3-030-55244-2_9

Lung" Cold Storage with Room Air); (4) avoidance of cardiopulmonary bypass and adoption of controlled slow ventilation and reperfusion at implantation; (5) preemptive initiation of venovenous Extracorporeal Membrane Oxygenation (vvECMO) rather than late venoarterial ECMO (vaECMO) in support of recipients developing severe PGD.

Table 9.1 Classical "Standard Criteria" of ideal donor lung

1. Age less than 55 years
2. ABO blood group compatible
3. Appropriate size match
4. Clear chest radiograph
5. PaO_2/FiO_2 ratio > 300 on 5 cmH_2O PEEP
6. Tobacco history of less than 20 pack years
7. Absence of chest trauma
8. No evidence of aspiration or sepsis
9. Absence of purulent secretions at bronchoscopy
10. Absence of organisms on sputum Gram stain
11. No history of primary pulmonary disease or active pulmonary infection

FiO_2 fraction of inspired oxygen, *PEEP* peak end expiratory pressure, *PaO_2* partial arterial oxygen tension

9.2 Definition, Incidence, Grading and Significance of PGD

PGD is a syndrome occurring within the first 72 h after lung transplantation characterized by progressive acute lung injury encompassing a spectrum of severity of mild to severe. PGD is characterized by inflammatory pulmonary edema with diffuse alveolar damage that manifests clinically as progressive hypoxemia with radiographic pulmonary infiltrates similar to Adult Respiratory Distress Syndrome (ARDS) [15].

Following ischemia and reperfusion, inflammatory and immunological injury-repair responses appear to be the key controlling mechanisms of PGD [15, 16]. Hypoxemia and parenchymal opacities in the chest x-ray (CXR) generally appear on postoperative day 1, peak by day 3, and subside afterward corresponding to the natural chronological progression and convalescence of the injury-repair response [1]. Since 2005, the International Society of Heart and Lung

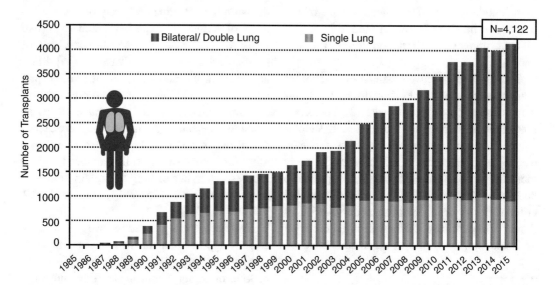

Fig. 9.1 Increasing numbers of lung transplantation worldwide. From Chambers DC, Yusen RD, Cherikh WS, Goldfarb SB, Kucheryavaya AY, Khusch K, et al. The Registry of the International Society for Heart and Lung Transplantation: Thirty-fourth Adult Lung And Heart-Lung Transplantation Report-2017; Focus Theme: Allograft ischemic time. The Journal of heart and lung transplantation: the official publication of the International Society for Heart Transplantation. 2017;36(10):1047–59 [10]. with permission

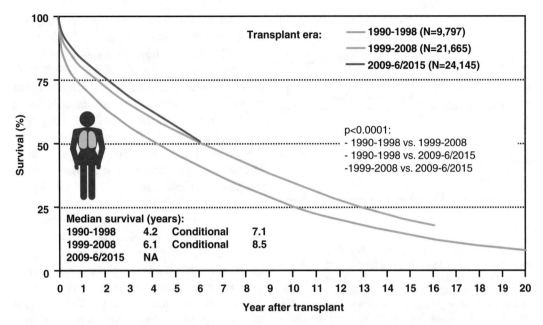

Fig. 9.2 Improving survival of lung transplantation worldwide. From Chambers DC, Yusen RD, Cherikh WS, Goldfarb SB, Kucheryavaya AY, Khusch K, et al. The Registry of the International Society for Heart and Lung Transplantation: Thirty-fourth Adult Lung And Heart-Lung Transplantation Report-2017; Focus Theme: Allograft ischemic time. The Journal of heart and lung transplantation: the official publication of the International Society for Heart Transplantation. 2017;36 (10):1047–59 [10]. with permission

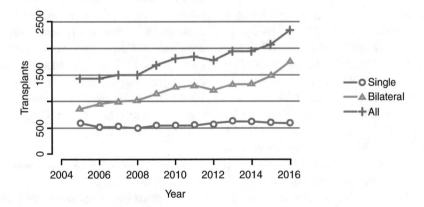

Fig. 9.3 Increasing numbers of lung transplantation in the U.S. . From Valapour M, Lehr CJ, Skeans MA, Smith JM, Carrico R, Uccellini K, et al. OPTN/SRTR 2016 Annual Data Report: Lung. American journal of trans-plantation: official journal of the American Society of Transplantation and the American Society of Transplant Surgeons. 2018;18 Suppl 1:363–433 [11]. with permission

Transplantation (ISHLT) definition and criteria of PGD has been utilized as a standardized taxonomy and grading system [17].

Incidence of the severe form of PGD (ISHLT Grade 3: partial arterial oxygen tension (PaO_2)/ fraction of inspired oxygen (FiO_2) <200 with radiographic pulmonary infiltrates) has been reported to range 15–35% at any time point in the first 72 h (ISHLT Grade 3 at T0-T72) and 10–20% between 48 and 72 h (ISHLT Grade 3 at T48–72) [18, 19].

Severe (Grade 3) PGD, especially at T48 to T72 has been reported to have significant impact on short- and long-term mortality, morbidity,

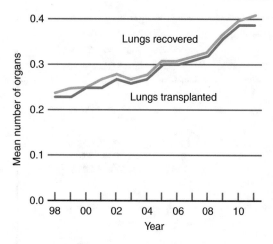

Fig. 9.4 Utilization rates in the U.S. Note that a count of recovered or transplanted lungs differs from the number of donor or procurement cases because lungs can be transplanted as either single or double. Currently about 70% double and 30% single lung transplantation performed in the U.S. From Valapour M, Paulson K, Smith JM, Hertz MI, Skeans MA, Heubner BM, et al. OPTN/SRTR 2011 Annual Data Report: lung. American journal of transplantation: official journal of the American Society of Transplantation and the American Society of Transplant Surgeons. 2013;13 Suppl 1:149–77 [13]. with permission

functional outcomes as well as incidence of bronchiolitis obliterans syndrome (BOS). [1] Short-term (30-day to 90-day) mortality has been reported 0–7% for Grade 0–2 PGD at T48-T72 vs 23–43% for Grade 3 PGD at T48-T72 with risk ratio (RR) of 4.8–6.95 accounting for up to 42% of all-cause mortality. Long-term outcome has been reported 87–89% 1-year survival, 60–66% 5-year survival and 35–38% 10-year survival for Grade 0–2 PGD at T48-T72 vs 66–73% 1-year, 44–51% 5-years and 11–19% 10-year survival for Grade 3 PGD at T48–72. Incidence of stage 1 BOS has been reported as 15% at 1 year, 59% at 5 years, 87% at 10 years for Grade 0–2 PGD at T48-T72 vs 22% at 1 year, 72% at 5 years and 91.5% at 10 years for Grade 3 PGD at T48-T72 (median time to BOS 3.4–3.9 years) [1]. Significant association of PGD with development of BOS has been reported in dose-dependent fashion with stage 1 BOS RR of 2.07 for Grade 1 PGD at T72, RR of 2.81 for Grade 2 PGD at T72 and RR of 4.25 for Grade 3 PGD at T72 and with Stage 2 and stage 3 BOS RR of 7.24 and 7.99 respectively for Grade 3 PGD at T72 [20–23].

A recent study of 1179 subjects using the Lung Transplant Outcomes Group (LTOG) data from 10 U.S. lung transplant centers re-evaluated the construct validity of the ISHLT PGD definition system and found significantly better mortality discrimination at any interval using ISHLT Grade 3 severe PGD (PaO_2/FiO_2 ratio <200 and positive CXR finding) at T48 to T72 (15.9% incidence) [24]. The authors fit a multivariable Cox proportional hazard model using potential confounding variables previously associated with PGD and mortality (donor smoking history, recipient diagnosis, recipient body mass index, recipient pulmonary artery pressure, transplant type, cardiopulmonary bypass use, and recipient reperfusion FiO_2) and demonstrated Grade 3 PGD at T48–72 hazard ratio of 2.05 (p-value of <0.001). The strongest lung injury biomarker previously associated with PGD (plasma plasminogen activator iBALnhibitor-1 level) was also used for testing divergent discrimination and demonstrated a dosage effect with moderate and severe injury. The effects of ventilator status and transplant procedure type (single vs bilateral) were also evaluated and found not to negatively affect discriminant validity. This study reinforces the concept that PGD is a graded syndrome of acute lung injury and inflammation. Increased severity of injury increases the risk of secondary effects such as other organ failure and infection leading to death [25].

9.3 Risk Factors and Pathogenesis of PGD

Much work has been done to identify significant risk factors for development of PGD [1]. During the lung transplantation process, there are sequential stages where injury to donor lungs may occur, including: (1) primary and secondary injuries occurring at the time of death, (2) procurement related injury, (3) ischemia-reperfusion injury (IRI) at implantation, (4) postoperative recovery and resuscitation. Table 9.2 illustrates consistently identified clinical risk factors for PGD, which are practically categorized as

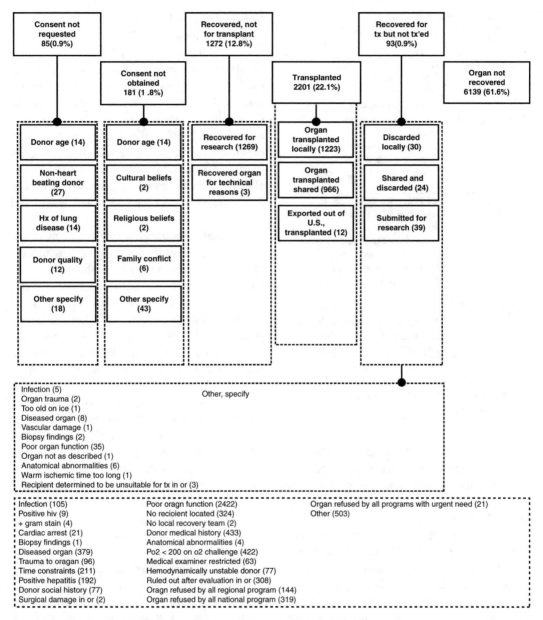

Fig. 9.5 Utilization of donor lungs in 2016. From Israni AK, Zaun D, Rosendale JD, Schaffhausen C, Snyder JJ, Kasiske BL. OPTN/SRTR 2016 Annual Data Report: Deceased Organ Donation. American journal of trans-plantation: official journal of the American Society of Transplantation and the American Society of Transplant Surgeons. 2018;18 Suppl 1:434–63 [14]. with permission

donor-inherent, donor-acquired, recipient, and procedural variables [26–28].

IRI is central to the pathogenesis of PGD [15, 16]. IRI results from the damage of ischemia, generation of reactive oxygen species (ROS) at reperfusion, and subsequent activation

of the damage-amplifying proinflammatory cascade. Experimental and clinical studies suggest that PGD develops in a biphasic pattern [29–31]. In the early phase, development of PGD appears to be dependent primarily on innate macrophages and lymphocytes present in the

Table 9.2 Risk factors for PGD

Category	Risk factors for PGD
Donor-inherent variables	Age > 45 yo and age < 21 yo African american race Female gender **History of smoking** > 20 py, >10 py, current, **any**
Donor-acquired variables	Prolonged mechanical ventilation Aspiration pneumonia Head trauma and/or brain death Hemodynamic instability Neurogenic and/or pulmonary edema
Recipient variables	**Obesity with BMI > 25** Diagnosis of idiopathic pulmonary fibrosis **Diagnosis of primary pulmonary hypertension** **Diagnosis of sarcoidosis** **Elevated pulmonary artery pressure**
Procedural variables	Prolonged ischemic time > 8 h **Use of cardiopulmonary bypass** **Blood transfusion > 1 little** **High FiO$_2$ > =0.4 at reperfusion**

Bold: More consistently reported factors for PGD
BMI Body Mass Index, *FiO$_2$* Fraction of Inspiratory Oxygen Concentration, *PGD* Primary Graft Dysfunction, *py* pack year, *yo* year old

alveolar site of donor lungs interacting with the endothelium. In the later phase, development of PGD appears to result from influx of recipient neutrophils and lymphocytes enhancing inflammatory responses.

Downstream effectors such as tumor necrosis factor (TNF)-α, interleukin (IL)-17 and other mediators of leukocyte, neutrophil and innate immune components have been implicated in the recipient response causing PGD [32]. A novel human prospective study using bronchoalveolar lavage (BAL) and tissue biopsy samples showed increased levels of IL-8 (neutrophil chemoattractant and activator) in the lung tissue and in the BAL fluid of brain-dead donor correlate with PGD severity and mortality in a dose-dependent manner. Immunolocalization staining of IL-8 and IL-8 messenger RNA expression in donor lung tissues also showed findings suggesting that alveolar macrophage

and epithelial cells were major sources of the widespread increase of IL-8 in the donor lungs that later functioned poorly [33].

Many investigations for clinical biomarkers, mediators, and genetic determinants of development of PGD have identified associated pathophysiological mechanisms of PGD: alveolar epithelial and endothelial injury, cytokines and chemokines, adhesion molecules, hypercoagulability and impaired fibrinolysis, vascular permeability, cell proliferation, intracellular assembly for homeostasis and signaling, and innate and acquired immunity [34, 35].

Alveolar epithelial injury (type 1 pneumocyte injury for gas exchange and type 2 pneumocyte injury for surfactant) has been shown to be an integral part of both ARDS and PGD. Plasma soluble form of the receptor for advanced glycation end products (RAGE: a marker for type 1 pneumocyte injury) in plasma of recipients after reperfusion as well as RAGE in BAL fluid of donors was shown to have significant association with PGD [36, 37].

Anti-type V collagen (a stimulant of IL17 dependent cellular innate immunity in the alveolus) antibody in plasma of recipients after reperfusion as well as pre-existing delayed-type hypersensitivity reaction to type V collagen in recipients was shown to have significant association with PGD [38, 39]. Delayed-type hypersensitivity reaction to type V collagen was also shown to have significant association with severe BOS [40].

Recent studies of genetic determinants for development of severe ISHLT Grade 3 PGD showed that genes in inflammasome-mediated innate immune pathways, genes in Toll-like receptors-mediated innate immune pathways, and genes in oxidant stress regulatory pathways have significant association [15, 41–43]. Targeted therapy on these in the alveolus and other subsequent mediators may be feasible for modifying injury-repair responses of donor lungs of severe PGD in the future [44–46]. In this perspective, ex-vivo lung perfusion is a prospective platform for such studies.

9.4   Management of PGD

9.4.1   No Effective Direct Treatment or Consensus Guideline Available for PGD

Due to its complexity and a lack of appropriately powered clinical studies, there is no consensus guidelines for the treatment and management of PGD [2]. There are no effective direct treatment for PGD available. However, advances in preventive strategy and supportive care have improved survival with steady increase of the number of lung transplantation. Similar to ARDS, supportive treatment is sufficient for mild to moderate PGD including lung protective ventilation, avoidance of excess fluid administration, diuresis and early mobilization [1]. Use of other medical adjuncts such as pulmonary vasodilators for severe PGD including inhaled Nitric Oxide or Prostaglandin I 2 (PGI 2) (prostacyclin: iloprost and epoprostenol) may be beneficial in recipients with right ventricular dysfunction with increased PVR (pulmonary vascular resistance), however, there is insufficient data to support the efficacy of these agents for hypoxia alone [47]. Retransplantation is generally not a recommended option due to poor outcomes in this indication [1].

Practically, a variety of other circulatory, mechanical, infectious, inflammatory, and immune pathologies of the lung can coexist in the management of PGD including ones carried over from donor before procurement as well as ones developed at and after implantation procedure. Therefore, simultaneous timely treatment of these pathologies based on a simple comprehensive checklist (Table 9.3) is helpful for the success of managing PGD and recipient's immediate post-surgical conditions. These pathologies were listed as exclusion criteria in the ISHLT PGD definition and grading system [17, 48].

Major significant pathologies on donor lungs are neurogenic pulmonary edema from brain death, aspiration and subsequent developing pneumonia, trauma, and pulmonary embolism. Circulatory, mechanical, infectious, and inflammatory control are the basic principle of surgery.

Table 9.3 Coexisting causes of inflammation and other pathological states of lungs mimicking PGD. These require simultaneous timely management at implantation surgery

- Aspiration pneumonia, lung trauma, pulmonary embolism that had occurred in donor lungs
- Cardiogenic pulmonary edema, volume overload (Circulation Control)
- Pulmonary venous anastomotic obstruction (Mechanical Control)
- Influence of cardiopulmonary bypass, bleeding, blood transfusion (Inflammation & Infection Control)
- Hyperacute rejection (Immunity Control)

PGD primary graft dysfunction

Immune control and management is specifically required for transplant surgery. Prompt recognition and correction of pulmonary venous anastomotic obstruction is critically important because a few hours of delay of correction leads to high mortality [49].

9.4.2   Systematic Prevention of PGD at Donor-Recipient Matching: Making Cautious Clinical Decision Based on Estimates of Severe PGD Probability

In view of the significant negative impact of severe PGD and its lack of effective medical treatment, systematic and comprehensive prevention strategies are of paramount importance (Table 9.4). Basic tenets are to mitigate risks by eliminating prohibitive risks and attenuating negative factors in the clinical context of donor lung conditions, recipient conditions, and procedural demands. Although there is no definitive prediction model for PGD, simplified donor assessment tools have been described by several groups including the Oto donor lung score and the University of Minnesota Donor Lung Quality Index [50, 51]. For a tool to be effective and popularized it needs to be simple, easily remembered, and give a reasonable accurate prediction.

A recent multicenter cohort study utilized recipient body mass index (BMI), diagnosis, and mean pulmonary artery pressure (mPA) and donor smoking history to define risk [52]. Data

Table 9.4 Systematic management strategy for PGD

- Donor lung management protocol
    - Lung protective ventilation
    - Lung protective fluid management
    - Hormone therapy for brain death
- Donor-recipient matching and surgical planning
- Donor lung evaluation and decision at procurement
    - Quantification of aspiration pneumonia and inflammation
- Protective and preservative measures at procurement
    - Lung protective ventilation
    - Total organ circulation control prioritizing heart, liver, kidney, and lung
    - Airway clearance and thorough recruitment at direct evaluation
    - Maintained recruitment on low tidal volume and PEEP
    - Topical hypothermia
    - PGE1, low potassium with dextran pulmonoplegia, antegrade and retrograde cold flush
    - "Open Lung" Cold Storage with room air
- Protective and supportive measures at reperfusion and implantation
    - Avoidance of cardiopulmonary bypass with cardiotomy reservoir if feasible
    - Maintenance of hypothermia of lungs while implanting
    - Controlled Slow Ventilation after gentle recruitment and Controlled Slow Reperfusion in the first 10 min at reperfusion
    - Total circulation control to vital organs including brain, heart, lung, liver, kidney, and blood cells
    - Preemptive initiation of vvECMO support benefitting lung protection and kidney circulation by pulmonary vasodilatory effect of higher oxygen
    - Lung protective ventilation
    - Fluid management to protect lungs and kidney

vvECMO venovenous Extracorporeal Membrane Oxygenation, *PEEP* positive end expiratory pressure, *PGD* Primary Graft Dysfunction, *PGE1* Prostaglandin E1

Table 9.5 Addition of donor smoking history significantly increases incidence of severe PGD in high-risk recipients but not in low-risk recipients

Severe PGD incidence	Donor smoking NO	Donor smoking YES
Low-risk recipients (BMI < 25, mPA < 25 mmHg, diagnosis of COPD or CF)	4–7%	4–11% (**no increase**)
High-risk recipients (all others)	15–18%	24–28% (significant increase)

CF Cystic Fibrosis, *COPD* Chronic Obstructive Pulmonary Disease, *BMI* Body Metabolic Index, *mPA* mean pulmonary artery pressure, *PGD* Primary Graft Dysfunction

included a derivation (n = 1255) and validation (n = 382) cohorts with a severe PGD 16.8% and 14.7%, respectively. A logistic regression identified body metabolic index (BMI) >25, any diagnosis other than Chronic Obstructive Pulmonary Disease (COPD) or cystic fibrosis (CF), and mPA > 40 mmHg (moderate pulmonary hypertension) as recipient predictors and any smoking history as donor predictors of severe PGD. In their prediction models, low-risk recipients who had absence of all three predictors had a pre-dicted severe PGD risk of 4–7% in contrast to 15–18% in all other recipients categorized as high-risk group. Matching donor lungs with any smoking history to a high-risk recipient group significantly increased severe PGD risk to 24–28%, although risk did not significantly change in low-risk recipients (4–11%) (Table 9.5).

In the derivation cohort, low risk recipients also had a lower risk of 90-day and 1-year mortality. The addition of a smoking donor did not significantly affect the predicted risk of 90-day or 1-year mortality. This study was limited by missing data, inaccuracy of smoke exposure history and quantification of smoke exposure, and relatively small numbers of subjects. Additional decision curve analysis showed that the utility of the predictive model could apply only for severe PGD incidences between 5 and 25%, which include average severe PGD incidence of the U.S. institutions. Despite these limitations, this study showed feasibility, validity, and reproducibility of a simple probability prediction model for severe PGD in additive fashion of recipient risk factors and in synergistic fashion of donor risk factors (Table 9.5 and Fig. 9.6). At the time of considering donor-recipient matching, having estimates of severe PGD probability can be useful for clinical decision by striking a balance between risk of staying on the waiting list and risk of accepting specific donor lungs with certain marginality [50, 53].

All of donor information including history, demographics, labs and examinations

\+

Objective Donor Smoking assessment by CXR & CT in advance of preliminary acceptance

\+

Qualification & Quantification of Infiltrations (areas of aspiration pneumonia) at procurement

\+

Estimates of transportation time and ischemic time

Recipient Diagnosis→Elevated PAP (mPA > 40, > 25)→Obesity (BMI > 25)→Procedure demands (BBB)

o	Primary Pulmonary Hypertension	--- Low Risk Donor Lungs or DCD Lungs
o	Sarcoidosis	---Low Risk Donor Lungs
o	Elevated PAP (mPA>40)	
	in IPF BMI > 25	--- Low to Moderate Risk Donor Lungs
	CF, COPD BMI ≤ 25	--- Low to Moderate Risk Donor Lungs
o	Moderately elevated PAP (40 > mPA > 25)	
	in IPF BMI > 25	--- Moderate Risk Donor Lungs
	CF, COPD BMI ≤ 25	--- Moderate Risk Donor Lungs
o	No elevated PAP (mPA < 25)	
	in IPF BMI > 25	--- Moderate Risk Donor Lungs
	CF, COPD & BMI ≤ 25	--- Donor Lungs with smoking > 20 py

Fig. 9.6 Key thought process of donor-recipient matching: Note that there is no perfectly suited organ available in reality, which underscores the importance of clinical decision. Note importance of "eye-balling" of CXR and Chest CT images by lung transplant physicians who know a specific clinical context and make important clinical decision of Donor-Recipient Matching. "Images = shadow": CXR and Chest CT should be interpreted in a specific clinical context. *BBB* Bypass-Bleeding-Blood Transfusion, *BMI* Body metabolic index, *CF* Cystic fibrosis, *COPD* Chronic obstructive pulmonary disease, *CXR* chest X-ray, *CT* computed tomography, *DCD* donation from determination of cardiac death, *IPF* Idiopathic pulmonary fibrosis, *mPA* mean pulmonary artery pressure (mmHg), *PAP* pulmonary artery pressure, *py* pack years

Almost all of donor lungs have some injury [54]. Major pathologies on donor lungs are neurogenic pulmonary edema from brain death and catecholamine storm, aspiration and subsequent developing pneumonia, trauma, and pulmonary embolism; Among them, most frequent and most formidable one is aspiration and subsequent pneumonia due to frequent cardiopulmonary resuscitation. Aspiration can be also frequently caused by an initial acute event such as drug intoxication, stroke, head trauma, and motor vehicle accident leading to brain death [27]. It is difficult to argue against the basic premise that acutely injured donor lungs can be continuously treated in a body of recipient and can be restored to function as healthy as before the event of brain death unless prohibitively severe PGD or other insults occur during the course of lung transplantation. This is the principle of successful use of donor lungs with some acceptable marginality [55].

There was little data to suggest that any single extension of the historical "standard donor criteria" (Table 9.1) impacts either short-term or long-term mortality. There were studies that evaluated the effects of multiple extended donor criteria with mixed results [9, 53, 54, 56–71]. These studies suggest that donor lungs with any single extended criteria can be safely usable for transplantation, but caution has to be exercised when

[[(Recipient Risk × Donor Risk) * (Cold Ischemic Time + Procedure Demands) = PGD Risk.   ]]

Currently 22-29% Lung Utilization from Donor in the U.S.	Recipient Risk High	Recipient Risk Low
Donor Lung Risk Prohibitively High with various extended donor lung criteria (about 70% of offer)	Currently contraindication	Currently contraindication
Donor Lung Risk High with multiple extended criteria depending on degree of aspiration pneumonia and donor smoking exposure (about 10% of offer)	Turned down at procurement	Turned down at procurement
	Sometimes need taking a chance with a planned preemptive vvECMO based on recipient's clinical urgency	back-up single lung candidates or back-up candidates tolerable for extended criteria or tolerable for size mismatch Cautiously explorable
Donor Lung Risk High with one extended criterion depending on degree of aspiration pneumonia and donor smoking exposure (about 5% of offer)	Cautiously explorable	Widely and safely explorable
Donor Lung Risk Low wit only one extended criterion (about 5% of offer)	Widely and safely explorable	Widely and safely explorable
Donor Lung "Standard" without any extended criteria (<10% of offer)	A chance	"Lotus Land" Rare but possible to encounter

PGD: Primary graft dysfunction, vvECMO: venovenous Extracorporeal Membrane Oxygenation
Procedure Demands: Risks for PGD at implantation including Bypass, Bleeding, and Blood Transfusion

Fig. 9.7 Exploring safe donor-recipient matching and organ suitability. *PGD* Primary graft dysfunction, *vvECMO* venovenous Extracorporeal Membrane Oxygenation. Procedure Demands: Risks for PGD at implantation including Bypass, Bleeding, and Blood Transfusion

donor lungs offered have more than one extended donor criteria (Fig. 9.7).

There are only less than 10% of donor lungs that are standard and perfectly clean. Therefore, the majority of successfully transplanted lungs had some marginality and would have been waisted if perfection is sought. Sound understanding, recognition, program consensus, and acceptance of estimated probability of PGD risk in each specific recipient to available donor lungs striking a balance between risk of staying on the waiting list and risk of accepting specific donor lungs with certain marginality forms the foundation of successful lung transplantation.

In view of frequency and clinical significance of "smoker donor lungs", effort to obtain objective findings of smoker lungs at preliminary matching decision is worthy of mention. There are obvious limitations of inaccuracy of smoke exposure history and quantification of smoke exposure. However, detailed objective findings of "smoker lungs" can be obtained by chest images. Therefore, importance of "eyeballing" of CXR and Chest CT (Computed Tomography) images by expert and experienced lung transplant physicians who make ultimate clinical decision in the complex clinical context cannot be underscored enough.

Focus should be on the degree of "smoker lungs" with the spectrum of anatomical emphysematous changes and existence of incidental nodules to rule out malignancy. Wide anatomical spectrum of emphysematous change chronically progressive in decades are similar to the wide spectrum of atherosclerotic changes of cardiovascular disease. Depressed level of the diaphragm below the tenth rib, hyperinflation of the lungs without high peak end expiratory pressure (PEEP), enlarged intercostal space, and narrowed cardiac contour ("drop heart shadow") are suggestive findings on CXR. Chest CT findings of kissing of both lungs in the middle of the anterior mediastinum, diffusely increased lucency (CT density) of lung parenchyma, large heterogeneous areas of different lucency gradation can be identified.

Detection of small (<3 mm) nodules abutting visceral pleura is limited on CT. It is important at procurement to carefully palpate each side of lungs thoroughly standing from the contralateral side of the donor in old donors (>35 years old) with smoking history. Detection of small blebs at the apex can be feasible on CT but detection of small blebs abutting visceral pleura second most frequent at the superior segment of the lower lobe is limited on CT but easily resectable to prevent spontaneous pneumothorax. Bullous lung disease in the "smoker lungs" with emphysematous changes is different from bullous emphysema in that bullous lung disease has bullae with structurally normal intervening lung, whereas bullous emphysema has bullae associated with more diffusely abnormal lung parenchyma in the advanced form of the emphysema spectrum. Discrimination and quantification of consolidation whether atelectasis, pneumonia, trauma, or pulmonary embolism is limited on CT unless clear air-bronchograms or peripheral wedge shape are identified. It is also difficult on CT taken within 2 days of the initial even to detect and qualify aspiration pneumonia which develops and establishes matured pneumonia in about 3–4 days.

9.4.3 Systematic Prevention of PGD at Making Cautious Clinical Decision on Organ Suitability

In a clinical context of certain recipient conditions and procedural demands, questions at procurement point toward how severe those acute injuries and inflammation are and how large areas are involved in those acutely injured lungs focusing especially on aspiration pneumonia [27]. Our guiding principle for the physical and functional evaluation of donor lungs at procurement is that "all precious donor lungs are usable for transplantation unless proved prohibitively injured."

Our current contraindications at procurement after airway clearance by bronchoscopy and direct recruitment are; (1) continuous repooling of purulent secretions in a large area (>2/3 lobe) corresponding to infiltrations at inspection, (2) a non-resectable large area (>1/2 lobe) of consolidation without aeration (organizing aspiration pneumonia, pulmonary infarct, and hemorrhagic parenchymal contusion), (3) poor compliance with peak inspiratory pressure (PIP) >28 cm H_2O at tidal volume (TV) of 10 ml/kg ideal body weight on PEEP of 5. Most of the infiltrations suggesting aspiration pneumonia are identified in the right and left lower lobes. Another contraindication is a finding of diffuse bronchial mucosal inflammation with mucosal erosions at bronchoscopy suggesting fulminant diffuse aspiration injuries and inflammation.

If one side of lungs is relatively intact, single lung transplantation is a meaningful and effective treatment for selected recipients who can back up the primary candidate [72]. Of note, there are frail recipients such as elderly recipients who would not securely tolerate bailout ECMO because of reduced reserved vital function including heart, liver, kidney, nutrition, blood, immunity, coagulation and fibrinolysis, vascular, brain, and musculoskeletal. In such cases, the decision should stay in a conservative side (Fig. 9.7).

Our current guidelines for comfortable and confident final acceptance for donor lungs with aspiration pneumonia are up to 2/3 areas of single lobe and complete aeration of the area of infiltrations at recruitment of Valsalva maneuver at 30–35 cm H_2O. How easily and how well areas of infiltrations with bogginess (moist areas without heaviness) are aerated and recruited is the most reliable finding from our experience. If it requires 40 cm H_2O of Valsalva pressure, generally suggests contraindication. These findings usually correspond to selective lobar pulmonary venous $PaO_2 > 300$ mmHg. Once decision is made, we try to tent the area of infiltrations and aspiration pneumonia with PEEP of 10 cm H_2O and TV of <7 ml/kg ideal body weight keeping PIP < 25 cm H_2O for protection (Table 9.4).

Poor compliance is worse warning finding than poor oxygenation. PaO_2 is condition-dependent with a wide range of values, though objective numbers are helpful to communicate. Partial arterial carbon dioxide tension ($PaCO_2$) constantly >45 mmHg with minute volume of 10 ml/kg ideal body weight is contraindication. A drop test is to test compliance of the lungs by sudden cessation of positive pressure mechanical ventilation and exposure to atmospheric pressure by disconnecting mechanical ventilation tube from endotracheal tube for 10–30 s to see the compliance, recoil, and air-trapping of the lungs. Because almost all donor lungs have some bogginess, slow recoil with 5–10 s to deflate, and some residual air up to 50% of lung volume at 10 ml/kg ideal body weight are acceptable. But, residual air >70% is our current contraindication. Caution needs to be exercised when oversized donor lungs have poor compliance (PIP 25–28 cm H_2O) and residual air (50–70%) because this combination pauses a technical difficulty at sewing bron-

chial anastomosis: a difficulty in keeping space to accommodate the lung and keeping exposure angle for approximating and sewing anastomosis of the main bronchus. Larger donor lungs with poor compliance is contraindicated to a recipient with smaller chest cavity.

9.5   Preventive Measures at Procurement

After acute leading event to brain death, donor lung management protocols before procurement have been shown effective in improving rates of donor lung utilization (from 27 to 43% in one study, from 27 to 54% in one study) without increasing incidence of PGD or early mortality [73, 74]. Many advances have been made in measures at procurement and during ischemic storage and transportation reducing incidence and severity of PGD; notably use of extra-cellular low-potassium dextran flush solution (Perfadex®), plostagrandin E1 (PGE1), and retrograde flush allowing up to 6–8 h cold ischemia safely [2, 16, 27].

9.5.1   Simple Implementation of Preventive Measures with more Attention to Protection from Alveolar Side at Procurement <<Hypothermia and Recruitment>>

Hypothermia with topical ice-cold saline, initial cold pulmonoplegia flush, and simple ice-cold immersion storage has been the gold standard of protective and preservative method for lungs up to 6–8 h, which has been the time-tested safe and reliable practice to prevent severe PGD. Attention and care need to be exercised to thermo insulating effect and floating effect of air uniquely inside of the lungs (Table 9.6). Hypothermia has its own well-known deleterious effect on lungs, however, warm ischemia causes tissue necrosis without any chance of recovery [2]. One basic study in 1993 showed that 10 degrees Celsius

Table 9.6 Lungs are unique solid organ at procurement

A. Maintain low oxygen metabolism from oxygen in the alveolar side during cold ischemia before reperfusion   <<Dual supply of oxygen from both alveolar and endothelial sides>>
B. Most vulnerable injured areas with infiltrations are NOT protected by antegrade pulmonoplegia   <<Intrinsic auto-vasoconstriction to keep VQ (ventilation-perfusion) matching>>
C. Contain air inside of lungs   <<Thermo insulating effect and floating effect of air>>.

storage provided better preservation for PGD [75]. Another basic study in 2014 showed that initial flush of room temperature solution and subsequent inflated storage on ice provided better preservation for PGD than cold preservation [76]. These are interesting findings warranted for further studies, but so far, no further evidences have been collected. Large gaps remain to be filled to extrapolate from small animal lungs with different thermo insulating effect of air to large human lungs clinically accompanied with aspiration and other various acute injuries [54]. There is a practical pitfall of getting warm ischemia of lungs during the anastomosis for 60–90 min with direct contact to chest wall and blood at warm body temperature if lungs are not cooled enough.

9.6 "Open Lungs" Cold Storage with Room Air

Lungs are unique organ with dual supply of oxygen from alveolar side as well as from circulation. Learned from successful practice of donation from determination of cardiac death (DCD) lung transplantation backed up with basic studies, lungs can be initially protected from cessation of circulation by topical cooling and continued ventilation with reduced oxygen demand [77–84]. Initial cold pulmonoplegia flush can be delayed up to 30-60 min, which reinforces the importance of hypothermia and recruitment with maintained low alveolar oxygen to protect donor lungs from PGD (Table 9.6).

Lungs are also unique organ which have strong ability to keep V/Q (ventilation-perfusion) matching with auto-vasoconstriction, which implies that acutely injured most vulnerable areas of donor lungs without recruitment and aeration, especially areas of infiltrated aspiration pneumonia, are not protected by initial antegrade cold pulmonoplegia flush in situ [85] (Table 9.6). Importance of recruitment of lungs before and at antegrade cold flush in situ especially in areas of non-aerated infiltrations can be visualized at the time of retrograde flush; larger amount of residual blood flushed back from the areas of non-aerated infiltrations. Recent experimental study in ventilation induced lung injury (VILI) in ARDS also suggested that in comparison to the "lung rest" strategy with residual atelectasis, the "open lung" strategy enhanced the protection from VILI-induced release of proinflammatory cytokines likely by protective apoptosis through the expression of mitogen-activated protein kinases (MAPKs) [86, 87] (Table 9.7).

Numerous experimental studies using intracellular component pulmonoplegia with high potassium in 1990s showed deleterious effects of deflated lung preservation with increased edema. Increased tendency of edema and barotrauma of fully inflated lung preservation was also shown,

Table 9.7 Keys to management of PGD

I. **Consistent Lung Protective Ventilation** (Airway Clearance + Recruitment + Low Tidal Volume + PEEP)
II. **Cautious Clinical Decision**—"Err on the side of Caution"
III. Quantification of **Aspiration Pneumonia** and **Inflammation** at organ decision
IV. **Hypothermia** and **Recruitment** ("Open Lung" Cold Storage with room air) plus **Pulmonoplegia**
V. **Controlled Slow Ventilation and Reperfusion** in the first 10 min
VI. Total Recipient Vital Organ Protection especially **Lung** and **Kidney**
VII. **Preemptive vvECMO** (to keep PIP < 35 cm H_2O, FiO_2 < 0.6) and Damage Control if necessary

FiO_2 fraction of inspired oxygen, *PEEP* peak end expiratory pressure, *PIP* peak inspiratory pressure, *PGD* primary graft dysfunction, *vvECMO* venovenous Extracorporeal Membrane Oxygenation

thus recommending inflation with 50% Total Lung Capacity (TLC) for preservation [16, 88, 89]. One recent animal study using current low potassium with dextran pulmonoplegia revisited optimal TV for preservation. It showed 75–100% of vital capacity (VC) had significantly better oxygenation with attenuated levels of IRI markers and significantly better preservation of lung surfactants in the alveolar space with caution of potential barotrauma [90]. In terms of optimal alveolar oxygen concentration for lung inflation at 8-h cold ischemia, one animal study in 2001 found that feasibly lowest oxygen concentration (5% in the study, practically 21% at room air) showed lowest mitochondrial dysfunction and lowest lipid peroxidation. Oxygen concentration of 5% resulted in better preservation of lung function from reperfusion injury than 0% and any other higher concentrations [91]. Table 9.4 summarizes our current approach for protection and preservation at procurement.

9.7 Preventive Measures at Implantation

9.7.1 Use of vaECMO Instead of Cardiopulmonary Bypass

Use of cardiopulmonary bypass at implantation has been one of the most impactful risk factors for PGD with a reported Odds Ratio (OR) of 3.4; 95% CI 2.2–5.3; P < 0.001 [26]. Cardiopulmonary bypass circuit lacks blood biocompatibility of the endothelium. Blood continuously contacts with materials and air leading to activation of the complement system by the classic and alternative pathways. Activation of the other systemic inflammatory responses also occur. As an alternative, ECMO with a heparin-coated circuit and new generation oxygen membrane without a cardiotomy reservoir has been gaining more utilization with improved outcomes [92]. With a lack of well-devised randomized controlled studies, there have been arguments that cardiopulmonary bypass is an associated event of sicker recipients rather than a causative relationship [93, 94]. Nonetheless, retrospective studies and a meta-analysis showed use of vaECMO at implant result in equivalent or better short-term survival and better outcomes than cardiopulmonary bypass in complications, PGD, and renal impairment [92, 95–99].

9.7.2 Controlled Ventilation Following Gentle Recruitment and Controlled Slow Reperfusion

Basic animal and clinical studies showed that lung graft function can be significantly improved using initial controlled slow reperfusion by lowering initial perfusion pressure by 50% with mPA < 20 mmHg and 200 ml/min for 10 min. Modifications of leukocyte depleted, buffered, hypocalcemic, nitroglycerin- or PGE1-added, and nutrient rich perfusate, if feasible, were reported effective [100–104]. Basic animal studies also showed that gentle recruitment to TLC keeping <25 cm H_2O for 2 min before reperfusion, keeping initial low ventilation volume with 20% of TV on PEEP of 5 cm H_2O, keeping initial low ventilation pressure < 15 cm H_2O, and keeping initial low ventilation concentration of oxygen <50% for the first 10 min of reperfusion can significantly reduce IRI after cold ischemia. Reperfusion with physiologic ventilatory pressures resulted in poor function, whereas a 50% reduction in ventilatory pressure for the first 10 min of reperfusion yielded function similar to non-ischemic controls [105–108] (Table 9.8).

Table 9.8 Recommended initial controlled slow ventilation and reperfusion

i.	Gentle recruitment to TLC keeping <25 cm H_2O for 2 min before reperfusion
ii.	Lowering initial reperfusion pressure by 50% with mPA < 20 mmHg and 200 ml/min for 10 min
iii.	Keeping initial low ventilation volume with 20% of TV on PEEP of 5 cm H_2O
iv.	Keeping initial low ventilation pressure < 15 cm H_2O
v.	Keeping initial low ventilation concentration of oxygen <50% for the first 10 min of reperfusion

mPA mean pulmonary artery pressure, *PEEP* positive end expiratory pressure, *TLC* total lung capacity, *TV* tidal volume

9.7.3 Preemptive Initiation of vvECMO for Severe PGD: Use of vvECMO not as a Salvage but a Preemptive Support to Protect Lungs as well as Other Vital Organs Especially Kidney

Historically, vaECMO was used for salvage from refractory hypoxemia and hemodynamic instability due to severe PGD following lung transplantation. Complications are common including bleeding, limb ischemia, stroke, infection, and multiple organ failure with non-survivors reported if initiated later than 24 h of lung transplantation [25]. Recently, vvECMO has gained popularity with potentially good survival if started early [109, 110]. In the past, a study showed that patients requiring vaECMO (45%) or vvECMO (55%) (7.6% of total recipients) had poor long-term survival with 30-day, 1-year, and 5-year survival of 55 vs 58%, 39 vs 42%, and 22 vs 29%, respectively [111]. However, the more recent development of a high-performance membrane oxygenator and heparin-coated circuit together with preemptive strategy has led to improved results [2, 112]. A study from Duke group showed that patients requiring vaECMO (65%) or vvECMO (35%) (4.4% of total 522 recipients in 1992–2004) had 30-day and 3-year survival of 7% vaECMO vs 88% vvECMO and 0% vaECMO vs equivalent to non-ECMO in vvECMO, respectively with less complications in vvECMO. Recipients with vvECMO showed significant reduced PVR and improved hemodynamic instability within 1–4 h. Most of the complications with vvECMO involved renal failure but by hospital discharge, recovery of renal function with normal creatinine values were found. Incidence of BOS and acute rejection was equivalent in patients with vvECMO to non-ECMO. However, peak FEV1 was significantly lower in vvECMO vs non-ECMO recipients with 1.71 L (1.28–2.39) vs 2.66 L (2.24–3.24) (P = 0.006) [109]. Preemptive timely initiation of vvECMO may reduce potential toxicity of high-grade supportive care: high concentration oxygen, high volume and pressure on mechanical ventilation, and high dose vasopressors compromising lungs and other vital organs especially kidney.

A follow-up study from Duke group showed that patients requiring vvECMO (5.35% of total 498 recipients in 2001–2009) had improved survival of 30-day, 1-year, and 5-year survival of 82%, 64%, and 49%, respectively. Initiating vvECMO support was considered when supporting ventilatory requirement reaches at PIP of 35 cm H_2O and FiO_2 content surpasses 0.60, or whenever copious pulmonary edema secretions develop. Freedom from BOS was 88% in vvECMO at 3 years and incidence of acute rejection was equivalent to non-ECMO but peak FEV1 was significantly lower with 2.0 L (58% predicted) in vvECMO vs 2.7 L (83% predicted) in non-ECMO recipients (P = 0.001). Strategies to improve lung allograft function in patients developing severe PGD are still needed [112].

A study using UNOS registry in 2015–2016 showed 5.3% (107 out of 2001) recipients requiring post lung transplantation ECMO were younger (56 vs 60 years old, P = 0.007) with higher BMI (27.2 vs 25.8, P = 0.012), increasing ischemic time, and pre-transplantation ECMO support and with 62.2% 6-month survival. Post-transplantation dialysis was associated with mortality. Six-month survival for recipients requiring post-transplantation ECMO with vs without dialysis was 25.8% vs 86.7% (P < 0.001) [113].

As severe PGD appears injury-repair response complicated with edema, bypass, bleeding, blood transfusion, and multiple organ dysfunction, the armamentarium of surgical damage control including open chest management is also fundamental to secure successful management of severe PGD [114] (Table 9.7).

9.8 Conclusion

PGD appears to be a spectrum of injury-repair response involving IRI as a central role in the complicated and integrated background of donor lung conditions, recipient conditions, procedural insults, and donor-recipient immunological interactions. Management of PGD has a pivotal role to the successful outcomes and efficient use of limited organ pool in lung transplantation. Due to its complexity and a lack of appropriately powered clinical studies, there is no consensus guidelines for the treatment and management of PGD.

Without effective direct treatment or consensus guidelines, management of PGD centers avoidance, prevention, and secure support by clinical decisions and measures scientifically and semi-empirically evidenced. Emphasis should be directed to cautious risk balance, simple comprehensive protective measures, and preemptive supportive measures for lungs as well as other vital organs especially kidney. With all considerable efforts in the field, safe expansional use of donor lungs with certain marginality has been successfully achieved, which steadily increased numbers of lung transplantation with improved outcomes.

In view of such critical significance of PGD, further studies warranted for many complicated facets of PGD. Above all, large gaps exist between current clinical practices with variously injured lungs and basic animal studies with lungs without background complex injuries. Well-devised randomized controlled clinical trials filling those gaps are essentially needed.

References

1. Suzuki Y, Cantu E, Christie JD. Primary graft dysfunction. Semin Respir Crit Care Med. 2013;34(3):305–19.
2. Van Raemdonck D, Hartwig MG, Hertz MI, Davis RD, Cypel M, Hayes D Jr, et al. Report of the ISHLT working group on primary lung graft dysfunction part IV: prevention and treatment: a 2016 consensus group statement of the international society for heart and lung transplantation. J Heart Lung Transplant. 2017;36(10):1121–36. The official publication of the international society for heart transplantation
3. Orens JB, Boehler A, de Perrot M, Estenne M, Glanville AR, Keshavjee S, et al. A review of lung transplant donor acceptability criteria. J Heart Lung Transplant. 2003;22(11):1183–200. The official publication of the international society for heart transplantation
4. Botha P, Rostron AJ, Fisher AJ, Dark JH. Current strategies in donor selection and management. Semin Thorac Cardiovasc Surg. 2008;20(2): 143–51.
5. Egan TM, Edwards LB. Effect of the lung allocation score on lung transplantation in the United States. J Heart Lung Transplant. 2016;35(4):433–9. The official publication of the international society for heart transplantation
6. Cypel M, Yeung JC, Liu M, Anraku M, Chen F, Karolak W, et al. Normothermic ex vivo lung perfusion in clinical lung transplantation. N Engl J Med. 2011;364(15):1431–40.
7. Schiavon M, Falcoz PE, Santelmo N, Massard G. Does the use of extended criteria donors influence early and long-term results of lung transplantation? Interact Cardiovasc Thorac Surg. 2012;14(2):183–7.
8. Zych B, Garcia Saez D, Sabashnikov A, De Robertis F, Amrani M, Bahrami T, et al. Lung transplantation from donors outside standard acceptability criteria--are they really marginal? Transplant Int. 2014;27(11):1183–91. Official journal of the European society for organ transplantation
9. Sommer W, Kuhn C, Tudorache I, Avsar M, Gottlieb J, Boethig D, et al. Extended criteria donor lungs and clinical outcome: results of an alternative allocation algorithm. J Heart Lung Transplant. 2013;32(11):1065–72. The official publication of the international society for heart transplantation
10. Chambers DC, Yusen RD, Cherikh WS, Goldfarb SB, Kucheryavaya AY, Khusch K, et al. The registry of the international society for heart and lung transplantation: thirty-fourth adult lung and heart-lung transplantation Report-2017; focus theme: allograft ischemic time. J Heart Lung Transplant. 2017;36(10):1047–59. The official publication of the international society for heart transplantation
11. Valapour M, Lehr CJ, Skeans MA, Smith JM, Carrico R, Uccellini K, et al. OPTN/SRTR 2016 annual data report: lung. Am J Transplant Off J Am Soc Transplant Am Soc Transplant Surg. 2018;18(Suppl 1):363–433.
12. Valapour M, Skeans MA, Heubner BM, Smith JM, Schnitzler MA, Hertz MI, et al. OPTN/SRTR 2012 annual data report: lung. Am J Transplant Off J Am Soc Transplant Am Soc Transplant Surg. 2014;14(Suppl 1):139–65.
13. Valapour M, Paulson K, Smith JM, Hertz MI, Skeans MA, Heubner BM, et al. OPTN/SRTR 2011 annual data report: lung. Am J Transplant Off J Am Soc Transplant Am Soc Transplant Surg. 2013;13(Suppl 1):149–77.
14. Israni AK, Zaun D, Rosendale JD, Schaffhausen C, Snyder JJ, Kasiske BL. OPTN/SRTR 2016 annual data report: deceased organ donation. Am J Transplant Off J Am Soc Transplant Am Soc Transplant Surg. 2018;18(Suppl 1):434–63.
15. Diamond JM, Wigfield CH. Role of innate immunity in primary graft dysfunction after lung transplantation. Curr Opin Organ Transplant. 2013;18(5):518–23.
16. de Perrot M, Liu M, Waddell TK, Keshavjee S. Ischemia-reperfusion-induced lung injury. Am J Respir Crit Care Med. 2003;167(4):490–511.

17. Christie JD, Carby M, Bag R, Corris P, Hertz M, Weill D. Report of the ISHLT working group on primary lung graft dysfunction part II: definition. A consensus statement of the international society for heart and lung transplantation. J Heart Lung Transplant. 2005;24(10):1454–9. The official publication of the international society for heart transplantation

18. Trulock EP. Lung transplantation. Am J Respir Crit Care Med. 1997;155(3):789–818.

19. Christie JD, Kotloff RM, Ahya VN, Tino G, Pochettino A, Gaughan C, et al. The effect of primary graft dysfunction on survival after lung transplantation. Am J Respir Crit Care Med. 2005;171(11):1312–6.

20. Kreisel D, Krupnick AS, Puri V, Guthrie TJ, Trulock EP, Meyers BF, et al. Short- and long-term outcomes of 1000 adult lung transplant recipients at a single center. J Thorac Cardiovasc Surg. 2011;141(1):215–22.

21. Daud SA, Yusen RD, Meyers BF, Chakinala MM, Walter MJ, Aloush AA, et al. Impact of immediate primary lung allograft dysfunction on bronchiolitis obliterans syndrome. Am J Respir Crit Care Med. 2007;175(5):507–13.

22. Huang HJ, Yusen RD, Meyers BF, Walter MJ, Mohanakumar T, Patterson GA, et al. Late primary graft dysfunction after lung transplantation and bronchiolitis obliterans syndrome. Am J Transplant Off J Am Soc Transplant Am Soc Transplant Surg. 2008;8(11):2454–62.

23. Whitson BA, Prekker ME, Herrington CS, Whelan TP, Radosevich DM, Hertz MI, et al. Primary graft dysfunction and long-term pulmonary function after lung transplantation. J Heart Lung Transplant. 2007;26(10):1004–11. The official publication of the international society for heart transplantation

24. Cantu E, Diamond JM, Suzuki Y, Lasky J, Schaufler C, Lim B, et al. Quantitative evidence for revising the definition of primary graft dysfunction after lung transplant. Am J Respir Crit Care Med. 2018;197(2):235–43.

25. Wigfield CH, Lindsey JD, Steffens TG, Edwards NM, Love RB. Early institution of extracorporeal membrane oxygenation for primary graft dysfunction after lung transplantation improves outcome. J Heart Lung Transplant. 2007;26(4):331–8. The official publication of the international society for heart transplantation

26. Diamond JM, Lee JC, Kawut SM, Shah RJ, Localio AR, Bellamy SL, et al. Clinical risk factors for primary graft dysfunction after lung transplantation. Am J Respir Crit Care Med. 2013;187(5):527–34.

27. de Perrot M, Bonser RS, Dark J, Kelly RF, McGiffin D, Menza R, et al. Report of the ISHLT working group on primary lung graft dysfunction part III: donor-related risk factors and markers. J Heart Lung Transplant. 2005;24(10):1460–7. The official publication of the international society for heart transplantation

28. Liu Y, Liu Y, Su L, Jiang SJ. Recipient-related clinical risk factors for primary graft dysfunction after lung transplantation: a systematic review and meta-analysis. PLoS One. 2014;9(3):e92773.

29. Eppinger MJ, Jones ML, Deeb GM, Bolling SF, Ward PA. Pattern of injury and the role of neutrophils in reperfusion injury of rat lung. J Surg Res. 1995;58(6):713–8.

30. Eppinger MJ, Deeb GM, Bolling SF, Ward PA. Mediators of ischemia-reperfusion injury of rat lung. Am J Pathol. 1997;150(5):1773–84.

31. Fiser SM, Tribble CG, Long SM, Kaza AK, Cope JT, Laubach VE, et al. Lung transplant reperfusion injury involves pulmonary macrophages and circulating leukocytes in a biphasic response. J Thorac Cardiovasc Surg. 2001;121(6):1069–75.

32. Sharma AK, Mulloy DP, Le LT, Laubach VE. NADPH oxidase mediates synergistic effects of IL-17 and TNF-alpha on CXCL1 expression by epithelial cells after lung ischemia-reperfusion. Am J Physiol Lung Cell Mol Physiol. 2014;306(1):L69–79.

33. Fisher AJ, Donnelly SC, Hirani N, Haslett C, Strieter RM, Dark JH, et al. Elevated levels of interleukin-8 in donor lungs is associated with early graft failure after lung transplantation. Am J Respir Crit Care Med. 2001;163(1):259–65.

34. Diamond JM, Christie JD. The contribution of airway and lung tissue ischemia to primary graft dysfunction. Curr Opin Organ Transplant. 2010;15(5):552–7.

35. Morrison MI, Pither TL, Fisher AJ. Pathophysiology and classification of primary graft dysfunction after lung transplantation. J Thorac Dis. 2017;9(10):4084–97.

36. Christie JD, Shah CV, Kawut SM, Mangalmurti N, Lederer DJ, Sonett JR, et al. Plasma levels of receptor for advanced glycation end products, blood transfusion, and risk of primary graft dysfunction. Am J Respir Crit Care Med. 2009;180(10):1010–5.

37. Pelaez A, Force SD, Gal AA, Neujahr DC, Ramirez AM, Naik PM, et al. Receptor for advanced glycation end products in donor lungs is associated with primary graft dysfunction after lung transplantation. Am J Transplant Off J Am Soc Transplant Am Soc Transplant Surg. 2010;10(4):900–7.

38. Bobadilla JL, Love RB, Jankowska-Gan E, Xu Q, Haynes LD, Braun RK, et al. Th-17, monokines, collagen type V, and primary graft dysfunction in lung transplantation. Am J Respir Crit Care Med. 2008;177(6):660–8.

39. Iwata T, Philipovskiy A, Fisher AJ, Presson RG Jr, Chiyo M, Lee J, et al. Anti-type V collagen humoral immunity in lung transplant primary graft dysfunction. J Immunol (Baltimore, Md: 1950). 2008;181(8):5738–47.

40. Burlingham WJ, Love RB, Jankowska-Gan E, Haynes LD, Xu Q, Bobadilla JL, et al. IL-17-dependent cellular immunity to collagen type V predisposes to obliterative bronchiolitis in human lung transplants. J Clin Invest. 2007;117(11):3498–506.

41. Cantu E, Suzuki Y, Diamond JM, Ellis J, Tiwari J, Beduhn B, et al. Protein quantitative trait loci analysis identifies genetic variation in the innate immune regulator TOLLIP in post-lung transplant primary graft dysfunction risk. Am J Transplant Off J Am Soc Transplant Am Soc Transplant Surg. 2016;16(3):833–40.

42. Cantu E, Shah RJ, Lin W, Daye ZJ, Diamond JM, Suzuki Y, et al. Oxidant stress regulatory genetic variation in recipients and donors contributes to risk of primary graft dysfunction after lung transplantation. J Thorac Cardiovasc Surg. 2015;149(2):596–602.

43. Cantu E, Lederer DJ, Meyer K, Milewski K, Suzuki Y, Shah RJ, et al. Gene set enrichment analysis identifies key innate immune pathways in primary graft dysfunction after lung transplantation. Am J Transplant Off J Am Soc Transplant Am Soc Transplant Surg. 2013;13(7):1898–904.

44. Ware LB. Targeting resolution of pulmonary edema in primary graft dysfunction after lung transplantation: is inhaled AP301 the answer? J Heart Lung Transplant. 2017;37(2):P189–91. The official publication of the international society for heart transplantation

45. Shaver CM, Ware LB. Primary graft dysfunction: pathophysiology to guide new preventive therapies. Expert Rev Respir Med. 2017;11(2):119–28.

46. Hamilton BC, Kukreja J, Ware LB, Matthay MA. Protein biomarkers associated with primary graft dysfunction following lung transplantation. Am J Physiol Lung Cell Mol Physiol. 2017;312(4):L531–l41.

47. Ramadan ME, Shabsigh M, Awad H. Con: inhaled pulmonary vasodilators are not indicated in patients undergoing lung transplantation. J Cardiothorac Vasc Anesth. 2017;31(3):1127–31.

48. Snell GI, Yusen RD, Weill D, Strueber M, Garrity E, Reed A, et al. Report of the ISHLT working group on primary lung graft dysfunction, part I: definition and grading-a 2016 consensus group statement of the international society for heart and lung transplantation. J Heart Lung Transplant. 2017;36(10):1097–103. The official publication of the international society for heart transplantation

49. Barr ML, Kawut SM, Whelan TP, Girgis R, Bottcher H, Sonett J, et al. Report of the ISHLT working group on primary lung graft dysfunction part IV: recipient-related risk factors and markers. J Heart Lung Transplant. 2005;24(10):1468–82. The official publication of the international society for heart transplantation

50. Oto T, Levvey BJ, Whitford H, Griffiths AP, Kotsimbos T, Williams TJ, et al. Feasibility and utility of a lung donor score: correlation with early post-transplant outcomes. Ann Thorac Surg. 2007;83(1):257–63.

51. Loor G, Radosevich DM, Kelly RF, Cich I, Grabowski TS, Lyon C, et al. The University of Minnesota Donor Lung Quality Index: a consensus-based scoring application improves donor lung use. Ann Thorac Surg. 2016;102(4):1156–65.

52. Shah RJ, Diamond JM, Cantu E, Flesch J, Lee JC, Lederer DJ, et al. Objective estimates improve risk stratification for primary graft dysfunction after lung transplantation. Am J Transplant Off J Am Soc Transplant Am Soc Transplant Surg. 2015;15(8):2188–96.

53. Snell GI, Westall GP, Oto T. Donor risk prediction: how 'extended' is safe? Curr Opin Organ Transplant. 2013;18(5):507–12.

54. Dark JH. What's new in pulmonary transplantation: finding the right lung for every patient. J Thorac Cardiovasc Surg. 2016;151(2):315–6.

55. Gabbay E, Williams TJ, Griffiths AP, Macfarlane LM, Kotsimbos TC, Esmore DS, et al. Maximizing the utilization of donor organs offered for lung transplantation. Am J Respir Crit Care Med. 1999;160(1):265–71.

56. Chaney J, Suzuki Y, Cantu E 3rd, van Berkel V. Lung donor selection criteria. J Thorac Dis. 2014;6(8):1032–8.

57. Whiting D, Banerji A, Ross D, Levine M, Shpiner R, Lackey S, et al. Liberalization of donor criteria in lung transplantation. Am Surg. 2003;69(10):909–12.

58. Alvarez A, Moreno P, Espinosa D, Santos F, Illana J, Algar FJ, et al. Assessment of lungs for transplantation: a stepwise analysis of 476 donors. Eur J Cardiothoracic Surg. 2010;37(2):432–9. Official journal of the European association for cardio-thoracic surgery

59. Moreno P, Alvarez A, Santos F, Vaquero JM, Baamonde C, Redel J, et al. Extended recipients but not extended donors are associated with poor outcomes following lung transplantation. Eur J Cardiothoracic Surg. 2014;45(6):1040–7. Official journal of the European association for cardio-thoracic surgery.

60. Aigner C, Seebacher G, Klepetko W. Lung transplantation. Donor selection. Chest Surg Clin N Am. 2003;13(3):429–42.

61. Pierre AF, Sekine Y, Hutcheon MA, Waddell TK, Keshavjee SH. Marginal donor lungs: a reassessment. J Thoracic Cardiovascular Surg. 2002;123(3):421–7. discussion, 7–8

62. Courtwright A, Cantu E. Evaluation and Management of the Potential Lung Donor. Clin Chest Med. 2017;38(4):751–9.

63. Somers J, Ruttens D, Verleden SE, Cox B, Stanzi A, Vandermeulen E, et al. A decade of extended-criteria lung donors in a single center: was it justified? Transplant Int. 2015;28(2):170–9. Official journal of the European society for organ transplantation

64. Reyes KG, Mason DP, Thuita L, Nowicki ER, Murthy SC, Pettersson GB, et al. Guidelines for donor lung selection: time for revision? Ann Thorac Surg. 2010;89(6):1756–64. discussion 64–5

65. Mulligan MJ, Sanchez PG, Evans CF, Wang Y, Kon ZN, Rajagopal K, et al. The use of extended criteria donors decreases one-year survival in high-risk lung recipients: a review of the united network of

organ sharing database. J Thoracic Cardiovasc Surg. 2016;152(3):891–8.e2.

66. Kurosaki T, Miyoshi K, Otani S, Imanishi K, Sugimoto S, Yamane M, et al. Low-risk donor lungs optimize the post-lung transplant outcome for high lung allocation score patients. Surg Today. 2018;48:928–35.

67. Whited WM, Ising MS, Trivedi JR, Fox MP, van Berkel V. Use of drug intoxicated donors for lung transplant: impact on survival outcomes. Clin Transpl. 2018;32(5):e13252.

68. Fisher AJ, Donnelly SC, Pritchard G, Dark JH, Corris PA. Objective assessment of criteria for selection of donor lungs suitable for transplantation. Thorax. 2004;59(5):434–7.

69. Levvey BJ, Whitford HM, Williams TJ, Westall GP, Paraskeva M, Manterfield C, et al. Donation after circulatory determination of death lung transplantation for pulmonary arterial hypertension: passing the toughest test. Am J Transplant Off J Am Soc Transplant Am Soc Transplant Surg. 2015;15(12):3208–14.

70. Bhorade SM, Vigneswaran W, McCabe MA, Garrity ER. Liberalization of donor criteria may expand the donor pool without adverse consequence in lung transplantation. J Heart Lung Transplant. 2000;19(12):1199–204. The official publication of the international society for heart transplantation

71. Bittle GJ, Sanchez PG, Kon ZN, Claire Watkins A, Rajagopal K, Pierson RN 3rd, et al. The use of lung donors older than 55 years: a review of the united network of organ sharing database. J Heart Lung Transplant. 2013;32(8):760–8. The official publication of the international society for heart transplantation

72. Kron IL, Tribble CG, Kern JA, Daniel TM, Rose CE, Truwit JD, et al. Successful transplantation of marginally acceptable thoracic organs. Ann Surg. 1993;217(5):518–22. discussion 22-4

73. Venkateswaran RV, Patchell VB, Wilson IC, Mascaro JG, Thompson RD, Quinn DW, et al. Early donor management increases the retrieval rate of lungs for transplantation. Ann Thorac Surg. 2008;85(1):278–86. discussion 86

74. Mascia L, Pasero D, Slutsky AS, Arguis MJ, Berardino M, Grasso S, et al. Effect of a lung protective strategy for organ donors on eligibility and availability of lungs for transplantation: a randomized controlled trial. JAMA. 2010;304(23):2620–7.

75. Date H, Lima O, Matsumura A, Tsuji H, d'Avignon DA, Cooper JD. In a canine model, lung preservation at 10 degrees C is superior to that at 4 degrees C. a comparison of two preservation temperatures on lung function and on adenosine triphosphate level measured by phosphorus 31-nuclear magnetic resonance. J Thorac Cardiovasc Surg. 1992;103(4):773–80.

76. Munneke AJ, Rakhorst G, Petersen AH, van Oeveren W, Prop J, Erasmus ME. Flush at room temperature followed by storage on ice creates the best lung graft preservation in rats. Trans Int. 2013;26(7):751–60. Official journal of the European society for organ transplantation

77. De Leyn PR, Lerut TE, Schreinemakers HH, Van Raemdonck DE, Mubagwa K, Flameng W. Effect of inflation on adenosine triphosphate catabolism and lactate production during normothermic lung ischemia. Ann Thorac Surg. 1993;55(5):1073–8. discussion 9

78. Kuang JQ, Van Raemdonck DE, Jannis NC, De Leyn PR, Verbeken EK, Flameng WJ, et al. Pulmonary cell death in warm ischemic rabbit lung is related to the alveolar oxygen reserve. J Heart Lung Transplant. 1998;17(4):406–14. The official publication of the international society for heart transplantation

79. Date H, Matsumura A, Manchester JK, Cooper JM, Lowry OH, Cooper JD. Changes in alveolar oxygen and carbon dioxide concentration and oxygen consumption during lung preservation. The maintenance of aerobic metabolism during lung preservation. J Thorac Cardiovasc Surg. 1993;105(3):492–501.

80. Suzuki Y, Tiwari JL, Lee J, Diamond JM, Blumenthal NP, Carney K, et al. Should we reconsider lung transplantation through uncontrolled donation after circulatory death? Am J Transplant Off J Am Soc Transplant Am Soc Transplant Surg. 2014;14(4):966–71.

81. Van Raemdonck DE, Jannis NC, Rega FR, De Leyn PR, Flameng WJ, Lerut TE. Extended preservation of ischemic pulmonary graft by postmortem alveolar expansion. Ann Thorac Surg. 1997;64(3):801–8.

82. Kutschka I, Sommer SP, Hohlfeld JM, Warnecke G, Morancho M, Fischer S, et al. In-situ topical cooling of lung grafts: early graft function and surfactant analysis in a porcine single lung transplant model. Eur J Cardio-thoracic Surg. 2003;24(3):411–9. Official journal of the European association for cardio-thoracic surgery

83. Novick RJ, Gehman KE, Ali IS, Lee J. Lung preservation: the importance of endothelial and alveolar type II cell integrity. Ann Thorac Surg. 1996;62(1):302–14.

84. Fukuse T, Hirata T, Nakamura T, Kawashima M, Hitomi S, Wada H. Influence of deflated and anaerobic conditions during cold storage on rat lungs. Am J Respir Crit Care Med. 1999;160(2):621–7.

85. Baretti R, Bitu-Moreno J, Beyersdorf F, Matheis G, Francischetti I, Kreitmayr B. Distribution of lung preservation solutions in parenchyma and airways: influence of atelectasis and route of delivery. J Heart Lung Transplant. 1995;14(1 Pt 1):80–91. The official publication of the international society for heart transplantation

86. Allen GB, Suratt BT, Rinaldi L, Petty JM, Bates JH. Choosing the frequency of deep inflation in mice: balancing recruitment against ventilator-induced lung injury. Am J Physiol Lung Cell Mol Physiol. 2006;291(4):L710–7.

87. Fanelli V, Mascia L, Puntorieri V, Assenzio B, Elia V, Fornaro G, et al. Pulmonary atelectasis during low

stretch ventilation: "open lung" versus "lung rest" strategy. Crit Care Med. 2009;37(3):1046–53.

88. Haniuda M, Hasegawa S, Shiraishi T, Dresler CM, Cooper JD, Patterson GA. Effects of inflation volume during lung preservation on pulmonary capillary permeability. J Thorac Cardiovasc Surg. 1996;112(1):85–93.

89. DeCampos KN, Keshavjee S, Liu M, Slutsky AS. Optimal inflation volume for hypothermic preservation of rat lungs. J Heart Lung Transplant. 1998;17(6):599–607. The official publication of the international society for heart transplantation

90. Tanaka Y, Shigemura N, Noda K, Kawamura T, Isse K, Stolz DB, et al. Optimal lung inflation techniques in a rat lung transplantation model: a revisit. Thorac Cardiovasc Surg. 2014;62(5):427–33.

91. Fukuse T, Hirata T, Ishikawa S, Shoji T, Yoshimura T, Chen Q, et al. Optimal alveolar oxygen concentration for cold storage of the lung. Transplantation. 2001;72(2):300–4.

92. Bermudez CA, Shiose A, Esper SA, Shigemura N, D'Cunha J, Bhama JK, et al. Outcomes of intraoperative venoarterial extracorporeal membrane oxygenation versus cardiopulmonary bypass during lung transplantation. Ann Thorac Surg. 2014;98(6):1936–42. discussion 42-3

93. Marczin N, Royston D, Yacoub M. Pro: lung transplantation should be routinely performed with cardiopulmonary bypass. J Cardiothorac Vasc Anesth. 2000;14(6):739–45.

94. McRae K. Con: lung transplantation should not be routinely performed with cardiopulmonary bypass. J Cardiothorac Vasc Anesth. 2000;14(6):746–50.

95. Biscotti M, Yang J, Sonett J, Bacchetta M. Comparison of extracorporeal membrane oxygenation versus cardiopulmonary bypass for lung transplantation. J Thorac Cardiovasc Surg. 2014;148(5):2410–5.

96. Machuca TN, Collaud S, Mercier O, Cheung M, Cunningham V, Kim SJ, et al. Outcomes of intraoperative extracorporeal membrane oxygenation versus cardiopulmonary bypass for lung transplantation. J Thorac Cardiovasc Surg. 2015;149(4):1152–7.

97. Ius F, Kuehn C, Tudorache I, Sommer W, Avsar M, Boethig D, et al. Lung transplantation on cardiopulmonary support: venoarterial extracorporeal membrane oxygenation outperformed cardiopulmonary bypass. J Thorac Cardiovasc Surg. 2012;144(6):1510–6.

98. Hoechter DJ, von Dossow V, Winter H, Muller HH, Meiser B, Neurohr C, et al. The Munich lung transplant group: intraoperative extracorporeal circulation in lung transplantation. Thorac Cardiovasc Surg. 2015;63(8):706–14.

99. Hoechter DJ, Shen YM, Kammerer T, Gunther S, Weig T, Schramm R, et al. Extracorporeal circulation during lung transplantation procedures: a meta-analysis. ASAIO J (Am Soc Artif Int Organs: 1992). 2017;63(5):551–61.

100. Bhabra MS, Hopkinson DN, Shaw TE, Hooper TL. Critical importance of the first 10 minutes of lung graft reperfusion after hypothermic storage. Ann Thorac Surg. 1996;61(6):1631–5.

101. Pierre AF, DeCampos KN, Liu M, Edwards V, Cutz E, Slutsky AS, et al. Rapid reperfusion causes stress failure in ischemic rat lungs. J Thorac Cardiovasc Surg. 1998;116(6):932–42.

102. Halldorsson AO, Kronon MT, Allen BS, Rahman S, Wang T. Lowering reperfusion pressure reduces the injury after pulmonary ischemia. Ann Thorac Surg. 2000;69(1):198–203. discussion 4

103. Schnickel GT, Ross DJ, Beygui R, Shefizadeh A, Laks H, Saggar R, et al. Modified reperfusion in clinical lung transplantation: the results of 100 consecutive cases. J Thorac Cardiovasc Surg. 2006;131(1):218–23.

104. DeCampos KN, Keshavjee S, Liu M, Slutsky AS. Prevention of rapid reperfusion-induced lung injury with prostaglandin E1 during the initial period of reperfusion. J Heart Lung Transplant. 1998;17(11):1121–8. The official publication of the international society for heart transplantation

105. DeCampos KN, Keshavjee S, Slutsky AS, Liu M. Alveolar recruitment prevents rapid-reperfusion-induced injury of lung transplants. J Heart Lung Transplant. 1999;18(11):1096–102. The official publication of the international society for heart transplantation

106. de Perrot M, Imai Y, Volgyesi GA, Waddell TK, Liu M, Mullen JB, et al. Effect of ventilator-induced lung injury on the development of reperfusion injury in a rat lung transplant model. J Thorac Cardiovasc Surg. 2002;124(6):1137–44.

107. Singh RR, Laubach VE, Ellman PI, Reece TB, Unger E, Kron IL, et al. Attenuation of lung reperfusion injury by modified ventilation and reperfusion techniques. J Heart Lung Transplant. 2006;25(12):1467–73. The official publication of the international society for heart transplantation

108. Silva CA, Carvalho RS, Cagido VR, Zin WA, Tavares P, DeCampos KN. Influence of lung mechanical properties and alveolar architecture on the pathogenesis of ischemia-reperfusion injury. Interact Cardiovasc Thorac Surg. 2010;11(1):46–51.

109. Hartwig MG, Appel JZ 3rd, Cantu E 3rd, Simsir S, Lin SS, Hsieh CC, et al. Improved results treating lung allograft failure with venovenous extracorporeal membrane oxygenation. Ann Thorac Surg. 2005;80(5):1872–9. discussion 9–80

110. Oto T, Rosenfeldt F, Rowland M, Pick A, Rabinov M, Preovolos A, et al. Extracorporeal membrane oxygenation after lung transplantation: evolving technique improves outcomes. Ann Thorac Surg. 2004;78(4):1230–5.

111. Bermudez CA, Adusumilli PS, McCurry KR, Zaldonis D, Crespo MM, Pilewski JM, et al. Extracorporeal membrane oxygenation for primary graft dysfunction after lung transplantation: long-term survival. Ann Thorac Surg. 2009;87(3):854–60.

112. Hartwig MG, Walczak R, Lin SS, Davis RD. Improved survival but marginal allograft function in patients treated with extracorporeal membrane oxygenation after lung transplantation. Ann Thorac Surg. 2012;93(2):366–71.

113. Mulvihill MS, Yerokun BA, Davis RP, Ranney DN, Daneshmand MA, Hartwig MG. Extracorporeal membrane oxygenation following lung transplantation: indications and survival. J Heart Lung Transplant 2017. S1053-2498(17)31880-6. The official publication of the international society for heart transplantation.

114. Shigemura N, Orhan Y, Bhama JK, D'Cunha J, Zaldonis D, Pilewski JM, et al. Delayed chest closure after lung transplantation: techniques, outcomes, and strategies. J Heart Lung Transplant. 2014;33(7):741–8. The official publication of the international society for heart transplantation

Kidney Transplantation

10

Hillary Braun and Nancy L. Ascher

10.1 History

There were numerous attempts at kidney transplantation before the first successful kidney transplant was performed in 1954 in Boston. In this procedure, a kidney was transplanted from one identical twin to another, providing proof of concept of the technical aspects of the kidney transplant. The recipient lived 8 years after transplantation without the use of immunosuppression drugs. The donor died 56 years later, suggesting that donation of a kidney does not compromise longevity. The exchange of nonidentical live donor kidneys and deceased donor kidneys awaited the development of immunosuppressive medications to ameliorate the rejection response.

In the United States (US), besides the development of immunotherapy as an important adjunct to the development of the field of kidney transplantation, two other developments were key: (1) the decision by the federal government to support the care of patients with end stage renal disease (this decision fostered both transplantation and renal replacement therapy), and (2) the development of the criteria for brain death. The implementation of the National Organ Transplant Act (NOTA) in 1984 established a central clearing house for organ placement and data collection furthered this development. In many countries, key legislative developments have fostered the growth of transplant activity. Examples include the support of the Spanish Government of the National Transplant Organization (ONT) and the Global Observatory which oversees Spanish transplant activity and serves as a repository of transplant data from around the world; Spain's emphasis has been on deceased donation with the development of a strong program of enhanced deceased donation that has served as a model and been adopted throughout the world. A second example is the collaborative approach in Iran between the medical community, the government and religious leaders, which has facilitated the establishment of an active deceased donor program that had little activity prior to 2010.

10.2 Global Burden of Disease

It is estimated that two million people die each year with end stage renal disease, and that more than 200 million people worldwide have chronic kidney disease (CKD). The exact number of patients with CKD is unknown; this highlights the reality that most patients with renal failure do not have access to renal replacement therapy. The highest rates of CKD are in Latin America, Asia and Sub-Suharan Africa [1]. In Mexico, CKD ranks second to isch-

H. Braun · N. L. Ascher (✉)
Department of Surgery, University of California, San Francisco, USA
e-mail: Hillary.braun@ucsf.edu;
Nancy.Ascher@ucsf.edu

© Springer Nature Switzerland AG 2021
N. Hakim et al. (eds.), *Transplantation Surgery*, Springer Specialist Surgery Series,
https://doi.org/10.1007/978-3-030-55244-2_10

emic heart disease in terms of life years lost and more than 50% of patients with CKD have diabetes [2]. There has been a transition in lower to middle income countries away from communicable diseases to noncommunicable chronic diseases which include ischemic heart disease, diabetes mellitus, chronic kidney disease, obesity and hypertension [3]. Renal replacement therapy is expensive and often available to only a small portion of a population unless there is support from the government or extensive insurance coverage. In the case of middle and high resourced countries, renal replacement therapies exist, but access depends on coverage. In low resourced countries, only a few individuals may have access to treatment. It is estimated that fewer than 5% of the half million new cases of ESRD in Sub-Suharan Africa gain access to even limited dialysis [1]. It has been reported that 100 countries which represent a population greater than 1 billion people have no provision for renal replacement therapy. The global estimate of the prevalence of CKD is 3–18%, with a female predominance, and a larger contribution by elderly adults. The approach of the ministries of health to the problem of chronic kidney disease has largely been to begin with support of renal replacement therapy. While this approach has short- term benefits in extending the lives of patients with chronic kidney disease, it has also fostered the proliferation of private renal replacement enterprises without the concomitant development of transplant capabilities (see national self-sufficiency below). In addition to having a positive effect on survival, kidney transplantation is cost effective when compared to renal replacement therapy.

10.3 Worldwide Kidney Transplantation Activity

In 2016 there were 126, 000 solid organ transplants performed globally [4]. It is estimated that this represents 10% of the global need. The majority of these transplants- 85,000 transplants- are kidney transplants, and were performed in 103 countries as reported to the Global Observatory in Transplantation [4]. There are two potential sources of kidney donors- living and deceased donors. Most countries have a combination of both deceased and live donors. For example, in the US, 40% of kidney transplants are performed using organs from live donors and 60% are done using kidneys from deceased donors. Other countries with mixed (live and deceased) donation include Korea and Iran. In other countries there is a preponderance of either live (Turkey, Pakistan, Philippines, Japan, and Mexico) or deceased (Spain and Croatia). For countries to realize self-sufficiency, it is likely they will need to develop both donor sources.

The results for live donor kidney transplant are superior to that from deceased donation. However, the use of live donors introduces the potential for donor harm or donor exploitation through forced donation or coercion. Success of a live donor program mandates careful evaluation of the donor, transparency of donor complications, and commitment to long term monitoring of the donor. The establishment of a deceased donor program, on the other hand, requires extensive governmental support to establish brain death legislation, organ procurement units, registries for patients awaiting transplantation, and transparent distribution algorithms. Robust deceased donor programs also require public trust and active community involvement in this identification of donors and support for donor families. Regardless of the donor source, long term recipient follow up and transparency regarding morbidity and mortality are essential. It is also clear that durable success in kidney transplantation requires long-term immunosuppression with concomitant toxicities and compliance challenges. Attempts to wean immunosuppression have been largely unsuccessful in kidney transplant; protocols for tolerance induction are being developed and may ultimately prove useful in avoiding or decreasing immunosuppression.

10.4 Technical Aspects of Kidney Transplantation

The principles behind the technical aspects of the kidney transplant operation are to provide optimal arterial inflow, venous outflow, and urinary drainage. Although simple in concept, the achievement of these goals may be challenging in specific patients. The standard operative approach is to perform the kidney transplant in the retroperitoneal approach with a right or left lower quadrant incision and development of the retroperitoneal space. Most commonly the iliac vessels are used for arterial inflow and venous outflow and the host bladder for urinary continence. The intraperitoneal approach is used in small children or in patients whose iliac vessels have been previously been used for transplant or for other procedures. Recently, a robotic approach has been suggested in transplantation of the obese or frail recipient which may lead to fewer wound complications and could subject patients to a less invasive procedure [5]. Typically an end to side renal artery to external artery anastomosis is fashioned; alternatively an end to end anastomosis to the internal iliac vessel may be done or the common iliac may be used for inflow. The choice for the inflow depends on the degree of calcification and caliber of the inflow vessel. In patients less than 10 kg, the aorta is used for inflow. A preoperative non-contrast CT scan may be used to assess the integrity of the iliac vessels and plan the operative approach.

A history of deep venous thrombosis, pulmonary embolism or finding of unilateral leg swelling may dictate a venogram or ultrasound to evaluate for venous obstruction or occlusion. Both the arterial and venous anastomoses are done with fine vascular suture and care to avoid strictures. Urinary continuity is usually accomplished by an ureteroneocystomy; if the bladder is very small or scarred, an ureteroureterostomy is fashioned using native ureter and a stent. Preoperative evaluation of the bladder and assurance that it empties may need to be performed if bladder function is in question. In patients with a neurogenic or inadequate bladder, an augmentation procedure or an ileal conduit may be necessary prior to consideration for transplantation. The ureteroneocystotomy is usually reinforced with an overlying muscle layer of bladder in an attempt to decrease the incidence of ureteral reflux. The donor operation for live donor kidney transplantation is generally done with a laparoscopic approach [6]. Most commonly the left kidney is used to benefit from its longer vein. If one kidney appears smaller or has other abnormalities (such as cysts), the less optimal kidney is used for donation. There are a few reports of the donor procedure performed with robotic technique.

10.5 Complications

After kidney transplantation, patients are susceptible to a variety of medical and surgical complications. As with any operation, routine complications in the immediate post-operative period include infection, venous thromboembolism, and bleeding. In the long term, due in part to side effects from the immunosuppression regimen required after transplantation, kidney transplant recipients may also develop medical conditions such as hypertension, hyperlipidemia, tremors, infections, and de novo diabetes. The subsequent discussion of complications after kidney transplantation will focus on those that are both specific to kidney transplantation and generally technical in nature.

10.5.1 Vascular

Inadequate hemostasis may lead to hematoma formation after kidney transplantation. While the majority of hematomas are small and incidental, re-operative intervention is indicated in the presence of hemodynamic instability, of compromised graft function related to compression of the graft secondary to hematoma, and for graft rupture. Anticoagulants such as heparin and antiplatelet agents such as aspirin and clopidigrel have been associated with a greater risk of hematoma formation after kidney transplantation [7]. Hematomas may also occur after biopsy of the transplanted kidney; cessation of antiplatelet agents has been shown to decrease the incidence of minor biopsy-associated complications [8].

Arterial complications include transplant renal artery thrombosis and stenosis. Renal artery thrombosis is rare and is most often due to technical complications such as kinking. Renal artery stenosis, on the other hand, is the most common vascular complication after kidney transplantation [7], occurring 3 months to 2 years after transplantation [9] with an incidence as high as 23%. The manifestations of transplant renal artery stenosis (TRAS) most commonly include worsening hypertension, with radiographic findings of arterial stenosis. Etiologies of TRAS include fibrosis (40%), donor artery atherosclerosis (27%), and renal artery kinking (21%) [10]. A stenosis of >70% warrants intervention [7], typically with angioplasty and stenting or surgical revision.

Unlike arterial complications, renal vein complications are almost immediately evident. Renal vein thrombosis is typically caused by kinking of a long left renal vein or compression of a short right renal vein and manifests as the abrupt onset oliguria followed by hematuria. If untreated, the sequalae associated with renal vein thrombosis can lead to life threatening graft rupture. Surgical correction is almost always mandated. The placement of a right renal graft with a short vein placed low in a patient with a narrow pelvis may increase the risk of renal vein thrombosis.

10.5.2 Lymphatic

Lymphocele formation after kidney transplantation is common, with an incidence ranging from 2–50%, and occurs as a result of leaking lymphatics which have been divided overlying the iliac vessels. It is thought that lymphocele formation after kidney transplantation might be due, in part, to immunosuppression which compromises the normal healing process and fails to seal any leaky lymphatic channels. Lymphoceles generally occur within 1 week to 6 months following transplantation and may be more common during rejection episodes. They may present in a variety of ways including urinary frequency, unilateral leg edema, deep vein thrombosis, and graft dysfunction secondary to compression. While often asymptomatic, structurally significant lymphoceles can result in graft compression and/or precipitate infection or rarely the development of a lymphocutaneous fistula, particularly within the wound bed. Generally, lymphoceles recur after percutaneous aspiration or drain placement. Either open or laparoscopic creation of a peritoneal fenestration to facilitate drainage and reabsorption into the intraabdominal cavity provides more durable therapy.

10.5.3 Ureteral

The incidence of urologic complications after kidney transplantation ranges from 1 to 15% and includes ureteral leaks, strictures and reflux in addition to urinary tract infections, hematuria, urinary calculi, obstruction, retention, and development of urologic malignancies. We will focus here on ureteral leaks, strictures and reflux.

The native ureter is supplied by both renal and pelvic vasculature, while the transplant ureter is supplied only by the renal artery anastomosis. As a result, the distal ureter is most prone to ischemia and extra care must be taken to preserve any superior or inferior pole arteries that could be the primary, or a significant, source of blood flow to the ureter.

Ureteral leaks have an incidence of 1–3%; early leaks (within the first 24 h) are most often a result of technical errors, while late leaks (within the first 14 days) are more often due to ischemia. Leaks often manifest as a cessation of urine output in association with wound drainage, increased drain output, or development of a new fluid collection. Diagnosis is confirmed by sending the fluid for creatinine; imaging with CT scan or MAG-3 study can also aid in the diagnosis. Nonoperative management consists of stenting and foley catheter placement. The approach to operative management depends on the extent of ureter necrosis. If no necrosis is observed and the leak appears due to a technical flaw with the anastomosis, the defect can be primarily repaired with interrupted sutures. However, any amount of necrosis mandates resection of the necrotic portion; a small resection can be followed by simple reimplantation, but if the necrosis is extensive and the anastomosis cannot be made tension free, a more extensive repair involving mobilization of the bladder is warranted.

The incidence of ureteral stenosis is approximately 3% [11]. These complications are thought to be caused by one of three mechanisms: (1) external compression; (2) intrinsic ischemia; (3) intraluminal obstruction [7]. Ureteral stenoses may occur at any time after kidney transplantation and have been associated with several risk factors including donor age, >2 renal arteries, and delayed graft function [12]. Ureteral stenosis manifests as a gradually increasing creatinine and hydronephrosis on ultrasound. Endoscopic stenting is typically the first line treatment modality. Recurrent strictures usually require open surgical revision. Ureteral reflux refers to urine passing from the bladder back into the ureter with bladder contraction. This reflux may lead to infection of the upper urinary tract with pyelonephritis. The overlay of the bladder muscle on top of the ureter as it enters the bladder at the time of transplant may prevent this complication. Urinary revision with an anti-reflux muscle tunnel may be indicated.

10.5.4 Rejection

The most important complication after kidney transplant is rejection. Acute rejection, manifested by rise in creatinine, decreased urine output, weight gain and hypertension may be the result of either a cellular mediated process or the development of antibody mediated rejection. A biopsy confirms the diagnosis and enables classification and grading of the process; this in turn dictates therapy and provides prognosis.

Severe acute rejection, with both interstitial and vascular involvement, carries a poor prognosis. Similarly, chronic rejection graft fibrosis, interstitial infiltrate, and the development of anti-donor antibodies carries a poor prognosis. Approximately 40% of grafts are lost due to immunological mechanisms and retransplantation for chronic rejection represents 20% of kidney transplants undertaken in the U.S. Compliance is an important issue in chronic graft loss. Noncompliance due to patient choice or to an inability to afford immunosuppression drugs is a major challenge for the field.

10.6 Immunosuppression

In the initial era of kidney transplantation in the 1960s, the mainstays of immunosuppression were azathioprine and corticosteroids. Azathioprine is an imidazolyl derivative of 6-mercaptopurine that inhibits DNA and RNA synthesis by suppressing purine synthesis and inhibits lymphocyte proliferation. Steroids were originally only used to treat episodes of acute rejection, but were quickly administered alongside azathioprine as immediate post-transplant immunosuppression. The precise mechanism of action of steroids remains incompletely understood, but they provide potent immunosuppressive and anti-inflammatory effects through suppression of IL-2 activity and monocyte inhibition, respectively. The use of steroids and azathioprine combination allowed kidney transplant to extend beyond identical twin transplants into other live donor sources as well as to deceased donors.

In the late 1970s, cyclosporine was discovered, which ushered in the era of calcineurin inhibitor therapy. Renal transplant results greatly improved with cyclosporine and allowed for transplant of other solid organs. Soon thereafter in the 1980s, monoclonal T-cell depleting antibody therapies became feasible, ultimately leading to the concept of induction immunosuppression. At the present time, the typical immunosuppression regimen following kidney transplantation begins with induction with a T cell depleting agent or an IL-2 receptor antagonist (IL2RA) followed by double or triple maintenance therapy with a calcineurin inhibitor, antiproliferative agent, and steroids.

10.6.1 Induction

The purpose of induction therapy is to minimize the risk of acute rejection, which has been associated with decreased graft survival. In the United States, lymphocyte depleting agents such as antithymocyte globulins (ATG) are used in the majority of kidney transplant recipients, while in Europe, induction with an IL2RA agent such as basiliximab is more prevalent.

Polyclonal antibody preparations include ATG derived from rabbits and horses. Because these preparations include a wide variety of antibodies, their mechanism of action is multifactorial and incompletely understood. It is believed that these antibodies act on multiple pathways including antigen recognition, adhesion, and costimulation [7].

Conversely, monoclonal antibodies focus on a single target. Muromonab (OKT3) was the initial monoclonal antibody used in kidney transplantation and targeted CD3. As of 2009 it is no longer commercially available in the United States due to an unfavorable side effect profile. IL2RA agents are also referred to as anti-CD25 agents. The two most common anti-CD25 drugs were daclizumab and basiliximab, however daclizumab is no longer commercially available. A widely cited Cochrane review published in 2010 by Webster et al. looked at randomized controlled trials comparing induction therapy with IL2RA versus placebo, no treatment, or other antibody therapy [13]. Compared with placebo, graft loss after IL2RA treatment was reduced by 25% at 6 months and 1 year, with concomitant reduction in biopsy-proven acute rejection (BPAR) at 1 year and a decrease in the incidence of CMV infection. When IL2RA treatment was compared with ATG, there was no difference in graft loss or clinical rejection, but ATG was associated with a decreased risk of BPAR, as well as an increased risk of malignancy and CMV infection [13].

The other primary monoclonal antibody therapy is rituximab, a chimeric anti-CD20 monoclonal antibody. CD20 is involved in B-cell activation, so rituximab is typically used as an induction agent in sensitized patients. More commonly, it is used as an adjunct therapy in treating antibody mediated rejection and as treatment for post-transplant lymphoproliferative disorder.

10.6.2 Maintenance

The purpose of maintenance therapy after kidney transplantation is to reduce the immune response to the allograft without generating the complement of side effects associated with intense immunosuppression used for either induction or rescue therapies. The mainstay of maintenance immunotherapy is treatment with calcineurin inhibitors.

Cyclosporine was developed in the 1970s and tacrolimus was clinically utilized beginning in the 1990s. Both act by inhibiting the phosphatase activity of calcineurin that prevents the translocation of nuclear factor of activated T cells, which in turn prevents IL-2 gene transcription and subsequently inhibits T cell activation. Cyclosporine binds to cyclophilin, while tacrolimus binds to an intracellular protein, FKBP-12. Both cyclosporine and tacrolimus have a narrow therapeutic index and require frequent monitoring. Unfortunately, both agents are also associated with a variety of side effects including nephrotoxicity, neurotoxicity, hypertension, hyperlipidemia, and diabetes.

Another cornerstone of maintenance immunosuppression is mycophenolate, an antiproliferative agent which has replaced azathioprine. Mycophenolate is a reversible, non-competitive inhibitor of inosine 5′-monophosphate dehydrogenase. This enzyme is the rate-limiting step in guanine nucleotide synthesis, so inhibition halts DNA synthesis and subsequently depresses T and B cell proliferation. Side effects are primarily gastrointestinal in nature (abdominal pain, diarrhea) and myelosuppression.

Steroid therapy was mentioned previously, and is often continued in a low dose for patients on triple maintenance immunosuppression. Some centers, however, are moving towards steroid free maintenance regimens, as a result of the significant side effect profile associated with long term steroid use.

More recently, the mammalian targets of rapamycin (mTOR) inhibitors sirolimus and everolimus have been used in addition to, or in place of, calcineurin inhibitors. Both sirolimus and everolimus act by binding to FK506-binding protein 12, which interferes with downstream signaling and cytokine activation, ultimately inhibiting lymphocyte growth and proliferation. While mTOR inhibitors have yet to replace calcineurin inhibitors in maintenance immunosuppression, they have been associated with a small but significant decrease in the development of overall post-transplant malignancy and in non-melanoma skin cancer specifically. Aside from proteinuria, the most concerning complication of mTOR inhibitors is their impact on wound healing. As a result, most recipients are transitioned to mTOR inhibitors in the first month or two following transplantation, when it is presumed that the anastomoses and wound are adequately healed.

Increasingly, the important role of antibody mediated rejection has been identified as an important factor in graft loss. There is great interest in its classification and treatment. The development of donor specific antibodies is a prognostic factor for graft loss. Rituximab and plasmapheresis may be used once a patient has developed donor specific antibodies.

10.7   National Self-Sufficiency

Organ shortage remains the most pressing issue in transplantation; in the US, nearly 7000 people die each year awaiting transplantation, and a similar phenomenon is observed in countries throughout the world. Since the early 2000s, the World Health Organization (WHO) has emphasized the importance of national self-sufficiency. The concept of self-sufficiency is that countries can meet the transplant needs of their citizens and residents through donors from their own population, and through regional collaboration. The importance of self-sufficiency is that it provides all the transplant needs from within a given country and eliminates the need to rely on the population or practices of another country as an organ source [14].

Self-sufficiency can realistically be obtained through robust deceased donor programs, as seen in countries such as the US, England, and Spain, but it can also be achieved through optimization of living donor transplants. For countries with robust deceased donor practices, utilization of marginal or high-risk donors has been one strategy used to increase the number of donor organs. In Spain, improved utilization of donation after cardiac death donors and older donors has led to an enormous overall increase in donor organs. In countries with fledgling deceased donor programs, however, increasing deceased donation can be difficult—often due to social, cultural, and religious beliefs. In Korea, implementation of a national reporting mechanism for all potential brain dead donors increased deceased donors significantly (from 148 deceased donors in 2007 to 408 deceased donors in 2012) [15]. Perhaps the best example of this transformation is in Iran. After brain death was officially recognized in 2000, the rate of deceased donors increased dramatically. Now, at Namazi hospital in Shiraz, more than 92% of kidney transplants are performed using organs from deceased donors. There is no monetary compensation for donation, but the families of the deceased are honored, the donor is buried in a martyr's graveyard, and family members also receive priority access to health care services [15].

In 2011, Delmonico, Dominguez-Gil and colleagues proposed that national self-sufficiency required five factors: (1) national legislation and regulatory oversight; (2) deceased donation practice integrated into the healthcare system; (3) ethical living donation system; (4) donation/transplantation practices aligned with international health organization standards; and (5) preventative medical practices to curtail the development of end stage organ failure [14]. The previously mentioned examples highlight the importance of tailoring efforts toward self-sufficiency according to the needs of individual countries. While international oversight from organizations such as the WHO and The Transplantation Society (TTS) is essential, strong advocates for self-sufficiency must come from within each country as well, in order to both identify and implement best practices.

10.8   Organ Trafficking

In 2004, the WHO issued a call to member states to "protect the poor and vulnerable from transplant tourism and to address the wider problem of international trafficking of human organs and tissues". In response, in 2008, TTS and the International Society of Nephrology (ISN) convened a summit in Istanbul to create a declaration defining organ trafficking and transplant tourism and to achieve consensus on principles of practice. This meeting generated the Declaration of Istanbul (DOI), which was endorsed by more than 135 professional societies and has served as an ethical compass for the transplant community for the past 10 years. The Declaration of Istanbul Custodian Group (DICG) was formed in 2010 and charged with promoting and implementing the principles of the declaration across the world. In 2017, the Pontifical Academy of Sciences (PAS) of the Vatican City convened the Summit on Organ Trafficking and Transplant Tourism. This gathering of international physicians, ethicists, and jurists culminated in the issuance of a statement officially condemning organ trafficking and recognizing it as a crime against humanity. In March 2018, the DICG called for increased investigation and reporting of patients who have traveled abroad for transplantation, in order to provide better care for this patient population [16]. And in June 2018, the DICG issued an updated edition of the DOI, with further detail and clarification of definitions and guiding principles.

The 2018 DOI defines organ trafficking as follows [17]:

(a) removing organs from living or deceased donors without valid consent or authorization or in exchange for financial gain or comparable advantage to the donor and/or a third person;

(b) any transportation, manipulation, transplantation or other use of such organs;

(c) offering any undue advantage to, or requesting the same by, a healthcare professional, public official, or employee of a private sector entity to facilitate or perform such removal or use;

(d) soliciting or recruiting donors or recipients, where carried out for financial gain or comparable advantage; or.

(e) attempting to commit, or aiding or abetting the commission of, any of these acts.

According to the WHO, over 125,000 transplants are performed each year and approximately 10% of transplants occur as part of international organ trade [18]. The majority of these are kidney transplants, and countries known to be engaging in various forms of organ trafficking include Pakistan, India, China, and the Phillipines [18]. Quantifying the exact burden of organ trafficking, identifying vulnerable populations of potential donors, and prosecuting the individuals and organizations that enable organ trafficking has remained challenging, due largely in part to the covert nature of these operations. As a result, the majority of information on organ trafficking comes from media reports or statement papers from societies such as the WHO, TTS, or PAS.

To circumvent this dearth of information, Delmonico published an overview of international organ trafficking activities in 2009 [19]. In this review, he described a variety of practices taking place throughout the world, including the use of organs from executed prisoners in China (a practice that has ceased as of the writing of this chapter), utilization of deceased donor livers in Columbia in excess of that required to support the Columbian population alone, living unrelated donor vendors in Iran, and travel largely from the United States and Canada for organ purchases abroad [19]. As evidenced by these examples, the DOI is violated in a variety of ways throughout the world, which adds an additional layer of complexity to implementing and upholding its principles.

While efforts to identify and eradicate organ trafficking internationally have continued over the past decade, a new area of interest has emerged in the United States: travel for transplantation. Travel for transplantation and transplant tourism are phenomena related to organ trafficking. Travel for transplantation is defined by the WHO and DOI as, "the movement of organs, donors, recipients or transplant professionals across jurisdictional borders for transplantation purposes" [20]. Travel for transplantation becomes transplant tourism when trafficking of persons is introduced or when the allocation of organs to non-resident patients undermines a country's ability to achieve self-sufficiency in organ transplantation [21]. Transplant tourism is internationally regarded as an unethical practice.

In the US, travel for transplantation comes occurs in both imports and exports: (1) imports: transplant of foreign nationals in the US, and (2) exports: US residents or citizens who travel abroad for transplantation. The latter is not well described, but the former has become increasingly discussed, particularly as organ allocation policies continue to evolve. Transplant centers are allowed to perform transplants in non-citizen, non-resident patients; historically, these cases were limited to 5% of the center's total transplant volume. In 2014, this policy changed and removed the 5% restriction but mandated reporting of whether recipients had traveled to the US specifically for the purpose of undergoing transplantation. In 2018, Ascher et al. examined the phenomenon of transplants performed in the US in non-resident, non-citizen recipients between 2013 and 2016 [22]; 1176 transplants were performed in this cohort, constituting 2% of the total transplant volume in the US during that time period. Approximately 50% of the non-resident, non-citizen patients who underwent transplantation during the study period had traveled to the US with the explicit purpose of undergoing transplantation. A subsequent study by Goldberg et al. examined outcomes after transplantation in foreign national patients and found that, compared with US residents, non-resident, non-citizen liver transplant candidates were less likely to die or be removed from the waitlist, had lower post-transplant mortality, and were more likely to be lost to follow up after transplantation [22].

Travel for transplantation, transplant tourism, and organ trafficking remain significant problems facing the international transplant community. In order to maintain the trust of the public, honor the gifts of both living and deceased donors, and safeguard the reputation of our field, we must remain engaged and vigilant with regard to these complex ethical, legal, and political issues.

10.9   Conclusion

Since the first successful transplant in 1954, kidney transplantation has driven the global development of the entire field of solid organ transplantation. This phenomenon is due to the global burden of kidney disease and to the immunogenicity of the kidney, which has propelled the study of rejection and tolerance and fueled the development of better immunosuppressants. In high income societies, the current focus in kidney transplantation is optimizing access, utilizing marginal donor organs to increase organ availability, and finding new ways to increase graft longevity. In lower income societies, however, fundamental issues such as access to transplantation and protection of donors and their families remain at the forefront. As we promote and encourage the implementation of self-sufficiency across the world, it is our hope that disparities in access to kidney transplantation and the exploitation of vulnerable donor populations will dissipate.

References

1. Ojo A. Addressing the global burden of chronic kidney disease through clinical and translational research. Trans Am Clin Climatol Assoc. 2014;125:229–43. discussion 243–226
2. Torres-Toledano M, Granados-Garcia V, Lopez-Ocana LR. Global burden of disease of chronic kidney disease in Mexico. Rev Med Inst Mex Seguro Soc. 2017;55(Suppl 2):S118–23.
3. Disease GBD, Injury I, Prevalence C. Global, regional, and national incidence, prevalence, and years lived with disability for 310 diseases and injuries, 1990–2015: a systematic analysis for the global burden of disease study 2015. Lancet. 2016;388(10053):1545–602.
4. Globa observatory on donation and transplantation. 2018. www.transplant-observatory.org.
5. Sood A, Ghosh P, Menon M, Jeong W, Bhandari M, Ahlawat R. Robotic renal transplantation: current status. J Minim Access Surg. 2015;11(1):35–9.
6. Ratner LE, Ciseck LJ, Moore RG, Cigarroa FG, Kaufman HS, Kavoussi LR. Laparoscopic live donor nephrectomy. Transplantation. 1995;60(9):1047–9.
7. Morris PJ, Knechtle SJ. Kidney transplantation: principles and practice. 7th ed. Philadelphia: Elsevier; 2014.

8. Mackinnon B, Fraser E, Simpson K, Fox JG, Geddes C. Is it necessary to stop antiplatelet agents before a native renal biopsy? Nephrol Dial Transplant. 2008;23(11):3566–70.

9. Hurst FP, Abbott KC, Neff RT, et al. Incidence, predictors and outcomes of transplant renal artery stenosis after kidney transplantation: analysis of USRDS. Am J Nephrol. 2009;30(5):459–67.

10. Voiculescu A, Schmitz M, Hollenbeck M, et al. Management of arterial stenosis affecting kidney graft perfusion: a single-Centre study in 53 patients. Am J Transplant. 2005;5(7):1731–8.

11. Shoskes DA, Hanbury D, Cranston D, Morris PJ. Urological complications in 1,000 consecutive renal transplant recipients. J Urol. 1995;153(1):18–21.

12. Karam G, Hetet JF, Maillet F, et al. Late ureteral stenosis following renal transplantation: risk factors and impact on patient and graft survival. Am J Transplant. 2006;6(2):352–6.

13. Webster AC, Ruster LP, McGee R, et al. Interleukin 2 receptor antagonists for kidney transplant recipients. Cochrane Database Syst Rev. 2010;1:CD003897.

14. Delmonico FL. The science and social necessity of deceased organ donation. Rambam Maimonides Med J. 2011;2(2):e0048.

15. Min SI, Ahn C, Han DJ, et al. To achieve national self-sufficiency: recent progresses in deceased donation in Korea. Transplantation. 2015;99(4):765–70.

16. Dominguez-Gil B, Danovitch G, Martin DE, et al. Management of Patients who Receive an organ transplant abroad and return home for follow-up care: recommendations from the declaration of Istanbul custodian group. Transplantation. 2018;102(1):e2–9.

17. Group DoIC. The declaration of Istanbul on organ trafficking and transplant tourism (2018 Edition). 2018.

18. Shimazono Y. The state of the international organ trade: a provisional picture based on integration of available information. Bull World Health Organ. 2007;85(12):955–62.

19. Delmonico FL. The implications of Istanbul declaration on organ trafficking and transplant tourism. Curr Opin Organ Transplant. 2009;14(2):116–9.

20. World Health Organization. Global glossary of terms and definitions on donation and transplantation. Geneva: WHO; 2009.

21. Summit SCotI. Organ trafficking and transplant tourism and commercialism: the declaration of Istanbul. Lancet. 2008;372:5–6.

22. Delmonico FL, Gunderson S, Iyer KR, et al. Deceased donor organ transplantation performed in the United States for noncitizens and nonresidents. Transplantation. 2018;102(7):1124–31.

Surgical Complications after Kidney Transplant

11

Mehmet Haberal, Fatih Boyvat, Aydincan Akdur, Mahir Kirnap, Ümit Özçelik, and Feza Yarbuğ Karakayali

11.1 Introduction

11.1.1 Intraoperative Complications of External Iliac Arterial Dissection

Traumatic external iliac artery dissection (EIAD) after renal transplant is a rare complication, but it should be treated immediately due to its devastating effects on graft and lower limb circulation. External iliac artery dissection is seen more in recipients with diabetes mellitus and comorbid diseases. Vascular atherosclerosis and cardiomyopathy are predisposing factors for EIAD. Besides senility, hypertension, dyslipidemia, smoking, and diabetes, many other risk factors (like anemia, microalbuminemia, and oxidative stress) may play a role in EIAD in patients with end-stage renal disease. External iliac artery dissection after renal transplant appears with

hypertension, sudden pain in lower limbs without pulse, oliguria, or anuria. Graft artery and femoral artery blood flow cannot be visualized by Doppler ultrasound. Recipients with EIAD should be treated immediately by percutaneous angioplasty or surgical reconstruction. In the literature, some cases have been treated by percutaneous angioplasty and stenting and/or endarterectomy [1]. The other treatment option is reconstruction with expanded polytetrafluoroethylene (ePTFE) graft. In our center, EIAD complications have occurred in only 2 patients. Both cases were due to vascular clamping, and we treated the patients with expanded polytetrafluoroethylene graft reconstruction technique (Fig. 11.1). The dissected part of the external iliac artery was resected and replaced with a 6- to 8-cm × 8-mm PTFE graft using 6/0 Prolene. The renal artery was then anastomosed to the PTFE graft with 7/0 Prolene continuously. Both patients were doing well at follow-up with normal kidney function (Fig. 11.2a and b).

11.2 Postoperative Vascular Complications

Vascular complications can result from renal graft vessels (renal artery thrombosis, renal vein thrombosis), the native vessels (iliac artery

M. Haberal (✉) · A. Akdur · M. Kirnap
Departments of General Surgery and Transplantation,
Başkent University, Ankara, Turkey
e-mail: rectorate@baskent.edu.tr

F. Boyvat
Departments of Interventional Radiology,
Başkent University, Ankara, Turkey

Ü. Özçelik · F. Y. Karakayali
Department of General Surgery and Transplantation,
Başkent University, Istanbul, Turkey

© Springer Nature Switzerland AG 2021
N. Hakim et al. (eds.), *Transplantation Surgery*, Springer Specialist Surgery Series,
https://doi.org/10.1007/978-3-030-55244-2_11

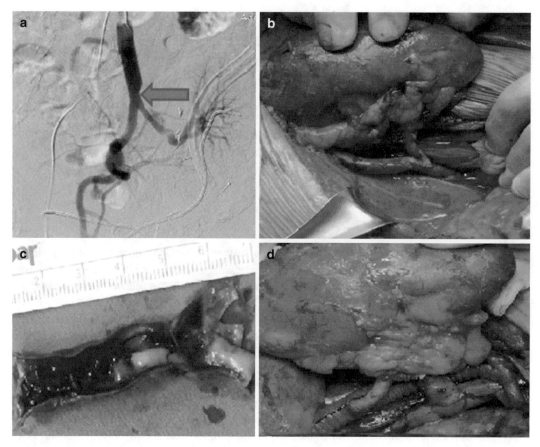

Fig. 11.1 (**a**) Dissection of Left Common Iliac Artery and Occlusion of the Dissected External Iliac Artery; (**b**) Dissected External Iliac Artery; (**c**) Inside of Dissected External Iliac Artery; (**d**) External Iliac Artery Is Replaced With Expanded Polytetrafluoroethylene Graft

thrombosis, pseudoaneurysms, deep venous thrombosis), or both.

Refinement of the operative technique for kidney transplant has greatly reduced surgical complications, morbidity, and mortality rates in recipients. In particular, significant progress has been made regarding methods of vascular anastomosis. The introduction of the Carrel patch vascular technique by Alexis Carrel in 1902 is considered one of the most important steps in transplant surgery [2]. Some vascular complications associated with renal transplant procedures can be managed with percutaneous techniques. Others call for urgent surgical intervention because of possible graft loss if treatment is not swift and appropriate. The incidence of vascular complications has been reported to be as high as

30% during early stages of transplant development, whereas currently the incidence rate is 0.8–6% [3].

According to Clarke and associates [4], Starzl (1964) mentioned 1 patient who survived removal of a pulmonary embolus and complications of the vena cava for 2 months, during which the kidney functioned, but at necropsy the renal vein was occluded by thrombus, which extended to its smallest branches. Another group (Smellie and associates, 1968) attempted to visualize the renal vein by pertrochanteric venography in 3 transplant recipients. In all 3 patients, the renal vein was thought to be patent, although only its terminal portion was demonstrated as such. Other groups reported by Clarke and associates included Walsh, who described arterial

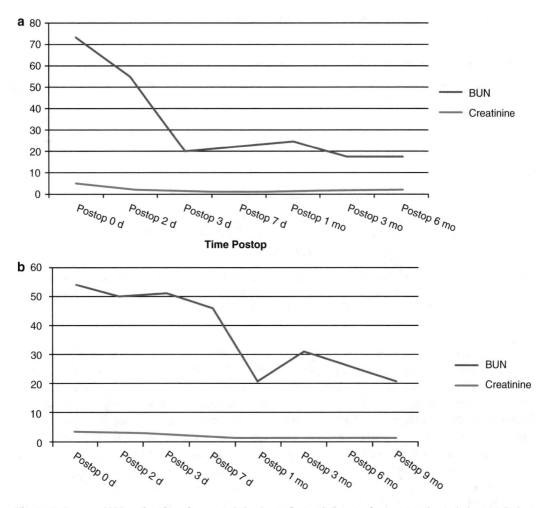

Fig. 11.2 Improved kidney function after expanded polytetrafluoroethylene graft reconstruction technique (**a**) Patient 1; (**b**) Patient 2. Abbreviations: *BUN* serum urea nitrogen, *Postop* postoperative

complications but did not mention thrombosis of the renal vein in 1969, and Khastagir and associates, who mentioned 2 patients in 1969 in which thrombosis of the renal vessels occurred as part of the rejection process, although the investigators did not specifically describe the renal veins. Finally, Owen in 1969 suggested that, if diagnosed early enough, it was worthwhile to explore thrombosed anastomoses but that it was not often possible to obtain a viable kidney.

In Turkey, the first living donor kidney transplant was performed by Haberal and team on November 3, 1975. Since 1975, Haberal has described different vascular anastomosis techniques. From November 1993 to December 2003,

his group performed end-to-side or end-to-end anastomoses using the 4 quadrant running suture technique [5]. After December 2003, he defined corner-saving renal artery anastomosis [6]. In his series, arterial complication rates are 0.35% for thrombosis and 0.7% for stenosis.

11.2.1 Postoperative Iliac Artery Dissection

The dissection of the iliac artery is a rare complication. A few cases have been reported in the literature [7–9], and one of our patients also presented with this complication. Seven days

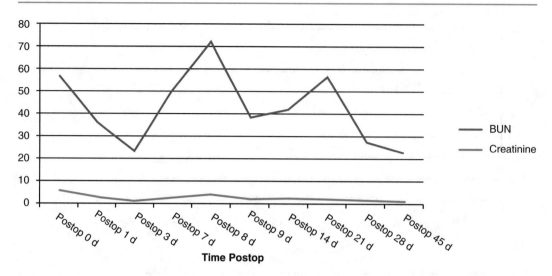

Fig. 11.3 Postoperative creatinine levels of patient. Kidney function decreased after postoperative day 7 due to external iliac artery dissection and improved after expanded polytetrafluoroethylene graft reconstruction. Abbreviations: *BUN* serum urea nitrogen, *Postop* postoperative

after transplant, immediate surgery was required. After exploration, the renal artery was separated from the external iliac artery. The kidney was then flushed with histidine-tryptophan-ketoglutarate solution via the renal artery, after a renal vein branch opening. Without opening the main renal vein anastomosis, we replaced the dissected section of the external iliac artery with a PTFE graft, and the graft kidney's artery was anastomosed to it. At last follow-up, the patient's kidney was functioning well (Fig. 11.3).

11.2.2 Renal Artery Thrombosis

Although vascular thrombosis is a rare complication, it has become a major cause of early graft loss, accounting for up to one-third of graft loss within 1 month and up to 45–47% within 2–3 months. In the pediatric North American Pediatric Renal Transplant Cooperative Study cohort from 1996 to 2001, thrombosis was the most common cause of early graft loss [2, 10].

Renal artery thrombosis usually occurs soon after transplant and is a catastrophic complication, usually resulting in graft loss. Its incidence is reported to range from 0.2 to 7.5% [2] or from 0.5 to 3.5% [11–13]. Children have a higher incidence

than adults. The most important sign of renal artery thrombosis is instantaneous cessation of urine outflow due to the absence of graft perfusion and the presence of worsening hypertension. In preemptive patients and patients who have preoperative urine output, this sign can be masked. In these patients, postoperative bedside Doppler ultrasonography is recommended [14]. The most common causes of renal artery thrombosis are technical complications, including faulty suture techniques producing incomplete intimal reapproximation with secondary intraluminal fibrosis.

Since November 1975, our transplant team has performed 2248 kidney transplants. We currently use the four-quadrant running suture technique or the corner-saving renal artery anastomosis for arterial anastomosis. During this period, 8 renal artery thromboses (0.35%) have been seen, with surgical exploration performed in 5 patients, which included thrombectomy, reperfusion, and reanastomoses. The other 3 patients who developed renal artery thrombosis were treated with percutaneous transluminal angioplasty, thrombolysis, and intraluminal stent placement. One of the 8 patients with renal arterial thrombosis died from a pulmonary embolism at 9 days after transplant. The remaining 7 patients had normal renal function (Fig. 11.4).

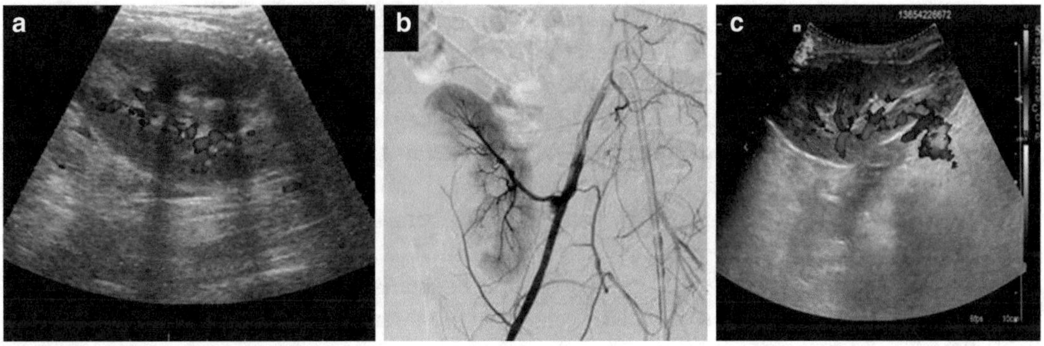

Fig. 11.4 Segmental renal artery thrombosis. (**a**) Doppler ultrasonography showing decreased perfusion of the anterior segmental branch. (**b**) Angiographic image revealing occluded segmental artery, with patient subsequently anti- coagulated with Coumadin. (**c**) Doppler ultrasonography showing normal perfusion at first year due to hypertrophy of the remaining renal parenchyma

Another surgical complication related to renal artery thrombosis is the possible development of endothelial damage during donor nephrectomy and/or perfusion. The other factors for thrombosis are kinking or twisting of the renal artery, postoperative hypotension, hypercoagulable state, atherosclerosis of the donor or recipient vessels, wide disparity in vessel size, increased intrarenal pressure resulting from acute tubular necrosis, hydronephrosis, or cellular rejection. In our center, 7 cases (0.3%) of renal artery kinking were seen, with patients treated via surgical exploration to rearrange the positions of their grafts. All patients had return of normal renal function.

Renal artery thrombosis is a surgical emergency and its diagnosis is made by color Doppler ultrasonography or surgical exploration. To save the transplanted kidney, immediate exploration with restoration of the blood flow to the kidney is needed. A few cases of graft salvage in transplant renal artery thrombosis with endovascular catheter-directed thrombolysis with or without angioplasty have been reported. More commonly, by the time diagnosis is confirmed, it is already too late, and graft nephrectomy is the only option left.

11.2.3 Renal Artery Stenosis

Renal artery stenosis represents the most common vascular complication, with an estimated incidence between 19 and 23% of all transplant recipients [15–17]. In our centers, the rates are 0.5–0.75%. Renal artery stenosis is diagnosed first using ultrasonography and then angiography. Our preferred and initial option for treatment is the interventional radiologic approach. However, in cases where this is not successful, we have resorted to surgical reconstruction [12–14, 17–21].

Transplant renal artery stenosis (TRAS) is a relatively frequent, potentially curable cause of refractory hypertension and allograft dysfunction that accounts for approximately 1–5% of cases of posttransplant hypertension (renal transplant arterial stenosis). In some series, the incidence of TRAS was reported to be 25%. It usually becomes apparent between 3 months and 3 years after renal transplant, but it can present at any time. Transplant renal artery stenosis can occur at the anastomosis, preanastomosis, or postanastomotic renal artery stage. About 50% are located at the anastomosis, and end-to-end anastomoses have a threefold higher risk than end-to-side anastomoses. It frequently presents with worsening or refractory hypertension and/or graft dysfunction in the absence of rejection, ureteric obstruction, or infection. Different locations and timing of disease onset may reflect different causes. Thus, an anastomotic stenosis is most likely related to trauma to the donor or recipient vessels during organ recovery, clamping, or suturing and usually arises early after transplant. Small, subtle intimal flaps or subintimal dissections of the vascular wall precede intimal scarring and hyperplasia that result in narrowing or occlusion of the lumen. The other predictors of TRAS include older donor and recipient age, expanded criteria donors (defined as any deceased donor over the age of 60 y or from a donor over the age of 50 y with 2 of the following: a history of hypertension, a terminal serum creatinine level $\geq$ 1.5 mg/dL, or death resulting from a cerebral vascular accident), delayed graft function, ischemic heart disease, and induction immunosuppression.

Evaluation of TRAS may be performed with both noninvasive and invasive imaging techniques. Color flow duplex ultrasonography and magnetic resonance angiography have now become the primary noninvasive imaging modalities for diagnosis of TRAS, although catheter-based angiography has conventionally been held as the criterion standard in evaluation of arterial stenosis.

Three different treatment options are feasible. If the kidney functions and Doppler ultrasonography finding are normal, the first option for treatment can be medical therapy. In these patients, angiotensin-converting enzyme inhibitors should be used to control blood pressure.

Intervention, either percutaneous or surgical, may be considered if refractory hypertension and/or worsening graft function as measured by increasing creatinine levels are present. Primary treatment with percutaneous transluminal angioplasty with or without stent placement have shown significant improvements in blood pressure and creatinine levels and can be considered as an initial treatment of choice (Figs. 11.5, 11.6 and 11.7).

11.2.4 Renal Vein Thrombosis

Renal vein thrombosis usually occurs within the first 7 days after transplant. The incidence of renal vein thrombosis ranges from 0.1 to 8.2%, and it usually causes graft lost in the early period of transplant [2, 4, 10]. Risk factors for renal vein thrombosis are surgical technical errors, hypercoagulopathy states such as deficiency of anti-

thrombin III, protein C, or protein S, right kidney transplant with kinking due to short renal vein, transplant in the left iliac fossa with kinking due to position of external iliac vein, dehydration, ipsilateral iliofemoral thrombophlebitis, deep femoral thrombosis, and vascular compression due to hematomas and lymphoceles. Clinical presentations of this condition include sudden oliguria or anuria accompanied by pain, hematuria, and life-threatening hemorrhage due to rupture of the graft. Depending on hemorrhage, patients may develop circulatory shock. For diagnosis, Doppler imaging studies are the best diagnostic tools [14, 17]. In our clinic, we routinely apply Doppler ultrasonography examinations on the postoperative third and seventh days for diagnoses of early vascular problems. Furthermore, Doppler ultrasonography must be performed during the immediate postoperative period on clinical suspicion and/or biochemical evidence of renal dysfunction. Evaluations of renal Doppler ultrasonography can confirm the increase in renal volume and absence of venous flow [13, 17, 20]. An arterial view can show reverse diastolic flow. Perinephric hematomas and lymphocele can also be seen with ultrasonography. External compression of the vessels (hematomas, lymphocele) produce vascular problems. These problems can be solved by percutaneous drainage.

Treatment includes emergency exploration for venous thrombectomy and to restore blood flow. If this treatment is not possible, nephrectomy is performed to save the patient. In our series, we had 4 patients (0.17%) who developed renal vein thrombosis after transplant, with all treated with urgent thrombectomy. Unfortunately, 2 of the treatments were unsuccessful, and the grafts were lost. One patient had a renal vein problem due to external iliac vein thrombosis. Interventional radiologists placed a self-expanding stent to the proximal external iliac vein, and the graft was rescued. At recent follow-up, all patients maintained good graft function (Fig. 11.8). In our center, 9 patients (0.4%) showed renal vein kinking, which was treated with surgical exploration to reposition the graft. At recent follow-up, all patients maintained normal renal function.

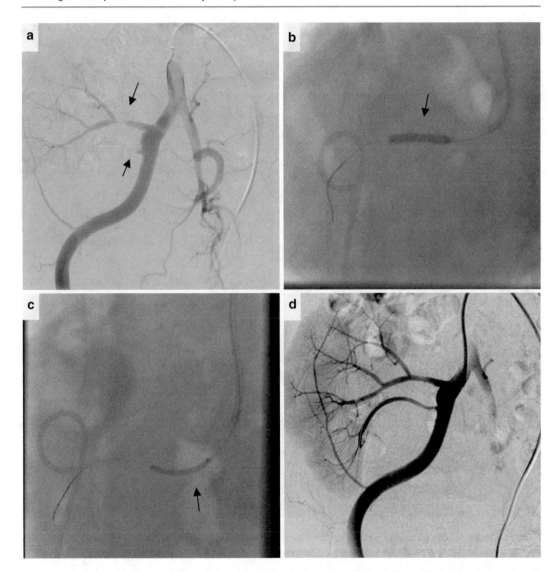

Fig. 11.5 Renal percutaneous transluminal angioplasty. (**a**) High-grade stenosis of the main and the polar arteries of transplanted renal artery. (**b** and **c**) Balloon dilation of both arteries. (**d**) Postballoon dilation showing good result after percutaneous transluminal angioplasty

11.3   Posttransplant Urologic Complications

Urologic complications are the most common surgical complications encountered after renal transplant, causing significant morbidity and mortality [22–24]. Rates of urologic complications after kidney transplant range between 2.5 and 30% of all recipients [22, 23, 25–27].

11.3.1   Urine Leakage

Urologic complications associated with the ureterovesical anastomosis after transplant may cause graft loss and mortality. Incidences of urinary leakage in different transplant centers have ranged from 0 to 8.9%, with incidences of ureteric stricture reported to range from 0.1 to 12.4%. Major urologic complications, for exam-

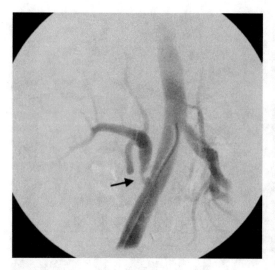

Fig. 11.6 Anastomotic stenosis of transplanted renal artery at 9 months after transplant

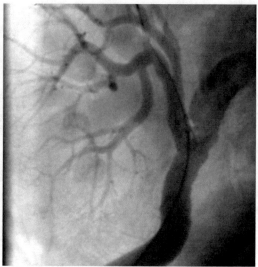

Fig. 11.7 Stent placement for stenosis

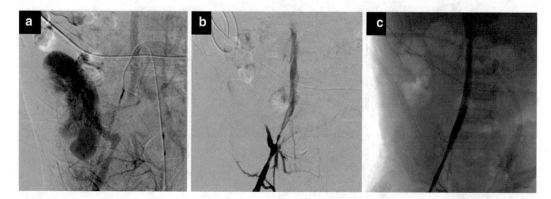

Fig. 11.8 Renal vein complications due to external iliac vein thrombosis. (**a** and **b**) External iliac vein is blocked and causing venous congestion of the renal vein. (**c**) Placement of self-expanding vascular stent in the external iliac vein

ple leakage and stenosis, are often related to the ureteroneocystostomy [25, 28]. To avoid urologic complications, clinicians at some transplant centers routinely prefer stenting as this maneuver avoids anastomotic tension, kinking, and ureteral narrowing. In our center, from 1975 to 1983, we performed ureteroneocystostomies using the modified Politano-Leadbetter technique [29]. Beginning in 1983, we began using the extravesicular Lich-Gregoir technique in combination with temporary ureteral stenting [29]. In September 2003, we began using the corner-saving ureteral reimplantation technique without stenting [30, 31]. Because the double J stent increases the risk of postoperative urinary infection and removal of this device requires an invasive procedure, we prefer not to routinely use a double J ureteral catheter. Although there are many disadvantages to the stent we do advocate its use in select patient groups such as those with thin graft kidney ureter walls or thin urine bladder walls, especially with transplants involving deceased donations. To evaluate complications early, we use ultrasonographic and scintigraphic findings from days 1, 3, and 7 and creatinine levels on day 7 and at 1 month after transplant. In our series, 1% of patients developed urine leakage after transplant.

Risk factors that contribute to the prevalence of urologic complications need to be determined. So far, many factors have been described in the literature, including several donor and recipient characteristics. Furthermore, problems encountered during graft recovery, prolonged ischemia times, type of ureteroneocystostomy, presence of accessory arteries, and stent placement may influence the incidence of urologic complications.

It has been suggested that urologic complications are caused by an insufficient blood supply to the ureter. Excessive dissection of the site known as "golden triangle" (the site confined by the ureter, kidney and renal artery) should therefore be avoided during graft procurement. Damage of this triangle may lead to necrosis of the distal ureter in 70% of cases.

In most cases, these complications require placement of a percutaneous nephrostomy (Fig. 11.9). Sometimes, even a surgical revision is required, leading to additional morbidity and costs.

11.3.2 Ureteral Obstruction

Ureteral obstruction occurs in 2–10% of renal transplant patients postoperatively, usually presenting within the first few weeks or the first year [26, 28]. Prompt diagnosis and remedial treatment are vital to prevent graft loss. Ureteric ischemia is the most common cause, accounting for around 90% of occurrences [26, 28]. The other causes are more than 2 arteries, long cold ischemia time, tumor, calculi, lymphocele, hematomas, abscess, kinking, and technical problems. Some occurrences of transplant ureteric stenosis may be associated with ureteric leak or necrosis (Fig. 11.10).

Percutaneous therapy of ureteral strictures consists of balloon dilatation with or without temporary stenting (Figs. 11.11 and 11.12). Balloon dilatation should be repeated to achieve adequate results, especially in patients with resistant strictures. A cut balloon also may be applied in fibrotic strictures in which a standard balloon dilatation would usually fail. After successful dilatation, most authors suggest temporary stenting of the ureter with a double J stent. Metallic stents have been used to treat ureteral stenoses after failed balloon dilatation, but uroepithelial ingrowth has been a major issue with these devices [24, 26, 28].

If all of these methods are unsuccessful, surgical treatment should be applied. The options are to perform either a ureteral reimplantation or a ureteroureterostomy using the native ureter (side-to-side or end-to-end) through an abdominal or a kidney incision.

There are 3 different surgical techniques for ureteral stricture management occurring after renal transplant: [1] proximal transections of the anastomosis after anastomosis stricture and making ureteroneocystostomy; [2] excision of the strictured part and end-to-end ureteroure-

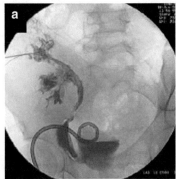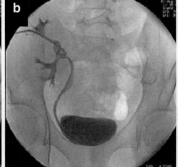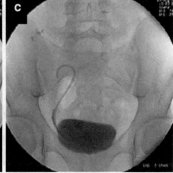

Fig. 11.9 (a) Postrenal transplant ureteral anastomosis leak; (b) Treatment With Percutaneous Nephrostomy and Double J Stent Replacement; (c) At 2-month Follow-Up, Leak Had Disappeared Completely and Nephrostomy Catheter Was Removed. Double J stent was also removed at 2-month follow-up. No sign of leakage after treatment was shown

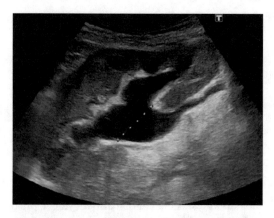

Fig. 11.10 Ultrasonographic image showing hydrone-phrosis due to distal ureteral stricture

terostomy; and [3] ureteroureterostomy using the native ureter (ipsilateral or contralateral native ureter). At our center, we have performed 4 revisions after urethra strictures. For 2 patients, the old ureteroneocystostomy was terminated and a ureteroneocystostomy was performed. In 1 patient, we performed native nephrectomy and end-to-side anastomosis between the native urethra and graft's renal pelvis (Fig. 11.13a and b). Figure 11.14 shows the same patients at postoperative 6-month evaluations. In the other patient, we performed end-to-side anastomosis between the graft's urethra and native urethra.

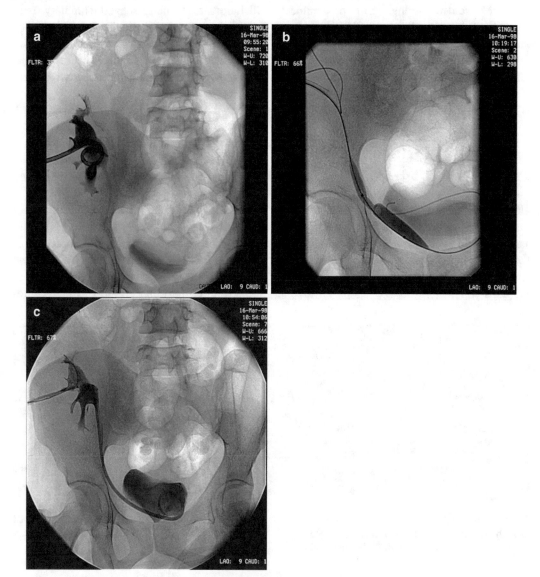

Fig. 11.11 (**a** and **b**) Distal Ureteral Stenosis and Balloon Dilation; (**c**) Double J Stent Placement

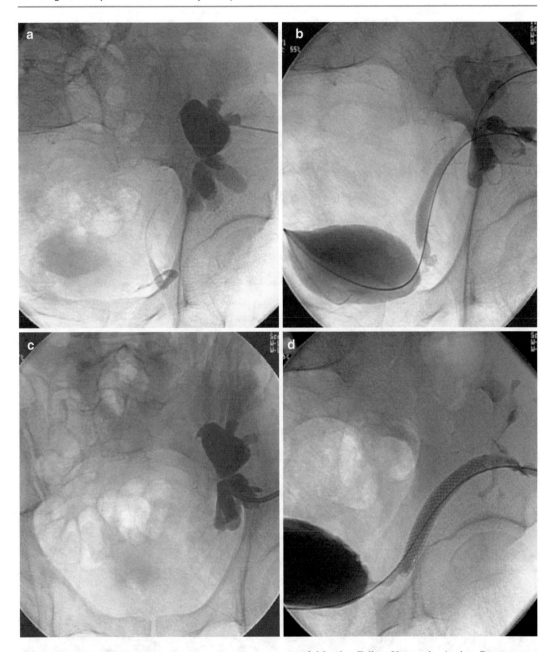

Fig. 11.12 (**a**) Hydronephrosis and Proximal Ureteral Stenosis; (**b**) After Balloon Dilation of Ureter, Infundibulum and Pelvis With 2 Percutaneous Access Points to the Kidney; (**c**) Complete Obstruction Developed at 2-Month Follow-Up and Again Percutaneous Nephrostomy Was Placed; (**d**) Resistant Stenosis of Ureteral Anastomosis, Treated With Metal Stenting

11.3.3 Lymphoceles

Another urologic complication in kidney transplant recipients is a lymphocele, which is a fluid collection between the kidney allograft and the bladder. This complication (rate of 0.6–40%) is caused primarily by extravasation of the lymph from the lymphatic vessels injured during preparation of the iliac vessels of the recipient and unligated lymphatic system from the renal hilum of the donor. Other factors such as acute rejection, urinary obstruction, and graft decapsulation

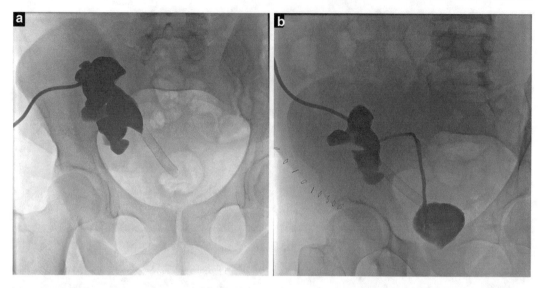

Fig. 11.13 (**a**) Antegrade Pyelography Was Performed Via Nephrostomy Catheter Revealing Occlusion of the Ureter (previously a metal stent had been placed and was also occluded); (**b**) Successful Surgical Result After Uretero-Ureterostomy Pyelography

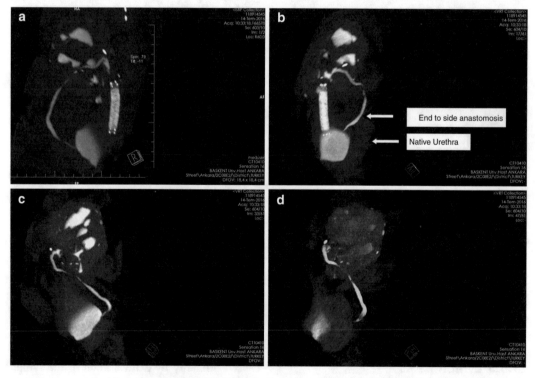

Fig. 11.14 (**a–d**) 6-Month Posttransplant Tomography Images of Patients With Native Nephrectomy and End-to-Side Anastomosis Between Native Ureter and Graft's Renal Pelvis. Ureteroureterostomy anastomosis seems normal, and preoperative pelvicaliceal dilatation has disappeared

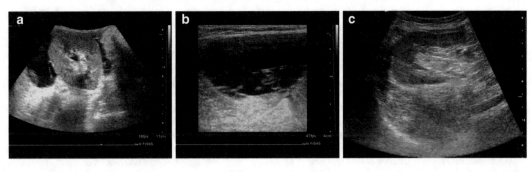

Fig. 11.15 (**a**) and (**b**) Ultrasonographic Examination Revealing Septated Fluid Collection Around Renal Transplant; (**c**) Lymphocele Treated With Percutaneous Drainage, With Control Ultrasonography Showing Complete Healing

may contribute to the development of lymphocele. Patients are usually asymptomatic, and spontaneous resolution occurs after a few months [32–36].

The incidence of symptomatic lymphoceles after kidney transplant in our center has been 4.2% (109/2594 total cases). This complication presented with elevated serum creatinine levels in 31 patients (28.4%), pain and abdominopelvic swelling in 53 patients (48.6%), and lower extremity edema in 25 patients (22.9%). Diagnosis of lymphocele was confirmed by ultrasonography. Percutaneous drainage was used for the treatment of lymphocele in 104 patients (95.4%) and for 66 patients (60.5%) who also received povidone iodine injection. In the remaining 5 patients (4.5%), the primary approach was surgical intraperitoneal drainage due to multiloculated collection and inappropriate access for percutaneous drainage. However, in our experience, percutaneous drainage is the most effective approach to treat this complication (Fig. 11.15).

Acknowledgments The authors declare that they have no sources of funding for this study, and they have no conflicts of interest to declare.

References

1. Tsai SF, Chen CH, Hsieh SR, Shu KH, Ho HC. Salvage of external iliac artery dissection immediately after renal transplant. Exp Clin Transplant. 2013;11(3):274–7. https://doi.org/10.6002/ect.2012.0152.
2. Keller AK, Jorgensen TM, Jespersen B. Identification of risk factors for vascular thrombosis may reduce early renal graft loss: review of recent literature. J Transp Secur. 2012;2012:793461–9. https://doi.org/10.1155/2012/793461.
3. Soliman SA, Shokeir AA, El-Hefnawy AS, et al. Vascular and haemorrhagic complications of adult and paediatric live-donor renal transplantation: a single-centre study with a long-term follow-up. Arab J Urol. 2012;10(2):155–61. https://doi.org/10.1016/j.aju.2011.12.002.
4. Clarke SD, Kennedy JA, Hewitt JC, McEvoy J, McGeown MG, Nelson SD. Successful removal of thrombus from renal vein after renal transplantation. Br Med J. 1970;1(5689):154–5.
5. Haberal M, Karakayali H, Bilgin N, Moray G, Arslan G, Büyükpamukçu N. Four-quadrant running-suture arterial anastomosis technique in renal transplantation: a preliminary report. Transplant Proc. 1996;28(4):2334–5.
6. Haberal M, Moray G, Sevmis S, et al. Corner-saving renal artery anastomosis for renal transplantation. Transplant Proc. 2008;40(1):145–7. https://doi.org/10.1016/j.transproceed.2007.11.071.
7. Merkus JW, Dun GC, Reinaerts HH, Huysmans FT. Iliac artery dissection after renal transplantation. Nephrol Dial Transplant. 1992;7(12):1242–5.
8. Khattab OS, Al-Taee K. Early post transplantation renal allograft perfusion failure due to intimal dissection of the renal artery. Saudi J Kidney Dis Transpl. 2009;20(1):112–5.
9. Esteban RJ, Sánchez D, González F, Bravo JA, Asensio C. Spontaneous iliac artery dissection in a kidney transplantation treated with and endovascular stent. Nephrol Dial Transplant. 1999;14(6):1610.
10. McDonald RA, Smith JM, Stablein D, Harmon WE. Pretransplant peritoneal dialysis and graft thrombosis following pediatric kidney transplantation: a NAPRTCS report. Pediatr Transplant. 2003;7(3):204–8. https://doi.org/10.1034/j.1399-3046.2003.00075.x.
11. Srivastava A, Kumar J, Sharma S, Abhishek, Ansari MS, Kapoor R. vascular complication in live related renal transplant: an experience of 1945 cases. Indian J Urol. 2013;29(1):42–7. https://doi.org/10.4103/0970-1591.109983.

12. Emiroglu R, Karakayali H, Sevmis S, Arslan G, Haberal M. Vascular complications in renal transplantation. Transplant Proc. 2001;33(5):2685–6.

13. Aktas S, Boyvat F, Sevmis S, Moray G, Karakayali H, Haberal M. Analysis of vascular complications after renal transplantation. Transplant Proc. 2011;43(2):557–61. https://doi.org/10.1016/j.transproceed.2011.01.007.

14. Drudi FM, Liberatore M, Cantisani V, et al. Role of color Doppler ultrasound in the evaluation of renal transplantation from living donors. J Ultrasound. 2014;17(3):207–13. https://doi.org/10.1007/s40477-014-0077-6.

15. Bruno S, Remuzzi G, Ruggenenti P. Transplant renal artery stenosis. J Am Soc Nephrol. 2004 Jan;15(1):134–41. https://doi.org/10.1097/01.ASN.0000099379.61001.F8.

16. Seratnahaei A, Shah A, Bodiwala K, Mukherjee D. Management of transplant renal artery stenosis. Angiology. 2011;62(3):219–24. https://doi.org/10.1177/0003319710377076.

17. Iezzi R, la Torre MF, Santoro M, et al. Interventional radiological treatment of renal transplant complications: a pictorial review. Korean J Radiol. 2015;16(3):593–603. https://doi.org/10.3348/kjr.2015.16.3.593.

18. Braga AF, Catto RC, Dalio MB, et al. Endovascular approach to transplant renal artery stenosis. Ann Transplant. 2015;20:698–706. https://doi.org/10.12659/AOT.894867.

19. Rajan DK, Stavropoulos SW, Shlansky-Goldberg RD. Management of transplant renal artery stenosis. Semin Intervent Radiol. 2004;21(4):259–69. https://doi.org/10.1055/s-2004-861560.

20. Libicher M, Radeleff B, Grenacher L, et al. Interventional therapy of vascular complications following renal transplantation. Clin Transpl. 2006;20(Suppl 17):55–9. https://doi.org/10.1111/j.1399-0012.2006.00601.x.

21. El Atat R, Derouiche A, Guellouz S, Gargah T, Lakhoua R, Chebil M. Surgical complications in pediatric and adolescent renal transplantation. Saudi J Kidney Dis Transpl. 2010;21(2):251–7.

22. Slagt IK, Ijzermans JN, Visser LJ, Weimar W, Roodnat JI, Terkivatan T. Independent risk factors for urological complications after deceased donor kidney transplantation. PLoS One. 2014;9(3):e91211. https://doi.org/10.1371/journal.pone.0091211.

23. Dalgic A, Boyvat F, Karakayali H, Moray G, Emiroglu R, Haberal M. Urologic complications in 1523 renal transplantations: the Baskent University experience. Transplant Proc. 2006;38(2):543–7. https://doi.org/10.1016/j.transproceed.2005.12.116.

24. Moray G, Yagmurdur MC, Sevmis S, Ayvaz I, Haberal M. Effect of routine insertion of a double-J stent after living related renal transplantation. Transplant Proc. 2005;37(2):1052–3. https://doi.org/10.1016/j.transproceed.2005.01.083.

25. Ali-Asgari M, Dadkhah F, Ghadian A, Nourbala MH. Impact of ureteral length on urological complications and patient survival after kidney transplantation. Nephrourol Mon. 2013;5(4):878–83. https://doi.org/10.5812/numonthly.10881.

26. Kumar S, Ameli-Renani S, Hakim A, Jeon JH, Shrivastava S, Patel U. Ureteral obstruction following renal transplantation: causes, diagnosis and management. Br J Radiol. 2014;87(1044):20140169. https://doi.org/10.1259/bjr.20140169.

27. Dinckan A, Tekin A, Turkyilmaz S, et al. Early and late urological complications corrected surgically following renal transplantation. Transpl Int. 2007;20(8):702–7. https://doi.org/10.1111/j.1432-2277.2007.00500.x.

28. Aytekin C, Boyvat F, Harman A, Ozyer U, Colak T, Haberal M. Percutaneous therapy of ureteral obstructions and leak after renal transplantation: long-term results. Cardiovasc Intervent Radiol. 2007;30(6):1178–84. https://doi.org/10.1007/s00270-007-9031-8.

29. Emiroğlu R, Karakayall H, Sevmiş S, Akkoç H, Bilgin N, Haberal M. Urologic complications in 1275 consecutive renal transplantations. Transplant Proc. 2001;33(1–2):2016–7. https://doi.org/10.1016/S0041-1345(00)02772-X.

30. Haberal M, Emiroglu R, Karakayali H, et al. A corner-saving ureteral reimplantation technique without stenting. Transplant Proc. 2006;38(2):548–51. https://doi.org/10.1016/j.transproceed.2005.12.112.

31. Haberal M, Karakayali H, Sevmis S, Moray G, Arslan G. Urologic complication rates in kidney transplantation after a novel ureteral reimplantation technique. Exp Clin Transplant. 2006;4(2):503–5.

32. Ranghino A, Segoloni GP, Lasaponara F, Biancone L. Lymphatic disorders after renal transplantation: new insights for an old complication. Clin Kidney J. 2015;8(5):615–22. https://doi.org/10.1093/ckj/sfv064.

33. Bailey SH, Mone MC, Holman JM, Nelson EW. Laparoscopic treatment of post renal transplant lymphoceles. Surg Endosc. 2003;17(12):1896–9. https://doi.org/10.1007/s00464-003-8814-5.

34. Giuliani S, Gamba P, Kiblawi R, Midrio P, Ghirardo G, Zanon GF. Lymphocele after pediatric kidney transplantation: incidence and risk factors. Pediatr Transplant. 2014;18(7):720–5. https://doi.org/10.1111/petr.12341.

35. Coursey Moreno C, Mittal PK, Ghonge NP, Bhargava P, Heller MT. Imaging complications of renal transplantation. Radiol Clin N Am. 2016;54(2):235–49. https://doi.org/10.1016/j.rcl.2015.09.007.

36. Brown ED, Chen MY, Wolfman NT, Ott DJ, Watson NE Jr. Complications of renal transplantation: evaluation with US and radionuclide imaging. Radiographics. 2000;20(3):607–22.

Long-Term Management of the Kidney Transplant Recipient

12

Heidi M. Schaefer

12.1 Introduction

Kidney transplantation remains the treatment of choice for patients with end-stage renal disease. With significant advances in short-term outcomes primarily driven by advances in immunosuppression with low acute rejection rates, a large percentage of patients are surviving long-term with functioning allografts. 3As of 2015 over 200,000 patients in the United States had functioning allografts [1]. These patients present with a particular and complex set of medical issues that require intensive management to allow for longevity of both the patient and the allograft. Due to constraints of the transplant center and a limited number of transplant nephrologists, it is important that the community nephrologist and primary care providers have an understanding of the complex and interacting medical issues these patients face. Common aspects of medical care of the transplant recipient will be discussed here.

H. M. Schaefer (✉)
Division of Nephrology, Department of Medicine, Vanderbilt University School of Medicine, Nashville, TN, USA

Vanderbilt University Medical Center, Nashville, TN, USA
e-mail: heidi.schaefer@vumc.org

12.2 Cardiovascular Disease

Although successful kidney transplantation confers a notable increase in life expectancy over dialysis therapy for patients with ESRD, the survival of kidney transplant recipients is significantly shortened by cardiovascular disease (CVD) [2, 3]. The annual risk of CVD death is 3.5–5% in kidney transplant recipients [4] and is the primary etiology of death with a functioning graft. The most common causes of cardiac death are cardiac arrest (45%), myocardial infarction (31%) and cardiac arrhythmia (13%) [5]. In addition to the CVD burden carried over from ESRD, transplant recipients encounter several factors in the post-transplant period that further accentuate the prevalence and severity of several CVD risk factors. It is well recognized that immunosuppressive agents have associated effects on hypertension, dyslipidemia and diabetes [3]. Aggressive management of these factors must be carried out by the treating physician (Table 12.1).

12.2.1 Hypertension

Hypertension is the most prevalent CVD risk factor in kidney transplant recipients, affecting up to 80% of patients [6]. In addition to essential hypertension, primary kidney disease, quality of donor organ, delayed graft function, acute rejection, calcineurin inhibitor therapy, glucocorticoids, trans-

Table 12.1 Cardiovascular risk factor management in the transplant recipient

Risk factor	Guideline	Goal of treatment	Treatment recommendations	Comments
Hypertension	K/DOQI	<130/80 mmHg	• Lifestyle modification • Calcium channel blocker • ACEI/ARB if proteinuria present • Beta-blocker if known h/o CAD	Avoid diltiazem/verapamil due to interactions with calcineurin inhibitors
Dyslipidemia	NCEP III	Total cholesterol <200 LDL <100 Triglycerides <150	• Lifestyle modification • Statins • Fibrates • Ezetimibe	Avoid bile acid sequestrants. Monitor for hepatitis, myositis and rhabdomyolysis when using statin/fibrate drugs
NODAT	KDIGO	Target HbA1C 7.0–7.5%	• Lifestyle modification • Oral agents • Insulin	Increased risk of lactic acidosis with use of metformin
Anemia	K/DOQI	Target Hgb 11–12 g/dL	• Iron (intravenous and oral) • Recombinant erythropoietin	Avoid liberal use of recombinant erythropoietin due to possible increased risk of thrombotic and vascular events
Obesity	KDIGO	BMI <35–40 kg/m^2	• Lifestyle modification • Referral to dietician • Bariatric surgery	
Tobacco abuse	KDIGO	Smoking cessation	• Behavioral counseling • Pharmacologic therapy	

K/DOQI Kidney Disease Outcome Quality Initiative, *NCEP III* National Cholesterol Education Program Report of the Expert Panel, *KDIGO* Kidney Disease Improving Global Outcomes, *ACEI* ace inhibitor, *ARB* angiotension receptor blocker, *LDL* low density lipoprotein, *HbA1C* hemoglobin A1C, *Hgb*, hemoglobin, *BMI* body mass index

plant renal artery stenosis and chronic allograft nephropathy all contribute to the pathogenesis of post-transplant hypertension [7]. Based on published guidelines, the recommended treatment goal for hypertension in transplant recipients is <130/80 mm Hg [8]. In addition to lifestyle modifications including weight loss, dietary sodium restriction and physical exercise, the majority of transplant recipients will require medical therapy to achieve goal blood pressure. Most classes of antihypertensive agents have been used and are effective in treating kidney transplant recipients but it is important to recognize that the pharmacologic management of hypertension in this population presents several unique issues related to potential drug interactions and side effects. Calcium channel blockers have been used as first line agents due to their vasodilatory properties that may counteract the vasoconstrictive effects of calcineurin inhibitors. It should be noted however

that verapamil and diltiazem significantly interact with and raise calcineurin inhibitor levels with potential for nephrotoxicity and should be avoided if possible. In those patients who have known CVD, beta-blockers are recommended as first line agents. If the transplant recipient has significant proteinuria and/or diabetes, angiotensin converting enzyme inhibitors or angiotensin receptor blockers should be instituted due to their potential reno-protective effects with close attention given to serum potassium levels.

12.2.2 Dyslipidemia

Post-transplant hyperlipidemia occurs in 60–80% of transplant recipients with immunosuppressive agents contributing significantly to lipid abnormalities [9]. Increases in total cholesterol and LDL are the most common abnormalities, with elevated triglyceride levels usually noted as well. All recipients should have at least one fasting lipid panel obtained within the first 2–3 months after transplant and then measured annually. Updated KDIGO guidelines no longer recommend specific LDL cholesterol treatment targets. Instead, the decision to initiate cholesterol-lowering treatment should be based on the absolute risk of coronary events [10] with kidney transplantation considered as a coronary heart disease equivalent risk. In addition to therapeutic lifestyle changes and dietary modification, it has been suggested that statin therapy be prescribed for all kidney transplant recipients >30 years of age regardless of baseline cholesterol level. In one of the few randomized controlled trials in transplantation, the Assessment of Lescol in Renal Transplant (ALERT) trial demonstrated a significant reduction in LDL cholesterol, incidence of myocardial infarction and cardiac death in those patients randomized to Fluvastatin [11]. For those patients with significant hypertriglyceridemia, fibric acid derivatives such as gemfibrozil are recommended [12]. Both statins and fibrate drugs can interact with calcineurin inhibitors and increase the risk of hepatitis, myositis and rhabdomyolysis with close monitoring of patients required after institution of these agents. Ezetimibe has been shown to be well tolerated and effective in lowering LDL cholesterol when used alone and in combination with statin therapy [13]. Specialist involvement is suggested for patients with fasting triglyceride levels >1000 mg/dL or LDL levels >190 mg/dL [10].

12.2.3 Diabetes

Diabetes after transplant is related to both insulin resistance and beta-cell dysfunction and is associated with worsening of graft function and increased morbidity and mortality, especially from CVD [14]. Identified risk factors for the development of post-transplant diabetes include increasing age, ethnic background, positive family history, viral infections, immunosuppressive medications including tacrolimus and sirolimus,

steroid therapy, obesity and hypertension [15]. All patients should be screened periodically with the diagnosis based on American Diabetes Association criteria including fasting plasma glucose levels ≥126 mg/dl or 2-h plasma glucose levels ≥200 mg/dl [16]. As with hyperlipidemia, dietary modification and exercise should be encouraged. In addition, modification of the immunosuppressive regimen should be considered with rapid taper of corticosteroids and reduction in exposure to tacrolimus and sirolimus. Chronic hyperglycemia management should follow the guidelines outlined by the ADA for the treatment of individuals with type 2 diabetes [17]. The physician should set blood glucose targets for each individual patient and adjust therapy according to a "treat to target" approach. If unable to reach target with the above discussed methods, oral glucose lowering monotherapy or combination therapy and/or insulin is recommended. There are no specific recommendations regarding choice of oral agent used but caution should be taken if prescribing metformin due to the possibility of life-threatening lactic acidosis, particularly in patients with renal failure, sepsis and cardiovascular compromise. Referral to a diabetologist may be of benefit and patients should be counseled regarding regular opthalmological evaluation and foot care.

12.3 CKD Care

12.3.1 Anemia

Anemia is a common complication post-transplant and is estimated to occur in 30–40% of patients [18]. The American Society of Transplantation (AST) defines anemia as hemoglobin <13 mg/dl for men and < 12 mg/dl for women [19]. Studies in kidney transplant recipients have demonstrated a biphasic patter of anemia with an initial phase of high post-transplant anemia prevalence in the first 3–6 months reaching a nadir at 1 year and then a subsequent rise in the prevalence over the ensuing years [20]. Both the use of erythrocyte stimulating agents and pre-emptive transplant has helped to provide kidney transplant recipients with higher post-operative hemoglobin levels. The causes of anemia are multifactorial. In addition to inadequate erythropoietin production and iron deficiency, surgical blood loss, frequent phlebotomy and allograft dysfunction may lead to continued anemia in the early post-operative period. In patients with well-functioning grafts, hemoglobin levels usually normalize within 6 months after transplantation. There are a multitude of additional factors that may lead to anemia in the late post-transplant period (≥ 6 months) including immunosuppressive agents (MMF, azathioprine, sirolimus) viral infections (parvovirus, EBV, CMV) and acute or chronic allograft dysfunction. Mycophenolate mofetil and azathioprine appear to have direct antiproliferative effects on the bone marrow, while mTOR inhibitors may have effects on iron hemostasis and increased erythropoietin resistance.

Transplant providers should screen all kidney transplant patients routinely for anemia. In those patients with anemia, follow-up testing should include iron studies, RBC indices, reticulocyte count, and occult blood for stool. If hemolytic anemia is suspected, bilirubin, haptoglobin, and lactate dehydrogenase should be measured. Although anemia has been shown to be an independent risk factor for post-transplant LVH and cardiovascular events [21], there is currently insufficient evidence to show that aggressive anemia management improves overall outcomes. It is recommended that the KDIGO guidelines for the management of anemia in CKD be followed in the transplant population [22], but until prospective, randomized trials are carried out determining optimal hemoglobin targets in kidney transplant recipients, liberal use of recombinant erythropoietin should be avoided.

12.3.2 Bone Metabolism

Post-transplant bone disease is a complex disorder and may lead not only to reduced bone quality or bone loss, which may result in fractures, but also to changes in mineral metabolism. There are many factors that contribute to post-transplant bone dis-

ease including pre-existing renal osteodystrophy, corticosteroid therapy, hormone deficiencies, persistent hyperparathyroidism and hypophosphatemia. Bone loss is greatest in the first 6–12 months after transplantation leading to an increased risk of fractures. The incidence has been variably reported but exceeds 40% in some studies [23]. A unique characteristic is that most of the fractures occur primarily in the appendicular skeleton, particularly the feet with diabetics being at increased risk. Additional risk factors include older age, female sex, receipt of dialysis before transplantation and previous history of fracture.

The prevention and management of bone disease post-transplant requires a multifactorial approach. Dual-energy X-ray absorptiometry (DXA) is recommended in the first 3 months after transplant in those patients who received corticosteroids or have general population risk factors for osteoporosis. Patients who are deemed to be high risk based on risk factors should be considered for steroid avoidance protocols. Laboratory evaluation should include measurement of calcium, phosphorus, intact parathyroid hormone, and 25-hydroxyvitamin D levels. Patients should have adequate calcium intake (1200 mg/d) and 25-hydroxyvitamin D repleted to levels above 30 ng/mL. Bisphosphonates have been shown to prevent early bone loss in kidney transplant recipients, but there are no controlled studies that demonstrate fracture prevention [24]. In addition, it is important to recognize that use of bisphosphonates has been associated with adynamic bone disease and should be used with caution in kidney transplant recipients. In addition to pharmacologic therapies, non-pharmacologic measures should be employed to prevent early bone loss. These include regular physical exercise, weight resistance training, and improving balance and mobility.

12.4   Transplant Related Care

12.4.1 Allograft Dysfunction

Despite significant advances in immunosuppression reducing early allograft loss, long term allograft loss rates have remained unchanged

[25]. It is important that allograft function be assessed at routine intervals post-transplant through laboratory monitoring as reduced kidney allograft function is associated with poor patient and graft outcomes [26]. In the late post-transplant period, patients may present with acute kidney injury or a slow decline over time in allograft function, termed chronic allograft dysfunction. Acute kidney injury most commonly is related to volume depletion, drugs (CNI, ACE-I, ARB, NSAIDS) and urinary tract infections. Acute rejection is rare in this period, but should be suspected if the treatment of other causes does not return the creatinine back to the previous baseline or if the patient admits to noncompliance with their immunosuppressive regimen. In these particular instances, allograft biopsy should be performed. Causes of chronic allograft dysfunction include chronic allograft nephropathy, calcineurin inhibitor nephrotoxicity, chronic active antibody mediated rejection, and recurrent or de novo glomerulonephritis. Chronic allograft nephropathy is associated with significant morbidity and mortality and is the main reason for returning to dialysis after transplantation [27]. It is defined as a condition of renal allograft dysfunction occurring at least 3 months after transplantation without evidence of active acute rejection, drug toxicity or other diseases. It is characterized clinically by gradual deterioration of graft function, increasing proteinuria and worsening hypertension. Treatment of chronic allograft nephropathy can be challenging but should focus on prevention of early acute rejection and in subsequent years, limitation of CNI exposure. In addition, several studies have suggested that ACE-I's and ARB's may have a beneficial effect in prolonging allograft survival in those recipients with CAN and proteinuria [28, 29]. Along with chronic allograft nephropathy, calcineurin inhibitor nephrotoxicity plays a significant role in progressive kidney dysfunction post-transplant with most allografts showing histopathologic signs of CNI toxicity by 10 years [30]. A variety of tactics have been employed to try to limit CNI toxicity through CNI avoidance, early withdrawal or minimization. Several systematic reviews have shown higher creatinine

clearance in those patients withdrawn from CNI and treated with sirolimus or belatacept based regimens [31–33]. Chronic antibody mediated rejection (AMR) is defined by the presence of donor specific antibodies in the recipient serum and C4d deposition in the peritubular capillaries. These patients present with significant proteinuria as a result of transplant glomerulopathy, a specific glomerular lesion felt to be the result of immune injury. Patients who are considered immunologic high risk at the time of transplant may benefit from DSA screening and subsequent adjustment of immunosuppression. Finally, glomerulonephritis both recurrent and de novo can occur at any time post-transplant and contribute to loss of the allograft. Focal and segmental glomerulosclerosis, membranoproliferative GN and hemolytic uremic syndrome are the disorders known to be most aggressive when they recur. Recurrent and de novo GN is associated with a two-fold increase in risk for graft loss [34] and should be considered in any patient presenting with proteinuria, hematuria and a decline in allograft function. Biopsy with both electron microscopy and immunofluorescence staining should be performed.

12.4.2 Infections

Infections occurring in the transplant recipient are common with the risk of infection determined primarily by the intensity of the immunosuppression and epidemiologic exposures of the individual (donor-derived infections, recipient-derived infections, nosocomial infections, and community infections). The incidence and severity of early post-transplant infections has been dramatically reduced by the use of antimicrobial prophylaxis. Most transplant centers use trimethoprim-sulfamethoxazole for prophylaxis against Pneumocystis jiroveci pneumonia for at least 6 months after surgery. In addition to PCP, the drug can prevent infections with common urinary, respiratory and gastrointestinal pathogens. Dapsone, atovaquone, and pentamidine are alternative agents that may be used in the case of sulfa allergy Cytomegalovirus prophylaxis should also be instituted with most centers using oral valganciclovir for at least 4 months post-transplant. Based on the results of the Improved Protection Against CMV in Transplant trial (IMPACT), those patients deemed highest risk (donor +/ recipient −) should receive 6 months of therapy [35]. Due to reduction in overall immunosuppression exposure, the risk of infection diminishes 6 months after transplant with the most common infections being community acquired respiratory illnesses. In addition, urinary tract infections are quite common, and some would argue for the routine surveillance of UTI with urine cultures obtained at each post-transplant visit. In those patients who receive increased immunosuppression due to acute rejection episodes, increased vigilance for opportunistic infections including Pneumocystis jiroveci, *Listeria monocytogenes*, Nocardia asteroids, *Cryptococcus neoformans*, and Aspergillus should be undertaken.

In addition to prophylactic therapy, all patients should be appropriately vaccinated to prevent infectious complications (Table 12.2) [36]. It is important to remember that live vaccines should be avoided in transplant recipients. Recipients should receive yearly influenza vaccination. All patients should receive both the 23-valent polysaccharide pneumococcal vaccine (PPV23) and the 13-valent pneumococcal conjugate vaccine (PCV13). Hepatitis B vaccination is recommended in all solid organ transplant candidates and if a suboptimal response is seen with negative titers following vaccination, the series should be repeated after transplantation. Hepatitis A is recommended in patients with liver disease. Meningococcal vaccine should be given to all patients with risk factors including those with a history of splenectomy and before treatment with eculizumab. Patients should be up to date with Haemophilus influenza, tetanus and acelluar pertussis vaccines. Recombinant zoster vaccine (Shingrix) is recommended for all organ transplant candidates and recipients ≥50 years old. Patients should be varicella zoster IgG positive and should wait at least 3 months post-transplant and 1 year from a shingles episode to receive the vaccine. Patients travelling overseas should receive appropriate counseling and vaccinations as needed prior to their trip [37].

12.4.3 Malignancy

Malignancy after transplant is a leading cause of death among transplant recipients. It has an incidence that is 2–4 times higher than general population. Cancers tend to be more aggressive and can be challenging to treat with worse prognosis. The most common cancers causing death in kidney transplant recipients are non-Hodgkin lymphoma and renal cell carcinoma.

Immunosuppression is felt to play a major role in the pathogenesis of post-transplant malignancy by lowering immunosurveillance mechanisms, directly damaging host DNA, and potentiating the effect of pro-oncogenic viruses, such as human herpes virus type 8 for Kaposi sarcoma, Epstein-Barr virus for post-transplant lymphoproliferative disorder (PTLD), and human papillomavirus for oropharyngeal and anogenital carcinomas. Additional risk factors include underlying disease, type of transplant, history of malignancy before transplant, and established risk factors such as age, sex, ethnicity, geographic location, and smoking [38].

Table 12.2 Immunizations following solid organ transplant

Recommended vaccines	Contraindicated vaccines
• Diptheria-pertussis-tetanus	• Bacillus Calette-Guerin (BCG)
• Haemophilus influenza B	• Smallpox
• Hepatitis A (travel, occupational risk, and endemic regions)	• Intranasal influenza
	• Live oral typhoid Ty21a
• Hepatitis B	• Measles (except during outbreak)
• Pneumococcal (PCV13, PPV23)	• Mumps
• Inactivated polio	• Rubella
• Influenza A and B (annually)	• Oral polio
• Meningococcal (if high risk)	• Live Japanese B encephalitis vaccine
• Typhoid V	• Yellow fever
• Inactivated varicella zoster	• Live varicella zoster

Nonmelanoma cancer is the most common malignancy post-transplant with an incidence of squamous cell carcinoma that is 60–250 times greater than in the general population [39]. It is expected that one third of all kidney transplant recipients will have a nonmelanoma skin cancer within 10 years of transplant. Risk factors for skin cancer include older age, male sex, skin type, sun exposure, and duration of immunosuppression. Kidney transplant recipients should undergo annual skin exams by an experienced physician or dermatologist and should be counseled regarding sun protective measures. In those patients with a primary skin cancer, conversion to an mTOR inhibitor should be considered as they have been shown to lower risk of the development of subsequent skin cancers [40].

PTLD is the second most common de novo malignancy after transplantation with 85% of B-cell origin. EBV plays a key role in the pathogenesis of PTLD with a higher incidence in children who are EBV negative prior to transplant. It usually presents in a bimodal pattern with the highest incidence in the first year and another peak after the fifth year [38]. The clinical presentation is variable with extranodal manifestations common. In several large series, PTLD frequently involved the gastrointestinal tract, solid allografts and the central nervous system [41]. Treatment includes reduction in immunosuppression, surgical excision and radiotherapy to localized disease, rituximab monotherapy, and chemotherapy. Rituximab has become standard treatment for those who do not respond to lowering of immunosuppression with chemotherapy reserved for those who do not develop remission with rituximab (Dierickx).

As cancer screening guidelines for organ transplant recipients are inconsistent and based on limited available evidence, it is recommended that physicians follow the guidelines for breast, colorectal, cervical, and prostate cancer available for the general population. Screening for lung and renal malignancies is not recommended among kidney recipients [42].

12.5 General Health Maintenance

12.5.1 Pregnancy

As fertility can be restored to normal soon after a kidney transplant, it is important for physicians caring for recipients to be able to inform the patient about the potential risks of pregnancy and offer contraception. If pregnancy is desired, optimal circumstances include: stable allograft function for at least 1 year post-transplant without rejection, good control of blood pressure and appropriate adjustment of immunosuppression and other known teratogenic medications prior to conception [43]. There have been no obvious associations with any congenital malformations with calcineurin inhibitors. On the other hand, mycophenolic acid products have been known to cause various deformities such as such as cleft lip and palate, microtia, absence of external auditory canals, and possible coloboma. In addition, distal limb, heart, esophagus, and kidney abnormalities have been seen. The miscarriage rate may be increased with exposure [44]. It is recommended that mycophenolic acid be discontinued at least 6 weeks prior to conception efforts. Limited data are available for pregnancies during mTOR inhibitor use. These drugs have been associated with impaired spermatogenesis and may reduce male fertility [45]. Safety of breastfeeding by mothers receiving immunosuppressants remains uncertain but small studies have shown no lingering effects to infants to infants who were breastfed while their mothers were taking calcineurin inhibitors, azathioprine, and/or prednisone [46].

In planning for pregnancy, one should discuss pregnancy outcomes and risks both to the mother and fetus. Studies show that transplanted women who are pregnant are more likely to have hypertension, are more often diagnosed with preeclampsia and have more Cesarean sections performed [44]. Pre-pregnancy hypertension is associated with intrauterine growth retardation, preterm delivery, miscarriage, and low birth weight. Current recommendations are to control BP to below 140/90 during pregnancy using acceptable agents including methyldopa, labetalol, and nifedipine. Hydralazine and thiazide diuretics have been safely used as adjunctive agents. One needs to have a high index of suspicion for preeclampsia as it may be difficult to distinguish from acute rejection. Although, rejection rates and graft loss in pregnant kidney transplant recipients are not reported to be higher than their non-pregnant counterparts, it is recommended that these patients be seen more frequently during pregnancy to have both kidney function and immunosuppression levels monitored closely. Post-kidney transplant pregnancies are considered high risk and should be managed in close conjunction with a high-risk obstetrician.

12.5.2 Preventive Care

Patients should be counseled on the need for lifestyle modification post-transplant. Many transplant patients gain excess weight due to increased caloric intake and lack of routine physical activity. Female, African American, low-income patients with type 2 diabetes are at highest risk for obesity [47]. Obesity may exacerbate the cardiovascular risk profile (hypertension, hyperlipidemia and diabetes) affecting negatively long-term allograft and patient outcomes. It is important that patients receive appropriate counseling regarding healthy dietary practices and may benefit from consultation with a transplant dietician. In addition to lifestyle modification, available pharmacologic and surgical options should be discussed with appropriate patients.

Along with obesity, smoking tobacco has also been shown to exacerbate the cardiovascular risk profile. Kidney transplant recipients should be strongly discouraged from smoking as it has been shown to contribute significantly to allograft loss [48]. Both behavioral counseling and pharmacologic therapy should be recommended to the transplant recipient to aid in smoking cessation.

12.6 Conclusion

Kidney transplant recipients present with a unique and complex set of medical issues. As patients survive longer with functioning allografts, the responsibility for their care will become increasingly dependent on the community nephrologist and primary care physicians. It is important that these providers have the necessary skills and knowledge to provide appropriate care to these recipients ensuring optimum health. Diligence and early intervention of transplant related complications and cardiovascular risk factors should be undertaken with assistance from published guidelines and the transplant centers with the hope of improving long-term outcomes.

References

1. US Renal Data System 2017 annual data report: epidemiology of kidney disease in the United States. AJKD. 2018 Mar;71(3):S1–S676.
2. Wolfe RA, Ashby VB, Milford EL, Ojo AO, Ettenger RE, Agodoa LY, et al. Comparison of mortality in all patients on dialysis, patients on dialysis awaiting transplantation, and recipients of a first cadaveric transplant. N Engl J Med. 1999 Dec;341(23):1725–30.
3. Kasiske BL. Ischemic heart disease after renal transplantation. Kidney Int. 2002 Jan;61(1):356–69.
4. Ojo AO. Cardiovascular complications after renal transplantation and their prevention. Transplantation. 2006 Sept;82(5):603–11.
5. Neale J, Smith AC. Cardiovascular risk factors following renal transplant. World J Transplant. 2015 Dec;5(4):183–95.
6. Campistol JM, Romero R, Paul J, Gutierrez-Dalmau A. Epidemiology of arterial hypertension in renal transplant patients: changes over the last decade. Nephrol Dial Transplant. 2004 Jun;19(Suppl 3):iii62–6.
7. Kasiske BL, Anjum S, Shah R, Skogen J, Kandaswamy C, Danielson B, et al. Hypertension after kidney transplantation. Am J Kidney Dis. 2004 Jun;43(6):1071–81.
8. Becker GJ, et al. Kidney disease: Improving global outcomes (KDIGO) blood pressure work group. KDIGO clinical practice guideline for the management of blood pressure in chronic kidney disease. Kidney Inter. 2012;2(Suppl):337–414.
9. Kobashigawa JA, Kasiske BL. Hyperlipidemia in solid organ transplantation. Transplantation. 1997 Feb;63(3):331–8.
10. Wanner C, Tonelli M, The Kidney Disease: Improving Global Outcomes Lipid Guideline Development Work Group Members. KDIGO clinical practice guideline for lipid management in CKD: summary of recommendation statements and clinical approach to the patient. Kidney Int, 2014 Jun;85(6):1303–9.
11. Jardine AG, Holdaas H, Fellstrom B, Cole E, Nyberg G, Gronhagen-Riska C, et al. Fluvastatin prevents car-

diac death and myocardial infarction in renal transplant recipients: post-hoc subgroup analyses of the ALERT study. Am J Transplant. 2004 Jun;4(6):988–95.

12. Kasiske B, Cosio FG, Beto J, Bolton K, Chavers BM, Grimm R Jr, et al. Clinical practice guidelines for managing dyslipidemias in kidney transplant patients: a report from the managing dyslipidemias in chronic kidney disease work group of the national kidney foundation kidney disease outcomes quality initiative. Am J Transplant. 2004;4(Suppl 7):13–53.

13. Puthenparumpil JJ, Keough-Ryan T, Kiberd M, Lawen J, Kiberd BA. Treatment of hypercholesterolemia with ezetimibe in the kidney transplant population. Transplant Proc. 2005 Mar;37(2):1033–5.

14. Sharif A, Cohney S. Post-transplantation diabetes: state of the art. Lancet Diabetes Endocrinol. 2016 Apr;4:337349.

15. Kasiske BL, Snyder JJ, Gilbertson D, Matas AJ. Diabetes mellitus after kidney transplantation in the United States. Am J Transplant. 2003 Feb;3(2):178–85.

16. Expert Committee on the Diagnosis and Classification of Diabetes Mellitus. Report of the expert committee on the diagnosis and classification of diabetes mellitus. Diabetes Care. 2003 Jan;26(Suppl 1):S5–20.

17. Wilkinson A, Davidson J, Dotta F, Home PD, Keown P, Kiberd B, et al. Guidelines for the treatment and management of new-onset diabetes after transplantation. Clin Transpl. 2005 Jun;19(3):291–8.

18. Vanrenterghem Y, Ponticelli C, Morales JM, Abramowicz D, Baboolal K, Eklund B, et al. Prevalence and management of anemia in renal transplant recipients: a European survey. Am J Transplant. 2003 Jul;3(7):835–45.

19. Kasiske BL, Vazquez MA, Harmon WE, Brown RS, Danovitch GM, Gaston RS, et al. Recommendations for the outpatient surveillance of renal transplant recipients. American society of transplantation. J Am Soc Nephrol. 2000 Oct;11(Suppl 15):S1–86.

20. Blosser CD, Bloom RD. Posttransplant anemia in solid organ recipients. Transplant Rev (Orlando). 2010 Apr;24(2):89–98.

21. Rigatto C. Anemia, renal transplantation, and the anemia paradox. Semin Nephrol. 2006 Jul;26(4):307–12.

22. KDIGO Anemia Work Group. KDIGO clinical practice guideline for anemia in chronic kidney disease. Kidney Int Suppl. 2012 Aug;2(4):279–335.

23. Naylor KL, Li AH, Lam NN, Hodsman AB, Jamal SA, Garg AX. Fracture risk in kidney transplant recipients: a systematic review. Transplantation. 2013 Jun;95(12):1461–70.

24. Versele EB, Van Laecke S, Dhondt AW, Verbeke F, Vanholder R, Van Biesen W, Nagler EV. Bisphosphonates for preventing bone disease in kidney transplant recipients: a meta-analysis of randomized controlled trials. Transplant Int. 2016 Feb;29(2):153–64.

25. Meier-Kriesche HU, Schold JD, Kaplan B. Long-term renal allograft survival: have we made significant progress or is it time to rethink our analytic and therapeutic strategies? Am J Transplant. 2004 Aug;4:1289–95.

26. Karthikeyan V, Karpinski J, Nair RC, Knoll G. The burden of chronic kidney disease in renal transplant recipients. Am J Transplant. 2004 Feb;4(2):262–9.

27. Halloran PF, Melk A, Barth C. Rethinking chronic allograft nephropathy: the concept of accelerated senescence. J Am Soc Nephrol. 1999 Jan;10(1):167–81.

28. Artz MA, Hilbrands LB, Borm G, Assmann KJ, Wetzels JF. Blockade of the renin-angiotensin system increases graft survival in patients with chronic allograft nephropathy. Nephrol Dial Transplant. 2004 Nov;19(11):2852–7.

29. Lin J, Valeri AM, Markowitz GS, D'Agati VD, Cohen DJ, Radhakrishnan J. Angiotensin converting enzyme inhibition in chronic allograft nephropathy. Transplantation. 2002 Mar;73(5):783–8.

30. Nankivell BJ, Borrows RJ, Fung CL, O'Connell PJ, Allen RD, Chapman JR. The natural history of chronic allograft nephropathy. N Engl J Med. 2003 Dec;349(24):2326–33.

31. Mulay AV, Hussain N, Fergusson D, Knoll GA. Calcineurin inhibitor withdrawal from sirolimus-based therapy in kidney transplantation: a systematic review of randomized trials. Am J Transplant. 2005 Jul;5(7):1748–56.

32. Mulay AV, Cockfield S, Stryker R, Fergusson D, Knoll GA. Conversion from calcineurin inhibitors to sirolimus for chronic renal allograft dysfunction: a systematic review of the evidence. Transplantation. 2006 Nov;82(9):1153–62.

33. Masso P, Henderson L, Chapman JR, Craig JC, Webster AC. Belatacept for kidney transplant recipients. Cochrane Database Syst Rev. 2014 Nov;11:CD010699.

34. Chadban S. Glomerulonephritis recurrence in the renal graft. J Am Soc Nephrol. 2001 Feb;12(2):394–402.

35. Humar A, Lebranchu Y, Vincenti F, Blumberg EA, Punch JD, Limaye AP, et al. The efficacy and safety of 200 days valganciclovir cytomegalovirus prophylaxis in high-risk kidney transplant recipients. Am J Transplant. 2010 May;10(5):1228–37.

36. Kumar D. Immunizations following solid-organ transplantation. Curr Opin Infect Dis. 2014 Aug;27(4):329–35.

37. Kotton CN, Ryan ET, Fishman JA. Prevention of infection in adult travelers after solid organ transplantation. Am J Transplant. 2005 Jan;5(1):8–14.

38. Doycheva I, Amer S, Watt KD. De novo malignancies after transplantation: risk and surveillance strategies. Med Clin North Am. 2016 May;100(3):551–67.

39. Mittal A, Colegio OR. Skin cancers in organ transplant recipients. Am J Transplant. 2017 Oct;17(10):2509–30.

40. Karia PS, Azzi JR, Heher EC, Hills VM, Schmults CD. Association of sirolimus use with risk for skin cancer in a mixed-organ cohort of solid-organ transplant recipients with a history of cancer. JAMA Dermatol. 2016 May;152(5):533–40.

41. Dierickx D, Habermann TM. Post-transplantation lymphoproliferative disorders in adults. NEJM. 2018 Feb;378(6):549–62.

42. Acuna SA, Huang JW, Scott AL, Micic S, Daly C, Brezden-Masley C, Kim SJ, Baxter NN. Cancer screening recommendations for solid organ transplant recipients: a systematic review of clinical practice guidelines. Am J Transplant. 2017 Jan;17(1):103–14.

43. McKay DB, Josephson MA, Armenti VT, August P, Coscia LA, Davis CL, et al. Reproduction and transplantation: report on the AST consensus conference on reproductive issues and transplantation. Am J Transplant. 2005 Jul;5(7):1592–9.

44. Josephson MA, McKay DB. Women and transplantation: fertility, sexuality, pregnancy, contraception. Adv Chronic Kidney Dis. 2013 Sept;20(5):433–40.

45. Zuber J, Anglicheau D, Elie C, Bererhi L, Timsit MO, Mamzer-Bruneel MF, Ciroldi M, et al. Sirolimus may reduced fertility in male renal transplant recipients. Am J Transplant. 2008 Jul;8(7):1471–9.

46. Constantinescu S, Pai A, Coscia L, Davison JM, Moritz MJ, Armenti VT. Breast-feeding after transplantation. Best Pract Res Clin Obstet Gynaecol. 2014 Nov;28(8):1163–73.

47. Potluri K, Hou S. Obesity in kidney transplant recipients and candidates. Am J Kidney Dis. 2010 Jul;56(1):143–56.

48. Sung RS, Althoen M, Howell TA, Ojo AO, Merion RM. Excess risk of renal allograft loss associated with cigarette smoking. Transplantation. 2001 Jun 27;71(12):1752–7.

Paul Johnson, Edward Sharples, Sanjay Sinha, and Peter J. Friend

13.1 Introduction

Since the first pancreas transplant by William Kelly and Richard Lillehei in 1966 at the University of Minnesota, transplantation of the pancreas has been fraught with challenges [1]. Although insulin independence was achieved in these early ventures, graft failure occurred quickly and commonly and the operation came with great morbidity for patients. Since then, with improvements in surgery, immunosuppression, antimicrobials, organ preservation and better understanding of donor selection, insulin-independence is now more frequent and more prolonged and patient outcomes much improved, such that whole-organ transplantation is now an established treatment option for selected patients with advanced diabetes.

Until recently this had led to an increase in popularity, but with stabilisation of the waiting list and the advent of more advanced exogenous insulin delivery systems, the number of pancreas transplants performed globally has stabilised or even decreased [2]. Certainly, there remains considerable risk in pancreas transplantation due to the sequelae to ischaemia-reperfusion injury, and thus pancreas transplantation remains reserved for selected patients where the benefits justify the intervention.

The first clinical islet transplant performed in 1974 by Paul Lacy but was also met with complications [3]. It was the isolation and transplantation protocol from Edmonton that that lead to a resurgence of enthusiasm and consistently successful results making islet transplantation more widely offered for selected patients [4]. Although islet transplantation can lead to insulin-independence, though at a lower rate than that after whole organ transplantation, success does not require this: the elimination of hypoglycaemia-unawareness is the definition of success in this group of patients. The procedure remains far less invasive than solid organ transplantation, and the indications for islet or whole organ transplant differ and therefore the choice between the procedures should be made on an individualised basis.

P. Johnson · P. J. Friend (✉)
Nuffield Department of Surgical Sciences, University of Oxford, Oxford, UK
e-mail: paul.johnson@nds.ox.ac.uk; peter.friend@nds.ox.ac.uk

E. Sharples · S. Sinha
Oxford University Hospitals NHS Trust, Oxford, UK
e-mail: Edward.Sharples@ouh.nhs.uk; Sanjay.Sinha@ouh.nhs.uk

13.2 Indications

There is a body of unequivocal evidence that good glycaemic control is beneficial in terms of the development and progression of the secondary complications of diabetes [5]. Most people with type 1 diabetes are able to manage their

© Springer Nature Switzerland AG 2021
N. Hakim et al. (eds.), *Transplantation Surgery*, Springer Specialist Surgery Series, https://doi.org/10.1007/978-3-030-55244-2_13

glycaemic control through a regime of exogenous insulin, delivered via basal bolus insulin injections or for some via a continuous subcutaneous infusion pump. For some with very brittle and difficult to control diabetes, exogenous insulin may result in regular dangerous swings from hyperglycaemia to hypoglycaemia, leading to loss of normal physiological reactions to hypoglycaemia or hypoglycaemic unawareness. This puts the patient at high risk of entering a potentially fatal hypoglycaemic coma and is an indication for islet or solid organ pancreas-alone transplantation. Even for those where this is not the case, many are unable to achieve sufficiently good glycaemic control with insulin therapy resulting in the development and progression over years of debilitating secondary complications, including nephropathy, retinopathy, neuropathy and cardiovascular disease. Where long-standing diabetes has resulted in end-stage diabetic nephropathy, patients are eligible for pancreas and kidney transplantation. In each of these cases, pancreas transplant aims to restore insulin-independence and normoglycaemia resulting in improved quality and quantity of life.

13.2.1 Renal Failure

Diabetic kidney disease leads to excessive morbidity and mortality for affected patients. While, renal dysfunction is associated with increased mortality in most populations, large national registry studies show that the effect on life expectancy is particularly marked in patients with diabetes. A long term population study in Finland showed that patients with type-1 diabetes mellitus had similar life expectancy to the general population in the absence of any evidence of diabetic kidney disease, but the presence of any manifestation of kidney disease (from albuminuria to impaired GFR) had significantly adverse effects on mortality [6]. Although evidence from large randomised controlled trials has led to increased use of angiotensin receptor antagonists, the incidence of end stage renal failure associated with diabetes continues to increase: indeed diabetes is now the most common cause

of end-stage renal failure. Furthermore, diabetes is associated with notably poor life-expectancy in dialysis patients: despite the overall improvements in patient survival observed over the past 20 years, patients with diabetes (of all age groups) continue to have a shorter life expectancy on dialysis than other groups, with a higher propensity to cardiovascular disease. In this group, transplantation has the potential to greatly improve life expectancy and is the treatment of choice for patients with diabetic kidney disease, and patients with renal failure therefore account for 75–80% of all those undergoing whole pancreas transplantation.

Transplant options for patients with diabetes and progressive kidney disease include simultaneous kidney pancreas transplantation (SPK), simultaneous islet and kidney (SIK), or kidney transplantation alone (KTA), potentially followed by whole organ pancreas transplant (PAK), or islet transplant (IAK). The addition of the pancreas graft undoubtedly increases peri-operative mortality and morbidity, but is justified by the benefit of normal metabolic control, with effects on patient survival, kidney graft survival and the risk of diabetic complications: importantly, the long-term complications of transplantation are almost entirely related to immunosuppression, and there is therefore no incremental effect of the pancreas in patients undergoing the combined procedure.

In the UK, and in line with patients referred for kidney transplantation for any reason, patients with insulin-dependent diabetes may be listed for SPK transplant with an eGFR below 20 ml/min/1.73 m^2. To be considered for the combined procedure, most centres would require the recipient to be non-obese with low insulin resistance (BMI <30 kg/m^2) and undergo cardiac functional testing with myocardial perfusion scanning, stress echocardiography and/or cardio-pulmonary exercise testing. For patients who fulfil these criteria, SPK enables them to benefit not only from the excellent glycaemic control offered by the pancreas transplant but also from excellent kidney function: not only is there evidence that a functioning pancreas transplant protects against diabetic nephropathy in the transplanted kidney, but also the organ allocation system prioritises SPK recipients for donor kidneys from younger, fitter donors and often shorter cold ischaemia times than they may have received if undergoing kidney transplant alone.

Living donor kidney transplantation should not be dismissed as an option for patients with type 1 diabetes, and should be considered alongside the work-up for the simultaneous kidney pancreas waiting list. Living donor transplantation has the advantage that the patient can receive a kidney transplant with minimal delay, whereas the wait for a combined operation is unpredictable. Living donor kidney transplantation can be achieved with significantly lower peri-operative mortality and this option will be more suitable for a proportion of patients with significant co-morbidities, especially established cardiovascular disease, or as an option to minimize the adverse effects of time spent waiting whilst on dialysis. This could be followed by pancreas after kidney transplantation in patients who are deemed fit enough for this. There is still some debate over the criteria for PAK or IAK transplantation, and whether they should match the criteria for pancreas transplant alone (i.e. the criterion of hypoglycaemia unawareness), in view of the additional surgical morbidity. Currently in the UK this is not part of listing requirements, on the (logical) basis that PAK/IAK patients are already immunosuppressed and the risk-benefit balance is different from pancreas transplant alone (PTA) patients. Nevertheless, the decision to proceed with a PAK must be balanced against the risks of a further procedure, the increased risk of immunological incident and the (poorly understood) inferior pancreas graft survival of PAK compared to SPK. For this reason, in the UK, history of glycaemia or chronic hyperglycaemia with HbA1c >53 mmol/mol is necessary for eligibility [7].

With the success of islet transplantation, the use of islets as part of simultaneous islet kidney, or islet after kidney transplantation is now available to be considered for some recipients. Importantly and in contrast to islet transplantation alone (ITA), severe hypoglycaemia is not an essential criterion for listing for SIK or IAK transplant, as the recipient meets the standard criteria for SPK, or PAK transplant. Islet transplantation is preferable if the recipient is not suitable for a solid organ PAK, which may be for a variety of recipient-related factors, including co-morbidities or anticipated technical difficulty in placing the organ,. In SIK, the islets from the same donor as the kidney are isolated, and administered 24 hours later irrespective of total islet yield (unlike ITA in which there is a minimum threshold). Insulin independence is not guaranteed, but results show benefits of beta cell replacement, at much lower morbidity. Several studies have compared long term outcomes in recipients of SIK/IAK and those receiving SPK transplant. Lehman et al demonstrated that the SIK recipients had a greater than 90% reduction in hypoglycaemic events, although few were insulin independent at 5 years. The rate of re-laparotomy, however, was four times more common in the SPK recipients [8]. Another, more recent, study by Gerber et al. compared SIK recipients with patients receiving SPK, IAK, or intensive insulin therapy following a failed pancreas graft. Glycated haemoglobin was significantly lower following SIK, or IAK, compared to levels with intensive insulin therapy. There was also a reduction in the incidence of severe hypoglycaemia, and lower insulin usage [9].

13.2.2 Recipients with Type 2 Diabetes Mellitus

The majority (90%) of SPK recipients have type 1 diabetes, although pancreas transplantation is an option for patients with type-2 diabetes mellitus requiring insulin therapy. The rate of simultaneous kidney pancreas transplantation in patients with type-2 diabetes has increased significantly from 6 to 9% over the last decade, while the rate of solitary pancreas transplants has remained stationary, both pancreas after kidney (PAK) and pancreas transplant alone (PTA). Although the popularity of pancreas transplantation in type-2 diabetes remains disproportionately lower than in type-1, previous data from multiple centres support the notion that pancreas transplantation in younger (<50 years old), insulin-dependent patients with minimal comorbidities, especially limited cardiovascular disease, lower BMI (<30 kg/m^2), and insulin requirement threshold (<1 iu/kg), is successful and outcomes are comparable to recipients of SPK transplants with type-1 diabetes. The clinical dilemma, however, remains triaging the appropriate T2DM patients to pancreas transplantation, to minimize perioperative complications and maximise chance of insulin independence, and while making best use of living donor transplantation if available. Despite the limitations described above, there is little or no evidence for restricting pancreas transplantation on the basis of Type 2 status or insulin requirement.

In an updated analysis of International Pancreas and Transplant Registry (IPTR) data, Gruessner et al. examined the outcomes of pancreas transplants in type-2 diabetes recipients between 1995 and 2015 [10]. From the data, 1514 pancreas transplants in patients with type-2 diabetes were identified, the majority of which were SPK (88%), with only 33 pancreas re-transplants performed. In the most recent cohort, significant improvement was noted for SPK patient survival, whereby the 1- and 3-year patient survival rates increased from 91.4 and 86.5%, to 97.6 and 95.8%. Risk factors with the greatest impact on patient mortality were failure of kidney or pancreas graft, recipient age over 43 years and being African–American. Pancreas graft survival also improved significantly, with 1- and 3-year pancreas graft function from 80.2 and 70.5%, to 89.0 and 83.3%. Importantly, the rate of early technical failures decreased over time.

13.2.3 Hypoglycaemic Unawareness

Patients with brittle, difficult to control diabetes in the absence of renal failure, who have experienced more than 2 severe hypoglycaemia-unawareness episodes within the last 2 years may be offered pancreas transplant alone or islet transplantation. In contrast to islet transplantation, the goal of whole organ transplantation is insulin independence, and this is frequently

achieved. This is, of course, at the expense of a surgical procedure with greater morbidity. While the results of islet transplantation continue to improve, the primary goal is not insulin-independence but rather reduction in the frequency, severity and symptoms of hypoglycaemia: this is frequently achieved in the context of reduced doses of insulin and thus enabling improved glycaemic control and greatly improved quality of life. Islets are infused via a percutaneous transhepatic approach into the portal vein: while complications may occur, the procedure is minimally invasive by comparison. Both islet and whole organ approaches come with the need for life-long immunosuppression, including the associated risks of opportunistic infection and malignancy, and while often compared, these two approaches are best considered complementary, with choice informed by patient preference.

13.3 Patient and Graft Survival

Overall, transplantation improves patient survival significantly when compared to the waiting list population. A retrospective analysis of the UNOS database and Social Security death master file over a twenty-five year period examined the life years gained with transplantation compared to those who remained on the waiting list. Simultaneous kidney pancreas transplantation was associated with median survival 14.5 years compared to 4.2 years on the waiting list [11]. In the presence of a functioning pancreas transplant, patient survival is prolonged beyond what might be expected with kidney transplant alone. Weiss et al. examined the SRTR database to compare patient and graft survival in patients transplanted between 1997 and 2005. Patient survival was significantly better in those patients with pancreatic function at one year after SPK transplant (88%) when compared to recipients in whom the pancreas had failed (73.9%), or patients who had undergone living donor kidney transplant (80.0%) [12]. This difference in survival was confirmed by multi-variate analysis and was not influenced by the take-up of pancreas after kidney transplantation. Kidney graft survival was also highest in the SPK cohort on unadjusted data. Recipients in whom the pancreas graft failed in the early post-op period did not gain this survival advantage.

There is debate about the optimal timing of transplantation. Outcomes of patients receiving pre-emptive transplantation are superior, and so the adverse effects of time spent on dialysis may outweigh any advantage of delaying the intervention, and pre-emptive SPK listing should be considered as standard. Differences in kidney graft survival have been attributed to the beneficial effect of the pancreas graft, although proper correction for donor demographics is critical to determine the factors responsible for the observed improvement. A recent re-assessment of this survival advantage following SPK transplant over kidney transplant alone has suggested that the difference in survival is significant, but possibly less than that suggested in earlier studies. Data from the SRTR was used to compare graft and patient survival in 7308 SPK recipients and 4653 recipients of kidney transplants, matched for a number of co-variants including transplant centre, BMI, recipient and donor age, from a cohort of adult patients with type 1 diabetes mellitus transplanted between 1998 and 2009. Mean restricted kidney graft survival and patient survival were superior: this survival benefit was primarily observed in younger patients [13].

Graft failure has typically been defined as a return to exogenous insulin therapy; although this may require review in light of the entrance to the market of non-insulin therapies for diabetes and the increased recognition of 'partial function'— the patient requiring injectable insulin despite ongoing endogenous insulin production. This has led to the specification by OPTN that the definition of transplant failure requires that insulin therapy should exceed 0.5 units/kg and continue for >90 consecutive days [14]. Studies examining the influence and importance of serum c-peptide levels have been performed at national levels and no correlation to graft failure has been found. As such, although c-peptide levels are often measured, these do not form part of diagnostic criteria. Conversely, for islet transplantation, insulin-independence is not considered necessary to achieve the desired outcome of eliminating hypoglycaemic awareness. Consistent c-peptide production is required and therefore does form part of defining graft failure in these cases. Freedom from hypoglycaemia unawareness is the primary criterion for success in this group of patients.

Using current definitions, the outcomes of both whole organ pancreas and islet transplantation have moved closer to the level of other solid organ transplantation [15]. Graft survival remains superior in simultaneous pancreas-kidney transplant compared to pancreas transplant alone, with pancreas graft survival rates now much improved to 96%, 89% and 81% for 1-, 3- and 5-year survival for SPK and 82%, 72% and 60% for pancreas only transplantation. The greatest improvement is graft outcomes has been achieved in the first 12 months, when graft loss rates are highest. This may be due to changes in donor selection, efforts to minimise cold ischaemia time or awareness and early management of the sequelae of graft pancreatitis. The reason for superior outcomes in SPK when compared to pancreas alone is not fully understood, but often attributed to the presence of a kidney from the same donor in the former allowing renal function to act as a surrogate biomarker for rejection in the pancreas. The kidney does have the advantage of having an easily measurable marker of function but also being amenable to biopsy, however in studies involving biopsy of both organs, discordance rates have been reported as high as 37% [16]. Recipients of SPK transplants are on average older than recipients of solitary pancreas transplants, and are at a later stage in their diabetes. Rises in auto and allo-antibodies are often seen after transplantation and it may be that a more immune-reactive environment in solitary pancreas transplant recipients may be a contributing factor.

The results of islet transplantation have also improved significantly over the last decade. Insulin-independence has been reported at 58% at 1-year compared to only 11% in the 1990s, albeit with a high rate of attrition thereafter with only 10% insulin-independent at 5 years. However 80% of these patients still retained c-peptide positivity and had well-controlled HbA1c [17]. The level of expertise at the isolating and transplanting centres does have an impact of islet graft survival rates, nevertheless, even in the best centres the longer-term outcomes of islet transplantation are inferior to those of whole organ transplantation. The lower morbidity does allow for repeat transplantation to take place, although this is as the risk of sensitising the recipient to HLA antigens, which may be problematic for patients that might require kidney transplantation at a later stage [18].

13.4 Donor Selection

The success of whole organ pancreas transplantation relies heavily on donor selection and the retrieval process. Donor organs for pancreas transplantation come predominantly from deceased donors declared dead by neurological (brain-stem death, DBD) or cardiovascular (circulatory death, DCD) criteria (formerly known as non-heart beating donation). Living pancreas donor transplantation has been carried out in small numbers in a very small number of centres: due to the associated morbidity for the donor (15–30%), this has not become standard practice internationally [19]. Most cases were performed at the University of Minnesota, and in Japan (where deceased donors are rarely available). Segmental pancreas transplantation (transplantation of the body and tail of the pancreas on the splenic vessels) is performed in these cases: no advantage in the recipient has been shown over deceased donation, and metabolic studies have detected significant subsequent abnormalities in the donor [20].

Most DBD or DCD donors who have been deemed as appropriate for cardiothoracic and other abdominal organ donation should be considered for pancreas donation. However, donor selection for pancreas donation remains more stringent than that for other solid organs: DBD donors comprise the majority. Comparable outcomes have been achieved using DCD donors; however, such donors are accepted with a very selective approach with regard to other risk fac-

tors. The criteria for quality assessment in donor and organ selection remain unclear, although there have been many attempts to identify donor features associated with adverse outcomes. The best tool is the Pancreas Donor Risk Index (PDRI) devised by Axelrod et al. which describes the relative cumulative impact of donor characteristics in a score relative to 1 [21]. Nevertheless, studies attempting to validate the PDRI as a predictive tool have provided mixed results [22, 23], and without recipient factors built into the model it is difficult to interpret in real-life scenarios. Thus the PDRI is seldom used in clinical practice, and instead a pragmatic and individualised approach is most often used to balance the commonly identified poor prognostic characteristics: advanced donor age (>45 years), high BMI (>30 kg/m^2), donation after circulatory death and prolonged cold ischaemia time (>12 h).

In the UK, two-thirds of donor pancreases meeting nationally-agreed criteria and offered for transplantation are declined as unsuitable [24]. Donors may be declined due to absolute contraindications specific to pancreas donation: these include a history of diabetes mellitus (Type 1, Type 2, or gestational), previous pancreatic surgery, significant pancreatic trauma, acute or chronic pancreatitis (active acute or chronic). Relative contraindications include alcohol abuse, severe atherosclerosis, fatty infiltration, or pancreatic oedema. Additional factors include a long anticipated cold preservation time, a recent history of IV drug abuse or high-risk sexual behaviour, severe obesity (> 150% ideal body weight [IBW], body mass index [BMI] > 30 kg/m^2) or sometimes an inexperienced organ retrieval team. Despite a selective approach to organ acceptance at the time of offering, even after a donor is accepted, the conversion rate from pancreas donor to transplant remains low: the pancreas is the organ most often discarded after organ retrieval. On visual inspection either in the donor or *ex vivo*, the pancreas is often found to be abnormal with macroscopic appearances of fibrosis or fatty infiltration. These features are broadly associated with severe reperfusion injury (reperfusion pancreatitis): given that there is not the same level of donor organ shortage for the pancreas as for other organs, most surgeons are reluctant knowingly to subject a recipient to any increased risk of high morbidity and early graft loss. However, visual inspection is highly subjective and the risk notoriously difficult to assess.

Organ allocation systems for whole organ pancreas transplantation and islet transplantation run in parallel in many countries since the preferred donor for islet transplant differs slightly to that of whole organ transplantation. For islet transplantation, older and higher-BMI donors are more acceptable whereas solid organ transplanters favour younger slim donors. However, intra-parenchymal fat or fibrosis may still hinder pancreas digestion. Cold ischaemia is limited to under 8 h for islet isolation (in the UK): for solid organ transplantation every effort is made to restrict cold ischaemia time to less than 12 h. These limitations are factored into the organ allocation arrangements.

13.5 Organ Retrieval

There are two retrieval strategies in DBD donation: (1) rapid dissection of vasculature and organs in the cold phase after flush-out (mandatory if the donor is unstable) or (2) warm dissection before cold perfusion [25]. The retrieval technique for DCD organs differs in the timing of the cross clamping, with 'super rapid recovery' through laparotomy and immediate cannulation of the aorta or by direct cannulation of the femoral artery. This to minimise the warm ischaemia time following cessation of cardiorespiratory function: there is an obligatory 5 min observation period following circulatory arrest, before any intervention is permissible. In a multi-organ retrieval procedure, if portal perfusion is to be performed then this must be either done via a completely transected portal vein or the portal circulation needs to be vented through the splenic or inferior mesenteric vein: this is to avoid back pressure, non-perfusion and congestion of the pancreas. The role of the retrieval surgeon to look after the interests of all organs is paramount. The assessment of the organ is best done on the bench rather than in the donor's body, since allows both visual and tactile assessment of the donor pancreas. Currently, assessment and decision-making in organ acceptance is multifactorial and largely subjective with significant inter-clinician and inter-centre variability. Macroscopic features of the pancreas such as the degree of inter- and intra-lobular pancreatic steatosis, fibrosis and calcification are important and may be associated with the likelihood of reperfusion pancreatitis and poorer long-term function.

Organ preservation is a key factor in the two major (and related) early complications of solid organ pancreas transplantation, vascular complications and reperfusion pancreatitis. Novel perfusion devices have been developed in recent years to enable the preservation and perfusion of visceral organs at hypothermic and normothermic temperatures. These have been tested in trials and have entered clinical practice in kidney, liver, heart and lung transplantation, with increasing evidence suggesting improved patient outcomes and better graft survival. Perversely, preservation techniques for the fragile pancreatic allograft have changed little [26] and, while there have been attempts at perfusion, the prospect of perfusing the whole pancreas remains far from realisation into clinical practice at the present time. Currently, static cold storage is the preferred approach, and has been the most widely used method for pancreas preservation for the last 30 years. University of Wisconsin solution (UWS) is the most commonly utilised preservation fluid, and is used for flushing the pancreas after explant and before implantation, as well as during transportation. An alternative to UWS is Histidine Tryptophan Ketoglutarate solution (HTK) and Celsior, however despite numerous trials no advantage over UWS has been shown [27].

13.6 Implantation Procedure

Back-table preparation of the pancreas graft must be undertaken with care: this is usually started as soon as the pancreas graft arrives in the implanting centre in order to minimise cold ischaemia time. The pancreas graft is assessed macroscopically for damage or fatty infiltration. If the graft is deemed suitable for transplant, the recipient is called to the operating theatre and anaesthetic procedures begin while the graft is prepared. The pancreas is a retro-peritoneal organ and requires considerable dissection with attention to haemostasis. The spleen and excess fat are removed and small vessels and lymphatics ligated, the mesenteric root is over-sewn and the attached donor duodenum shortened, restapled and also over-sewn. The dual arterial input of the pancreas is reconstructed to a single point of inflow, using a Y-graft of donor iliac vessels to the superior mesenteric artery and splenic artery. The graft is flushed with University of Wisconsin fluid before being replaced in static cold storage until time for implantation. As mentioned, attempts at perfusing the pancreas ex vivo have not been successful and thus static cold storage and minimising cold ischaemia times remains the primary focus in clinical practice.

Implantation is usually (although not in all centres) performed through a midline incision with the pancreas graft placed in the right iliac fossa with arterial inflow from the recipient right common iliac artery via the Y-graft, and venous outflow from the donor portal vein into the recipient inferior vena cava or right common iliac vein. In a minority of centres, portal venous drainage (to the portal or superior mesenteric veins) has been employed with the aim of achieving more physiological insulin drainage. However this approach has not been supported by any evidence of benefit [28].

After perfusion of the pancreas and careful haemostasis, the donor duodenum is anastomosed to an accessible section of recipient jejunum. Historically, drainage of the exocrine secretions of the pancreas has been seen as the 'Achilles heel' of pancreas transplantation, and various methods have been adopted, including drainage into the bladder, jejunum or duodenum, with or without a Roux-en Y loop. Enteric drainage of secretions is clearly more physiological but with loss of the potential benefit of monitoring urinary amylase with bladder-drainage.

Islet transplantation is far less invasive involving the infusion of isolated islets into the liver via the portal vein. This is usually performed via a percutaneous radiologically-guided transhepatic approach, however, may also be performed through cannulation of a mesenteric vessel reached laparoscopically or through a mini-laparotomy. The principle challenge in islet transplantation, is in the isolation (a process of pancreas digestion combining enzymatic and mechanical dissociation and islet purification using density-gradient separation). In terms of the utilisation of donor organs, this is relatively inefficient, with only 30% of isolations resulting in transplantable yields. Islet isolation requires specialised expertise and many programmes are based on a hub-and-spoke model.

13.7 Immunosuppression

Immunosuppression in islet and pancreas transplantation follows a similar pattern to other solid organ transplantation. Biological antibody induction (thymoglobulin, alemtuzumab or basiliximab) is used perioperatively to reduce the immediate cell-mediated immune response, with maintenance therapy comprising tacrolimus and mycofenolate mofetil to block T-cell activation and expansion. Mycofenolate has been shown to be associated with lower rates of graft rejection [29] compared to azathioprine and there was a reduction in severe rejection and 3 year graft loss in the EUROSPK 001 trial comparing an immunosuppression regime including tacrolimus to the same with cyclosporine [30]. There is a recent trend towards the use of steroid-free regimens: the avoidance of long-term steroid use is desirable in terms of minimising insulin insensitivity and risk of wound infection [31].

13.8 Complications

Whole organ pancreas and islet transplantation carry similar long term risks with respect to immunosuppression (opportunistic infections, specific drug side effects and malignancy). Islet-specific complications are rare and usually fall into either portal vein thrombosis or bleeding.

Solid organ pancreas transplantation is associated with a much higher number of potential complications. Like any operation, there is the risk of general anaesthesia, bleeding and infection, and, as with other organ transplants, there are also risks of delayed graft function, primary non-function, thrombosis, rejection (acute or chronic), in addition to other complications of immunosuppression. One in four pancreas recipients will require further surgery, most commonly for bleeding or the management of graft pancreatitis. Because the pancreas is not an organ that is immediately essential for life, severe complications are more commonly managed by removal of the graft than in other types of transplant. Early graft failure necessitating graft pancreatectomy may occurs in the context of thrombosis (usually venous). Non-occlusive venous thromboses are frequently identified by in radiological assessment, with incidence reported as being 10–35%: this may be associated with ischaemia-reperfusion injury and reperfusion pancreatitis in this very sensitive organ. The vascular flow in the major vessels (especially the splenic vessels) is much lower than in normal physiology due the removal of the spleen, and low velocity combined with endothelial injury due to organ preservation constitute a substantially increased risk of thrombosis. Because of this, careful attention is given to anticoagulation, often with frequent monitoring using methods such as thromboelastography. Another devastating, much later, vascular complication is that of mycotic pseudoaneurysm, usually occurring years after transplantation: it is thought that vascular suture line infection may be caused by contamination at the time of transplantation. To avoid this antifungal treatment is given routinely: in any patient who presents with gastrointestinal bleeding the possibility of this diagnosis is entertained.

13.8.1 Rejection and Biopsy

Acute rejection of the pancreas graft is difficult to diagnose, which creates a challenge since treatment is far more likely to be successful before hyperglycaemia is apparent. Attempts to salvage rejecting organs once serum glucose rises are unlikely to be fruitful. Rejection rates have been described in the literature as between 5 and 25%, with definitions being based on a number of factors.

Various biomarkers have been used in monitoring protocols with the aim of providing earlier warning of impending pancreas rejection, but these are based on limited evidence. In the case of bladder-drained pancreases, urinary amylase has been used: a drop in urinary amylase has been shown to precede evidence of endocrine dysfunction [32]. However, bladder drainage is associated with considerable morbidity for recipients and has been abandoned in most centres. Serum amylase has not been shown to correlate well with pancreas graft rejection, and lipase is used in many centres in preference, since it shows a quicker peak that can prompt more timely intervention, however the evidence base for this is also limited [33]. The emergence of donor-specific HLA antibodies and diabetic auto-antibodies have been shown to be associated with poor pancreas outcomes and undoubtedly relate to underlying inflammatory processes [34]. However, it is not clear if these arise in advance of the event sufficiently to be useful. Pancreas biopsies are only performed in a few centres: these may be performed at open surgery, laparoscopically, via endoscopy or radiologically guided. Although features of rejection have been described and based on histological findings [35], experience in interpreting pancreas biopsies is limited. The biopsy procedure is associated with a risk of bleeding, fistulation and graft loss, as well as a high rate of procedural failure, making biopsies challenging to justify without clear clinical indication.

13.8.2 Pancreatitis

Ischaemia-reperfusion injury is manifest in the transplanted pancreas as graft pancreatitis. There is no specific biochemical test to make the diagnosis of graft pancreatitis, which is therefore made on a combination of clinical and radiological findings. Clinically patients experience pain, often with ileus and failure to progress, with on-going raised inflammatory markers. Radiological assessment may show an oedematous pancreas graft often associated with fluid collection and thrombosis. The recipients are likely then have a prolonged length of stay, often requiring repeated operations to wash-out amylase rich collections and inspect the pancreas. Without intervention, patients may progress to sepsis and multi-organ failure: if progress is not made in the individual case, early pancreatectomy must be considered.

Severe graft pancreatitis is a complication much feared by clinicians, and is the major contributor to early graft loss. This leaves the recipient having been through the trauma of surgery and sepsis without reaping any of the benefits of pancreas transplantation. In addition also patients are potentially sensitised to HLA antigens, making attempts at retransplantation more challenging. The single greatest need in the field of pancreas transplantation is to understand better the aetiology of pancreatitis and develop the means to abrogate this devastating complication.

13.9 Graft Function and Surveillance

Successful pancreas transplantation achieves insulin independence, with normalisation of blood glucose and HbA1c, but monitoring after pancreas (and islet) transplantation remains a challenge. The natural history of functional decline after pancreas transplantation and the mechanisms that lead to graft failure are not understood. Unlike the kidney, there is no easily measurable marker of function to monitor and, even in those centres where it is carried out, biopsy of the pancreas is a means of diagnosis rather than surveillance. As a result, graft failure appears to occur suddenly with little opportunity for graft salvage. It is often presumed that this is a result of rejection; however other underlying mechanisms have been postulated including recurrence of autoimmunity and development of type 2 diabetes [36].

Most centres follow monitoring protocols including regular laboratory and possibly radio-logical testing, with measurement of serum amylase, lipase, insulin, c-peptide and glucose. HbA1c and oral glucose tolerance testing may also be employed. In the past, bladder-drainage of exocrine secretions enabled monitoring of urinary amylase levels which was used as a biomarker and early warning of impending graft failure and prompt further investigation and intervention [37]. However, this approach is not used widely partly as bladder-drainage was associated with metabolic and urological complications that resulted in frequent hospital admissions and renal impairment. In simultaneous pancreas-kidney transplantation, kidney function may be used as a surrogate however disconcordance rates of rejection between the two organs are too high to make this robust [16]. Nevertheless, this may be one factor in the superior outcomes of the combined procedure over pancreas transplant alone.

In islet transplantation, there have been several useful metabolic scores introduced to provide an objective assessment of graft function, including the beta-score and HYPO score [38]. These are not applicable to whole organ transplantation due to systemic drainage of insulin and the high incidence of renal dysfunction. To date, in whole organ transplantation there is no easily applicable method for measuring graft function sequentially and monitoring remains a challenge. Existing metabolic assessment tools are invasive and laborious, radiological and radioisotopic methods to measure beta-cell mass are of experimental interest but are not in clinical use and have not been shown to correlate with graft function. Immunological monitoring may give warning of an immunological reaction but interpretation and intervention are both challenging. Novel interventions such as the use of a vascularised donor sentinel skin flap to allow for protocol biopsies have been studied but are not yet part of routine clinical practice.

13.10 Diabetic Complications

Diabetes is associated with other devastating secondary complications in addition to nephropathy. Good glycaemic control is known to reduce decline in renal function, which is particularly important in the context of lifelong immunosuppression with nephrotoxic calcineurin inhibitors. This benefit is best realised with stable function beyond 10 years, by which time studies of non-uraemic pancreas transplant alone recipients have shown stabilisation of early functional decline and improvements in glomerular structure to normal [39, 40]. Browne et al. compared 2776 PAK and 13,635 kidney alone recipients and confirmed that these histological and functional improvements translated into improved graft survival, thereby endorsing the additional benefit of the pancreas in this situation [41].

Whether pancreas transplantation conveys benefit with respect to other complications is less clearly established. Although there has been some evidence of stabilisation of diabetic neuropathy after transplantation, large and robust studies have been limited by the lack of a 'gold standard' outcome measure [42]. Diabetic retinopathy is the leading cause of blindness in young people, however most patients already have established advanced retinopathy at the time of transplant limiting the potential for benefit. Indeed, rejection episodes have been shown to be associated with a deleterious effect [43]. While neuropathy and retinopathy lead to great morbidity for patients, cardiovascular disease is the main cause of death. While data do show that SPK is associated with lower rates of cardiac death, this is in the context of stringent pre-operative cardiac screening and optimisation [44]. Further research is needed to clearly define the impact of pancreas transplantation and graft function on the development and progression of diabetic complications.

13.11 Interventions and Further Research

Although there have been significant technological advances in insulin-delivery systems, with continuous glucose monitoring enabling insulin pumps to deliver insulin responsively in systems described as the 'artificial pancreas', islet transplantation is still likely to have a role for those who are not able to control their very brittle dia-

betes in this manner. Meanwhile, whole organ pancreas transplantation remains the only treatment for diabetes to normalise glucagon in what is now understood to be a bi-hormonal disease.

Currently, the risk of pancreas transplantation and its associated complications limits its risk-benefit and restricts its use to a selected group of patients. New methods to prevent and minimise morbidity, particularly that of graft pancreatitis, will expand the criteria for transplantation and increase the access to transplantation. With the donor population becoming progressively more marginal, and the risks associated with ischaemia-reperfusion injury driving increasingly conservative donor selection, there is a need to improve organ utilisation with new approaches to organ retrieval, preservation, assessment and the control of ischaemia-reperfusion injury. There is a pressing need for more effective graft monitoring, perhaps by immunological or biochemical biomarkers, to aid early identification of rejection and other causes of graft dysfunction, enabling improved graft survival. There is much interest in alternative methods of generating functional beta-cells or better islets, but this technology is still a considerable distance away from clinical practice.

References

1. Kelly WD, Lillehei RC, Merkel FK, Idezuki Y, Goetz FC. Allotransplantation of the pancreas and duodenum along with the kidney in diabetic nephropathy. Surgery. 1967;61(6):827–37.
2. Kandaswamy R, Stock PG, Gustafson SK, Skeans MA, Urban R, Fox A, et al. OPTN/SRTR 2017 annual data report: pancreas. Am J Transplant. 2019;19(Suppl 2):124–83.
3. Karl RC, Scharp DW, Ballinger WF, Lacy PE. Transplantation of insulin-secreting tissues. Gut. 1977;18(12):1062–72.
4. Shapiro AM, Lakey JR, Ryan EA, Korbutt GS, Toth E, Warnock GL, et al. Islet transplantation in seven patients with type 1 diabetes mellitus using a glucocorticoid-free immunosuppressive regimen. N Engl J Med. 2000;343(4):230–8.
5. Lasker RD. The diabetes control and complications trial. Implications for policy and practice. N Engl J Med. 1993;329(14):1035–6.
6. Skupien J, Smiles AM, Valo E, Ahluwalia TS, Gyorgy B, Sandholm N, et al. Variations in risk of end-stage

renal disease and risk of mortality in an international study of patients with type 1 diabetes and advanced nephropathy. Diabetes Care. 2019;42(1):93–101.

7. Accessed March 2013. http://odt.nhs.uk/pdf/advisory_group_papers/PAG/Standard_%20listing%20_criteria_summary.pdf

8. Lehmann R, Graziano J, Brockmann J, Pfammatter T, Kron P, de Rougemont O, et al. Glycemic control in simultaneous islet-kidney versus pancreas-kidney transplantation in type 1 diabetes: a prospective 13-year follow-up. Diabetes Care. 2015;38(5):752–9.

9. Gerber PA, Hochuli M, Benediktsdottir BD, Zuellig RA, Tschopp O, Glenck M, et al. Islet transplantation as safe and efficacious method to restore glycemic control and to avoid severe hypoglycemia after donor organ failure in pancreas transplantation. Clin Transplant. 2018;32(1).

10. Gruessner AC, Laftavi MR, Pankewycz O, Gruessner RWG. Simultaneous pancreas and kidney transplantation-is it a treatment option for patients with type 2 diabetes mellitus? An analysis of the international pancreas transplant registry. Curr Diab Rep. 2017;17(6):44.

11. Gruessner RW, Sutherland DE, Gruessner AC. Mortality assessment for pancreas transplants. Am J Transplant. 2004;4(12):2018–26.

12. Weiss AS, Smits G, Wiseman AC. Twelve-month pancreas graft function significantly influences survival following simultaneous pancreas-kidney transplantation. Clin J Am Soc Nephrol. 2009;4(5):988–95.

13. Sung RS, Zhang M, Schaubel DE, Shu X, Magee JC. A reassessment of the survival advantage of simultaneous kidney-pancreas versus kidney-alone transplantation. Transplantation. 2015;99(9):1900–6.

14. Access March 2019. https://optn.transplant.hrsa.gov/media/1116/03_pa_graft_failure_definition.pdf

15. Kandaswamy R, Stock PG, Skeans MA, Gustafson SK, Sleeman EF, Wainright JL, et al. OPTN/SRTR 2011 annual data report: pancreas. Am J Transplant. 2013;13(Suppl 1):47–72.

16. Troxell ML, Koslin DB, Norman D, Rayhill S, Mittalhenkle A. Pancreas allograft rejection: analysis of concurrent renal allograft biopsies and posttherapy follow-up biopsies. Transplantation. 2010;90(1):75–84.

17. Shapiro AM, Ricordi C, Hering BJ, Auchincloss H, Lindblad R, Robertson RP, et al. International trial of the Edmonton protocol for islet transplantation. N Engl J Med. 2006;355(13):1318–30.

18. Naziruddin B, Wease S, Stablein D, Barton FB, Berney T, Rickels MR, et al. HLA class I sensitization in islet transplant recipients: report from the Collaborative Islet Transplant Registry. Cell Transplant. 2012;21(5):901–8.

19. Kirchner VA, Finger EB, Bellin MD, Dunn TB, Gruessner RW, Hering BJ, et al. Long-term outcomes for living pancreas donors in the modern era. Transplantation. 2016;100(6):1322–8.

20. Robertson RP, Sutherland DE, Seaquist ER, Lanz KJ. Glucagon, catecholamine, and symptom responses to hypoglycemia in living donors of pancreas segments. Diabetes. 2003;52(7):1689–94.

21. Axelrod DA, Sung RS, Meyer KH, Wolfe RA, Kaufman DB. Systematic evaluation of pancreas allograft quality, outcomes and geographic variation in utilization. Am J Transplant. 2010;10(4):837–45.

22. Mittal S, Lee FJ, Bradbury L, Collett D, Reddy S, Sinha S, et al. Validation of the pancreas donor risk index for use in a UK population. Transpl Int. 2015;28(9):1028–33.

23. Blok JJ, Kopp WH, Verhagen MJ, Schaapherder AF, de Fijter JW, Putter H, et al. The value of PDRI and P-PASS as predictors of outcome after pancreas transplantation in a large European Pancreas Transplantation Center. Pancreas. 2016;45(3):331–6.

24. Accessed March 2019. https://nhsbtdbe.blob.core.windows.net/umbraco-assets-corp/12300/transplant-activity-report-2017-2018.pdf

25. Brockmann JG, Vaidya A, Reddy S, Friend PJ. Retrieval of abdominal organs for transplantation. Br J Surg. 2006;93(2):133–46.

26. Maglione M, Ploeg RJ, Friend PJ. Donor risk factors, retrieval technique, preservation and ischemia/reperfusion injury in pancreas transplantation. Curr Opin Organ Transplant. 2013;18(1):83–8.

27. Stewart ZA, Cameron AM, Singer AL, Dagher NN, Montgomery RA, Segev DL. Histidine-tryptophanketoglutarate (HTK) is associated with reduced graft survival in pancreas transplantation. Am J Transplant. 2009;9(1):217–21.

28. Sollinger HW, Odorico JS, Becker YT, D'Alessandro AM, Pirsch JD. One thousand simultaneous pancreas-kidney transplants at a single center with 22-year follow-up. Ann Surg. 2009;250(4):618–30.

29. Stegall MD, Simon M, Wachs ME, Chan L, Nolan C, Kam I. Mycophenolate mofetil decreases rejection in simultaneous pancreas-kidney transplantation when combined with tacrolimus or cyclosporine. Transplantation. 1997;64(12):1695–700.

30. Saudek F, Malaise J, Boucek P, Adamec M, Euro SPKSG. Efficacy and safety of tacrolimus compared with cyclosporin microemulsion in primary SPK transplantation: 3-year results of the Euro-SPK 001 trial. Nephrol Dial Transplant. 2005;20 Suppl 2:ii3–10, ii62.

31. Gruessner RW, Sutherland DE, Kandaswamy R, Gruessner AC. Over 500 solitary pancreas transplants in nonuremic patients with brittle diabetes mellitus. Transplantation. 2008;85(1):42–7.

32. Sibley RK, Sutherland DE. Pancreas transplantation. An immunohistologic and histopathologic examination of 100 grafts. Am J Pathol. 1987;128(1):151–70.

33. Sugitani A, Egidi MF, Gritsch HA, Corry RJ. Serum lipase as a marker for pancreatic allograft rejection. Transplant Proc. 1998;30(2):645.

34. Mittal S, Page SL, Friend PJ, Sharples EJ, Fuggle SV. De novo donor-specific HLA antibodies: biomarkers of pancreas transplant failure. Am J Transplant. 2014;14(7):1664–71.

35. Drachenberg CB, Odorico J, Demetris AJ, Arend L, Bajema IM, Bruijn JA, et al. Banff schema for grading pancreas allograft rejection: working proposal by a multi-disciplinary international consensus panel. Am J Transplant. 2008;8(6):1237–49.

36. Vendrame F, Pileggi A, Laughlin E, Allende G, Martin-Pagola A, Molano RD, et al. Recurrence of type 1 diabetes after simultaneous pancreas-kidney transplantation, despite immunosuppression, is associated with autoantibodies and pathogenic autoreactive CD4 T-cells. Diabetes. 2010;59(4):947–57.

37. Prieto M, Sutherland DE, Goetz FC, Rosenberg ME, Najarian JS. Pancreas transplant results according to the technique of duct management: bladder versus enteric drainage. Surgery. 1987;102(4):680–91.

38. Ryan EA, Shandro T, Green K, Paty BW, Senior PA, Bigam D, et al. Assessment of the severity of hypoglycemia and glycemic lability in type 1 diabetic subjects undergoing islet transplantation. Diabetes. 2004;53(4):955–62.

39. Fioretto P, Steffes MW, Sutherland DE, Goetz FC, Mauer M. Reversal of lesions of diabetic nephropathy after pancreas transplantation. N Engl J Med. 1998;339(2):69–75.

40. Mauer M, Fioretto P. Pancreas transplantation and reversal of diabetic nephropathy lesions. Med Clin North Am. 2013;97(1):109–14.

41. Browne S, Gill J, Dong J, Rose C, Johnston O, Zhang P, et al. The impact of pancreas transplantation on kidney allograft survival. Am J Transplant. 2011;11(9):1951–8.

42. Navarro X, Kennedy WR, Loewenson RB, Sutherland DE. Influence of pancreas transplantation on cardiorespiratory reflexes, nerve conduction, and mortality in diabetes mellitus. Diabetes. 1990;39(7):802–6.

43. Scheider A, Meyer-Schwickerath E, Nusser J, Land W, Landgraf R. Diabetic retinopathy and pancreas transplantation: a 3-year follow-up. Diabetologia. 1991;34(Suppl 1):S95–9.

44. La Rocca E, Fiorina P, di Carlo V, Astorri E, Rossetti C, Lucignani G, et al. Cardiovascular outcomes after kidney-pancreas and kidney-alone transplantation. Kidney Int. 2001;60(5):1964–71.

Small Bowel Transplantation: The New Frontier in Organ Transplantation

14

Ruy J. Cruz, Robert M. Esterl, and Abhinav Humar

14.1 Background

The first experimental intestinal transplant was performed by Alexis Carrel in 1901, when he implanted a segment of bowel into the neck of a dog. The first human intestinal transplants occurred in the 1960s, but these transplants were suspended at that time because of dismal graft and patient survival due to lack of effective immunosuppressive protocols. The widespread introduction of calcineurin inhibitors (Cyclosporine in the 1980s and Tacrolimus in the 1990s) renewed interest in intestinal transplantation as a viable surgical option for patients with intestinal failure requiring total parenteral nutrition (TPN). Newer immunosuppressive regimens, advances in organ preservation, better donor and recipient selection, refinement in surgical techniques, earlier detection and treatment of infections and improved postoperative critical

R. J. Cruz (✉)
Intestinal Rehabilitation and Transplant Center, University of Pittsburgh, Pittsburgh, PA, USA
e-mail: cruzrj2@upmc.edu

R. M. Esterl
The University of Texas Health Science Center at San Antonio, San Antonio, TX, USA
e-mail: esterl@uthscsa.edu

A. Humar
Division of Transplant Surgery, Thomas Starzl Transplantation Institute, University of Pittsburgh, Pittsburgh, PA, USA
e-mail: humara2@upmc.edu

care management have all played significant roles in the success of intestinal transplants since the mid-1990s. Although intestinal transplants remain the least frequent of all transplants, one year graft survival rates have significantly improved and now approach those of other extrarenal transplants. As graft losses due to technical reasons have diminished greatly, immunologic and infectious issues remain primary challenges facing the field today. As the largest lymphoid organ in the human body and a host for potential infectious pathogens, the small bowel continues to be the most difficult solid organ to transplant [1–10].

14.2 Pretransplant Evaluation

Intestinal failure is defined as the inability of the intestine to maintain nutrition or fluid and electrolyte balance without long term TPN [2, 4, 6–8]. Causes of intestinal failure can be divided into 2 broad groups: (1) SBS (insufficient bowel length) and (2) functional disorders (impaired intestinal motility or absorption with an otherwise sufficient intestinal length and surface area). Currently an intestinal transplant is indicated for patients suffering from irreversible SBS who present with life-threatening complications secondary to TPN or underlying medical disease [6]. Centers for Medicare and Medicaid Services have approved coverage for intestinal transplants

© Springer Nature Switzerland AG 2021
N. Hakim et al. (eds.), *Transplantation Surgery*, Springer Specialist Surgery Series,
https://doi.org/10.1007/978-3-030-55244-2_14

in patients with SBS on TPN with these complications: (1) thrombosis of major venous access sites, (2) frequent central line infections and sepsis requiring hospitalization (more than two episodes per year), (3) impending or overt liver failure related to TPN, and (4) severe and frequent electrolyte imbalance and/or dehydration despite intravenous fluid supplementation in addition to TPN [3, 8, 11]. Many feel that patients who are stable on TPN without such complications are usually not considered intestinal transplant candidates, because their estimated annual survival rate may be higher with TPN.

The most common cause of SBS requiring an intestinal transplant includes extensive surgical resection of the small intestine. Uncommon indications for intestinal transplant in patients with intestinal failure but without SBS are (1) severe gastrointestinal myopathy or neuropathy (hollow visceral myopathy, total intestinal aganglionosis, pseudo-obstruction syndrome), (2) gut malabsorption syndromes (microvillous inclusion disease, radiation enteritis, selective autoimmune enteropathy), (3) neoplastic syndromes involving the root of the mesentery (neuroendocrine and desmoid tumors, often associated with familial adenomatous polyposis or Gardener's syndrome), and (4) diffuse portomesenteric thrombosis with high risk of gastrointestinal hemorrhage [2, 4, 7–9].

The causes of intestinal failure are different in adult versus pediatric populations. Gastroschisis, necrotizing enterocolitis, malrotation with midgut volvulus, and atresias are the most common causes in pediatric patients; mesenteric arterial thrombosis/embolism, trauma, Crohn's disease, and adhesions are the most frequent causes in adult patients [10]. Most patients (53%) who wait for an intestinal transplant have an underlying diagnosis of SBS [9]. The development of SBS depends not only on the resected length of bowel, but also on the location of the resection, and on the retainment (or not) of the ileocecal valve and/or the colon. As a rough guideline, most patients can tolerate up to 50% resection of their intestine

with subsequent adaptation, avoiding the need for long-term TPN. Loss of greater than 70% of intestine, however, usually necessitates some type of parenteral nutritional support. The development of TPN-induced liver failure is much more rapid in children when compared to adults. For these reasons pediatric patients with SBS should be referred for isolated intestinal transplant evaluation before the development of irreversible TPN-induced liver injury [2, 5, 7, 12].

The pretransplant evaluation is not too different from that for other transplants. The typical laboratory evaluation includes ABO type, HLA type, panel reactive antibody, complete blood count, comprehensive basic metabolic profile and coagulation profile. Serology studies should be performed for HIV, hepatitis B and C, CMV and EBV. A clear picture of the anatomy of the patient's gastrointestinal tract is essential [2]. An upper gastrointestinal tract contrast series and abdominal and pelvic CT scan are always necessary in order to plan gastrointestinal tract reconstruction during the transplant. It is important to estimate actual bowel length and function (transit time with upper gastrointestinal series). Hepatic function should be evaluated carefully and a transjugular or percutaneous liver biopsy is often required. If there is evidence of significant liver dysfunction, a combined liver-intestine or multivisceral transplant may be indicated [5, 12]. Duplex sonography of the liver and intraabdominal vascular system can be useful. Patients with thrombotic disorders need specific hematologic tests to define hypercoagulable states (such as protein C and S deficiency, prothrombin G20210 A and factor V Leiden mutation, and hyperhomocysteinemia) [2]. Conventional abdominal visceral angiography and a comprehensive evaluation of the upper and lower central venous system are mandatory in high-risk patients and those with thrombotic disorders. Absolute contraindications such as advanced malignancy, severe systemic disease, active infection, and marked cardiopulmonary insufficiency must be ruled out [2, 6].

14.3 Surgical Procedure

Unfortunately the nomenclature to describe the technical aspects of intestinal transplantation has not been consistent in the literature, particularly when other organs are transplanted with the intestinal graft [8]. The three most common types of intestinal transplants include: (1) isolated intestinal transplant, (2) combined liver–intestine transplant, and (3) multivisceral transplants (Fig. 14.1) [1–8]. The most common intestinal transplant is the isolated intestinal graft which includes the entire deceased donor jejunum and ileum, and is used in patients with intestinal failure that is limited to the small bowel. The arterial anastomosis is based on the recipient superior mesenteric artery or using a jump graft from the infrarenal aorta. Venous outflow is usually achieved with the anastomosis of the superior mesenteric vein to the native superior mesenteric vein or splenic vein; however, in some cases systemic venous drainage to inferior vena cava is

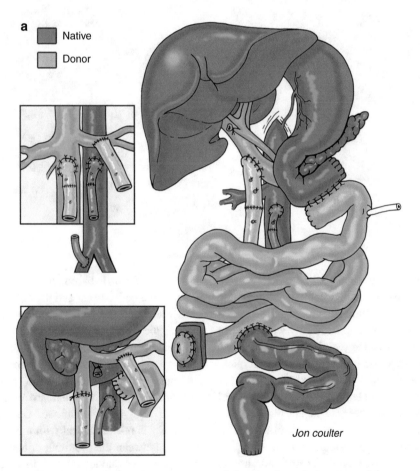

Jon coulter

Fig. 14.1 Types of visceral transplant. Native organs are coloured dark reddish brown and donor organs are light brown. (**a**) Isolated intestinal transplantation. Vascular inflow from native infrarenal aorta through an interposition graft and outflow into native portal vein through an interposition graft. Inset images show alternate options for vascular anastomoses: Chimney ileostomy allows easy endoscopic access to obtain periodic biopsies and jejunostomy tube for decompression and early enteral feeding. (**b**). Liver-intestine transplantation. Arterial anastomoses of the Carrel patch (segment of donor aorta with its branches including SMA and Celiac axis) to native infrarenal abdominal aorta and venous outflow of segment of donor IVC anastomosed in a piggy back fashion to native IVC. (**c**) Full multivisceral transplantation. Vascular anastomoses are similar to the liver-intestinal allograft. Gastrointestinal continuity is achieved by proximal end-to-end anastomosis between native stomach and donor stomach; distal end-to-side anastomosis between donor ileum and native sigmoid colon

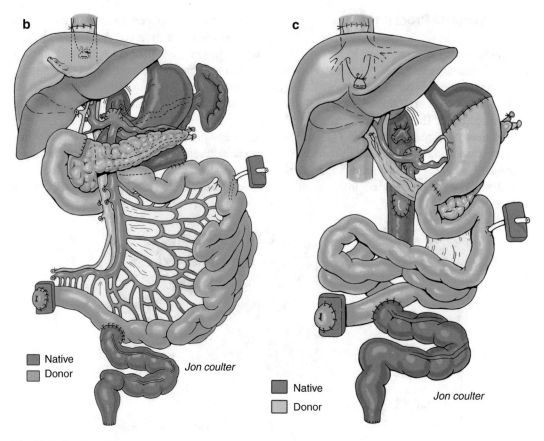

Fig. 14.1 (continued)

required. Gastrointestinal continuity occurs with a primary anastomosis between the recipient and donor proximal jejunum and the creation of a distal Bishop-Koop or loop ileostomy with or without anastomosis to the recipient colon. In living donation or in a case of severe donor-to-recipient size mismatch (deceased donor adult to pediatric recipient), a 200-cm length of distal small bowel is used; inflow to the graft is via the ileocolic artery, and outflow is via the ileocolic vein. In patients with combined pancreatic dysfunction (i.e., cystic fibrosis, type I diabetes and chronic pancreatitis) the inclusion of the pancreas should be considered with the intestinal transplant.

The second most common technique combines the liver and pancreas organs with the intestinal transplant [1–8]. The liver, pancreas and intestine (including the duodenum) are procured en bloc from the donor and are transplanted on bloc in the recipient. In the en bloc donor allograft

the arterial inflow is based an aortic conduit that includes the celiac trunk and the superior mesenteric artery and the venous outflow is based on the hepatic veins or inferior vena cava. In the recipient operation an arterial anastomosis occurs between the donor aortic conduit and the recipient suprarenal or infrarenal aorta; a vena caval anastomosis occurs via standard caval replacement or piggyback technique. Gastrointestinal continuity is re-established with a primary anastomosis between the proximal donor and recipient jejunum or duodenum and distal creation of the Bishop-Koop or loop ileostomy with or without connection to the recipient colon. In this type of transplant there is a need of portocaval shunt for venous outflow of the remaining native organs (i.e. stomach, pancreas, duodenum and spleen).

The third type of transplant including the intestine is the multivisceral transplant. In the multivisceral transplant additional gastrointestinal organs can be transplanted in continuity with the intestine including the donor stomach, duodenum, pancreas, colon with or without the liver. The common indications for multivisceral transplant include, but are not limited to, hollow visceral myopathy or neuropathy, pseudo-obstruction syndrome, extensive GI polyposis, neuroendocrine tumors, and symptomatic total splanchnic vascular thrombosis. The operation involves complete splanchnic evisceration and en bloc transplantation of stomach, duodenum, pancreas, liver, and small bowel, and on occasion, the right and transverse colon (full multivisceral transplant). If the stomach is involved in the upper abdominal evisceration, gastrointestinal continuity is achieved by connecting the donor stomach to the recipient distal esophagus or small gastric remnant. In patients with preserved liver function, the native liver is left intact (modified multivisceral transplant). In patients with chronic or impending renal failure, a renal graft (usually right kidney) can also be included in the multivisceral transplant.

Early series suggested that inclusion of the colon increases the risk of infectious complications, but recent reports describe that inclusion of the colon is not only safe, but may lead to better absorption of water from stool, resulting in fewer episodes of dehydration and hospital readmissions [8]. The inclusion of the stomach is also a controversial topic, in that some centers universally apply this technique and other centers rarely or never do. Evidence regarding the benefit or risk to include the stomach in the multivisceral transplant is limited [8].

The recipient operation can be a challenging procedure due to the presence of abdominal adhesions from multiple previous operations, stomas, gastrojejunostomies, reduced abdominal space, and, in some cases, considerable portal hypertension (if the patient requires a liver transplant). The loss of abdominal domain is a unique problem with intestinal transplants unless the patient has significant ascites from liver failure or hollow visceral myopathy or neuropathy (i.e. pseudo-obstruction syndrome). Loss of domain has been addressed with several innovative techniques including transplantation of the abdominal wall, placement of tissue expanders, staged closure of the abdominal wall and musculocutaneous free flaps [8].

Gastrojejunostomy tubes are almost always placed intraoperatively, permitting gastric decompression and enteral nutrition in the early postoperative period [2, 6, 13]. A Bishop–Koop or loop ileostomy is used to decompress the terminal ileum and to facilitate enteroscopy/biopsy, which is the only reliable method to monitor the allograft and diagnose acute rejection. These ileostomies are usually taken down within one year after transplantation if there is little need to continue monitoring of the intestine for rejection. Of note, a prophylactic (donor or native) appendectomy and (donor or native) cholecystectomy are performed in all cases to avoid postoperative infectious complications. Finally, in multivisceral transplants a donor pyloroplasty should be performed to facilitate gastric emptying.

Several factors should be considered in appropriate matching of the donor and the recipient for an intestine transplant. Usually ABO-identical grafts are used; ABO nonidentical but compatible grafts are usually avoided because of a higher risk of graft-versus-host disease. Donors are typically young, hemodynamically stable, brain-dead but heart-beating donors. Donors should usually be of similar or smaller size than the recipients, as the latter usually have contracted peritoneal cavities, so that a smaller graft may be more appropriate because of space constraints. Selective bacterial and fungal decontamination of the gut (amphotericin B, polymyxin B, and gentamicin) through a nasogastric tube should be attempted in all donors. Cytomegalovirus (CMV) enteritis can be a devastating problem in intestinal transplant recipients, and so, if possible, CMV seronegative recipients should receive CMV seronegative intestinal grafts. If possible, similar viral matching should be performed for Epstein Barr virus, if possible, because of the risk for post transplant lymphoproliferative disorder (PTLD) [2].

14.4 Postoperative Care

The early post transplant care is, in many ways, similar to that of other transplant recipients. The postoperative care in intestinal transplant recipients can be difficult and complicated, especially in those recipients who present with deterioration/malnutrition and various organ system failures, when sequellae can persist postoperatively even with improving allograft function. Postoperative management often requires an aggressive, interprofessional approach by medical, nursing and ancillary health care providers [2]. Initial care is usually in a critical care setting, so that vital signs, urine output, fluid and electrolytes, and blood product replacement can be carefully monitored. Serial hemoglobin measurements are performed to monitor for any evidence of hemorrhage. Serum pH and lactate should also be followed for evidence of intestinal ischemia or injury. In patients who received liver-intestine, or multivisceral allografts, pancreatic enzymes and liver function tests should be assessed daily to track organ functional status. Selective bacterial and fungal gut decontamination through a nasogastric tube or gastrojejunostomy tube postoperatively until enteral nutrition begins. Broad-spectrum antibiotics against bacteria and fungi are routinely administered given the high risk for infectious complications. Routine prophylaxis should also be administered against CMV, EBV and Pneumocystis carinii infection [2]. In Pneumocystis carinii prophylaxis, patients with allergies/intolerance to sulfa medication should receive monthly inhaled pentamidine.

Postoperative nutritional support initially occurs by resumption of standard TPN solutions. When the gastrointestinal function begins to recover and upper gastrointestinal contrast studies confirm the integrity of gastrointestinal anastomoses, enteral nutrition is initiated via the gastrojejunostomy tube. Most tube feedings are polymeric formulas containing whole complex components instead of a pre-digested product which can be switched to fiber-containing formulas if significant diarrhea develops [13]. This switch from parenteral to enteral nutrition is gradual and usually occurs in the first 2 weeks after transplant. Tube feeding is slowly decreased and removed, while oral intake is increased proportionately to an unrestricted diet except in patients with a chylous leak who should receive a low fat diet. All patients receive antiulcer prophylaxis with proton pump inhibitors, and some patients require anti-diarrheal (loperamide, diphenoxylate hydrochloride and atropine sulfate, opiates, or soluble fiber supplements) or prokinetic agents (metoclopramide or erythromycin) to modulate stool or stoma output, once rejection or enteritis is ruled out [2].

Most patients can be weaned from TPN and remain TPN free after an intestinal transplant [8]. Matarese reported that enteral nutrition began through a jejunostomy tube at a mean 10.3 days after transplant, that TPN was discontinued at a mean 30.8 days after transplant and that most patients achieved a regular oral diet at a mean 57 days after transplant [13]. In the early postoperative period some patients who receive multivisceral transplants do not take appropriate oral nutrition. This eating disorder, usually seen in the pediatric population, is caused by many etiologies, including: (1) some patients never had the opportunity to eat food before the transplant and never learned the mechanics of food consumption, (2) some patients have associated the act of food consumption with disagreeable and distasteful sentiments with accompanying nausea, vomiting, diarrhea, and abdominal distension and pain, and (3) some patients develop a hypergag reflex evoked by food consumption [2]. Many of these are learned behaviors, and these patients require cognitive redirection of their beliefs and perceptions around food consumption. They need regular emotional support and nutritional guidance after the intestinal transplant. They often require very slow introduction of new foods. The use of small frequent meals, prokinetic and antidiarrheal agents and use appetite stimulants aid in the transition to regular diets for patients with early satiety, diarrhea or anorexia [13].

Some intestinal recipients exhibit renal dysfunction in the postoperative period due to inadequate intraoperative resuscitation, dehydration from diarrhea/increased stomal output and high dose tacrolimus immunotherapy. All patients in the immediate postoperative period have a urinary catheter to monitor the adequacy of resuscitation and appropriate urine output. The increased use of induction immunotherapy for intestinal transplants has led to delayed introduction/decreased target levels for tacrolimus which hopefully translates to recovery of renal function in the immediate postoperative period and preserved long term renal function [8].

Immunosuppression should be initiated in the immediate postoperative period [2]. A number of different immunosuppressive protocols have been described. The OPTN/SRTR 2013 Annual Data Report noted that 54% of intestinal recipients received T cell depleting agents and 11% received interleukin-2 receptor antagonists for induction therapy, yet 38% received no induction therapy. In this report the most common initial maintenance immunosuppressive medications were tacrolimus (95%), steroids (73%), mycophenolate (35%) and mTOR inhibitors (15%). Seventy percent of recipients were still maintained on oral steroids one year after the intestinal transplant. Target trough levels for tacrolimus in the whole blood are typically 12–15 ng/ml in the first postoperative month, followed by levels of 8–12 ng/ml in the next three months.

Regardless of the immunosuppressive regimen, intestinal transplants clearly have a high risk of rejection. The ORPN/SRTR 2013 Annual Data Report indicates that the incidence of a first rejection episode increases over time. In adult recipients of isolated intestinal transplants 45% experience an episode of acute rejection within the first year and 53% within the second year. Although the use of induction agents and tacrolimus-based maintenance therapy have reduced episodes of acute rejection in intestinal transplants, the consequences of steroid resistant rejection carry a 50% mortality in adult intestinal transplant recipients mainly due to sepsis [8, 14].

Although traditional treatment for acute rejection aims to control the T-cell mediated response in the intestinal graft with steroid bolus or antilymphocyte therapy, recent attention has been paid to the role of antibody-mediated mechanisms in intestinal graft rejection [8]. Antibody mediated rejection continues to be a problem in intestinal transplant, because it is relatively resistant to corticosteroid therapy, but donor specific antibodies in particular are becoming recognized as causes of chronic rejection and late graft loss [15]. This recognition has followed the widespread introduction and implementation of new immunological technologies, namely single antigen fluorescent bead assays to detect donor specific antibodies. The presence of preformed donor specific antibody and/or increased panel reactive antibody correlate with rejection and graft loss [8, 15]. Both preformed and de novo donor specific antibodies have been associated with antibody mediated rejection and decreased graft survival; patients with donor specific antibodies before and after the intestinal transplant appear to have the lowest long term graft survival, due not only to episodes of acute rejection but also chronic allograft enteropathy. Important features of chronic allograft enteropathy are mucosal atrophy and ulceration, mesenteric lymphoid depletion, and mesenteric fibrosis and sclerosis, caused by mesenteric vasculopathy which is highly dependent of donor specific antibodies [15]. The presence of CD4 and direct evidence of other antibody and complement activity in mesenteric vasculopathy associated with chronic allograft enteropathy may be lacking in the literature, largely because they are best seen on full thickness intestinal biopsies and not the typical mucosal biopsies. Finally complement activation appears to play a significant role in the development of late dysfunction and chronic allograft enteropathy [15]. Donor specific antibodies can bind to the C1q component of complement, activating the full complement cascade. Of note, inclusion of the liver along with the intestine seems to protect the recipient from intestinal rejection, either by inducing a tolerogenic state in the antigen presenting cells in the liver, or providing a reservoir to sequester sensitized T cells and/or antibodies against the intestine. Large studies are necessary to define the use of immunosuppressive medications/therapies to target these various mediators of rejection: preformed donor specific antibodies (plasmapheresis and immunoglobulin), cytokines (infliximab), B cells (rituximab), plasma cells (bortezomab) and early activation of the complement cascade (eclizumab) [8, 15].

In a patient with intestinal dysfunction, it is very important to differentiate enteritis (mostly caused by *Clostridium difficile*, adenovirus, cytomegalovirus and calicivirus) from rejection, since both conditions may be characterized by low grade fever, abdominal distension and pain, and diarrhea (or increased stoma output). The stoma if present should be carefully examined for color, texture and friability; in the face of rejection the stoma may appear edematous, erythematous, pale, congested, dusky or friable. Endoscopy should be performed for inspection of the mucosa and for purposes of biopsy of the most suspicious areas. Endoscopy with biopsy is the primary method to diagnose allograft rejection. Careful evaluation of an intestinal biopsy by an experienced pathologist is always necessary [2].

Because surveillance and diagnostic endoscopy and biopsy are costly and invasive procedures, there is increased interest to identify potential biomarkers of intestinal rejection [8]. Recent studies have shown that several molecules, namely calprotectin and citrulline, measured in the stool/ileostomy effluent and blood respectively, are reliable markers of moderate and severe intestinal rejection. Calprotectin is an S100 protein released by infiltrating neutrophils and macrophages into the gut lumen; increased calprotectin levels have been noted prior to the onset of histological changes of acute rejection and normal levels are consistently seen with normal intestine graft biopsies [8, 16]. Citrulline is an amino acid found almost exclusively in enterocytes, so decreased levels in the blood reflect decreased functional mass of enterocytes [16]. Hibi et al. noted that citrulline levels were inversely proportional to the severity of acute cellular rejection [17]. Negative predictive values for any type of acute cellular rejection (cut off was 20 lmol/L) and moderate/severe acute cellular rejection (cut off, 10 lmol/L) were 95% and 99%, respectively. Subgroup analysis showed a strong correlation between citrullene levels (obtained up to one week prior to biopsy) and severity of acute rejection on intestinal biopsy; as the citrulline level decreased, the grade of rejec-

tion on biopsy worsened. Other potential markers of intestinal graft dysfunction could include adipsin, C-reactive protein (an inflammatory marker used clinically in Crohn's Disease) and lathosterol (fecal marker of bile malabsorption when intestinal mucosa is dysfunctional) [16]. Larger studies are needed on all of these potential biomarkers in order to be widely used in clinical practice. Girlanda et al. used liquid chromatography to examine the metabolomic profile of ileostomy effluent in patients who had intestinal graft rejection vs. no rejection [18]. These investigators noted the highest fold change in the proinflammatory mediator leukotriene E4 in patients with rejection, and high fold changes in taurocholate and water soluble vitamins B2, B5 and B6 in patients with rejection. Metabolomic analysis could be a promising tool to characterize the pathophysiological mechanisms of intestinal graft rejection and to identify some potential early noninvasive biomarkers of graft dysfunction.

Short-term results have improved dramatically, mainly due to improvements in surgical techniques and in immunosuppression regimens. Nonetheless, intestinal transplants are still associated with fairly high surgical complication rates. Potential complications include enteric leaks with generalized peritonitis, localized intraabdominal abscesses, chylous ascites, biliary leakage and/or stricture (in liver-intestine aod full multivisceral allografts), vascular thrombosis/ stenosis, and life-threatening intraoperative and postoperative hemorrhage [2].

Infectious complications are, unfortunately, very common in intestinal transplant recipients and are a frequent cause of morbidity/mortality and hospital readmissions [2, 8]. There are several factors that contribute to this issue. The intestinal graft itself is a significant source of bacteria, and any process which compromises containment of these bacteria (intraoperative spillage of gastrointestinal contents or postoperative anastomotic leak) can lead to a localized abscess or systemic infection. Because of the higher risk of rejection, intestinal transplant recipients generally receive higher levels of immunosuppression compared with other organ recipients and they are at greater risk for severe infections including transplant associated infections (CMV, EBV) and community-acquired pathogens (RSV or influenza). The presence of uncorrected surgical/technical/mechanical problems (e.g., biliary leak or stricture in liver transplant, gastrointestinal anastomotic leak, vesicoureteral reflux in kidney transplant) may predispose intestinal recipients to recurrent infections [19]. If rejection causes disruption of the intestinal mucosal barrier, bacteria and fungi can translocate across the graft directly into the peritoneal cavity, leading to spontaneous bacterial peritonitis. Bacteria can also spread directly into the portal circulation, and subsequently disseminate to distant sites. Patients with indwelling catheters (central catheters for TPN, gastrojejunostomy tubes for enteral nutrition) are at increased risk for infectious complications until the need for the catheter is no longer necessary [19]. Finally, immunosuppression attenuates the native immune response to vaccines in the postoperative period; when higher levels of immunosuppression are required for intestinal transplants (i.e., rejection treatment), it puts pediatric patients at significantly higher risk for vaccine-associated diseases. Live viral vaccines remain a contraindication in intestinal recipients in the postoperative period, placing pediatric patients at risk for varicella in addition to measles, mumps and rubella if they have exposure to such viruses [19].

Bacterial infections are extremely common in the immediate postoperative period after an intestinal transplant. In a study of 40 adult intestinal recipients Premeggia et al. reported a 30 day postoperative infection rate of 58% with a mean time to first infection of 11 days [20]. In this study twenty three patients developed 36 bacterial infections; of patients with infections, 57% developed one infection, 30% developed two infections, and 13% developed three infections. The most common site of infection was the abdomen, followed by infections in the blood, urine, lung and surgical site. Of the microbial isolates 49% were gram-negative bacteria, 39% were gram-positive bacteria and 11% were fungi. The most common bacterial isolates included Pseudomonas (19%), Enterococcus (15%) and

Escherichia coli (13%). Of note 47% of these infections were caused by multidrug resistant pathogens. Postoperative bacterial infections remain important complications in intestinal recipients, and multidrug resistant pathogens have emerged as significant clinical challenges in intestinal transplants.

Fungal infections remain important infectious complications after intestinal transplants, but data particularly in pediatric recipients are lacking in the literature. In a series of 98 pediatric intestinal recipients Florescu et al. reported that 25 patients developed 59 episodes of Candida infections and four episodes of invasive Aspergillus infections [21]. Of the Candidal species, 37% were *C. albicans* and 63% were non-albicans. Of all fungal infections 66% were in the blood, 28.8% were in the intra-abdominal space, 3% were in the urinary tract and 2% were in the pleural space. Of the Candida intra-abdominal infections, 41% developed in the first postoperative month, while 80% of fungemia developed after more than six months. Median time from intestinal transplant to fungal infection was nine days for intra-abdominal infections versus 163 days for fungemia. Fungal infections occurred in approximately 25% of pediatric intestinal recipients and *Candida albicans* was the most common species. Intra-abdominal fungal infections occurred much earlier than fungemia after pediatric intestinal transplants.

In addition to bacterial infections, viral infections are also common in intestinal transplant recipients, of which CMV and EBV receive the most attention in the literature [2, 8, 22]. CMV is the most important viral infection in intestinal recipients. Not only does CMV cause tissue-invasive disease, it is also an independent risk factor for secondary bacterial and fungal infections and post-transplant lymphoproliferative disorder. It can also induce intestinal graft injury and rejection through indirect immunomodulatory causes. The patients who are at highest risk for CMV infection are CMV-negative recipients who receive CMV-positive intestinal organs. CMV-positive recipients are also at risk of CMV infections due to reactivation of latent virus. Anti-lymphocyte induction therapy only further enhances the risk of CMV infections. In patients who receive no prophylaxis, CMV occurs most often within the first three months after intestinal transplant, and can present as an asymptomatic infection or as a syndrome including fever, leukopenia, encephalitis, retinitis, pneumonitis, hepatitis or enteritis/graft involvement. Antiviral therapy is effective in the prevention and treatment of CMV. For prevention of CMV patients can receive either universal prophylactic therapy or preemptive therapy. Most experts recommend universal prophylaxis for CMV-negative recipients who receive CMV-positive intestinal organs, and universal prophylaxis or preemptive therapy for CMV-positive recipients for 3 to 6 months postoperatively or during intensified immunosuppressive treatments for rejection. CMV-negative recipients who receive CMV-negative intestinal organs are at the lowest risk of CMV infection and many experts recommend no CMV-specific antiviral prophylaxis [22]. Historical reports noted CMV to occur in 24% of intestinal recipients, but in a recent study of pediatric intestinal transplants Florescu et al. reported an 11% incidence of CMV viremia and a 7% incidence of CMV disease; in those patients with CMV disease, there was a high rate of CMV disease relapse and 11 fold increased risk of postoperative mortality [23]..

EBV is also an important viral infection especially in pediatric patients who receive intestinal transplants [2, 8, 22]. Like CMV patients with the highest risk for EBV infections are EBV-negative recipients who receive EBV-positive intestinal organs. EBV-positive recipients are at increased risk for reactivation of the latent virus which occurs 2 to 3 months postoperatively. EBV typically causes a syndrome which can include fever, leukopenia, thrombocytopenia, hepatitis, pneumonitis or PTLD. PTLD can present as a spectrum of diseases ranging from infectious mononucleosis to frank lymphoma that can be nodal or extranodal, localized or disseminated. A positive PCR for EBV in a patient with signs/symptoms of PTLD suggests the diagnosis, but tissue biopsy is confirmatory. Decreasing the immunosuppression by approximately 50% is the primary treatment which can result in lesion

regression. Other treatment options can include surgical resection and radiation therapy for local disease, in addition to rituximab (if CD20 positive) and chemotherapy for disseminated disease. Some centers use antiviral prophylaxis for EBV-negative recipients who received EBV-positive intestinal organs [22].

There is some evidence that intestinal transplantation improves quality of life compared to chronic TPN. In a study of 33 patients on chronic TPN vs. 22 patients with intestinal transplants, Pironi et al. noted that the intestinal recipients had better scores on treatment-specific quality of life questionnaires in the following categories: ability to vacation/travel, fatigue, gastrointestinal symptoms, stoma management/bowel movements, and global health status/quality of life. Subgroup analysis of patients who were employed showed that intestinal recipients had better scores in the ability to secure and maintain employment and emotional function. These data would suggest that a successful intestinal transplant was associated with less uncertainty about an employment situation and consequently less anxiety and/or depression [24].

14.5 Number of Transplants and Outcomes

The UNOS Database reported that approximately 2500 intestinal transplants have been performed in the United States over the last 25 years [10]. The OPTN/SRTR 2013 Annual Data Report indicated that only 23 centers performed pediatric intestinal transplants, and only 24 centers performed adult intestinal transplants in the United States [9]. According to this report the most common cause for intestinal failure was short gut syndrome (53%), caused by a host of etiologies. In this report approximately 170 new candidates were added to the waitlist for an intestinal transplant in 2013; of these candidates 49% waited for a liver-intestinal transplant and 51% waited for an intestinal transplant. Since 2008 candidates listed for an intestinal transplant outnumbered candidates listed for a liver-intestinal transplant. In the last decade the age distribution of listed

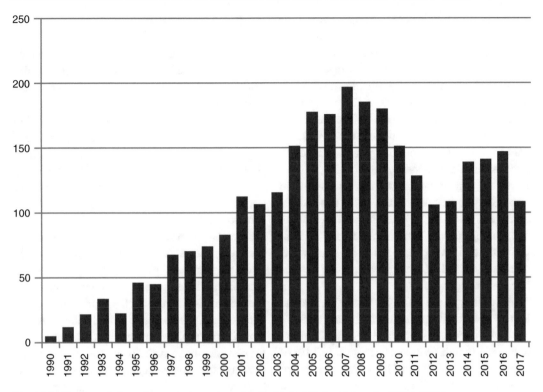

Fig. 14.2 Number of visceral transplants performed in the United States of America (1990–2017)

candidates shifted from a pediatric to an adult population, but the race or cause of disease distributions did not change over that time period.

Despite advances in the field, a significant reduction of the number of visceral transplants in the US since 2007 has been observed (Fig. 14.2). Some of the factors which have contributed to this decrease over the last decade include: inadequate reimbursement, the improved ability of intestinal failure units to avoid or resolve intestinal failure-associated liver disease, frequent social and/or psychiatric problems of this specific population, narrow risk-benefit ratio for small bowel transplantation in an era of improving outcomes with long-term TPN, and development of new drugs for treatment of patients with short gut syndrome (i.e. GLP-2 analog), among others [25].

According to the 2013 OPTN/SRTR Annual Report mortality on the waitlist decreased significantly for all age groups over the last decade [9]. Pretransplant mortality was higher for adult candidates than for pediatric candidates, and was higher for candidates who waited for a liver-intestinal transplant than for an intestinal transplant. This decrease in mortality was likely due to a greater proportion of candidates listed for an intestinal transplant than a liver-intestinal transplant (sicker liver failure patients), improved medical therapies for intestinal failure and improved organ allocation policies. Regarding three-year outcomes of intestinal candidates, 69% received an intestinal transplant, 8% were removed from the waitlist, 5% died on the list and 19% continued to wait on the list. Regarding three-year outcomes of liver-intestinal candidates, 66% received a liver-intestinal transplant, 11% were removed from the waitlist, 11% died on the list, and 12% still continued to wait on the list. Among candidates listed in 2012–2013, the median time to adult liver-intestinal transplant, adult intestinal transplant, and pediatric liver-intestinal transplant was 11 months, four months and seven months respectively. Among pediatric candidates listed in 2008–2009, the median wait time to intestinal transplant was 19 months.

In the 2013 OPTN/SRTR Annual Report the overall number of liver-intestinal transplants and intestinal transplants decreased steadily since 2009 [9]. It was noteworthy that in 2013 the overall of number of adult intestinal transplants was more than double the number of pediatric intestinal recipients. Moreover liver-intestinal transplant recipients were younger than intestinal transplant recipients, were more likely to have a diagnosis of necrotizing enterocolitis or congenital short gut syndrome and were likely to be hospitalized at the time of the transplant. In 2013, 52% recipients received an intestinal graft with another organ, and 19% of liver-intestinal recipients received a previous intestinal transplant compared to only 2% of intestinal recipients.

According to the 2013 OPTN/SRTR Annual Report intestinal graft survival has steadily improved over the last decade [9]. Graft failure within the first three months occurred in 14% of intestinal transplants and 11% of liver-intestinal transplants. For all intestinal transplants in 2008, the one and five-year graft survival rates were 73% and 62% respectively for pediatric recipients and 76% and 38% for adult recipients. One and five-year graft survival rates were 79% and 48% respectively for all intestinal recipients and 71% and 49% for all liver-intestinal recipients. The number of recipients who were alive with a functional intestinal graft steadily increased over the last decade. The incidence of acute rejection increased in the postoperative period approaching 53% at 2 years. For transplants which occurred from 2001 to 2011, 10% of intestinal recipients and 7% liver-intestinal recipients developed PTLD with 5 years postoperatively; and the incidence was highest in EBV-negative intestinal recipients. Regardless of recipient age, patient survival was better in intestinal recipients than in liver-intestinal recipients. Pediatric intestinal recipients had the highest one and five-year patient survival rates at 89% and 81% respectively, whereas adult liver-intestinal recipients had the lowest one and five year patient survival rates at 69% and 46% respectively.

14.6 Conclusion

Intestinal transplantation is a viable option for patients who suffer irreversible, life-threatening intestinal failure. The causes of intestinal failure vary greatly in the pediatric compared to the adult population. Evaluation of a patient who requires an intestinal transplant is similar to other solid organs, but a very clear picture of the patient's gastrointestinal tract and vascular system is essential. It is important to rule out whether the patient also has hepatic, pancreatic or renal dysfunction that warrants deeper investigation. There are several surgical options available to patients, including the isolated intestinal transplant, the liver-intestinal transplant and the multivisceral transplant. These operations can be complex and challenging with potential for significant medical and surgical postoperative complications. A systematic interprofessional approach is mandatory to manage these patients in the preoperative, intraoperative and postoperative settings. Despite significant improvements in immunosuppressive therapy, acute rejection in the intestinal graft remains a significant complication. Greater attention has been given to the role of donor specific antibodies and complement in causes of chronic allograft enteropathy and graft loss, and in potential noninvasive biomarkers to diagnose acute allograft rejection. Because intestinal recipients require increased immunosuppression to prevent rejection, they are at increased risk for bacterial, fungal and viral infections. Multidrug resistant bacteria, Candida, CMV and EVB can particularly problematic in the postoperative period. The demographics of the intestinal transplants have changed significantly over the last decade with an increased age of recipient and frequency of isolated intestinal transplants. With improved graft and patient survival after intestinal transplantation it does seem counterintuitive that the numbers of intestinal transplants have decreased over the last few years. With so few US centers performing pediatric or adult intestinal transplants, there could be issues of access to care and financial coverage of medical care/surgical procedures. In conclusion intestinal transplants will become an attractive alternative option to long-term maintenance therapy with TPN. The future for intestinal transplants will likely see improvements in surgical techniques and newer medications to treat rejection and infections, which translate into better graft and patient survival. Care of these patients in the critical perioperative period remains a crucial aspect of ensuring a successful outcome.

References

1. Abu-Elmagd KM, Costa G, Bond GJ, et al. Five hundred intestinal and multivisceral transplantations at a Single Center. Ann Surg. 2009;250(4):567–81.
2. Scotti-Fogelieni CL, Mariano IR, Cillo U, et al: Human intestinal and multivisceral transplantation. Three years clinical experience at the Pittsburgh Transplantation Institute. Date unknown, 41 pages.
3. Middleton SJ, Jamieson NV. The current status of small bowel transplantation in the UK and internationally. Gut. 2005;54:1650–7.
4. Arruda Pecora RA, David AI, Lee AD, et al. Small bowel transplantation. ABCD Arq Bras Cir Dig. 2013;26(4):223–9.
5. Gondolesi GE, Almau HM. Intestinal transplantation outcomes. Mt Sinai J Med. 2012;79:246–55.
6. Moon J, Iyer K. Intestinal rehabilitation and transplantation for intestinal failure. Mt Sinai J Med. 2012;79:256–66.
7. Fishbein TM. Intestinal transplantation. N Engl J Med. 2009;361:998–1008.
8. Sudan D. The current state of intestinal transplantation: indications, techniques, outcomes and challenges. Am J Transplant. 2014;14:1976–84.
9. Smith JM, Skeans MA, Horslen SP, et al. OPTN/SRTR 2013 annual data report: intestine. Am J Transplant. 2015;15(Suppl 2):1–16.
10. http://optn.transplant.hrsa.gov. Accessed on May 29, 2015.
11. CMS: Medicare national coverage determinations: intestinal and mutlivisceral transplantation, 2006. Available at www.cms.hhs.gov/transmittals/downloads/R58NCD.pdf
12. Diamanti A, Gambarara M, Marcellini M. Prevalence of liver complications in pediatric patients on home nutrition: indications for intestinal or combined liver-intestinal transplantation. Transplant Proc. 2003;35(8):3047–9.
13. Matarese LE. Nutrition interventions before and after adult intestinal transplantation: the Pittsburgh experience. Pract Gastroenterol. 2010;35(11):11–26.
14. Lauro A, Bagni C, Zanfi S, et al. Mortality after steroid-resistant acute cellular rejection and chronic rejection episodes in adult intestinal transplants: report from a single center in induction/preconditioning era. Transplant Proc. 2013;45:2032–3.
15. Berger M, Zeevi A, Farmer DG, et al. Immunologic challenges in small bowel transplantation. Am J Transplant. 2012;12:S2–8.
16. Christians U, Klawitter J, Klawitter J, et al. Biomarkers of immunosuppressant organ toxicity after transplantation-status, concepts and misconceptions. Expert Opin Drug Metab Toxicol. 2011;7(s):175–200.
17. Hibi T, Nishida S, Garcia J, et al. Citrulline level is a potent indicator of acute rejection in long term following pediatric intestinal/multivisceral transplantation. Am J Transplant. 2012;12:S27–32.
18. Girlanda R, Cheema AK, Kaur P, et al. Metabolics of human intestinal transplant rejection. Am J Transplant. 2012;12:S18–26.
19. Green M, Michaels MG. Infections in pediatric solid organ transplant recipients. J Pediatric Infect Dis Soc. 2012;1(2):144–51.
20. Primeggia J, Matsumoto CS, Fishbein TM, et al. Infection among adult small bowel and multivisceral transplant recipients in the 30-day postoperative period. Transpl Infect Dis. 2013;15:441–8.
21. Florescu DF, Islam KM, Grant W, et al. Incidence and outcome of fungal infections in pediatric small bowel recipients. Transpl Infect Dis. 2010;12:497–504.
22. Grim SA, Clark NM. Management of infectious complications in solid-organ transplant recipients. Clin Pharmacol Ther. 2011;90(2):333–42.
23. Florescu DF, Langnas AN, Sandkowsky U. Opportunistic viral infections in intestinal transplantation. Expert Rev Ant Infect Ther. 2014;11:367–81.
24. Pironi L, Baxter JP, Lauro A, et al. Assessment of the quality of life on home parental nutrition and after intestinal transplantation using treatment-specific questionnaires. Am J Transplant. 2012;12:S60–s66.
25. Grant D, Abu-Elmagd K, Mazariegos G, et al. Intestinal transplant registry report: global activity and trends. Am J Transplant. 2015;15(1):210–9.

Living Donor Liver Transplantation

15

Rauf Shahbazov and Daniel Maluf

15.1 Introduction

Liver transplantation is the most effective therapy for patients with end-stage liver disease [1]. However, for nearly half of patients on the waiting list, transplantation will not be an option as a result of the perennial shortage of available grafts from deceased donors [2, 3]. In recent years, a coordinated effort has been made to expand the donor pool including, living donor liver transplantation (LDLT), extended criteria donors (ECDs), including aged donor (>70 years old) [4], obese donors [5], and donation after cardiac death (DCD) [6]. Furthermore, recent advances in organ preservation with normothermic and hypothermic machine perfusion techniques have added new tools to the transplant field [7].

In recent decades, LDLT has emerged as a safe lifesaving alternative to deceased donor liver transplantation (DDLT). LDLT is the predominant form of liver transplantation in Asia, where cultural and religious beliefs do not allow deceased donation. LDLT accounts for 60–90% of all liver transplants in Asian countries [8]. In the US, where deceased donor liver grafts are more widely available and the main source of grafts for transplantation, LDLT accounts for less than 5% of liver transplants, mainly due to risks on the healthy donor [9, 10]. Historical events are described in Table 15.1.

15.2 Indications and Patient Selection

Nowadays, indications to LDLT patients are the same or similar to DDLT patients with cirrhosis, with few exceptions [21]. Deceased donor livers are prioritized to patients with the highest Model for End-Stage Liver Disease (MELD) scores [22]. Since 2002, when MELD scores were adopted by the United Network for Organ Sharing (UNOS), there has been a significant reduction in waiting list mortality [22]. For patients at the high end of the MELD scale, risks of liver transplantation are outweighed by the mortality of remaining on the waiting list. In contrast, the benefits of transplantation are not evenly distributed across all MELD scores [23]. LDLT is most beneficial for transplant candidates with low priority for a deceased graft but high risk of death while waiting for one. In the current liver allocation system, these patients include those with low to mid MELD scores [22–38] and those who do not meet UNOS approved MELD exception points (e.g., primary sclerosing cholangitis and

R. Shahbazov
Department of Surgery, Transplant Division, Upstate Medical University, Syracuse, NY, USA
e-mail: shahbazr@upstate.edu

D. Maluf (✉)
University of Maryland Health System, Baltimore, MD, USA
e-mail: DMaluf@SOM.umaryland.edu

© Springer Nature Switzerland AG 2021
N. Hakim et al. (eds.), *Transplantation Surgery*, Springer Specialist Surgery Series,
https://doi.org/10.1007/978-3-030-55244-2_15

Table 15.1 Milestones of living donor liver transplantation

Thomas Starzl (1967)	First successful liver transplantation	[11]
Henri Bistmuth (1984)	First reduced-size graft liver transplantation	[12]
Rudolf Pichmayr (1984)	First ex situ reduced-size graft liver transplantation	[13]
Raia et al. (1988)	First adult left lateral liver graft into a 4-year-old child with a 6-day survival	[14]
Strong et al. (1989)	Successfully transplanted an adult left lateral liver graft into a 17-month-old child	[15]
Hashikura et al. (1993)	Successful living-related partial liver transplantation to an adult patient	[16]
Yoshio Yamaoka (1994)	First right lobe living donor liver transplantation	[17]
Lo et al. (1996)	Adult-to-adult living donor liver transplantation using extended right lobe grafts	[18]
Lee et al. (2001)	Adult-to-adult living donor liver transplantations using dual grafts	[19]
Cherqui et al. (2002)	First fully laparoscopic left lateral liver graft for pediatric LDLT	[20]

Table 15.2 Indication for living donor liver transplantation [39]

Type of transplant	Country	Common indications	Other common indications	Less common indications
Elective	USA	NASH	Alcoholic liver disease HCC	Cholestasis liver diseases (PBC, PSC)
	Europe	Alcoholic liver	HCC	HCV, other cholestatic liver diseases
	Asia	HCC	Hepatitis B	
Emergency	USA	Drug induced ALF	Viral hepatitis	Autoimmune hepatitis or Wilson disease
	Europe	Drug induced ALF	Viral hepatitis Seronegative hepatitis	
	Asia	Hepatitis B	Autoimmune hepatitis, Viral hepatitis	

recurrent biliary sepsis). Especially, patients with hyponatremia, refractory ascites or recurrent variceal bleeding when trans jugular intrahepatic portosystemic shunt (TIPS) is contraindicated. Despite that, for patients with high MELD scores (>30) and acute fulminant liver failure (UNOS Status 1 or 1A) who have a higher chance of receiving a graft from a deceased donor, the use of LDLT is controversial as it may be associated with poor survival [24].

The use of LDLT in patients with acute liver failure (ALF), is controverted due to the short time between evaluation and transplant and may compromise donor altruism [25]. However, many studies in the US and other parts of the world have reported LDLT as a safe option in selected patients with ALF [26]. Since the first LDLT, various innovation and techniques have expanded the application of LDLT with contrasting impact in Eastern and Western countries (Table 15.2) [27].

Hepatitis C Virus In recent years, well-tolerated, 12-week interferon-free oral protease inhibitor hepatitis C virus (HCV) treatment regimens have revolutionized sustained virologic response rates—viral cures—to patients infected with HCV both pre-transplantation and post-transplantation [6]. Early concerns of more rapid HCV recurrence and graft failure in recipients infected with HCV undergoing LDLT were dispelled by a prospective single-center study examining liver biopsy tissue histology in patients infected with HCV [28, 29]. The study revealed no difference in recurrent HCV between recipients of LLDT and DDLT. More recent data by the multi-center Adult-to-Adult Living Liver Transplantation (A2ALL) cohort reported similar results, especially when LDLT was performed at high-volume centers [30]. Therefore, patients infected with HCV and in need of transplantation, should not be denied LDLT if a suitable living donor is available. Diabetes mellitus, older age ($\geq$55 years of age) and cirrhosis at the time of sustained virologic response are associated with a hepatocellular cancer risk and warrants mandatory surveillance.

Hepatocellular Carcinoma Liver transplantation is an established option for patients with unresectable hepatocellular carcinoma (HCC). In the US, MELD exception points are limited to patients with HCC that are within the Milan criteria [31]. The Milan criteria allows transplantation in patients who have one tumor up to 5 cm in diameter or no more than three tumors, each measuring up to 3 cm [32]. For patients with HCC outside the Milan criteria, LDLT can be the only option [33]. Findings from the A2ALL study reported an association between LDLT recipients and increased HCC recurrence compared to DDLT recipients, even after adjusting for tumor characteristics for the entire cohort [34]. In the LDLT patients with early recurrence, the tumor characteristics were consistent with an aggressive phenotype. One hypothesis suggests that the rapidity of liver regeneration after partial hepatectomy promotes growth of residual tumor cells, leading to higher HCC recurrence. In contrast, studies reported from other institutions showed no difference between HCC recurrence rates after LDLT and DDLT [35–37]. In recent years, LDLT has expanded its indication for some other tumors such as cholangiocarcinoma (CCA) [38] and nonresectable colorectal cancer [40], that if proven successful may significantly impact the need for living donors [41].

Frailty When patients are being considered for liver transplantation, it is important to assess their frailty [42]. Frailty associated with sarcopenia can be objectively measured with a CT scan of intramuscular adipose tissue content (IMAC) and psoas muscle mass index (PMI). Studies have reported low skeletal muscle quality and mass as strong predictors for post-LDLT mortality [43–46]. Findings from a pilot study measuring cross-sectional areas of psoas muscle via CT revealed with Cox regression models a strong association between psoas area and post-transplant mortality [43]. Another study from a Japanese transplant center revealed high IMAC and low PMI were independent risk factors for death after LDLT [47]. Despite these findings, the current MELD scoring system does not factor sarcopenia into the score. A recent report by Kim YR et al. reported the risk of tumor recurrence after LDLT in patients with advanced HCC was significantly higher in patients with psoas muscle wasting [48]. In this context, preoperative nutritional and exercise therapy should be required of transplant candidates to improve sarcopenic status and post-transplant outcomes.

15.3 Donor Evaluation and Selection

Potential adult liver donor evaluation is not significantly different between North America and Asia, but some specifications exist due to availability of living donors as well as cultural differences [39, 49]. Strict adult liver donor evaluation and selection are important to ensure both donor safety and recipient outcome. One of the primary goals of the living donor evaluation is to make sure the potential donor can make a decision that is informed, voluntary and without coercion. In 2015, the UNOS/OPTN implemented policy requirements to specify a minimum set of tests and procedures for the medical and psychological evaluation of potential liver donors in the US [10]. Beyond OPTN guidelines, which define absolute contraindications, transplant centers rely on their judgement and experience to evaluate potential donors on a case by case basis. A step-wise donor evaluation protocol is presented in Table 15.3.

Donor evaluation starts with a candidate contacting a liver transplant center through a dedicated live donor coordinator. This initiation reduces the element of coercion. In the first stage, all potential donors undergo routine physical tests and psychosocial evaluation. Potential donors can be excluded in the preclinical screen based on ABO incompatibility, obesity (BMI >35 kg/m^2), age (>60), substantial medical comorbidities or upper abdominal surgical histories [50]. However, these are relative contraindications and donor

Table 15.3 The step by step evaluation of donors before transplantation

Step 1	Living donor candidate contacts transplant center. Assessments of ABO compatibility, full information to potential donor, schedules blood work, evaluates donor history and performs routine physical tests, evaluation and social work interview with potential donor.
Step 2	Schedules lab work, radiological tests, angiography and biopsy of liver if necessary.
Step 3	Evaluation and social work interview with potential donor. First surgeon informed consent from donor obtained.
Step 4	Schedule operation date. Potential donor reviewed and reinforced. Second surgeon informed consent from donor is obtained. Statement of unsuitability offered to donor.

elimination is ultimately left up to the selection criteria of a given center. In Asia, experienced centers have developed innovative protocols to overcome the barrier of ABO-incompatible donation [51]. Those centers have adopted low-morbidity, highly effective ABO-incompatible LDLT protocols centered on rituximab, plasma exchange and intravenous immunoglobulin administration [52]. Similar protocols have been developed for kidney recipient desensitization [53]. Donor age is another important factor in determining transplant success. Although age cutoffs vary among centers, most avoid donors older than 55–60 years [54]. Transplant centers in Asia have pushed this limit, with some studies reporting equivalent outcomes after LDLT between carefully selected donors older than 55 when compared with younger donors [55, 56].

Medical Evaluation The medical evaluation includes donor history, physical exam, general laboratory and imaging tests, transmissible disease screening, cancer screening, liver-specific tests and liver anatomic assessment. Laboratory tests, such as liver function test, genetic disorder tests and thrombophilia workup, screen for undiagnosed liver disease and other extrahepatic conditions. Chest radiography, EKG, echocardiography are performed routinely. Additional tests such as pulmonary function and cardiac assessment are administered based on donor medical condition and age. In addition, centers are performing thrombophilia and genetic tests for donors and recipients, as it lowers the risk of thrombotic vascular morbidity [57–59].

Psychosocial Evaluation The goal of the psychosocial evaluation is to assess mental health and provide donors with the appropriate preoperative psychological support. Although donors understand that surgery will likely save the recipient's life, the prospect of a long recovery can cause anxiety, stress and depressive symptoms prior to or after surgery [60]. Therefore, psychological assessments are conducted to ensure the potential donor understands the donation process, is free of coercion, and identifies candidates who are emotionally vulnerable. Reluctant donors can be turned down at this point. Initially, living donors were most often genetically related to their recipient. But over time this relationship has evolved due to an increase in biologically unrelated donors, often referred to as nondirected or altruistic donors [61]. These donors typically require more consideration during the psychosocial evaluation to identify motivating factors for donation and to assess for signs of coercion or financial gain. Once potential donors have completed the preclinical screen and medical evaluation, a thorough informed consent is obtained as mandated in the US by UNOS.

The Independent Living Donor Advocate Any center performing LDLT is required to have an independent living donor advocate (ILDA), a person with no conflict of interest with the recipient's medical care and decision-making. The position was established in response to concerns that donor evaluation and recruitment were conducted by the same transplant team, which might be influenced by the recipient's needs. It is the responsibility of the ILDA to advocate on the donor's behalf and to supply unbiased information for the patient's informed consent. They also serve as a resource throughout the donation process and are responsible for assessing the donors' understanding of the potential risks [62].

The surgical evaluation includes detailed explanation of the transplant procedure, evaluation by the transplant surgeon and surgeon-informed consent. The transplant surgeon must discuss possible morbidity and mortality [10]. A multidisciplinary selection committee, composed of the complete evaluating team and the ILDA, meets to discuss all components of the donor evaluation for final approval.

Preoperative imaging is a critical step in donor evaluation to identify any intraparenchymal abnormalities, visualize vascular and biliary anatomy and determine the size of the whole liver. Evaluation by magnetic resonance imaging (MRI), MR angiography, MR cholongiography or triple phase computed tomography (CT) scans (based on center preference or software's used) provides important information about liver anatomy, presence of steatosis and volumetric assessments that are key to safe LDLT [63]. Use of MRI during liver volume assessment, combined with coeliac angiography and portal phase assessment, is typically enough to identify important hepatic vascular variants. MRCP is a specialized MRI scan used routinely to evaluate biliary anatomy, including multiple ducts, trifurcation, accessory right hepatic duct or dorsocaudal branch of the right hepatic duct coming off the left hepatic duct, that can lead to donor exclusion. Graft-to-recipient body weight ratio (GRWR) and future donor liver remnant are calculated based on liver volume. Donor remnant volume >35% is thought to be safe [28], but some centers will consider less remnant volume in certain situations [29]. On the recipient, a liver graft with ≥0.8% GRWR and graft weight >40 of standard liver mass is widely accepted for optimal outcomes [64]. Some experienced LDLT centers have expanded this criteria by using liver grafts from two donors [19, 65]. Once a donor is accepted for right or left lobe donation, some LDLT centers continue to rely on intraoperative cholangiography to mark and delineate the biliary tract division in the operative room. Liver biopsies may be required for potential donors with abnormal liver function tests, BMI >28–30 kg/m^2 or steatosis on imaging [21]. Donor steatosis increases the risk of post-transplant graft dysfunction and increases donor risk of complications. The degree of acceptable macrosteatosis depends on the transplant center, with some Asian centers accepting donors with steatosis up to 30% [66, 67].

Donor evaluation continues in the operative room when the surgeon performing the operation judges the anatomy in situ. In some circumstances, donor surgery is aborted intraoperatively due to unexpected findings [68]. Medical contraindication rates are quite high in LDLT and vary from center to center. The high donor rejection rate is likely due, in part, to low tolerance for donor risk [69].

15.4 Donor Operation

Donor hepatectomy techniques have evolved over the past 20 years [24]. A better understanding of liver anatomy and physiology, coupled with improved anesthesia techniques and widespread use of intraoperative ultrasound or liver surgery mapping, have led to virtually "bloodless" donor surgery [70]. Technological innovations have expanded the list of liver parenchymal transection devices and hemostatic agents. Use of each device or agent has a learning curve, and undoubtedly every experienced liver surgeon has his or her personal preferences. In addition, the development of sophisticated liver surgery planning software (Fig. 15.1) and improvements in 3D printing have demonstrated the ability to print synthetic exact replicas of patient livers. Having accurate anatomical reproductions of donor livers allows better preoperative surgical planning, thereby improving donor safety [71]. Furthermore, increased use of computer-assisted, or GPS, techniques are gaining interest and may became a vital tool for future liver surgery [72].

15.5 Steps in Standard Donor Hepatectomies

A fundamental understanding of liver anatomy is vital for any surgeon performing donor surgery. Each hepatic resection can be broken down into a series of steps. The key to being a proficient hepatic surgeon is not to operate swiftly but rather to accomplish the operation by completing

Fig. 15.1 Software's are useful for anatomy assessments and liver surgery planning

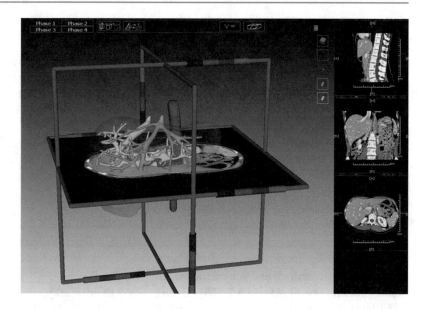

the steps in an orchestrated fashion. Mastery of operative steps, coupled with knowledge of liver anatomy and common anatomic variants, provides the foundation for safe donor surgery. Although there are many different techniques and sequences for accomplishing each of the donor operations, we present the most standardized and our preferred approach for right hepatic lobectomy, left hepatic lobectomy, and left lateral segmentectomy (left lateral sectionectomy).

15.6 Steps Common to All Open Donor Hepatectomy

1. Make the skin incision—midline or right subcostal with or without a partial or complete left subcostal extension across the midline, depending on the patient's habitus and surgeon's experience.
2. Open and explore the abdomen. Position a self-sustaining retractor (e.g., Thompson or OMNI).
3. Examine the liver with bimanual palpation. Access the liver for suitability for donation. Perform a liver ultrasound and confirm the operation can be performed. Perform a biopsy if there are concerns of graft steatosis or liver disease.

4. Take down the round and falciform ligament and expose the anterior surface of the hepatic veins.
   - *For left hepatectomy.* Divide the left triangular ligament.
   - *For right hepatectomy.* Mobilize the right lobe from the right coronary and divide triangular ligaments.
5. Open the gastrohepatic ligament, palpate the porta hepatis, and assess for accessory or replaced hepatic arteries.
6. Perform a cholecystectomy. Leave the gallbladder with the cystic duct intact to perform intraoperative cholangiogram.

15.7 Right Hepatic Lobectomy (Right Hepatectomy or Hemihepatectomy)

1. Mobilize the liver from the anterior aspect of the IVC in "piggyback" fashion. Ligate the short hepatic veins up to the right hepatic vein (RHV). Dissect and identify the RHV. Preserve any vein larger than 5 mm for recipient reimplantation to achieve optimal outflow.
2. Perform a right hilar dissection—gently lower the hilar plate, then isolate the right hepatic artery (RHA) with the vessel loop,

superior to the right side of the common bile duct.

3. Dissect and isolate a replaced or accessory RHA with the vessel loop, if present.

4. Expose the portal vein and identify the right and left branches. Often times a small lateral portal vein branch off the right portal vein (RPV) to the caudate lobe is present and needs to be controlled and ligated to allow exposure of additional length on the RPV. Dissect and isolate the RPV with a vessel loop.

5. Dissect the avascular tissue along the suprahepatic vena cava between the middle hepatic vein (MHV) and RHVs. Pass a silastic tube of a Jackson-Pratt drain through the RHV-MHV gap.

6. Notch or divide the caudate process crossing to the right hepatic lobe, and bring the drain up and through this notch behind the isolated RHA and RPV (in preparation for the "Hanging Maneuver").

7. Hang the liver over the drain by pulling up as you divide through the liver parenchyma.

8. Repeat the ultrasound and confirm the transection plane, staying to the right of the MHV.

9. Cauterize approximately 1 cm into the liver parenchyma, then switch to a hydro-jet dissection device or CUSA in combination with Bovie electrocautery and suture ligation.

10. Continue parenchymal division until the RHV is encountered. During this time, identification, careful control, and transection of the right hepatic duct (RHD) according to preoperative MRCP and intraoperative cholangiogram are obtained late in the parenchymal transection process to reduce bile duct injury.

11. The right hepatic lobectomy is completed with vascular clamping and transection of the right portal vein, right hepatic artery, following right bile duct. The RHV is then divided between vascular clamps. The graft is delivered and subjected to further flushing in the back bench with HTK or UW and possible reconstruction according to any findings.

12. Suture stamp the RHA, RPV, RHV with appropriate size monofilament Proline suture material and right bile duct with 6/0 PDS.

13. Examine the transected liver edge for bleeding. If bleeding is encountered, place a figure-of-eight ligating vascular suture.

14. Ensure hemostasis of the transected liver edge with an argon beam coagulator and suture ligation.

15. Inspect the transection surface for bile leaks or bleeding. These should be clipped or suture ligated. Apply a dilute solution of propofol or methylene blue to facilitate visualization of bile leaks.

16. Inspect the IVC and right retroperitoneal space for -hemostasis.

17. Fix the proximal falciform ligament back to the diaphragm side with figure-of-eight sutures to avoid donor hemi-graft torsions.

18. Apply tissue sealant to the cut surface of the liver, and place a Jackson-Pratt drain in the right subphrenic space. Close the abdomen in standard fashion.

Although some liver surgeons advocate a one-step division of the right bile duct with ligation and transection, the key is to perform intraoperative cholangiogram with different angles and compare to the preoperative MRCP for proper mapping and transection. Centers use different approaches to identify the proper area of transection of bile duct which may include metallic clips, radiopaque wires, rubber band or metallic instruments per surgeon preference (Fig. 15.2).

It is also important to get accurate ultrasound visualization and mapping of the MHV and to stay just to the right of it. Weaving in and out or bisecting the MHV can lead to major complications.

15.8 Left Hepatic Lobectomy (Left Hepatectomy or Hemihepatectomy)

1. Widely open the gastrohepatic ligament flush with the undersurface of the left lateral section and the caudate lobe.

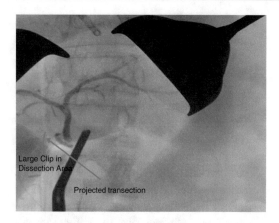

Fig. 15.2 Intraoperative Cholangiogram: Shows main, right and left bile ducts. Large Clip place to demarcate right CBD planned area of transection

2. Check for a replaced or accessory left hepatic artery (LHA). If present, dissect and isolate with a vessel loop.
3. Clamp the round ligament (ligament teres) and pull it anteriorly, like a handle, to expose the left hilum.
4. Divide any existing parenchymal bridge between the RHV and MHV.
5. Dissect the left hilum at the base of the umbilical fissure and lower the hilar plate anterior to the left portal pedicle.
6. Incise the peritoneum overlying the hilum from the left side, to dissect and isolate the LHA (after test clamping and confirming a palpable pulse in the RHA).
7. Dissect and isolate the portal vein with a vessel loop at the base of the umbilical fissure.
8. Expose the portal vein and identify the right and left branches. Identify and control the small portal vein branch off the LPV to the caudate lobe to allow exposure of additional length.
9. Ligate and divide the ligamentum venosum caudally.
10. Identify the long extrahepatic course of the left hepatic duct (LHD) behind the portal vein. Perform intraoperative cholangiogram to map extra and intra hepatic tree of bile ducts.
11. Fold the left lateral segment up and back to the right, exposing the window at the base of the MHV as it enters the IVC. This is facili-

tated by dividing any loose areolar tissue overlying the ligamentum venosum, which is divided proximally.

12. Carefully dissect until you pass a large, blunt right-angle clamp in the window between the RHV and the MHV. Hug the back of the MHV, aiming for the deep edge of the LHV. Do not force or perforate the IVC or MHV.
13. Once the venous branches (short veins) of segment one are dissected off and the left liver is separated from the IVC, pass the silastic tube of a Jackson-Pratt drain through this window.
14. Notch or divide the caudate process crossing to the left hepatic lobe and bring the drain up and through the notch.
15. Hang the liver over the drain by pulling up as you divide through the liver parenchyma.
16. Repeat the ultrasound and confirm the transection plane on the anterior surface, staying close to the demarcated line. Do not bisect the MHV as it passes tangentially from the left to the right lobe.
17. Cauterize down approximately 1 cm in the liver parenchyma, then switch to a CUSA or hydro-jet dissection device in combination with Bovie electrocautery and suture ligation.
18. Continue parenchymal division until the left/middle hepatic veins are encountered.
19. When the recipient side is ready to accept the liver graft, the left hepatic lobectomy is completed with clamping and transection of the left portal vein, left hepatic artery, following left bile duct. The left hepatic vein is then divided between vascular clamps. The graft is delivered and subjected to further flushing with HTK or UW at the back bench and reconstruction when needed. Carefully oversaw the stumps of the LHV, -MHV, on IVC, left postal vein, LHA with Prolene sutures and the stump of the left bile duct with PDS sutures. End of surgery colangiogram is performed in some centers or if concern exist.
20. Check the transected edge of the liver for surgical bleeding; ensure hemostasis of the

transected edge with an argon beam coagulator and suture ligation.

21. Inspect the transection surface for bile leaks. These should be clipped or suture ligated. Apply a dilute solution of propofol or methylene blue to facilitate visualization of bile leaks.

22. Apply tissue sealant to the transected surface of the liver. Place a Jackson-Pratt drain in the left subphrenic space and close the abdomen.

Because the right posterior duct arises from the left hepatic duct (LHD) in approximately 20% of cases and the right anterior duct arises from the LHD in approximately 5% of cases, it is vital to divide the LHD according to an exact previous mapping plan. The left lobe of the liver will be well demarcated after the left vascular inflow has been temporarily clamped, which guides the transection plane on the anterior surface. In general, the transection plane should be close to the demarcation line to minimize the amount of devascularized liver remaining. When dividing the LHV and MHV, the surgeon should keep in mind they have a common trunk approximately 90% of the time. If it is not easy to open the window deep to the MHV and LHV, then division of the MHV and LHV can be accomplished after the parenchymal transection.

15.9 Left Lateral Segmentectomy (Left Lateral Sectionectomy)

1. Widely open the gastrohepatic ligament flush with the undersurface of the left lateral section and the caudate lobe.

2. Identity, and isolate the replaced or accessory LHA, if present.

3. Clamp the round ligament and pull it anteriorly like a handle to expose the left hilum.

4. Divide any existing parenchymal bridge between segments III and IVB.

5. Carry the dissection down from the end of the round ligament, and the segment III pedicle will be encountered.

6. Incise the peritoneal reflection on the left side of the round ligament as it inserts into the umbilical fissure. When encircling the segment II pedicle, take care to avoid injury to the caudate inflow vessels coming off the LPV.

7. Divide the liver parenchyma, staying on the right side of the falciform ligament using Bovie electrocautery.

8. The LHV can be isolated before the liver transection or as the parenchymal transection is complete.

9. When the recipient side is ready to accept the liver graft, the left lateral sectionectomy is completed by transecting the left portal vein, left hepatic artery, following left bile duct. The left hepatic vein is then divided between vascular clamps. The delivered graft is subjected to additional flushing with HTK or UW at the bench back and possible reconstruction according to any findings.

15.10 Minimal Invasive Donor Hepatectomies

Minimally invasive surgery has the advantage of reducing operative morbidity, post-operative pain, and recovery time. Groups in Europe and Asia have described such approaches in the form of pure laparoscopic, hybrid hand-assisted and robotic-assisted techniques [73–76]. The first fully laparoscopic left lateral liver graft for pediatric LDLT was reported by Cherqui and colleagues in 2002 [77]. Since then, the procedure has been slow to be accepted, most likely due to the technical complexities of the procedure and the surgical expertise required. Early studies comparing minimally invasive living donor hepatectomy (MILDH) to open living donor hepatectomy (OLDH), have found donor morbidity rates, wound-related complications, hospital stays and analgesia use were reduced in MILDH [78, 79]. Blood loss and operative times were comparable between patients undergoing MILDH and OLDH. Despite current challenges, MILDH has the potential to replace open hepatectomy in the future [80], however continued progress will ultimately depend on accumulation of experiences, outcomes, center volumes to secure ultimately donor safety.

15.11 Donor Outcomes

Donor hepatectomy is a major operation with potential risks for serious complications [50]. The A2ALL consortium analyzed 760 living liver donors and reported a 40% complication rate for right lobe donors, with multiple complications occurring in 19% of patients [50]. In studies that included both right and left liver lobe donors, the overall complication rates were on the order of 21% [81]. Reported complication rates and type of complications in donors of hepatic lobes vary widely among centers [82, 83]. Common complications include bile leaks, bacterial infections, incisional hernia, pleural effusion and donor depression. Liver failure requiring rescue transplantation is extremely rare but frequently fatal [84]. The risk of death is estimated at 0.2% in western countries [85–87]. Using the Clavien system to classify severity of complications, approximately 50% are minor, defined as Clavien grade 1. Serious complications, defined as Clavien grade 3 or 4, are rare (1.1%), but include death or permanent disability [24, 50]. Most complications occur within 3 months of surgery, but psychological difficulties and hernias tend to develop later but within the first 3 years [88]. Despite some complications, over 95% of liver donors report satisfaction with the donation experience and say they would make the decision to donate again [89].

15.12 Recipient Operation

Due to shorter vessels and bile duct obtained in a living donor liver graft, hepatectomy is different from that for a DDLT [90, 91]. Usually bilateral subcostal incision, with if necessary upward midline extension, is adequate for good exposure. Meticulous hilar dissection is necessary to preserve the portal triads in preparation for the

reconstruction. Dissection and isolation of the right, middle, and left hepatic arteries is carried out till liver parenchymal level. Dissection of the common hepatic duct should start at the hilum to avoid excessive skeletinization and to preserve its blood supply [92]. Right and left hepatic ducts are severed by sharp dissection, and bleeding from feeding arteries on the distal stumps are controlled by using fine PDS sutures. The main, right and left portal veins are dissected and isolated. After controlling the main portal vein with a vascular clamp, the right and left portal veins are divided close to the liver hilum. Unlike a DDLT, the recipient's inferior vena cava needs to be preserved in a LDLT. Therefore, it is necessary to mobilize the caudate lobe from the inferior vena cava (IVC) by dissecting and dividing all the short hepatic veins. The hepatic veins (RHV, MHV, and LHV) are individually isolated and divided with a vascular stapler. In order to have optimal hepatic vein anastomosis, circumferential isolation and cross-clamping of the IVC is preferable, if tolerated, but not necessary. Once hemostasis is achieved, the IVC is partially occluded with a Satinsky clamp. The RHV stump is reopened (in the case of a Right lobe graft), and the lumen of the retrohepatic IVC is flushed with heparinized normal saline. The longitudinal orifice of the RHV is enlarged by transversely incising across the anterior wall of the IVC to fashion a triangular (or V) venotomy opening that matches the size and shape of the hepatic vein venoplasty cuff in the graft.

The implantation of the graft starts with anastomosis of the hepatic vein cuff with the recipient IVC opening, performed in a triangular fashion using 4–0 polypropylene. Several venoplasty techniques have been described [93] with the goal of achieving optimal graft outflow. Running sutures are applied, starting with the base of the triangle and continuing forward along the two sides and joined at the apex. After completion of the hepatic vein anastomosis, the portal vein stump is inspected for correct orientation. Portal anastomosis is performed with 6–0 polypropylene running sutures with a growth factor of about two thirds the diameter of the portal vein. The clamp on the IVC is released, and the systemic venous return is restored. The selection of the appropriate recipient hepatic artery for arterial reconstruction is based on length, caliber, and orientation. Most centers perform hepatic artery anastomosis under high magnification loupes. The use of microscopes has gained popularity and when performed by a dedicated microvascular surgeon, the complication rate drops below 2% [94]. Before using multiple interrupted stitches with 9–0 nylon monofilament sutures for anastomosis, it is important to check that both recipient and graft hepatic arteries have adequate size and length to allow rotating the vessels for placement of sutures on the posterior wall. After completion of arterial anastomosis, it is important to perform Doppler ultrasonography to ensure patency of all vascular anastomoses and correct doppler signal of the hepatic artery [95].

Reconstruction of the biliary ducts are performed either duct-to-duct or hepaticojejunostomy. Duct-to-duct anastomosis is the preferred technique except in cases where the recipient bile duct is not healthy, such as patients with primary sclerosing cholangitis. Duct-to-duct anastomosis is performed between the graft hepatic duct and the recipient common hepatic duct. One pitfall to avoid in biliary reconstruction is preserving a common hepatic duct in the recipient that is too long, with an ischemic end that may end up developing ischemic anastomotic stricture or bile leakage. The anastomosis is performed using 6–0 absorbable sutures, with continuous sutures for the posterior wall and interrupted ones for the anterior wall [96]. If more than one hepatic duct in the graft are close together, the adjacent ductal orifices are approximated to form a single cuff, and a single duct-to-duct anastomosis is performed incorporating the hilar plate. In some cases, ductoplasty is associated with a higher incidence of stricture and is not advisable. Some centers use an internal or external stents, but there is not agreement in the benefit of either approaches. Abdominal drains are placed in sub hepatic and supra hepatic areas.

15.13 Results of Living Donor Liver Transplantation

The care of a recipient after LDLT is similar to that after DDLT [97]. However, some differences are expected and require expertise and careful attention since the living donor liver graft is a partial graft and may develop early dysfunction, defined as small-for size syndrome (SFSS) [98]. SFSS represents a common complication in LDLT [99]. Accurate management of intravenous fluid replacement is necessary to avoid venous congestion, or systemic hypotension. Ultrasound/Doppler studies are performed daily to verify satisfactory vessel patency [100]. Due to the technical complexity of LDLT, the overall complication rates are higher in LDLT recipients compared with DDLT. Common early post-operative complications include bleeding and hepatic artery thrombosis (HAT) [101]. In LDLT, the risk of HAT remains high due to the smaller caliber of the vessels [102]. Significant post-operative intra-abdominal bleeding requires operative intervention. Reoperation for thrombectomy and revision of arterial anastomosis may be successful in early HAT, if diagnosed early by screening ultrasound. Primary nonfunction (PNF) is not commonly reported in LDLT compared to DDLT, presumably due to the quality of the graft and relatively short cold ischemia time [103]. Rejection rates are lower in related donor LDLT [24] and can be treated using similar immunosuppression protocols. Billiary complications, including bile leaks, bilomas, early and late bile duct strictures, are higher in LDLT [104, 105]. Infection rates are also higher after LDLT, likely due to higher rates of biliary complications leading to biloma and intra-abdominal abscess [104]. Biliary leak rates track closely with center experience. Management of a biliary leak includes biliary track drainage via ERCP, PTC or operative revision. Late biliary strictures are more common in LDLT than in DDLT and are more complex to treat due to multiple donor bile ducts and shorter length.

Recurrent disease also can impact long term outcomes of both DDLT and LDLT Hepatocellular carcinoma (HCC) is one of the most common indications for LDLT. Early studies show HCC recurrence after LDLT is higher than DDLT [34], but more recent series have demonstrated similar outcomes [35]. Primary sclerosing cholangitis, primary biliary cirrhosis, autoimmune hepatitis, alcohol, and nonalcoholic steatohepatitis recurrence rates are similar between LDLT and DDLT. LDLT is a complex and demanding procedure, to achieve the best recipient outcome all steps in the donor and recipient operation must be perfect.

15.14 Conclusion

LDLT is an available and safe alternative to DDLT and provides the same, or better short and long term allograft and patient survival [90]. To maximize safety and increase efficacy for both donors and recipients, requires the experience of a multidisciplinary team, careful selection and evaluation of donors, acceptable donor BMI, safe donor remnant liver mass of no less than 30–35% of native normal liver total mass and excellent peri-operative medical management. However, LDLT patients have more biliary complications, higher initial hospital costs and a longer hospital length of stay (LOS). Furthermore, center concerns on donor safety and potential psychosocial, surgical and medical complications have stagnated its further development in the US and Europe [106]. On the other hand, LDLT has flourished in the east [9, 39]. Reasons are multifactorial and include availability of deceased donors, cultural and religious reasons [9, 39].

The National Institutes of Health funded the Adult-to-Adult Living Donor Liver Transplantation Cohort Study (A2ALL) in 2004 to study the impact of liver donation on the health of the donor in the US [107]. These efforts demonstrated that LDLT outcomes are similar to DDLT, waitlist mortality is reduced, and complication rates improve with center experience [107–109]. The continued progress in surgical approaches and innovative techniques will enable better care and utilization of living liver donor and optimal LDLT practice.

Disclosure The authors declare no conflicts of interest.

References

1. Burra P, Germani G. Liver transplantation: indications and outcomes. Minerva Gastroenterol Dietol. 2018;64(2):124–5.
2. Kim WR, Lake JR, Smith JM, Schladt DP, Skeans MA, Harper AM, et al. OPTN/SRTR 2016 annual data report: liver. Am J Transplant. 2018;18(Suppl 1):172–253.
3. Tieleman M, van den Berg AP, van Hoek B, Polak WG, Dubbeld J, Porte RJ, et al. 'Will I receive a liver transplant in time?'; chance of survival of patients on the liver transplant waiting list. Ned Tijdschr Geneeskd. 2018;162:D2159.
4. Jimenez-Romero C, Caso Maestro O, Cambra Molero F, Justo Alonso I, Alegre Torrado C, Manrique Municio A, et al. Using old liver grafts for liver transplantation: where are the limits? World J Gastroenterol. 2014;20(31):10691–702.
5. Vinaixa C, Selzner N, Berenguer M. Fat and liver transplantation: clinical implications. Transpl Int. 2018;31(8):828–37.
6. Miller CM, Durand F, Heimbach JK, Kim-Schluger L, Lee SG, Lerut J, et al. The international liver transplant society guideline on living liver donation. Transplantation. 2016;100(6):1238–43.
7. Dirkes MC, Post IC, Heger M, van Gulik TM. A novel oxygenated machine perfusion system for preservation of the liver. Artif Organs. 2013;37(8):719–24.
8. Chen CL, Fan ST, Lee SG, Makuuchi M, Tanaka K. Living-donor liver transplantation: 12 years of experience in Asia. Transplantation. 2003;75(3 Suppl):S6–11.
9. Pinheiro RS, Waisberg DR, Nacif LS, Rocha-Santos V, Arantes RM, Ducatti L, et al. Living donor liver transplantation for hepatocellular cancer: an (almost) exclusive Eastern procedure? Transl Gastroenterol Hepatol. 2017;2:68.
10. OPTN: Organ Procurement and Transplantation Network Policies. 2018.
11. Starzl TE, Groth CG, Brettschneider L, Penn I, Fulginiti VA, Moon JB, et al. Orthotopic homotransplantation of the human liver. Ann Surg. 1968;168(3):392–415.
12. Bismuth H, Houssin D. Reduced-sized orthotopic liver graft in hepatic transplantation in children. Surgery. 1984;95(3):367–70.
13. Pichlmayr R, Brolsch C, Wonigeit K, Neuhaus P, Siegismund S, Schmidt FW, et al. Experiences with liver transplantation in Hannover. Hepatology (Baltimore, MD). 1984;4(1 Suppl):56s–60s.
14. Raia S, Nery JR, Mies S. Liver transplantation from live donors. Lancet (London, England). 1989;2(8661):497.
15. Strong RW, Lynch SV, Ong TH, Matsunami H, Koido Y, Balderson GA. Successful liver transplantation from a living donor to her son. N Engl J Med. 1990;322(21):1505–7.
16. Hashikura Y, Makuuchi M, Kawasaki S, Matsunami H, Ikegami T, Nakazawa Y, et al. Successful living-

related partial liver transplantation to an adult patient. Lancet (London, England). 1994;343(8907):1233–4.

17. Sugawara Y, Makuuchi M. Advances in adult living donor liver transplantation: a review based on reports from the 10th anniversary of the adult-to-adult living donor liver transplantation meeting in Tokyo. Liver Transplant. 2004;10(6):715–20.

18. Lo CM, Fan ST, Liu CL, Wei WI, Lo RJ, Lai CL, et al. Adult-to-adult living donor liver transplantation using extended right lobe grafts. Ann Surg. 1997;226(3):261–9; discussion 9–70.

19. Lee SG, Hwang S, Park KM, Kim KH, Ahn CS, Lee YJ, et al. Seventeen adult-to-adult living donor liver transplantations using dual grafts. Transplant Proc. 2001;33(7–8):3461–3.

20. Cherqui D, Soubrane O, Husson E, Barshasz E, Vignaux O, Ghimouz M, et al. Laparoscopic living donor hepatectomy for liver transplantation in children. Lancet (London, England). 2002;359(9304):392–6.

21. Knaak M, Goldaracena N, Doyle A, Cattral MS, Greig PD, Lilly L, et al. A donor body mass index greater than 30 is not a contraindication for live liver donation. Am J Transplant. 2016.

22. Wiesner R, Edwards E, Freeman R, Harper A, Kim R, Kamath P, et al. Model for end-stage liver disease (MELD) and allocation of donor livers. Gastroenterology. 2003;124(1):91–6.

23. Berg CL, Merion RM, Shearon TH, Olthoff KM, Brown RS Jr, Baker TB, et al. Liver transplant recipient survival benefit with living donation in the model for endstage liver disease allocation era. Hepatology. 2011;54(4):1313–21.

24. Abu-Gazala S, Olthoff KM. Status of adult living donor liver transplantation in the united states: results from the adult-to-adult living donor liver transplantation cohort study. Gastroenterol Clin N Am. 2018;47(2):297–311.

25. Abdeldayem H, Kashkoush S, Hegab BS, Aziz A, Shoreem H, Saleh S. Analysis of donor motivations in living donor liver transplantation. Front Surg. 2014;1:25.

26. Goldaracena N, Spetzler VN, Marquez M, Selzner N, Cattral MS, Greig PD, et al. Live donor liver transplantation: a valid alternative for critically ill patients suffering from acute liver failure. Am J Transplant. 2015;15(6):1591–7.

27. Dar FS, Bhatti ABH, Qureshi AI, Khan NY, Eswani Z, Zia HH, et al. Living donor liver transplantation in South Asia: single center experience on intermediate-term outcomes. World J Surg. 2017.

28. Facciuto M, Contreras-Saldivar A, Singh MK, Rocca JP, Taouli B, Oyfe I, et al. Right hepatectomy for living donation: role of remnant liver volume in predicting hepatic dysfunction and complications. Surgery. 2013;153(5):619–26.

29. Chaubal G, Borkar VV, Shetty G, Chattopadhyay S, Bahure U, Badhe R, et al. Estimation of liver volume in the western Indian population. Indian J Gastroenterol. 2016;35(4):274–9.

30. Terrault NA, Shiffman ML, Lok AS, Saab S, Tong L, Brown RS Jr, et al. Outcomes in hepatitis C virus-infected recipients of living donor vs. deceased donor liver transplantation. Liver Transpl. 2007;13(1):122–9.

31. Rahimi RS, Trotter JF. Liver transplantation for hepatocellular carcinoma: outcomes and treatment options for recurrence. Ann Gastroenterol. 2015;28(3):323–30.

32. Mazzaferro V, Regalia E, Doci R, Andreola S, Pulvirenti A, Bozzetti F, et al. Liver transplantation for the treatment of small hepatocellular carcinomas in patients with cirrhosis. N Engl J Med. 1996;334(11):693–9.

33. Lo CM, Fan ST, Liu CL, Chan SC, Wong J. The role and limitation of living donor liver transplantation for hepatocellular carcinoma. Liver Transpl. 2004;10(3):440–7.

34. Kulik LM, Fisher RA, Rodrigo DR, Brown RS Jr, Freise CE, Shaked A, et al. Outcomes of living and deceased donor liver transplant recipients with hepatocellular carcinoma: results of the A2ALL cohort. Am J Transplant. 2012;12(11):2997–3007.

35. Sandhu L, Sandroussi C, Guba M, Selzner M, Ghanekar A, Cattral MS, et al. Living donor liver transplantation versus deceased donor liver transplantation for hepatocellular carcinoma: comparable survival and recurrence. Liver Transpl. 2012;18(3):315–22.

36. Bhangui P, Vibert E, Majno P, Salloum C, Andreani P, Zocrato J, et al. Intention-to-treat analysis of liver transplantation for hepatocellular carcinoma: living versus deceased donor transplantation. Hepatology. 2011;53(5):1570–9.

37. Ninomiya M, Shirabe K, Facciuto ME, Schwartz ME, Florman SS, Yoshizumi T, et al. Comparative study of living and deceased donor liver transplantation as a treatment for hepatocellular carcinoma. J Am Coll Surg. 2015;220(3):297–304 e3.

38. Resch T, Esser H, Cardini B, Schaefer B, Zoller H, Schneeberger S. Liver transplantation for hilar cholangiocarcinoma (h-CCA): is it the right time? Transl Gastroenterol Hepatol. 2018;3:38.

39. Shukla A, Vadeyar H, Rela M, Shah S. Liver transplantation: east versus west. J Clin Exp Hepatol. 2013;3(3):243–53.

40. Gorgen A, Muaddi H, Zhang W, McGilvray I, Gallinger S, Sapisochin G. The new era of transplant oncology: liver transplantation for nonresectable colorectal cancer liver metastases. Can J Gastroenterol Hepatol. 2018;2018:9531925.

41. Uskudar O, Raja K, Schiano TD, Fiel MI, del Rio MJ, Chang C. Liver transplantation is possible in some patients with liver metastasis of colon cancer. Transplant Proc. 2011;43(5):2070–4.

42. Yadav SK, Choudhary NS, Saraf N, Saigal S, Goja S, Rastogi A, et al. Nutritional status using subjective global assessment independently predicts outcome of patients waiting for living donor liver transplant. Indian J Gastroenterol. 2017;36(4):275–81.

43. Englesbe MJ, Patel SP, He K, Lynch RJ, Schaubel DE, Harbaugh C, et al. Sarcopenia and mortality after liver transplantation. J Am Coll Surg. 2010;211(2):271–8.

44. Kaido T, Ogawa K, Fujimoto Y, Ogura Y, Hata K, Ito T, et al. Impact of sarcopenia on survival in patients undergoing living donor liver transplantation. Am J Transplant. 2013;13(6):1549–56.

45. Hamaguchi Y, Kaido T, Okumura S, Fujimoto Y, Ogawa K, Mori A, et al. Impact of quality as well as quantity of skeletal muscle on outcomes after liver transplantation. Liver Transpl. 2014;20(11):1413–9.

46. Masuda T, Shirabe K, Ikegami T, Harimoto N, Yoshizumi T, Soejima Y, et al. Sarcopenia is a prognostic factor in living donor liver transplantation. Liver Transpl. 2014;20(4):401–7.

47. Umemura A, Takahara T, Nitta H, Hasegawa Y, Sasaki A. Is sarcopenia a prognostic factor after living donor liver transplantation? Hepatobiliary Surg Nutr. 2017;6(4):258–9.

48. Kim YR, Park S, Han S, Ahn JH, Kim S, Sinn DH, et al. Sarcopenia as a predictor of post-transplant tumor recurrence after living donor liver transplantation for hepatocellular carcinoma beyond the Milan criteria. Sci Rep. 2018;8(1):7157.

49. Miller CM, Quintini C, Dhawan A, Durand F, Heimbach JK, Kim-Schluger HL, et al. The international liver transplantation society living donor liver transplant recipient guideline. Transplantation. 2017;101(5):938–44.

50. Abecassis MM, Fisher RA, Olthoff KM, Freise CE, Rodrigo DR, Samstein B, et al. Complications of living donor hepatic lobectomy – a comprehensive report. Am J Transplant. 2012;12(5):1208–17.

51. Kim SH, Lee EC, Shim JR, Park SJ. A simplified protocol using rituximab and immunoglobulin for ABO-incompatible low-titre living donor liver transplantation. Liver Int. 2017.

52. Lee CF, Cheng CH, Wang YC, Soong RS, Wu TH, Chou HS, et al. Adult living donor liver transplantation across ABO-incompatibility. Medicine (Baltimore). 2015;94(42):e1796.

53. Tyden G, Kumlien G, Genberg H, Sandberg J, Lundgren T, Fehrman I. ABO-incompatible kidney transplantation and rituximab. Transplant Proc. 2005;37(8):3286–7.

54. Renz JF, Diaz GC. The impact of adult-to-adult living donor liver transplantation on transplant center outcomes reporting. Clin Transplant. 2017;31(11).

55. Yoshida K, Umeda Y, Takaki A, Nagasaka T, Yoshida R, Nobuoka D, et al. Living donor liver transplantation for acute liver failure: comparing guidelines on the prediction of liver transplantation. Acta Med Okayama. 2017;71(5):381–90.

56. Kim SH, Lee EC, Shim JR, Park SJ. Right lobe living donors ages 55 years old and older in liver transplantation. Liver Transpl. 2017;23(10):1305–11.

57. Bustelos R, Ayala R, Martinez J, Martin MA, Toledo T, Grande S, et al. Living donor liver transplantation: usefulness of hemostatic and prothrombotic screening in potential donors. Transplant Proc. 2009;41(9):3791–5.

58. Mas VR, Fisher RA, Maluf DG, Wilkinson DS, Garrett CT, Ferreira-Gonzalez A. Hepatic artery thrombosis after liver transplantation and genetic factors: prothrombin G20210A polymorphism. Transplantation. 2003;76(1):247–9.

59. Maluf DG, Stravitz RT, Cotterell AH, Posner MP, Nakatsuka M, Sterling RK, et al. Adult living donor versus deceased donor liver transplantation: a 6-year single center experience. Am J Transplant. 2005;5(1):149–56.

60. Wang SH, Lin PY, Wang JY, Huang MF, Lin HC, Hsieh CE, et al. Mental health status after living donor hepatectomy. Medicine (Baltimore). 2017;96(19):e6910.

61. Jendrisak MD, Hong B, Shenoy S, Lowell J, Desai N, Chapman W, et al. Altruistic living donors: evaluation for nondirected kidney or liver donation. Am J Transplant. 2006;6(1):115–20.

62. Rudow DL, Swartz K, Phillips C, Hollenberger J, Smith T, Steel JL. The psychosocial and independent living donor advocate evaluation and post-surgery care of living donors. J Clin Psychol Med Settings. 2015;22(2–3):136–49.

63. Sahani D, Mehta A, Blake M, Prasad S, Harris G, Saini S. Preoperative hepatic vascular evaluation with CT and MR angiography: implications for surgery. Radiographics. 2004;24(5):1367–80.

64. Ikegami T, Yoshizumi T, Sakata K, Uchiyama H, Harimoto N, Harada N, et al. Left lobe living donor liver transplantation in adults: What is the safety limit? Liver Transpl. 2016.

65. Chan AC, Chok KS, Sin SL, Dai WC, Cheung TT, Chan SC, et al. Simultaneous implantation of bilateral liver grafts in living donor liver transplantation with fusion venoplasty. Liver Transpl. 2016;22(5):686–8.

66. Adam R, Reynes M, Johann M, Morino M, Astarcioglu I, Kafetzis I, et al. The outcome of steatotic grafts in liver transplantation. Transplant Proc. 1991;23(1 Pt 2):1538–40.

67. Urena MA, Ruiz-Delgado FC, Gonzalez EM, Segurola CL, Romero CJ, Garcia IG, et al. Assessing risk of the use of livers with macro and microsteatosis in a liver transplant program. Transplant Proc. 1998;30(7):3288–91.

68. Guba M, Adcock L, MacLeod C, Cattral M, Greig P, Levy G, et al. Intraoperative 'no go' donor hepatectomies in living donor liver transplantation. Am J Transplant. 2010;10(3):612–8.

69. Trotter JF, Wisniewski KA, Terrault NA, Everhart JE, Kinkhabwala M, Weinrieb RM, et al. Outcomes of donor evaluation in adult-to-adult living donor liver transplantation. Hepatology. 2007;46(5):1476–84.

70. Tulla KA, Jeon H. Living donor liver transplantation: technical innovations. Gastroenterol Clin N Am. 2018;47(2):253–65.

71. Zein NN, Hanouneh IA, Bishop PD, Samaan M, Eghtesad B, Quintini C, et al. Three-dimensional

print of a liver for preoperative planning in living donor liver transplantation. Liver Transpl. 2013;19(12):1304–10.

72. Radtke A, Nadalin S, Sotiropoulos GC, Molmenti EP, Schroeder T, Valentin-Gamazo C, et al. Computer-assisted operative planning in adult living donor liver transplantation: a new way to resolve the dilemma of the middle hepatic vein. World J Surg. 2007;31(1):175–85.

73. Koffron AJ, Kung R, Baker T, Fryer J, Clark L, Abecassis M. Laparoscopic-assisted right lobe donor hepatectomy. Am J Transplant. 2006;6(10):2522–5.

74. Scatton O, Katsanos G, Boillot O, Goumard C, Bernard D, Stenard F, et al. Pure laparoscopic left lateral sectionectomy in living donors: from innovation to development in France. Ann Surg. 2015;261(3):506–12.

75. Suh KS, Yi NJ, Kim T, Kim J, Shin WY, Lee HW, et al. Laparoscopy-assisted donor right hepatectomy using a hand port system preserving the middle hepatic vein branches. World J Surg. 2009;33(3):526–33.

76. Choi HJ, You YK, Na GH, Hong TH, Shetty GS, Kim DG. Single-port laparoscopy-assisted donor right hepatectomy in living donor liver transplantation: sensible approach or unnecessary hindrance? Transplant Proc. 2012;44(2):347–52.

77. Cherian PT, Mishra AK, Kumar P, Sachan VK, Bharathan A, Srikanth G, et al. Laparoscopic liver resection: wedge resections to living donor hepatectomy, are we heading in the right direction? World J Gastroenterol. 2014;20(37):13369–81.

78. Zhang B, Pan Y, Chen K, Maher H, Chen MY, Zhu HP, et al. Laparoscopy-assisted versus open hepatectomy for live liver donor: systematic review and meta-analysis. Can J Gastroenterol Hepatol. 2017;2017:2956749.

79. Nagai S, Brown L, Yoshida A, Kim D, Kazimi M, Abouljoud MS. Mini-incision right hepatic lobectomy with or without laparoscopic assistance for living donor hepatectomy. Liver Transpl. 2012;18(10):1188–97.

80. Chen KH, Siow TF, Chio UC, Wu JM, Jeng KS. Laparoscopic donor hepatectomy. Asian J Endosc Surg. 2018;11(2):112–7.

81. Olthoff KM, Smith AR, Abecassis M, Baker T, Emond JC, Berg CL, et al. Defining long-term outcomes with living donor liver transplantation in North America. Ann Surg. 2015;262(3):465–75; discussion 73–5.

82. Goldberg DS, French B, Abt PL, Olthoff K, Shaked A. Superior survival using living donors and donor-recipient matching using a novel living donor risk index. Hepatology (Baltimore, MD). 2014;60(5):1717–26.

83. Rossler F, Sapisochin G, Song G, Lin YH, Simpson MA, Hasegawa K, et al. Defining benchmarks for major liver surgery: a multicenter analysis of 5202 living liver donors. Ann Surg. 2016;264(3):492–500.

84. Hafeez Bhatti AB, Dar FS, Qureshi AI, Khan NY, Zia HH, Khan EUD, et al. Failure to rescue in living donor liver transplantation: patterns and predictors. Int J Surg. 2017;44:281–6.

85. Reddy MS, Narasimhan G, Cherian PT, Rela M. Death of a living liver donor: opening Pandora's box. Liver Transplant. 2013;19(11):1279–84.

86. Muzaale AD, Dagher NN, Montgomery RA, Taranto SE, McBride MA, Segev DL. Estimates of early death, acute liver failure, and long-term mortality among live liver donors. Gastroenterology. 2012;142(2):273–80.

87. Grewal HP, Thistlewaite JR Jr, Loss GE, Fisher JS, Cronin DC, Siegel CT, et al. Complications in 100 living-liver donors. Ann Surg. 1998;228(2):214–9.

88. Dew MA, Butt Z, Liu Q, Simpson MA, Zee J, Ladner DP, et al. Prevalence and predictors of patient-reported long-term mental and physical health after donation in the adult-to-adult living-donor liver transplantation cohort study. Transplantation. 2018;102(1):105–18.

89. Rudow DL, Chariton M, Sanchez C, Chang S, Serur D, Brown RS Jr. Kidney and liver living donors: a comparison of experiences. Prog Transplant. 2005;15(2):185–91.

90. Samstein B, Smith AR, Freise CE, Zimmerman MA, Baker T, Olthoff KM, et al. Complications and their resolution in recipients of deceased and living donor liver transplants: findings from the A2ALL cohort study. Am J Transplant. 2016;16(2):594–602.

91. Manas D, Burnapp L, Andrews PA. Summary of the British transplantation society UK guidelines for living donor liver transplantation. Transplantation. 2016;100(6):1184–90.

92. Abu-Gazala S, Olthoff KM, Goldberg DS, Shaked A, Abt PL. En Bloc Hilar dissection of the right hepatic artery in continuity with the Bile Duct: a technique to reduce biliary complications after adult living-donor liver transplantation. J Gastrointest Surg. 2016;20(4):765–71.

93. Lo CM, Fan ST, Liu CL, Wong J. Hepatic venoplasty in living-donor liver transplantation using right lobe graft with middle hepatic vein. Transplantation. 2003;75(3):358–60.

94. Uchiyama H, Shirabe K, Morita M, Kakeji Y, Taketomi A, Soejima Y, et al. Expanding the applications of microvascular surgical techniques to digestive surgeries: a technical review. Surg Today. 2012;42(2):111–20.

95. Segel MC, Zajko AB, Bowen A, Bron KM, Skolnick ML, Penkrot RJ, et al. Hepatic artery thrombosis after liver transplantation: radiologic evaluation. AJR Am J Roentgenol. 1986;146(1):137–41.

96. Cigna E, Curinga G, Bistoni G, Spalvieri C, Tortorelli G, Scuderi N. Microsurgical anastomosis with the 'PCA' technique. J Plast Reconstr Aesthet Surg. 2008;61(7):762–6.

97. Levy GA, Selzner N, Grant DR. Fostering liver living donor liver transplantation. Curr Opin Organ Transplant. 2016;21(2):224–30.

98. Goldaracena N, Echeverri J, Selzner M. Small-for-size syndrome in live donor liver transplantation-Pathways of injury and therapeutic strategies. Clin Transplant. 2017;31(2).

99. Govil S, Reddy MS, Rela M. Has "small-for-size" reached its "sell-by" date. Transplantation. 2016;100(11):e119.

100. Koh PS, Chan SC. Adult-to-adult living donor liver transplantation: operative techniques to optimize the recipient's outcome. J Nat Sci Biol Med. 2017;8(1):4–10.

101. Luo Y, Zhao D, Zhang M, Zhou T, Qiu BJ, Zhang JJ, et al. Hepatic artery reconstruction using 3-in-1 segmental resection in pediatric living donor liver transplantation: a case report and literature review. Transplant Proc. 2017;49(7):1619–23.

102. Tzeng YS, Hsieh CB, Chen SG. Continuous versus interrupted suture for hepatic artery reconstruction using a loupe in living-donor liver transplantation. Ann Transplant. 2011;16(4):12–5.

103. Pomposelli JJ, Goodrich NP, Emond JC, Humar A, Baker TB, Grant DR, et al. Patterns of early allograft dysfunction in adult live donor liver transplantation: the A2ALL experience. Transplantation. 2016;100(7):1490–9.

104. Baker TB, Zimmerman MA, Goodrich NP, Samstein B, Pomfret EA, Pomposelli JJ, et al. Biliary reconstructive techniques and associated anatomic variants in adult living donor liver transplants: the A2ALL experience. Liver Transplant. 2017.

105. Chok KS, Lo CM. Systematic review and meta-analysis of studies of biliary reconstruction in adult living donor liver transplantation. ANZ J Surg. 2017;87(3):121–5.

106. Nadalin S, Malago M, Radtke A, Erim Y, Saner F, Valentin-Gamazo C, et al. Current trends in live liver donation. Transpl Int. 2007;20(4):312–30.

107. Olthoff KM, Abecassis MM, Emond JC, Kam I, Merion RM, Gillespie BW, et al. Outcomes of adult living donor liver transplantation: comparison of the Adult-to-adult Living Donor Liver Transplantation Cohort Study and the national experience. Liver Transpl. 2011;17(7):789–97.

108. Freise CE, Gillespie BW, Koffron AJ, Lok AS, Pruett TL, Emond JC, et al. Recipient morbidity after living and deceased donor liver transplantation: findings from the A2ALL Retrospective Cohort Study. Am J Transplant. 2008;8(12):2569–79.

109. Olthoff KM, Merion RM, Ghobrial RM, Abecassis MM, Fair JH, Fisher RA, et al. Outcomes of 385 adult-to-adult living donor liver transplant recipients: a report from the A2ALL Consortium. Ann Surg. 2005;242(3):314–23, discussion 23–5.

Expanded Criteria for Hepatocellular Carcinoma in Liver Transplant

16

Mehmet Haberal, Aydincan Akdur, Gökhan Moray, Gülnaz Arslan, Figen Özçay, Haldun Selçuk, and Handan Özdemir

16.1 Introduction

Hepatocellular carcinoma (HCC) is a common cancer with a dismal prognosis. It is the sixth most common cancer worldwide and the third highest cause of death related to malignancy. Because of its typically late diagnosis, the median survival following HCC diagnosis is approximately 6–20 months, and 5-year survival rate is less than 12%. Hepatocellular carcinoma typically arises in the background of cirrhosis. Liver transplant is regarded as an optimal radical therapy for selected patients with HCC [1, 2]. This treatment modality can be offered to patients with unresectable HCC regardless of the patient's liver function. It can also treat the underlying liver disease and consequently decrease the risk of de novo HCC [3].

The Milan criteria are often used to determine which patients will benefit from liver transplant. However, Milan criteria are normally applied to those with early-stage tumors, with many centers having center-based criteria for transplant for advanced-stage patients. In this study, we describe our expanded criteria for patients with unresectable HCC and evaluate the long-term results of liver transplant in these patients.

M. Haberal (✉) · A. Akdur · G. Moray
Department of General Surgery, Division of Transplantation, Baskent University, Ankara, Turkey
e-mail: rectorate@baskent.edu.tr

G. Arslan
Department of Anesthesiology, Baskent University, Ankara, Turkey
e-mail: agurman@baskent.edu.tr

F. Özçay
Department of Pediatric Gastroenterology, Baskent University, Ankara, Turkey

H. Selçuk
Department of Gastroenterology, Baskent University, Ankara, Turkey

H. Özdemir
Department of Pathology, Baskent University, Ankara, Turkey

16.2 Materials and Methods

Between December 8, 1988, and January 1, 2017, we performed 552 liver transplants at our center. For this study, we retrospectively reviewed our liver transplant results in patients with HCC. At our center, our expanded criteria for liver transplant in HCC candidates includes patients regardless of tumor size and number, those without major vascular invasion and without distant metastasis, and those with negative cytology (if the patient has ascites) (Table 16.1). We found that 61 liver transplant procedures were performed for HCC (52 male and 9 female patients),

N. Hakim et al. (eds.), *Transplantation Surgery*, Springer Specialist Surgery Series, https://doi.org/10.1007/978-3-030-55244-2_16

and 36 patients were transplanted according to the Baskent University expanded criteria.

Before transplant, all patients were evaluated radiologically (computed tomography, magnetic resonance imaging, or positron emission tomography-computed tomography) for tumor metastasis. Biopsies of suspicious lesions were performed. In addition to liver transplant, patients also received interventional radiology for down-staging. Liver transplant was considered for patients with HCC if the tumor was determined unresectable because of its location or concomitant liver disease. Tumor staging was determined according to the American Liver Tumor Study Group Modified tumor-node-metastasis staging system for HCC. During follow-up, in addition to routine laboratory tests, patients had alpha-fetoprotein tests and ultrasonography examina-

Table 16.1 Baskent University expanded criteria for liver transplant for hepatocellular carcinoma

Independent of tumor size and number of nodules
No extrahepatic invasion
No major vascular invasion
No ascites containing tumor cells
Exploratory laparotomy and histopathologic examination as factors important in the final decision for transplant

tions every 3 months and computed tomography or magnetic resonance scans done every 6 months.

16.3 Results

Sixty-one patients had liver transplants for HCC (52 male and 9 female patients). Of these patients, 11 were children and 50 were adults. Forty-one patients had living-donor liver transplants(10 pediatric and 31 adult patients), and 20 patients had deceased-donor liver transplants (1 pediatric and 19 adult patients). Eighteen patients received down-staging therapy before liver transplant. We diagnosed HCC incidentally at pathologic examination in 6 patients (10.1%; 4 children and 2 adults). All 6 patients with incidental HCC diagnosis were still alive without HCC recurrence at 75–140 months.

Thirty-six patients received transplants according to the Baskent University expanded criteria, which included 11 children (30.5%) and 25 adults (69.5%). In the adult group, the most common cause of the liver disease was hepatitis B virus (HBV) infection (n = 16; 64%) (Table 16.2); in the pediatric group, the most common cause of liver disease was tyrosinemia type 1 (n = 5; 45.4%) (Table 16.3).

Table 16.2 Adult patients

Patient	Transplant date	Age at trans-plant, y	Cause of Liver Failure	Tumor properties	Source of liver	Neoadjuvant treatment	Follow-up, mo	Recurrence	Status
1	01/14/2004	52	HBV	Stage IVA, multifocal	DD	TACE	156	No	Alive
2	03/31/2004	64	HCV	Stage IVA, multifocal	LD		153	No	Alive
3	08/18/2004	55	HCV	Stage IVA, multifocal	LD	TACE	45	Yes	Died
4	09/29/2004	55	HCV	Stage IVA, multifocal	LD	TACE	73	No	Deceased
5	10/20/2004	58	HCV	Stage IVA, multifocal	LD		70	No	Deceased
6	02/23/2005	49	HBV	Stage III, 6 cm	LD	TACE+AI	23	No	Deceased
7	05/05/2005	56	HBV	Stage IVA, multifocal	DD	AI	64	Yes	Deceased
8	05/30/2005	59	Alcoholic hepatitis	Stage IVA, multifocal	DD	AI	64	No	Deceased
9	03/21/2006	50	HBV	Stage IVA, multifocal	DD	TACE+AI	14	Yes	Deceased

Table 16.2 (continued)

Patient	Transplant date	Age at transplant, y	Cause of Liver Failure	Tumor properties	Source of liver	Neoadjuvant treatment	Follow-up, mo	Recurrence	Status
10	01/30/2007	56	HBV	Stage IVA, multifocal	LD		121	Yes	Alive
11	03/05/2007	64	HBV	Stage IVA, multifocal	DD	TACE+AI	7	No	Deceased
12	04/17/2007	54	HBV	Stage IVA, multifocal	DD	TACE	4	Yes	Deceased
13	06/20/2007	65	HCV	Stage IVA, multifocal	DD		116	Yes	Alive
14	10/30/2007	56	HBV	Stage IVA, multifocal	LD	RFA + AI	112	No	Alive
15	02/20/2008	40	HBV	Stage IVA, multifocal	LD		1	No	Deceased
16	03/04/2008	62	HBV	Stage IVA, multifocal	LD		108	No	Alive
17	03/14/2008	57	HBV	Stage IVA, multifocal	LD		2	No	Deceased
18	05/14/2008	42	HBV	Stage III, multifocal	LD		105	No	Alive
19	10/02/2008	53	Alcoholic hepatitis	Stage III, 7 cm	DD	TACE	101	No	Alive
20	12/02/2008	52	HBV	Stage III, 6 cm	LD	RFA	15	No	Deceased
21	02/10/2009	56	HBV	Stage IVA, multifocal	LD		96	Yes	Alive
22	03/10/2009	49	HCV	Stage IVA, multifocal	LD	TACE+RFA	95	No	Alive
23	10/15/2009	54	HCV	Stage IVA, multifocal	DD		88	No	Alive
24	03/12/2013	64	HBV	Stage IVA, multifocal	LD	RFA	47	No	Alive
25	01/16/2015	61	HBV	Stage IVA, multifocal	LD	RFA	24	No	Alive

Abbreviations: *AI* alcohol injection, *DD* deceased donor, *HBV* hepatitis B virus, *HCV* hepatitis C virus, *LD* living donor, *RFA* radiofrequency ablation, *TACE* transcatheter arterial chemoembolization

Table 16.3 Pediatric patients

Patient	Transplant date	Age at transplant, y	Cause of liver failure	Tumor properties	Source of liver	Neoadjuvant treatment	Follow-up, mo	Recurrence	Status
1	07/21/2004	1	PFIC-2 (Byler)	Stage III, 6 cm, 2 cm	LD		152	No	Alive
2	09/03/2004	12	Tyrosinemia type 1	Stage IVA, multifocal	LD	Chemo-therapy	150	No	Alive
3	11/03/2004	14	Tyrosinemia type 1	Stage IVA, multifocal	LD	Chemo-therapy	148	No	Alive
4	01/12/2005	10	Tyrosinemia type 1	Stage III, multifocal	LD	Chemo-therapy	146	No	Alive
5	02/09/2005	1	PFIC-2 (Byler)	Stage III, multifocal	LD		145	No	Alive

(continued)

Table 16.3 (continued)

Patient	Transplant date	Age at trans-plant, y	Cause of liver failure	Tumor properties	Source of liver	Neoadjuvant treatment	Follow-up, mo	Recurrence	Status
6	11/15/2005	13	Wilson disease	Stage III, 5 cm, 4 cm	LD		136	No	Alive
7	05/12/2006	13	*Cryptogenic Cirrhosis*	Stage IVA, multifocal	LD		87	Yes	Deceased
8	05/24/2006	14	PFIC-3	Stage IVA, multifocal	LD		129	No	Alive
9	01/08/2007	16	HBV	Stage III, 7 cm	LD		122	No	Alive
10	11/07/2007	9	Tyrosinemia type 1	Stage IVA, multifocal	LD		112	Yes	Alive
11	08/21/2009	7	Tyrosinemia type 1	Stage IVA, multifocal	DD		90	No	Alive

Abbreviations: *DD* deceased donor, *HBV* hepatitis B virus, *LD* living donor, *PFIC-2* progressive familial intrahepatic cholestasis type 2, *PFIC-3* progressive familial intrahepatic cholestasis type 3

We found that 16 patients (4 pediatric and 12 adult patients) were within the Baskent University expanded criteria both radiologically and pathologically before transplant. The other 20 patients (7 pediatric and 13 adult patients) were within Milan criteria radiologically before transplant; however, after liver transplant, when pathologic specimens were evaluated, they were found to be within the Baskent University expanded criteria.

During follow-up, 9/36 patients (25%) had HCC recurrence (7 adult and 2 pediatric patients) (Tables 16.2 and 16.3). In 2 patients, we performed surgical resection for recurrence; the other patients were treated with interventional radiologic techniques.

In the pediatric group, 1 patient died due to HCC recurrence and liver failure (Table 16.3).In the adult group, 12 patients died, with 4 because of HCC recurrence and liver failure. The causes of death in the other patients included sepsis in 5 patient, cranial hemorrhage in 1 patient, and acute myocardial infarction in 2 patients (Table 16.2).

In the pediatric group, 5-year and 10-year survival rates of patients were 90%; in the adult group, the 5-year survival rate was 58.7% and the 10-year survival rate was 49.7% (Fig. 16.1). The overall 5-year survival was 71.7%, and the overall 10-year survival rate was 62.7% (Fig. 16.2).

16.4 Discussion

The first surgical treatment choice for HCC is resection. Because of the underlying liver disease, only 10–30% of patients have curative liver resection, although their 5-year survival rates range from 25 to 30% [1]. Liver transplant, which is a treatment option for cirrhosis and HCC, is now an established surgical treatment for patients with HCC [4].

Liver transplant for HCC according to the Milan criteria has been performed for many recipients with adjustments according to center-based selection methods. Since the landmark report of the Milan criteria by Mazzaferro and associates, which demonstrated comparable outcomes of patients with HCC having a single tumor smaller than 5 cm in diameter or up to 3 tumors smaller than 3 cm in diameter with no vascular invasion or extrahepatic disease determined by preoperative imaging studies, deceased-donor liver transplant has become an established treatment for cirrhotic patients with HCC [5]. We published our early report about expanded criteria in 2006 [6]. In that study, we showed that expanded-criteria liver transplant in patients with HCC, especially when donation from a living related donor is possible, appears to inhibit disease recurrence and improve outcomes.

Fig. 16.1 Survival rates of pediatric and adult patients. Abbreviations: *Cum* cumulative, *Ped* pediatric

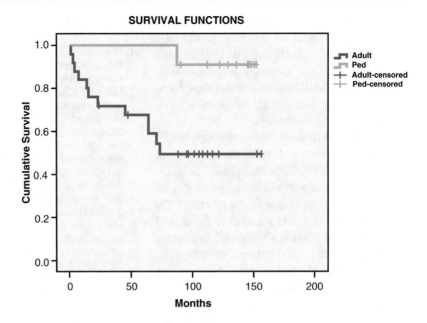

Fig. 16.2 Survival rates of all patients. Abbreviations: *Cum* cumulative

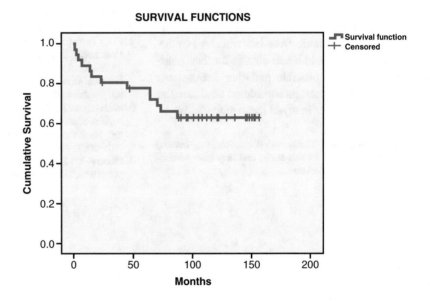

The annual incidence of HCC in the United States is 0.8 per one million children between the ages of 0 and 14 years and 1.5 per one million adolescents from 15 to 19 years old [7]. The 5-year overall survival rate is 42% for children and adolescents with HCC [8]. In pediatric patients, the most common cause of HCC is congenital or metabolic liver disease [9]. Similar to the literature, in our pediatric patients, only 1 had

HBV and the others had metabolic disease. In our series, pediatric patients had 5-year and 10-year survival rates of 90%, which were better than those shown in adults (5-year survival rate of 58.7% and 10-year survival rate of 49.7%).

In Turkey, most HCC develops in patients with cirrhosis. Turkey also has high rates of HBV and HCV seropositivity (HBV, 10%–40%; HCV, 7–10%) [10]. In our adult group, the most common cause of liver failure was HBV. Patients with HBV infection received antiviral prophylaxis with 6 doses of anti-HBs antibody (Hepatect, Biotest AG, Dreieich, Germany) and lamivudine (100 mg/d). Anti-HBs antibody levels were maintained at greater than 100 IU by means of periodic antibody bolus infusions.

In Turkey, as in many other countries, family members of patients with HCC are often willing to serve as donors for liver transplant. The availability of living donors allows surgeons to perform liver transplant with more liberal criteria for tumor staging. Whenever possible, living related donors who can provide a segmental liver graft, freely and without social pressure or obligation, are preferred for recipient with large and/or numerous tumors of the liver, poor hepatic function, and no other chance for treatment.

In conclusion, careful evaluation of recipients before transplant plays a critical step in curative treatment. We carefully expanded the Milan criteria in our center. We believe that patients with HCC and a cirrhotic liver but without extrahepatic disease should be candidates for liver transplant whenever possible and that living-donor liver transplant must be considered an alternative rescue therapy for many of these individuals.

Acknowledgments The authors declare that they have no sources of funding for this study, and they have no conflicts of interest to declare.

References

1. Haberal M, Emiroglu R, Karakayali H, et al. Expanded criteria for hepatocellular carcinoma and liver transplantation. IntSurg. 2007;92(2):110–5.
2. Ma KW, Cheung TT. Surgical resection of localized hepatocellular carcinoma: patient selection and special consideration. J Hepatocell Carcinoma. 2016;4:1–9.
3. Lee HW, Suh KS. Liver transplantation for advanced hepatocellular carcinoma. Clin Mol Hepatol. 2016;22(3):309–18.
4. Akamatsu N, Cillo U, Cucchetti A, et al. Surgery and hepatocellular carcinoma. Liver Cancer. 2016;6(1):44–50.
5. Mazzaferro V, Regalia E, Doci R, et al. Liver transplantation for the treatment of small hepatocellular carcinomas in patients with cirrhosis. N Engl J Med. 1996;334(11):693–9.
6. Karakayali H, Moray G, Sozen H, Dalgic A, Emiroglu R, Haberal M. Expanded criteria for liver transplantation in patients with hepatocellular carcinoma. Transplant Proc. 2006;38(2):575–8.
7. Howlader N, Noone AM, Krapcho M, et al Childhood cancer by the ICCC. SEER cancer statistics review, 1975–2009 (vintage 2009 populations). Bethesda, MD: National Cancer Institute; 2012, section 29.
8. PDQ Pediatric Treatment Editorial Board Web site. Childhood liver cancer treatment (PDQ): health professional version (2016 Sep 30). Bethesda, MD: National Cancer Institute; 2002. http://www.ncbi.nlm.nih.gov/books/NBK65790/. Accessed 28 Feb 2017.
9. Palaniappan K, Borkar VV, Safwan M, et al. Pediatric hepatocellular carcinoma in a developing country: is the etiology changing? Pediatr Transplant. 2016;20(7):898–903.
10. Haberal M, Dalgic A. New concepts in organ transplantation. Transplant Proc. 2004;36(5):1219–24.

Allogeneic Haemopoietic Stem Cell Transplantation

17

Eduardo Olavarria

17.1 Introduction

The field of allogeneic haemopoietic stem cell transplantation (HSCT) and, increasingly the use of cellular therapy, have continued to evolve since its origins in the early 1900's. Results are improving constantly mainly due to a combination of better understanding of the underlying biological background and major advances in supportive care. New diseases and indications have been developed and with the advent of reduced toxicity conditioning, this treatment modality has been extended to older patients and to patients who in previous times would have been considered ineligible for transplantation.

With increasing knowledge of the immunobiology of allogeneic transplantation and the development of more precise techniques for tissue typing and characterisation of the human histocompatibility genes, the use of alternative donors such as mismatched family members, matched or mismatched unrelated volunteers or cord blood stem cells has become widely accepted.

E. Olavarria (✉)
Imperial College London, Hammersmith Hospital, London, UK
e-mail: e.olavarria@nhs.net, e.olavarria@imperial.ac.uk

17.2 Historical Background

In the first half of the twentieth century, there had been attempts to use bone marrow tissue for its therapeutics effects in anaemia and leukaemia by oral, intramuscular or intravenous routes [1, 2]. In 1922, a Danish investigator, Fabriciuos Moeller, noted that guinea pigs, whose legs were protected from total body lethal irradiation, were able to survive this procedure and did not developed thrombocytopenia a haemorrhagic diathesis [3]. Although this findings were ignored for some years, until the mid 1950's when Jacobson showed that lethally irradiated mice could be protected by intraperitoneal injection of spleen cells (a haematopoietic organ in the mouse) or intravenous infusion of bone marrow [4].

Although initial consideration was given to a humoral factor, by the end of the decade, several reports had shown that the protection was due to the presence of donor cells in the bone marrow of the irradiated mice [1, 5, 6]. Ford et al. designated an animal that carried a mixture of own and foreign haematopoietic cells as a radiation chimera [7].

During the first years of experimental marrow transplantation, the emphasis was on radiation protection. However, subsequent studies focusing on the ultimate fate of the transplanted animals showed that many animals initially survived but later died of severe diarrhoea, weight loss and skin lesions [1, 8]. These observations rapidly led

© Springer Nature Switzerland AG 2021
N. Hakim et al. (eds.), *Transplantation Surgery*, Springer Specialist Surgery Series,
https://doi.org/10.1007/978-3-030-55244-2_17

to the description of a "secondary disease" initially term as runting syndrome [9]. This runt disease was in fact graft versus host disease and by the late 1960's it was clear that this was caused by the lymphocytes in the infused graft and that it was mediated by alloantigens present in the host but absent in the donor [8, 9].

The following step was the discovery of tolerance induced by marrow transplantation. Main and Prehn reported that mice surviving allogeneic marrow transplantation following TBI were able to permanently accept skin grafts from the original donor strain [10]. This was also demonstrated for xenografts using mice and rats [11]. Later on animal models of malignant disease were produced and studies showed that TBI followed by infusion of bone marrow cells was able to produce long-term cure although most animals still perished following the development of GVHD. Some studies suggested that lymphohaemopoietic tumours were more susceptible to the antitumour effect than sarcomas and carcinomas, perhaps due to the relative richness of transplantation alloantigens in these malignancies.

Although the Major Histocompatibility Complex (MHC) had been known since the late 1930's, it was not until the late 1960's and early 1970's that the concept of histocompatibility was fully established in allogeneic haemopoietic cell transplantation. However, in 1957 Thomas reported that large amounts of human marrow cells could be infused safely and described the first (albeit transient) marrow graft in patients affected of acute leukaemia [12]. In 1959, Mathé and co-workers attempted to treat six patients who had been exposed to high doses of radiation during an accident in Vinca, Serbia [13]. Several groups in USA and Europe started bone marrow transplant programmes with disappointing results. Most of these patients had end-stage acute leukaemia, were frequently severely infected at the time of transplant and died before proper assessment could be done. The following decade was fraught with frustration and when patients survived the initial phase of the transplant with apparently successful engraftment of the donor marrow cells, they often died of severe GVHD or late infections. It is worth mentioning that many of these transplants were performed without any tissue typing or using techniques that were found later to be unreliable.

In 1977 the Seattle group reported the results of HLA identical sibling bone marrow transplants in 100 patients with end-stage acute leukaemia [14]. This classical study confirmed the curative potential of marrow transplantation in acute leukaemia with 13 very long-term disease-free survivors. However, the initial enthusiasm about these remarkable results was tempered by the actuarial relapse rate of nearly 70% and the high incidence of transplant-related deaths [14]. The authors hypothesised that transplants performed in early remission stages would fare better and in 1979 they reported that of 19 patients transplanted from HLA identical siblings in first complete remission of their acute leukaemia, 10 of them were alive and leukaemia free [15]. It is generally accepted that the modern era of bone marrow transplantation began in the 1970's when reliable HLA typing was available and when patient with acute leukaemia were transplanted in early remission.

Only 30–40% of patients who are candidates for bone marrow transplantation, will have an HLA identical sibling. There are now well over 26 Million bone marrow volunteer donors in the different international registries. As always, the use of alternative donors was marked by advances in molecular typing of the different HLA genes and the improvement in the management of post transplant complications. Currently, more than 15,000 allogeneic stem cell transplants are carried out each year worldwide demonstrating the important role that this treatment modality plays in the managements of haematological malignancies.

17.3 The Role of HLA in HSCT

Tissue compatibility is determined by genes of the major histocompatibility complex (MHC), known as the HLA system in man, which are clustered on the short arm of chromosome 6. The HLA region is a multigenic system that encodes structurally homologous cell surface glycoproteins characterized by a high degree of allelic polymorphism within human populations. Immune responses against incompatible HLA Ag represent a major barrier to HSCT. The accuracy of histocompatibility testing and matching criteria will therefore have important consequences on graft outcome. This is particularly true in the case of transplantation with HSC from unrelated donors (UD), where serologically hidden incompatibilities may account for the increased rate of post-transplant complications.

The homologous HLA class I (HLA-A, -B, -C) and class II (HLA-DR, -DQ, -DP) antigens are codominantly expressed and differ in their structure, tissue distribution and characteristics in peptide presentation to T cells [16]. The biological function of HLA molecules is to present peptide Ag to T cells, thereby playing a key role in T cell-mediated adaptive immunity.

HLA class I molecules are expressed on most nucleated cells. They are composed of an alpha-chain (encoded in the MHC) non covalently associated with Beta-2-microglobulin (encoded on chromosome 15). Peptides (usually of 8–10 aminoacids.) presented by class I molecules are derived from proteolytic degradation of cytoplasmic proteins by the proteasome, transported across the endoplasmic reticulum where they bind to class I Ag. Pathogen-derived peptides presented to class I Ag are usually recognized by CD8+ CTL [16]. HLA class II Ag are expressed on a subset of cells of the immune system comprising dendritic cells, B-cells, activated T cells, macrophages, collectively referred to as Ag presenting cells (APC). They are heterodimers composed of two membrane-bound chains that are encoded by two genes that co-localize in the MHC. The peptide-binding pocket is formed by the most distal domains of the two chains. Extracellular Ag internalised by endocytosis/phagocytosis are degraded in an endocytic compartment into peptides of 10–30 aminoacids that bind class II molecules. HLA class II-peptide complexes expressed on the membrane are usually recognised by CD4+ T-helper cells [16].

The HLA system comprises 12 genes located on a 3.6 Mb segment of the short arm of chromosome 6. Three HLA class I genes (A,B,C) encode respectively for the heavy chains of HLA-A, -B and -C antigens. HLA class II Ag (DR, DQ, DP) are heterodimers encoded by an alpha-chain and a beta-chain gene (e.g. DRA/DRB1 or DQA1/DQB1) that co-localize at the centromeric part of the MHC [16, 17]. The HLA-DR subregion presents an additional complexity level since a second DRB gene may be present, i.e. DRB3 in DR11/DR12/DR13/DR14/DR17/DR18 haplotypes, DRB4 in DR4/DR7/DR9 haplotypes, and DRB5 in DR15/DR16 haplotype. Because of the codominant expression of HLA genes, a heterozygous individual may express up to 12 different HLA Ag.

In the early 1990's the role of HLA matching was hampered by the poor resolution achieved by HLA typing, particularly for HLA class I alleles. Based on high resolution typing methods more recent studies [18–22] reached the almost general consensus that allele-level matching does improve transplant outcome. However the relative importance of individual loci still remains under investigation.

Graft failure: The role of HLA-A/B/C/DR mismatches has been shown by several studies. The total number of disparities influences the risk of graft failure [18–20]. A comparison of serological versus allele class I mismatches in CML patients suggested that qualitative differences may influence the risk of graft failure, with a higher risk in serotype-mismatched patients [19].

GVHD: Multiple class I, or class II, or combined class I and II mismatches correlated with an increased risk of GVHD [19]. In the Japanese Marrow Donor Program (JMDP) study [20], HLA-A/B/C/DRB1 mismatches were found to be significant risk factors for grades III-IV acute GVHD, whereas the American NMDP data revealed a DRB1 effect with no contribution of HLA-DQ/DP [21], or HLA-B/C [22] mismatches. A few studies reported an association of HLA-DP disparities with an increased rate of acute GVHD.

Survival: HLA-A/B/C/DRB1, but not DQ/DP mismatches decreased survival in the NMDP study [21, 22], whereas in the JMDP study only A/B/DRB1 disparities were associated with mortality [20]. In CML patients from the Seattle study a single class II mismatch was well tolerated whereas single class I or multiple mismatches were associated with lower survival [18, 19]. Differences between studies may involve selection criteria of each transplant centre, patients age or other pre-transplant risk factors, experience in treating GVHD, as well as the relevance of the GvL effect in CML patients. In the largest cohort of CML patients studied so far [23], HLA-AB-serology/DRB1-allele "matched" unrelated HSCT were compared to matched sibling donor HSCT patients. Multivariate analysis revealed lower 5-years SRV rates after "matched" unrelated vs. matched sibling donor HSCT. Such decreased survival possibly results, at least in part, to the presence of undisclosed HLA-A/B/C allele mismatches in the so-called "matched" unrelated donors.

17.4 Sources and Procurement of Allogeneic Haematopoietic Stem Cells

The preferred source of progenitor cells for HSCT has changed over the years. Traditionally, cells were harvested from the iliac crests under general anaesthesia, but recently G-CSF mobilised peripheral blood (PBSC) have been increasingly used. Unmanipulated cord blood (CB) cells collected and cryopreserved at birth have been used both in related and unrelated HLA matched and mismatched allogeneic transplants in children and more recently in adults. It has become evident that there are many quantitative and qualitative differences between these cell sources (Table 17.1).

In 1995, 3 pivotal studies demonstrated the safety and feasibility of using G-CSF mobilized PB allografts [24]. Patients experienced prompt engraftment with an incidence of GVHD similar to that of BM recipients. In addition, no serious short-term complications of G-CSF mobilised PB harvesting were observed in the donors [24–26]. Direct comparison of PB and BM in allogeneic sibling donor transplantation has been reported in at least 8 randomised trials [25–32]. Most of them did not show a survival benefit (Table 17.2). The incidence of acute GVHD was

Table 17.1 Advantages and disadvantages in the search and identification Process of BM and CB unrelated donor

	Bone Marrow	Cord blood
Information on A + B + DRB1(DNA) type	16–56%	50–80%
Median search time	3–6 months	<1 month
Donors identified but not available	30%	< 1%
Rare haplotypes represented [a]	2%	29%
Major limiting factors to graft acquisition	HLA match	Cell Dose
Ease of rearranging date of cell infusion	Difficult	Easy
Potential for second HSC graft or DLI	Yes	No from the same donor
Potential—for viral transmission	Yes	No
—for congenital diseases	No	Yes
Risk to donor	Yes	No

similar in all but one of the studies, but an increase (statistically significant or a trend) in the incidence of overall and extensive chronic GVHD was demonstrated in recipients of PBSC allografts. The magnitude of this observation and its effect on relapse, survival and recipient quality of life is less clear. In unrelated transplant recipients, matched cohort comparisons of UD BMT and PBSCT reported faster haematological recovery among PB recipients with no difference in either acute GVHD or chronic GVHD.

While results of randomised studies are pending, the use of PB allografts in UD HSCT has varied among transplant centres and countries. Some registries of unrelated marrow donors have permitted the collection of allografts from the PB whereas others have not. Transplant centres may request a PB or a BM graft but the collection centre and wishes of the donor also determine which product is ultimately collected. Because of the absence of definitive data comparing both sources of cells, there is no indication to prefer either source of cells except perhaps in patients with advanced disease where chronic GVHD and subsequent GvL might decrease relapse and improve survival or, in a situation where a high number of

Table 17.2 Relapse incidence (RI) and survival after allo-PBSCT compared to allo-BMT in different randomised studies

Reference	Source	n	RI	Survival	
Bensinger	BM	91	25%	54%	– Early status: 72 vs. 75% p = ns
	PBSC	81	14% p = 0.04	66% p = .06	– Advanced: 33 vs. 57%, p = .04
Blaise	BM	52		65%	
	PBSC	48	ns	67% p = ns	
Heldal	BM	30			
	PBSC	28	ns	p = ns	
Powles	BM	19	0%	63%	
	PBSC	18	37%	70% p = ns	
Schmitz	BM	166			
	PBSC	163	ns	ns	
Vigoritto	BM	19			
	PBSC	18	ns	ns	

cells is necessary for engraftment, for example after non-myeloablative conditioning or if TCD is planned for a HLA mismatched transplant.

17.5 Principles of Conditioning Regimens

The diversity of today's conditioning regimens is based on its historical development (Table 17.3). The effects of TBI on BM provided a concept for BMT experiments in animals and man. It became possible to eliminate a diseased haematopoietic system without causing irreversible, other organ damage. TBI was intended to be an equivalent to surgical removal in solid organ transplantation. Therefore the term to "condition" meant the preparation of the recipient to accept a new organ in place of the diseased haematopoietic system [33].

There are three main objectives: space-making, immunosuppression and disease eradication. The first of these is a somewhat controversial concept which originated from the belief that immature progenitor cells occupy defined niches within the marrow stroma in order to obtain the necessary support for proliferation and differentiation. To allow access to these niches, existing host stem cell cells must be eradicated in order for donor engraftment to occur. Immunosuppression is required to prevent rejection of the incoming donor cells by residual host haematopoiesis. The probability of rejection is increased in situations of increasing HLA-disparity, e.g. volunteer UD and family mismatched transplants or in situations where the recipient has been "pre-sensitised" by the administration of multiple blood products prior to HSCT. It is also increased in T-cell depleted (TCD) HSCT. On the other hand, rejection (and relapse) is decreased by reduced GVHD prophylaxis, high stem cell dose and high T-cell dose. The ultimate role of the conditioning regimen is long-term disease control. This is a clear objective in the haematological malignancies, but it is also of vital importance in diseases characterised by hyperplastic bone marrows, e.g. thalassaemia. Partial engraftment may be sufficient in situations where only a "specific product" is required, e.g. B-cells in some immunodeficiency states.

Until recently, it was thought that the mechanism of cure of the malignancy was entirely due to the conditioning therapy, and that the HSCT itself was merely a supportive measure designed to allow the patient to receive so-called supra-lethal treatment without experiencing permanent bone marrow aplasia. However, the observation that disease recurrence was more frequent after TCD HSCT identified the "graft versus leukaemia" effect (GVL). Although GVL is important in the maintenance of remission, this effect cannot be solely responsible for the durable disease free remission seen in recipients of syngeneic and autologous HSCT. Reduced intensity conditioning (RIC) HSCT have been recently devel-

Table 17.3 Common conditioning regimens

Regimen	Total Dose	Daily Dose	Administration	Days
Conventional "old" regimens				
Cy/TBI				
Cyclosphosphamide	120 mg/kg	60 mg/kg	IV in 1 hour	−6, −5
Total Body Irradiation	12–14.4 Gy	2–2.4 Gy (2x/day)		−3,−2,−1
Bu/Cy				
Busulfan	16 mg/kg	4 mg/kg*	p.o. q 6 hour	−9,−8,−7,−6
Cyclophosphamide	200 mg/kg	50 mg/kg	IV in 1 hour	−5,−4,−3,−2
BACT				
BCNU	200 mg/m^2	200 mg/m^2	IV in 2 hours	−6
ARA-C	800 mg/m^2	200 mg/m^2	IV in 2 hours	−5,−4,−3,−2
Cyclophosphamide	200 mg/kg	50 mg/kg	IV in 1 hour	−5,−4,−3,−2
6-Tioguanina	800 mg/m^2	200 mg/m^2	p.o	−5,−4,−3,−2
Alternative "standard" regimens				
TBI/VP				
Total Body irradiation	12–13.2 Gy	2–2.5 Gy		−7,−6,−5,−4
Etoposide	60 mg/kg	(2x/day) 60 mg/kg	IV in 2 hours	−3
AC/TBI				
Ara-C	36 g/m^2	3 g/m^2	IV q 12 hours in 2 h	−9,−8,−7,−6-
Total Body irradiation	12 Gy	2 Gy (2x/day)		5,−4 −3,−2,−1
MEL/TBI				
Melphalan	110	110–140 mg/m^2	IV in 1 hour	−3
Total Body Irradiation	140 mg/m^2 10–14.85 Gy	2 Gy (2x day)		−2,−1,0
Bu/Cy (Tuschka)				
Busulfan	16 mg/kg	4 mg/kg*	p.o. q 6 hours	−7,−6,−5,−4,
Cyclophosphamide	120 mg/kg	60 mg/kg	IV in 1 hour	−3,−2
Bu/MEL				
Busulfan	16 mg/kg	4 mg/kg*	p.o. q 6 hours	−5,−4,−3,−2
Melphalan	140 mg/ m^2	140 mg/m^2	IV in 1 hour	−1
Intensified regimens				
Cy/VP/TBI				
Cyclophosphamide	120 mg/kg	60 mg/kg	IV in 1 hour	−6,−5
Etoposide	30–60 mg/kg	30–60 mg/kg	IV in 2 hours	−4
Total Body Irradiation	12–13.75 Gy	2–2.25 Gy (2/day)		−3,−2,−1
TBI/TT/Cy/ATG				
Total Body Irradiation	13.75 Gy	1.25 Gy (3x/day)		−9,−8,−7,−6
Thiotepa	10 mg/kg	5 mg/kg	IV in 1–2 hours	−5,−4
Cyclophosphamide	120 mg/kg	60 mg/kg	IV in 1 hour	−3,−2
ATG	120 mg/kg	30 mg/kg	IV in 5–6 hours	−5,−4,−3,−2
Bu/Cy/MEL				
Busulfan	16 mg/kg	4 mg/kg*	p.o. q 6 hours	−7,−6,−5,−4
Cyclophosphamide	120 mg/kg	60 mg/kg	IV in 1 hour	−3,-2
Melphalan	140 mg/m^2	140 mg/m^2	IV in 1 hour	−1
Reduced Intensity regimens				
TBI/Fluda				
Total Body	2 Gy	2 Gy		0
Irradiation Fludarabine	90 mg/m^2	30 mg/m^2	IV in 30 min	−4,−3,−2
Fluda/Bu/ATG				
Fludarabine	180 mg/m^2	30 mg/ m^2	IV in 30 min	−10 to −5
Busulfan	8 mg/kg	4 mg/kg*	p.o. q 6 hours	−6,−5
± ATG	40 mg/kg	10 mg/kg	IV in 8–10 hours	−4,−3,−2,−1

oped in the hope of reducing toxicity and mortality. Its goal is not tumour eradication or destruction of host haematopoiesis by cytotoxic therapy but via immune mediated effects. The immunosuppressive potential of the approach is based on several components; initial conditioning, graft composition, post transplant rejection prevention and use of donor lymphocyte infusions (DLI) in case of incomplete chimerism at specified time points. Many of these regimens require double immunosuppression with both CsA and MMF post transplant.

17.6 Early Complications After HSCT

The high dose chemo-radiotherapy included in conditioning regimens (see above) affects all organs and tissues, producing early and late secondary effects of variable intensity.

Haemorrhagic cystitis (HC): HC after HSCT can be produced by direct toxicity of the conditioning regimen on the urothelium or by viral infections affecting the urinary tract. Usually, HC due to conditioning appears early after HSCT (several days after receiving CT agents) while viral CH appears later (usually after day +30) [1]. The most frequent viruses involved are Human Polyomavirus type BK or JC, Adenovirus type 11 (less frequent) and CMV (exceptional). The incidence of HC related to conditioning without prevention is up to 70% but with prevention with mesna, hyperhydration and sometimes bladder irrigation, it can be reduced to 1% to 25%. The treatment of HC includes forced hydration and aggressive platelet support. In case of clots or vesical pain, then continuous irrigation, IVIG, cystoscopy and removal of clots, selective arterial embolisation, suprapubic cystostomy and cystectomy [34, 35].

Early complications of vascular origin: the injury of the vascular endothelium seems to be the most important initial event of several complications with imprecise diagnostic criteria and overlapping clinical features, which are observed within the first 30–60 days after HSCT. The best defined syndromes resulting from this endothe-

lial injury are: sinusoidal obstruction syndrome of the liver, capillary leak syndrome, engraftment syndrome, diffuse alveolar haemorrhage, thrombotic microangiopathy and idiopathic pneumonia syndrome.

Sinusoidal obstruction syndrome (SOS) of the liver is the term used to designate the symptoms and signs that appear early after HSCT as a consequence of the direct hepatic toxicity of the conditioning regimen. This syndrome, formerly termed veno-occlusive disease of the liver (VOD), is characterized by the development of: jaundice, fluid retention, weight gain, and hepatomegaly, usually painful [36–43]. The pathogenesis is not well-known, but the probable succession of events is as follows [36, 37]: In the first phase there is hepatic accumulation of toxic metabolites (e.g. acrolein) produced by the metabolism of certain drugs by the cytochrome P-450 enzymatic system and decreased transformation of these toxic metabolites to stable metabolites by an inadequate glutathione enzymatic system (due to previous liver disease or the action of agents as Busulfan, BCNU or TBI). Toxic metabolites are predominantly located in area 3 of the acinus (around centrilobular veins) because this area is rich in P-450 and poor in glutathione, producing damage of hepatocytes and sinusoidal endothelium. After endothelial damage and the procoagulant events there is a reduction of the hepatic venous outflow causing painful hepatomegaly, postsinusoidal intrahepatic portal hypertension and ascites. Due to unclear mechanisms, this is followed by a reduction of renal excretion of sodium and fluid retention, causing oedema, weigh gain and worsening ascites.

The diagnosis is mainly based on clinical criteria [36–38]. The Seattle criteria include two or more of the following in the first 20 days after HSCT: bilirubin >2 mg/dL; hepatomegaly or pain in the right-upper quadrant and weight gain (>2% basal weight). The Baltimore criteria requires a bilirubin >2 mg/dL + ≥ 2 of the following: painful hepatomegaly, ascites or weight gain (>5% basal weight). Other complementary studies include abdominal ultrasound, haemodynamic supra hepatic studies with a HVGP of 10 mmHg or greater and liver biopsy showing the classical changes of VOD such as concentric non-thrombotic narrowing of the lumen of small intrahepatic veins; eccentric narrowing of the venular lumen; phlebosclerosis; sinusoidal fibrosis and hepatocyte necrosis. The treatment is mainly symptomatic with restriction of salt and water intake, diuretics and support of the intravascular volume and renal perfusion by means of albumin, plasma expanders and transfusions (to maintain an haematocrit >30%). Direct measures include defibrotide, low dose dopamine, TIPS (transvenous intrahepatic portosystemic shunt), surgical shunt and, if indicated, liver transplantation [39, 42, 43].

The clinical manifestations of the thrombotic microangiopathy associated with HSCT include microangiopathic haemolytic anaemia (MHA) (anaemia, fragmented red cells >5%, increased LDH and other markers of haemolysis), thrombocytopenia or increase in requirement for platelet transfusions, fever of non-infectious origin and renal insufficiency or neurological changes [44]. The incidence is around 10–15% depending on the series and risk factors include use of cyclosporine or tacrolimus, GVHD, infections (CMV, fungal) or prior TBI. Several clinical forms are described:

- Nephrotoxicity due to CsA with MHA: occurs early after HSCT and is reversible after stopping CsA
- Neurotoxicity due to CsA with MHA: similar to the previous one but with CNS disturbances (cortical blindness, seizures, typical images in CNS scan). Good evolution if it improves quickly when stopping CsA
- Haemolytic uraemic syndrome: characterised by renal impairment, MHA, hypertension and thrombocytopenia. Occurs mainly in children and has no relation with high CsA levels. Low mortality and good response to plasmapheresis
- Fulminating multifactorial: Very early after HSCT and characterised by progressive renal failure, CNS disturbances, hypertension, MHA, and thrombocytopenia. Quickly fatal, usually no response to treatment

17.7　Graft vs. Host Disease

The principal complication of allo-HSCT is GVHD, which can occur despite aggressive immunosuppressive prophylaxis even when the donor is a "perfectly" matched (HLA-identical) sibling. It is a consequence of interactions between Ag-presenting cells of the recipient and mature T-cells of the donor. There is convincing evidence that T-cells contained in the donor graft or subsequently derived from donor stem cells react to host APC, causing target organ damage that is recognised as clinical manifestations of GVHD [45, 46]. Donor T-cells are infused into a host that has been profoundly damaged by underlying disease, infections and particularly by the conditioning regimen, all of which result in activation of host cells with secretion of proinflammatory cytokines such as TNF-α and IL-1 [46]. As a consequence, expression of MHC Ag and adhesion molecules is increased, thus enhancing the recognition of host alloantigens. The second step of the afferent phase of GVHD is characterised by donor T-cell interaction with host APCs and subsequent proliferation, differentiation and secretion of cytokines. Cytokines such as IL-2 and IFN-γ enhance T-cell expansion, induce CTL and NK cell responses, and prime additional mononuclear phagocytes to produce TNF-α [45]. These inflammatory cytokines in turn stimulate production of inflammatory chemokines, thus recruiting effector cells into target organs. The efferent phase of GVHD is a complex cascade of multiple effectors such as CTLs and NK cells, and inflammatory effectors such as TNF-α, IL-1 and nitric oxide (NO). The effector functions of mononuclear phagocytes are triggered via a secondary signal provided by lipopolysaccharide (LPS) that leaks through the intestinal mucosa damaged during the initial phase. This mechanism may result in the amplification of local tissue injury. Finally, the inflammatory response, together with the CTL and NK components, leads to target tissue destruction, via target cell apoptosis, in the transplanted host [46].

The median incidence of clinically significant (grade II-IV) acute GVHD (AGVHD) is about

40% but ranges from 10% to 80% according to risk factors [47]. By convention, AGVHD develops within the first 100 days of transplant [48]. A maculo-papular rash, often involving the palms and soles usually marks the onset of AGVHD. Lesions may be pruritic and/or painful. The rash then spreads and can involve the entire body surface. As the rash intensifies, it is often associated with papules. In more severe cases, bullae can form and surface areas can desquamate, leading to extremely painful denudation associated with protein loss and risk of superinfection. Liver involvement results in cholestatic hepatopathy, with or without jaundice, in which the cholestatic enzymes are substantially raised whilst the transaminases show only non-specific changes. The clinical diagnosis of AGVHD of the liver is difficult since distinguishing liver impairment due to therapy-associated hepatotoxicity, infection, VOD (SOS) or GVHD is not always possible. Involvement of the GI tract primarily manifests as nausea and green watery diarrhoea. The enteral fluid loss is used as a measure of gut involvement. Severe abdominal pain, bloody diarrhoea and massive enteral fluid losses accompany advanced disease. A variant of mild enteric GVHD involving only upper GI tract has been described. Symptoms include anorexia and nausea without diarrhoea and this usually responds very well to immunosuppressive therapy.

The overall grade of AGVHD usually predicts the clinical course [48, 49]. In general, grade I AGVHD has a favourable prognosis. Grade II is a moderately severe disease. Grade III is a severe, multi organ GVHD and grade IV is life threatening or fatal (Table 17.4).

Chronic GVHD (CGVHD) is defined by symptoms occurring afterwards, either de novo, or following AGVHD. It is a result of a later phase of alloreactivity. It is well recognised that CGVHD is the main determinant of long-term outcome after allo-HSCT. Similarities in the clinical features of CGVHD and several autoimmune diseases have been observed. The skin is the most frequently involved organ (80%). The clinical manifestations include depigmentation, lichenoid papules, and dermal and subcutaneous fibrosis with alopecia. Oral involvement (70%) includes lichen planus,

Table 17.4 Acute GVHD grading

Stage	Skin/Maculo-papular rash	Liver/Bilirubin	GI/Diarrhoea
(a) Grading system: stage for each organ			
+	<25%of body surface	34–50 μmol/lL	> 500 mL
++	25–50% of body surface	51–102 μmol/L	>1000 mL
+++	Generalised erythroderma	103–255 μmol/L	> 1500 mL
++++	Generalised erythroderma with bullous formation and desquamation	> 255 μmol/L	Severe abdominal pain with or without ileus
(b) Overall grading system (Glucksberg)			
Grade of AGVHD	Degree of organ involvement		
I	Skin: + to ++		
II	Skin: + to +++ Gut and/or liver: + Mild decrease in clinical performance		
III	Skin: ++ to +++ Gut and/or liver: ++ to +++ Marked decrease in clinical performance		
IV	Skin: ++ to ++++ Gut and/or liver: ++ to ++++ Extreme decrease in clinical performance		

ulcerations, atrophy and dryness. The commonest ocular symptom is also dryness (50%), which may evolve into kerato-conjunctivitis sicca. Other clinical manifestations are less frequent, including chronic sinusitis, obliterans bronchiolitis, and weight loss with or without anorexia and chronic diarrhoea, myositis, tendinitis and fasciitis. Immune deficiency due to CGVHD itself and/or to its treatment is associated with an increased susceptibility to late infections and an increased risk of late morbidity and mortality.

CGVHD was classified in 1980 by Schulman [50] according to the extent of the disease in 20 long term Seattle patients. With time, the spectrum of abnormalities observed in CGVH has changed, as a result of earlier diagnosis and greater efficacy of immunosuppressive treatments and of the limitations of this classification system has become apparent [51]. Although it is highly reproducible among transplant centres, the traditional grading system is of limited utility because it does not stratify patients for outcome (Table 17.5).

Table 17.5 Chronic GVHD Grading

(a) Limited
1. Abnormality of buccal cavity with a (+) lip or skin biopsy without other signs of CGVHD
2. Moderate modification of liver function tests with a (+) lip or skin biopsy without other signs of CGVHD
3. Less than 6 papulo-squamous plaques or a limited skin rash or depigmentation <20% of body surface with a (+) skin biopsy without other signs of CGVHD.
4. Ocular dryness (Schirmer ≤5 mm), with a (+) lip or skin biopsy without other signs of CGVHD
5. Vulvar or vaginal lesions with a (+) skin biopsy without other signs of CGVH

(b) Extensive
1. Manifestations on ≥2 organs with symptoms of CGVHD with a (+) biopsy
2. Weight loss <15% with a contribute biopsy on any organ.
3. Skin more than defined in limited CGVHD with a (+) biopsy
4. Scleroderma or morphea.
5. Onycholysis or onychodystrophia with a (+) biopsy on any organ
6. Fasciitis.
7. Contractures due to CGVH.
8. Bronchiolitis obliterans.
9. (+) liver biopsy and abnormal liver function tests
10. Gut (+) biopsy.

Prevention of GVHD involves immunosuppressive therapy and T-cell depletion (TCD). Cyclosporine A (CsA) appeared in the early 80s [52]. In contrast to the non-specific cytotoxic effect of MTX, CsA was the first molecule that specifically inhibits T-cell proliferation and IL2 production. The limitation of the therapy is mainly due to its nephrotoxicity. Other frequent adverse effects include hypertension, liver cholestasis, tremors, hirsutism and CNS disturbances. The "gold standard" regimen for the prevention of GVHD was established in 1986, based on a randomised study performed in Seattle [52]. MTX given at a dose of 15 mg/m^2 on day +1 and 10 mg/m^2 on days +3, +6 and +11 (referred to as short course MTX) was combined with IV CsA 3 mg/kg/d from D−1 to D+30 followed by oral treatment until D+180. This combination led to a significant decrease in the incidence and severity of AGVHD and to a significant improvement in the survival, compared to either CsA or MTX alone. This regimen is largely used in patients with "standard risk" leukaemia and a genoidentical donor. More recently, particularly for patients with high risk factors for GVHD, i.e. in MUD transplants, new immunosuppressive drugs have been tested. Tacrolimus (Prograf) is an immunosuppressive macrolide lactone which blocks the earliest steps of T-cell activation by inhibiting the calcium-dependent signal transduction pathway. Although the mechanism of action, pharmacokinetics and side effects profile of Tacrolimus are similar to those of CsA, its immunosuppressive potency in vitro is greater. Phase II and phase III studies have shown that Tacrolimus in combination with a short course of MTX appears active in preventing AGVHD after MUD transplantation [53]. Mycophenolate Mofetil (Cellcept) is a derivative of mycophenolic acid. It blocks T- and B cell proliferation and down regulates expression of adhesion molecules. The efficacy of MMF associated with CsA has been studied mainly after RIC regimen. The major toxicities are neutropenia and gut ulcerations.

T-cell depletion of grafts is an effective method for prevention of GVHD [54]. However, the limitations associated with this method are the occurrence of graft failure and/or relapse. In MUD transplants, several randomised or comparative studies have been performed comparing in vitro TCD to CsA + MTX, but so far, it has not been conclusively established whether TCD can improve survival [15]. In vitro positive selection of CD34(+) stem cells is the preferred technique for TCD. The CD34(−) fraction that contains T-cells can be frozen, making possible a delayed T cell add back if indicated. Several studies showed effectiveness of in vivo TCD, using ATG or MoAb (Campath, Alemtuzumab), as prophylaxis of GVHD after MUD transplantation. Unfortunately the strong immunosuppressive effect of this treatment is associated with an increased risk of severe infections and a higher TRM. Randomised studies are needed in order to evaluate long term DFS in large cohorts of patients.

The treatment of GVHD is based on Methyl-Prednisolone, at a dose of 2 mg/kg/d. This treatment, associated with CsA, is given for two weeks, and then tapered slowly if there is a complete response to therapy. The response of acute GVHD to initial therapy is of particular importance for the prognosis. Failure of therapy is usually defined as progression after 3 days, or no change after 7 days, or incomplete response after 14 days. Patients in whom initial therapy has failed will receive a second-line treatment. The rate of partial and complete response to second line therapy varies from 35 to 70%, but the 6–12 months survival is low because of infectious complications or recurrence of GVHD. Corticosteroid refractory AGVHD have received a variety of salvage regimens, including an association of Tacrolimus and MMF; high dose Methyl-Prednisolone: 5 to 20 mg/kg; various MoAb, such as OKT3, anti IL2-receptor (Dacluzumab), anti-TNF-α (Infliximab), ATG and Campath. Unfortunately, none of these therapies has been consistently successful in salvaging patients, pointing to the need for new approaches to improve outcome. The possible efficacy of Sirolimus (Rapamycin) has still to be evaluated.

Various approaches have been developed for patients with CGVHD not responsive to first line therapy with corticosteroids, including low dose total lymphoid irradiation, PUVA therapy, extracorporeal photochemotherapy, MMF, Tacrolimus and Thalidomide. All these treatments have been reported to improve clinical manifestations [55]. Long-term treatment with high-dose prednisolone is associated with a high risk for morbidity. Complications prominently include avascular necrosis, glucose intolerance requiring administration of insulin, infections, hypertension, changes in body habitus, cutaneous atrophy, cataracts, osteoporosis, emotional lability, interference with sleep, and growth retardation in children.

17.8 Immune Reconstitution After HSCT

Assessment of the host immune status is becoming a key issue in allo-HSCT, especially in the long-term follow-up of these patients, because severe post-transplant infections, relapse or secondary malignancies may be directly related to persistent immune defects. Immune deficiency leading to an increased susceptibility to infections lasts for more than a year. In relation to the occurrence of infections, the post-transplant period is subdivided in different phases. Although infections that occur in the first month mostly result from a deficiency in both granulocytes and mononuclear cells (MNC), later post-engraftment infections are due to a deficiency in MNC subsets, primarily CD4 T cells and B cells. T-cell reconstitution has been extensively studied because of the central role of T-cells in mediating both GVHD, evidenced by the reduced incidence of this complication following TCD, and a GvL effect as shown by donor lymphocyte infusions (DLI). DLI may cure 20–80% of patients with post-transplant relapsed leukaemia and lymphoma depending on the type and extent of the disease. This is one of the most important breakthroughs in HSCT in the last years illustrating the powerful anti-leukaemia effect mediated by allogeneic lymphocytes and the potential of immunotherapy in the treatment of malignant diseases.

In transplants performed following myeloablative conditioning regimens, immune reconstitution (IR) will depend upon the ability of the haematopoietic graft to generate de novo lymphoid and myeloid lineage cells and on the function of mature cells contained in the graft [56]. Post-transplantation, the different MNC populations reconstitute at different tempos. The first cells to reconstitute (within first 100 days) are those of the innate immune response, granulocytes, monocytes, macrophages and NK cells. In contrast, T and B lymphocytes remain severely reduced and their function is impaired for several months or years after HSCT [56].

B-lymphocytes (CD19+ B-cells) normalize by one year after transplant. B-cell regeneration may be associated with transient appearance of monoclonal or oligoclonal B-cell expansions [57]. After a decline in the first several months after HSCT, levels of specific antibodies to protein Ag frequently encountered after transplantation (e.g., CMV) return to pretransplantation levels within 1 year. In contrast, antibodies to proteins

Ag unlikely to be encountered after HSCT (e.g. tetanus, measles, polio) continue to decline. This supports the recommendation of post-HSCT vaccination. Antibody levels in the first year are affected primarily by pre-HSCT antibody levels in the recipient [57]. A persistent defect in IgA, especially in patients with CGVHD explains mucosal infections of the respiratory and digestive tracts. IgG2 and IgG4 subclasses are also deficient in the case of GVHD, accounting for the increased susceptibility to infections, primarily those due to encapsulated bacteria (e.g. *Streptococcus pneumoniae* or *Haemophilus influenzae*). PBSC recipients do not have higher antibody levels than BM recipients. Vaccinations with inactivated or conjugated vaccines should be initiated when CD4 and B lymphocyte counts are sufficient to expect efficacy, usually from 6 months post-transplant onwards.

NK cells are lymphocytes that act early in the immune response against infection and tumour-transformed cells. Based on phenotyping (CD16 and CD56), they are the first lymphocyte subpopulation to be reconstituted in all graft settings, usually within 3 months [58]. Memory T cells are the first to expand after HSCT; they may be either of donor origin in the case of a non-TCD BM or, in the case of a TCD, originate from host T cells that have survived the conditioning regimen [59]. They respond quickly to previously encountered pathogens, are easier to trigger, faster to respond and enter tissues more readily than naive T cells. They are frequently directed towards periodically reactivated herpes viruses, CMV or EBV, which they keep under control. They constitute the majority of oligoclonal T cell expansions found in healthy adults, especially in the CD8+ population. They are also less dependent than naive T cells upon recognition of self MHC-peptide complexes in their survival and expansion in the periphery. Finally, some of these probably account for recognition of host MHC-peptide complexes during GVHD as cross-reactive allorecognition and viral-specific immune responses have been evidenced, at least in vitro. In the long term, broad immune responses need the reconstitution of a naive T cell repertoire able to respond to a broad range of pathogens encoun-

tered by the host and to tumour antigens. Reconstitution of this compartment is an ongoing process which requires a functional thymus for the recovery of a complete T cell ontogeny [60]. As stated above, naive T cells also seem more dependent than memory T cells upon recognition of self MHC-peptide complexes for their survival in the periphery. Therefore, MHC mismatches may be considered detrimental for immune reconstitution in many respects, including impairment in thymic selection but also in the homeostasis of the naive T cell compartment.

17.9 Infections After HSCT

Despite considerable progress in the management of HSCT complications, infection remains an important cause of morbidity and mortality after HSCT. Major advances in the management of infectious complications have come from the understanding of the mechanisms of the complex immunosuppression observed during the first months after transplant, their role in the predisposition to given infections, and also from well-designed therapeutic trials.

After allo-HSCT following a conventional (myeloablative) conditioning regimen, the pattern of infections can be divided into three periods: (a) aplastic phase following the conditioning regimen until neutrophil recovery, (b) a second period from initial marrow engraftment to at least the third or fourth month, which is characterized by cell-mediated immune deficiency with decreased number and function of specific and non-specific cytotoxic cells, and (c) a late post-transplantation period from the fourth month onwards where immune reconstitution is mainly influenced by the presence and severity of CGVHD. Most patients have Ig deficiency, particularly of IgG2, which is responsible for a decrease in the response to polysaccharide Ag.

17.9.1 Bacterial Infections

Because of the hospital environment and its resistant bacteria, the physical environment of transplant patients is specifically designed to decrease the risk of nosocomial infection. Different measures can be implemented. The easiest is simple reverse nurse barrier isolation including mask, gloves, and gowns, and strict hand washing to prevent cross-transmission. The control of room air quality through filtration (HEPA) is the main measure used to decrease the risk of aspergillosis.

The second measure is the prevention of bacterial infection by gut decontamination with oral quinolones and/or non-absorbable antibiotics (neomycin, colistin) and a low microbial diet.

The third measure is the management of central IV lines. Catheters may be the source of bacteraemia with significant morbidity, and potential mortality. During the neutropenic phase, it is controversial whether a catheter should be left in *situ* if blood cultures have documented a pathogen, except in the case of methicillin resistant *S. aureus*, *Candida* sp., *Bacillus* sp. and corynebacterium JK, and any hospital-acquired resistant pathogen, such as *P. aeruginosa* or *Acinetobacter* sp., where the catheter should definitely be removed [61].

17.9.2 Fungal Infections

Aspergillus is the most worrisome fungal infection after HSCT [62], and also the most common cause of infectious death after allo-HSCT [63]. Reported incidences vary from 5% to 20% of transplants; the most common site is the lung and GVHD is the main risk factor. A first peak of incidence occurs during the neutropenic period, particularly in leukaemic patients who had been previously colonised. A second peak in incidence is seen between the second and third months, in patients with severe GVHD. Aspergillus infection may also occur at any time after transplant, particularly when corticosteroids have been used for prolonged periods. Recurrence may also occur in one third of the patients with previous Aspergillus infection [8]. New effective antifungal agents decrease mortality. Voriconazole has been shown to improve the survival for patients with aspergillosis when compared to a control group treated with conventional amphotericin B [64]. Echinocandins have been studied in refractory aspergillosis with encouraging results. Despite these improvements, the mortality of aspergillus in allo-HSCT patients remains over 50% in recent series. PCR and galactomannan antigenemia may early detect aspergillus infections. Candida infection is rare since the advent of azole prophylaxis and has a similar presentation in transplant patients when compared to other haematology patients, including candidemia, hepato-splenic candidiasis and pneumonia.

17.9.3 Viral Infections

Viral infections are frequent after HSCT. They may be life threatening, especially when affecting lung, liver, or CNS. The availability of new antiviral agents and results of comparative trials, has allowed a better control of herpes virus infections. However, due to the subsequent decrease in CMV infections and diseases, new viral infections have emerged, especially due to respiratory viruses and adenovirus.

HSV infections are extremely common, due to reactivation in sero(+) patients. The main early manifestation is mucosal lesions, difficult to distinguish from chemotherapy-induced mucositis in the absence of viral documentation. These lesions are painful and may be the portal of entry of bacteria from the gut. Treatment with IV acyclovir is usually effective. Acyclovir resistance is rare in HSCT patients, but this possibility must be considered in case of HSV disease documented during prophylaxis.

CMV disease has historically been a main cause of death in allo-HSCT patients other than in cases with both donor and recipient are sero(−). Since the demonstration that CMV infection usually precedes CMV disease, and considering the poor prognosis of CMV disease, a pre-emptive strategy has been adopted by most units. The quantification of viral load by PCR seems to be important since high levels of CMV DNA are indicators for a higher risk of CMV disease. Although first line pre-emptive strategies have been mainly studied with ganciclovir, foscarnet has been shown, in an EBMT comparative trial, as effective and no more toxic than ganciclovir [65]. Both can be used as first-line treatment of CMV infection, for an initial duration of 2 weeks. If CMV is still detected after 2 weeks of therapy, an additional course of 2 weeks should be given. Cidofovir has been studied only in uncontrolled trials and because of its toxicity profile; its use should be reserved for second line pre-emptive therapy. CMV prophylaxis includes transfusion policies to avoid acquisition of CMV through blood products, especially for CMV sero(−) recipients of sero(−) donors. These patients must receive blood products either from CMV sero(−) donors exclusively, or leukocyte-depleted products.

VZV infections occur frequently after allogeneic HSCT. Primary varicella may be severe. High dose intravenous acyclovir is the therapy of choice.

HHV6 infections after allo-HSCT has been associated with pneumonia, delayed marrow engraftment, and particularly with prolonged thrombocytopenia and encephalitis. HHV6-DNA is frequently detected in the blood during the first months after transplant, so that its implication in clinical symptoms is difficult to establish, except in encephalitis when HHV6-DNA is detected in cerebro-spinal fluid.

EBV associated lymphoproliferative disease (EBV-LPD) is a life-threatening complication occurring after allo-HSCT. The monitoring of the EBV viral load by quantitative PCR permits the early detection of EBV reactivation that may lead to EBV-LPD. Recipients of a TCD SCT are at higher risk of EBV-LPD. Preemptive therapy of EBV reactivation with Rituximab has been shown to improve the outcome. The infusion of EBV-specific cytotoxic T cells has also been studied in high-risk patients with elevated EBV-DNA levels. In the absence of prospective trials, the exact indication for pre-emptive therapy based on EBV-viral load for preventing EBV-LPD is not clearly established; and very much depends on the transplant population.

Respiratory viruses, including respiratory syncytial virus (RSV), parainfluenza virus, rhinovirus, and influenza virus, appear to be more frequent than CMV in causing pneumonitis. A prospective study from the EBMT in 1998 showed an incidence of respiratory virus pneumonia of 2.1% [66]. Most cases in this series were due to RSV or influenza A. The mortality of these infections also varies among series, and with the time after transplant and the degree of immunosuppression, but it may be as high as 80% in RSV pneumonia. Few data are available in the literature on the efficacy of antiviral drugs in RSV pneumonia. Due to the risk of spread in the transplant unit, it is important to diagnose these patients very early, and to provide adequate prevention of transmission in the ward.

Adenovirus can be a cause of severe disseminated infections in allo-HSCT recipients. Patients receiving mismatched or UD HSCT, or with severe AGVHD, or with viral isolation from multiple sites, and from blood, are at high risk of developing adenovirus organ involvement. There are currently no established regimens for prophylaxis or treatment of adenovirus disease. A recent retrospective study by the IDWP has showed that cidofovir was effective in 10/16 patients with invasive adenovirus disease [67].

17.9.4 Other Infections

Toxoplasmosis occurring after HSCT has been mainly investigated in Europe, due to a higher seroprevalence of the disease when compared to US [68]. Patients at risk are those who are sero(+) for toxoplasmosis before transplant, irrespectively of donor serology. Blood PCR allows an early detection of toxoplasma reactivation. A recent prospective study from the EBMT on toxoplasma reactivation documented by blood PCR shows a frequency of reactivation of 8%. Most reactivations occur in patients with GVHD, when trimethoprim-sulfamethoxazole has been stopped for side effects, and replaced by aerosolised pentamidine for prophylaxis of *P. jiroveci* (previously *P. carinii*). It is not yet clear whether asymptomatic toxoplasma infection documented by blood PCR should be treated. Pneumocystis jiroveci pneumonia must be prevented in allo-HSCT recipients from engraftment to at least 6 months post-transplant, even longer in case of prolonged immunosuppression. The best option is trimethoprim-sulfamethoxazole. In case of intolerance, alternatives are dapsone or aerosolised pentamidine.

17.9.5 Post Transplant Immunisation

Active immunisation to tetanus, poliovirus, and diphtheria is highly recommended in all transplant populations, due to the usual loss of specific immunity after both auto- and allo-HSCT. This is the only way to allow transplanted patients to have relatively normal immunity to these pathogens Immunisation with live vaccines is classically prohibited in immunocompromised patients. However, transplant patients may require active immunisation with vaccines that only exist in a live form, i.e. measles, mumps, or yellow fever. The current recommendations form the EBMT are summarised in Table 17.6.

Table 17.6 EBMT recommendations for immunisations after allogeneic HSCT

Vaccine	Allo-HSCT recipients	Auto-HSCT recipients	Time for immunisation (months)
Tetanus toxoid	++	++	6–12
Diphtheria toxoid	++	++	6–12
Inactivated polio	++	++	6–12
Pneumococci (23 valent)	+/− (S)	+/− (S)	6–12
H Influenzae	++	+ (S)	4–6
Measles, Rubella (attenuated)	+/− (S, R)	+/− (S, R)	Individual*
Influenza	+	+ (S)	6 #

++: Strongly recommended for all patients (benefit > > risk). +: Recommended (benefit > risk). +/−: Individual recommendation (benefit and risk must be weighed in individual cases). S: Might have particular benefit in subgroups of patients. R: regional variations depending on the epidemiological situation * Not earlier than 24 months after allo-HSCT # Season dependent

17.10 Indications and Results

Allogeneic HSCT remains the best therapy for the control of many malignant and non-malignant diseases. Table 17.7 shows the current indications from the EBMT.

17.10.1 Results in Children

HSCT represents an attractive option for children with high-risk (HR) acute leukaemia, defined as children who have a low cure rate expectancy with conventional therapies. The first treatment of choice is HLA identical sibling HSCT. Because 80% of children lack this kind of donor, the pros and cons of alternative approaches must be carefully weighed on a case-by-case basis: auto-HSCT can be used in selected cohorts of children with ALL or AML; in another 30–40% of cases, a matched unrelated donor (MUD) may be available in a short period of time; finally, the last few years have seen rise in the use of alternative options, such as unrelated cord blood stem cell donors or HLA-mismatched relatives.

The prognosis of AML in children has significantly improved over the past two decades: with intensive chemotherapy 80–90% of children achieve CR and 30–70% are cured if they receive post induction chemotherapy [68, 69]. HLA identical sibling HSCT in CR1 results in 45–64% long-term survival and is an attractive strategy for children who have an HLA-matched donor. Berlin-Frankfurt-Munster Group (BFM) trials 83 and 87 defined a HR group comprising 68% of patients with a 5-years EFS of 30–32% [70]. More recently, the Italian Association for Paediatric Haematology and Oncology (AIEOP) identified, on the basis of cytogenetic findings and poor early response, a HR group with similar results. In these patients there is an absolute indication for HSCT [71]. HSCT in CR1 has proven to be more efficient than chemotherapy alone in most comparative studies, with an EFS ranging from 55% to 72% in children given a sibling HSCT in CR1 [68].

Indications for HSCT for children with acute lymphoblastic leukaemia in CR1 are limited to

Table 17.7 Indications for allogenic HSCT: EBMT guidelines

Disease	Disease status	Sibling donor	Well-matched unrelated/1 ag related	Mm unrelated/>1 ag related
AML	CR1 (low risk[a])	CO	D	GNR
	CR1 (intermediate or high risk[a])	S	CO	D
	CR2/CR3/Relapse	S	CO	D
	M3 Molecular persistence-CR2	S	CO	GNR
ALL	CR1 (low risk[a])	D	GNR	GNR
	CR1 (high risk[a])	S	S	CO
	CR2, incipient relapse	S	S	CO
	Relapse or refractory	CO	GNR	GNR
CML	First chronic phase (CP)	S	S	GNR
	Accelerated phase or > first CP	S	S	CO
	Blast crisis	GNR	GNR	GNR
Myeloproliferatie disorders		CO	CO	D
Myelodysplastic syndrome	RA, RAEB	S	S	CO
	RAEBt, sAML in CR1 or CR2	S	CO	CO
CLL	Poor risk disease	S	S	D
Diffuse large cell NHL	CR1 (intermediate/high IPI at dx)	GNR	GNR	GNR
	Chemosensitive relapse; CR2	D	D	GNR
	Refractory	D	D	GNR
Mantle cell lymphoma	CR1/CR2/Relapse	D	D	GNR
	Refractory	D	D	GNR
Lymphoblastic and Burkitt's lymphoma	CR1	D	GNR	GNR
	Chemosensitive relapse; CR2	CO	D	GNR
	Refractory	D	D	GNR
Follicular B-cell NHL	CR1 (intermediate/high IPI at dx)	GNR	GNR	GNR
	Chemosensitive relapse; CR2	CO	CO	GNR
	Refractory	D	D	GNR
T-cell NHL	CR1	D	GNR	GNR
	Chemosensitive relapse; CR2	D	D	GNR
Hodgkin lymphoma	CR1	GNR	GNR	GNR
	relapse; CR2	D	D	D
	Refractory	D	D	GNR
Myeloma	All stages	CO	D	GNR
Amyloidosis		CO	D	GNR
SAA	Newly diagnosed	S	GNR	GNR
	Relapsed/Refractory	S	S	CO

S = standard of care, generally indicated in suitable patients; CO = clinical option, can be carried after careful assessment of risks and benefits; D = developmental, further trials are needed; GNR = Generally not recommended; CR1, 2, 3 = first, second, third complete remission; RA = refractory anaemia; RAEB = refractory anaemia with excess blasts; sAML = secondary acute myeloid leukaemia

[a]Categories are based mainly on number of white blood cells, cytogenetics at diagnosis, and time to achieve remission according to international trials

only 8–10% of children, who constitute a subpopulation of very HR ALL [72]. Most study groups define these patients as having an estimated EFS of less than 50%. SCT from a sibling cures more than 50% of patients who failed first line chemotherapy. Studies by the AIEOP show that the EFS of patients after sibling HSCT following an early BM relapse is significantly better compared to patients receiving chemotherapy (33 vs. 16%), whereas the difference does not reach statistical significance in patients undergoing HSCT following a late relapse (55 vs. 40%) [73].

SCID consists of a group of genetic disorders characterised by profoundly defective T-cell differentiation, with or without abnormal B cell differentiation, which lead to early death in the absence of HSCT. The overall frequency has been estimated at between 1:50,000 to 1:100,000 live births [74–76]. SCID is a paediatric emergency that needs to be treated as soon as possible once diagnosis is confirmed. The treatment of choice is an allo-HSCT which provides the missing progenitor of T cells and allows a survival rate of more than 90% when carried out shortly after birth [77–79]. In the presence of an HLA identical sibling donor, HSCT can be performed without any conditioning regimen and its course is characterised by the absence of GVHD and by the rapid development of the T cell function post transplant. In the European experience (1968–1999) for the EBMT/ESID group, the 3-year survival with evidence of sustained engraftment and improvement of the immunodeficiency disorder was 77% with a significant improvement over time from 62% in 1968–1985 up to 82% in 1999 [77].

Bone marrow failure (BMF) syndromes in children group several distinct entities including idiopathic and post hepatitis SAA that are not very different from the syndrome found in adults and several hereditary disorders which must be excluded before any attempt of treatment. Fanconi anaemia (FA) is a rare autosomal recessive disease characterized by congenital abnormalities, progressive BMF, chromosome breakage, and cancer susceptibility. At least 9 genes have been involved in the disease, which products functionally interact within the FA/BRCA biochemical pathway. HSCT is currently the only treatment that definitively restores normal haematopoiesis. FA anaemia cells are hypersensitive to DNA cross-linking agents. Cellular exposure to toxic agents including Cy, Bu or irradiation increases chromosome breaks and tissue damage. GVHD induces severe tissue damage and absence of repair. Therefore, standard conditioning must not be used. In a recent series of FA patients, conditioned with low dose

Cy and TLI, 5-years survival was 85% but the probability of head and neck carcinoma increased with time. The absence of irradiation in the conditioning regimen did not abolish the risk of secondary tumours, which are likely also to be related to the specific genetic defect present and to the environment, as shown by different phenotypic expression of the disease in homozygous twins [80].

β-Thalassemia and sickle cell disease (SCD) represent the most frequent haemoglobinopathies worldwide. Although supportive therapies can ameliorate their symptoms, HSCT represents the only cure for these diseases. In the last few years the outcome of HSCT for haemoglobinopathies has progressively improved thanks to the development of better conditioning regimens and supportive therapies. While the role of HSCT for β-thalassemia has been increasingly better defined, the use of this therapeutic strategy for SCD is still controversial and requires further investigation [81].

17.10.2 Results in Adults

For adult patients with acute leukaemia (AL), HSCT is the treatment associated with the lowest relapse incidence. AL is classified in two groups: Acute Myeloid Leukaemia (AML) and Acute Lymphoblastic Leukaemia (ALL). Both are treated with chemotherapy at the beginning of the disease to induce remission. The treatment plan involves a remission induction phase aimed at establishing a CR and a post-induction phase aimed at eradicating/reducing residual disease. Combination chemotherapy induces CR in an average of 60% to 80% of adults aged less than 60 years. In general, HSCT is performed after 2 or 3 courses of CT.

AML patients can be stratified according to three risk groups [82–84]:

1. For good risk patients in first CR, chemotherapy seems not inferior to transplant strategies. These patients include those with favourable cytogenetics such as t(8;21) and Inv16 and patients with acute promyelocytic leukaemia

(APL, AML-M3), which is characterised by the PML-RARA fusion gene arising from the t(15;17).

2. For poor risk patients and for all other patients who relapse, the chance of surviving without a transplant is very low. Poor risk includes patients not achieving CR after 1–2 courses of chemotherapy or patients with unfavourable cytogenetics such as abnormalities of chromosome 3, 5 or 7, 11q23 rearrangements (MLL gene), t(9;22) or complex karyotype. For those patients an early transplant strategy should be organised.

3. The remaining patients, including those with normal cytogenetics are considered intermediate risk. For intermediate risk patients with an HLA compatible sibling, allo-HSCT remains the best option. However, 30% of patients with no cytogenetic abnormality have an abnormality of the FLT3 gene, either an internal tandem duplication (ITD) or a point mutation. These patients may benefit from early transplantation from the best available donor.

In all studies which have tried to compare chemotherapy vs. allo-HSCT, allogeneic HSCT has never been shown to be inferior and was often superior [85–87]. However such studies have not so far completely clarified the situation. Patients under 55 years. in the UK MRC AML 10 trial who entered CR were tissue typed (n = 1063). 419 had a matched sibling donor and 644 had no match. When compared on a donor vs. no donor basis the relapse incidence (RI) was reduced in the donor arm (36% vs. 52%; p = 0.001) and the DFS improved (50% vs. 42%; p = 0.01), but OS was not different (55% vs. 50%). Sixty-one per cent of patients with a donor underwent HSCT. A significant benefit in DFS was seen in the intermediate-risk cytogenetic group (50 vs. 39%; p = 0.004). Allo-HSCT given after intensive chemotherapy was able to reduce RI in all risk and age groups. However, due to the competing effects of procedural mortality and an inferior response to CT if relapse does occur, there was a survival advantage only in patients of intermediate risk [84].

Results with unrelated donors show for patients in first CR, second CR and advanced phase a TRM of 20%, 42% and 48%, a relapse rate of 33%, 29% and 60% and a leukaemia-free survival of 50%, 42% and 28% respectively [88]. Using Eurocord registry data a matched pair analysis was performed in order to compare the results of UD-CBT versus UD-BMT in adults with AL [89]. The incidence of AGVHD was 32% after UD-CBT compared to 41% after UD-BMT (p = 0.05) and the incidence of CGVHD at 2 years was not statistically different (p = 0.53). Kaplan-Meier estimates of transplant related mortality (TRM) at day 100 and 2-years were respectively 37% and 66% after UD-CBT compared to 27% (p = 0.08) and 46% (p = 0.12) after UD-BMT 2 year. RI and survival were similar in both groups of patients. These data suggest that despite increased HLA disparities, the probabilities of relapse, OS and LFS after UD-CBT are comparable to those observed after UD-BMT. Therefore UD-CBT with a high number of infused cells ($>1.0 \times 10^7$/kg) and no more than 2 HLA disparities should be considered an acceptable alternative for adults with AL [89].

Haplo-identical transplant has been pioneered by the Perugia group [90–93]. Their most recent publications report the results in 33 AML patients transplanted with a median age of 38 (9–62) years. All were at high risk because of relapse at transplant, or second or later CR, or CR1 but with unfavourable prognostic features. Positively selected CD34+ cells were used and no post-transplant immunosuppressive therapy was given. Leukaemia relapse was largely controlled in AML recipients whose donor was NK alloreactive, with only 2 out of 16 relapsing. To date, 13 of 18 AML (72%) who were in any CR at transplant survive disease-free while 4 of the 15 patients (27%) in relapse at transplant survive.

There are only a few comparative prospective trials evaluating the best post-remission therapy for adult ALL patients. In the French LALA87 study, patients aged 15 to 40 who achieved a CR and had a matched related donor were assigned to allo-HSCT [94, 95]. The intention-to-treat analysis found an advantage for allografting vs chemotherapy (10 years OS = 46 vs. 31%). High-risk patients (Ph(+), age > 35, WBC >30,000/µL at diagnosis, or time to achieve CR > 4 weeks) benefited more from allo-HSCT (10 years OS = 44 vs. 11%) [95]. The MRC UKALL XII / EGOG 2993 study [96], which is the largest prospective randomised trial designed to evaluate post-remission therapy in adult ALL, has currently accrued 1500 patients, including over 1000 patients with Ph(−) ALL. Ninety-three percent of Ph(−) ALL patients achieved CR. Interim analysis of this study shows a significantly reduced RI in Ph(−) patients assigned to allograft (n = 190), compared with those assigned to chemotherapy (n = 253) (5 years RI = 23 vs. 61%, p = 0.001). There was a tendency for improved EFS in all patients assigned allograft, (5 years EFS = 54 vs. 34% p = 0.04), most noticeably in standard risk patients (5 years EFS =64 vs., 46%, p = 0.05). A retrospective comparative analysis by Horowitz et al. (on behalf of the IBMTR) reported the outcome of adult ALL patients (aged 15–45 years) treated with chemotherapy vs. allo-HSCT in CR1 [97]. The RI was significantly reduced after allograft compared to chemotherapy (26 vs. 59%). However, DFS was not different (44 vs. 38%), reflecting the higher mortality rate after allo-HSCT. However, a re-examination of this issue using more recently treated patients demonstrated superior DFS with allo-HSCT for patients <30 years [98].

The Philadelphia chromosome occurs in 20–30% of adult ALL patients. Although more then 60% of these patients succeed in achieving CR, most of them will relapse, and less then 10% will remain alive 5 years. after diagnosis. The poor outcome with conventional chemotherapy makes allogeneic HSCT an attractive option for patients with Ph(+) ALL. Dombret et al. [99], have recently reported the outcome of 154 patients with Ph(+) ALL who were entered into the prospective multicentre LALA-94 trial between 1994–2000. All patients who entered remission and had a matched related/unrelated donor were assigned to allo-HSCT, whereas those without a donor had an autologous HSCT. The existence of a donor and absence of MRD pre-transplantation were both associated with a longer DFS and OS. The ongoing MRC

UKALL XII /ECOG 2993 has recently reported the outcome in 167 Ph(+) ALL patients who were treated between 1993–2000 [92]. As expected, the 5 years. EFS and OS were higher in the allogeneic recipients, and approached 36% and 42% respectively, compared with 17% and 19% in non-allogeneic transplanted patients.

17.11 Final Considerations

Allogeneic haemopoietic stem cell transplantation is a well established treatment modality in malignant and non-malignant haematological disorders. Years of experience and prospective randomised clinical trials have shown that it can result in cure in a significant proportion of cases. Until a few years ago, this was the main focus of stem cell therapy. However, cellular therapy has experience a remarkable transformation with the discovery of the functional plasticity of human stem cells. These include haemopoietic stem cells but also stem cells from different origins: embryonic and somatic. Following a phase of excitement and rapid accumulation of results demonstrating the regenerative potential, research in this field is currently undergoing verification studies and prospective phase III trials. This has opened a new era in regenerative medicine.

References

1. Van Beckum DW, de Vries JJ. Radiation Chimeras. London: Logos; 1967.
2. Santos GW. Bone marrow transplantation. In: Stollerman GH, editor. Advances in internal medicine. Chicago: Year Book Publishers; 1979. p. 157–82.
3. Fabricious MJ. Experimental studies of Hemorrhagic diathesis from X-ray sickness. Levin and Munskgaard: Copenhagen; 1922.
4. Jacobson LO, Simmoms EL, Marks EK, Eldredge JH. Recovery from irradiation injury. Science. 1951;113:510–1.
5. Nowell PC, Cole LJ, Habermeyer JG, Roan PL. Growth and continued function of rat marropw cells in X-irradiated mice. Cancer Res. 1956;16:258–61.
6. Mitchinson NA. The colonization of irradiated tisuue by transplanted spleen cells. Br J Exp Pathol. 1956;37:239–47.

7. Ford CE, Hamerton JL, Barnes DWH, Loutit JF. Cytological identification of radiation chimeras. Nature. 1956;177:239–47.

8. Billingham RE. The biology of graft versus host disease. Harvey Lect. 1967;62:21–78.

9. Gowans JL. The fate of the parental strain small lymphocytes in F1 hybrid rats. Ann NY Acad Sci. 1962;99:432–55.

10. Main JM, Prehn RT. Successful skin homografts after the administration of high dosage X-radiation and homologous bone marrow. J Natl Cancer Inst. 1955;15:1023–9.

11. Santos OW, Garver RM, Cole LJ. Acceptance of rat and mouse lung grafts by radiation chimeras. J Natl Cancer Inst. 1960;24:1367–87.

12. Thomas ED, Lochte HL, Lu WC, Ferrebee JW. Intravenous infusion of bone marrow in patients receiving radiation and chemotherapy. N Engl J Med. 1957;257:491–6.

13. Mathe G, Jammet H, Pendic B, et al. Transfusions et graffes de moelle osseuse homologue chez des humains irradies a haute dause accidentellement. Revue Francaise Etudes Cliniques et Biologiques. 1959;4:226–38.

14. Thomas ED, Buckner CD, Banaji M, et al. 100 patients with acute leikemia treated by chemotherapy, total body irradiation and allogeneic marrow transplantation. Blood. 1977;49:511–33.

15. Thomas ED, Buckner CD, Clift RA, et al. Marrow transplantation for acute non-lymphoblastic leukaemia in first remission. New Engl J Med. 1979;301:597–9.

16. Klein J, Sato A. The HLA system. First of two parts. New Engl J Med. 2000;343:702–9.

17. Marsh SGE, Albert ED, Bodmer WF, et al. Nomenclature for factors of the HLA system, 2002. Tissue Antigens. 2002;60:407–64.

18. Petersdorf EW, Gooley TA, Anasetti C, et al. Optimizing outcome after unrelated bone marrow transplantation by comprehensive matching of HLA class I and II alleles in the donor and recipient. Blood. 1998;92:3515–29.

19. Petersdorf EW, Anasetti C, Martin PJ, Hansen JA. Tissue typing in support of unrelated hematopoietic cell transplantation. Tissue Antigens. 2003;61:1–11.

20. Morishima Y, Sasazuki T, Inoko H, et al. The clinical significance of human leukocyte antigen (HLA) allele compatibility in patients receiving a marrow transplant from serologically HLA-A, HLA-B, and HLA-DR matched unrelated donors. Blood. 2002;99:4200–6.

21. Petersdorf EW, Kollman C, Hurley CK, et al. Effect of HLA class II gene disparity on clinical outcome in unrelated donor hematopoietic cell transplantation for chronic myeloid leukemia: the US National Marrow Donor Program Experience. Blood. 2001;98:2922–9.

22. Flomenberg N, Baxter-Lowe LA, Confer D, et al. Impact of HLA class I and class II high resolution matching on outcomes of unrelated donor. Blood. 2001;98:813a.

23. Weisdorf DJ, Anasetti C, Antin JH, et al. Allogeneic bone marrow transplantation for chronic myelogenous leukemia: comparative analysis of unrelated versus matched sibling donor transplantation. Blood. 2002 Mar 15;99(6):1971–7.

24. Couban S, Barnett M. The source of cells for allografting. Biol Blood Marrow Transplant. 2003;9:669–73.

25. Champlin RE, Schmitz N, Horowitz MM, et al. Blood stem cells compared with bone marrow as a source of hematopoietic cells for allogeneic transplantation. Blood. 2000;95:3702–9.

26. Bensinger WI, Martin PJ, Storer B, et al. Transplantation of bone marrow as compared with peripheral blood from HLA identical relatives in patients with hematologic cancers. New Engl J Med. 2001;344:175–81.

27. Blaise D, Kuentz M, Fournier C, et al. Randomized trial of bone marrow versus lenogastrim-primed blood cell allogeneic transplantation in patients with early stage leukemia: a report from the Société Française de Greffe de Moelle. J Clin Oncol. 2000;18:537–46.

28. Gorin NC, Labopin M, Rocha V, et al. for the acute leukemia working party (ALWP) of the European Cooperative group for Blood and Marrow Transplantation (EBMT) Marrow versus peripheral blood for geno-identical allogeneic stem cell transplantation in acute myelocytic leukemia: influence of dose and stem cell source shows better outcome with rich marrow Blood 2003; 102: 3043-3051.

29. Ringden O, Remberger M, Runde V. Peripheral blood stem cell transplantation from unrelated donors: a comparison with marrow transplantation. Blood. 1999;94:455–64.

30. Remberger M, Ringden O, Blau IW, et al. No difference in graft versus host disease, relapse and survival comparing peripheral blood stem cells to bone marrow using unrelated donors. Blood. 2001;98:1739–45.

31. Ringden O, Labopin M, Bacigalupo A, et al. Transplantation of peripheral blood stem cells as compared with bone marrow from HLA identical siblings in adult patients with acute myeloid leukemia and acute lymphoblastic leukemia. J Clin Oncol. 2002;20:4655–64.

32. Rocha V, Cornish J, Sievers EL, et al. Comparison of outcome of unrelated bone marrow and umbilical cord blood transplants in children with acute leukemia. Blood. 2001;97:2962–71.

33. Thomas, et al. A history of bone marrow transplantation. In: Blume KG, Forman SJ, Appelbaum FR, editors. Thomas' hematopoietic cell transplantation. 3rd ed. Oxford: Blackwell Publishing; 2004. p. 4–8.

34. Sencer SF, Haake RJ, Weisdorf DJ. Hemorrhagic cystitis after bone marrow transplantation. Risk factors and complications. Transplantation. 1993;56:875–9.

35. Gine E, Rovira M, Real I, Burrel M, Montana J, Carreras E, Montserrat E. Successful treatment of severe hemorrhagic cystitis after hemopoietic cell-transplantation by selective embolization of the vesical arteries. Bone Marrow Transplant. 2003;31:923–5.

36. McDonald GB, Hinds MS, Fisher LD, et al. Veno-occlusive disease of the liver and multiorgan failure after bone marrow transplantation: a cohort study of 355 patients. Ann Intern Med. 1993;118:255–67.

37. Carreras E, Bertz H, Arcese W, et al. Incidence and outcome of hepatic veno-occlusive disease (VOD) after blood and marrow transplantation (BMT): a prospective cohort study of the European group for Blood and Marrow Transplantation (EBMT). Blood. 1998;92:3599–604.

38. Lee JL, Gooley T, Bensinger W, et al. Veno-occlusive disease of the liver after busulfan, melphalan, and thiotepa conditioning therapy: incidence, risk factors, and outcome. Biol Blood Marrow Transplant. 1999;5:306–15.

39. Carreras E-Veno-occlusive disease of the liver after hematopoietic cell transplantation. Eu J Haematol. 2000;64:281–91.

40. DeLeve LD, Shulman HM, McDonald GB. Toxic injury to hepatic sinusoids: sinusoidal obstruction syndrome (veno-occlusive disease). Semin Liver Dis. 2002;22:27–42.

41. Carreras E, Grañena A, Navasa M, Bruguera M, Marco V, Sierra J, et al. Transjugular liver biopsy in BMT. Bone Marrow Transplant. 1993;11:21–6.

42. Or O, Nagler A, Shpilberg O, Elad S, Naparstek E, Kapelushnik J, et al. Low molecular weight heparin for the prevention of veno-occlusive disease of the liver in bone marrow transplantation patients. Transplantation. 1996;61:1067–71.

43. Richardson PG, Murakami C, Jin Z, et al. Multi-institutional use of defibrotide in 88 patients after stem cell transplantation with severe veno-occlusive disease and multisystem organ failure: response without significant toxicity in a high-risk population and factors predictive of outcome. Blood. 2002;100:4337–43.

44. Daly AS, Xenocostas A, Lipton JH. Transplantation-associated thrombotic microangiopathy: twenty-two years later. Bone Marrow Transplant. 2002;30:709–15.

45. Billingham RE. The biology of graft versus host reactions. Harvey Lect. 1966-1967;62:71–8.

46. Reddy P, Ferrara JLM. Immunobiology of acute graft-versus-host disease. Blood Rev. 2003;17:187–94.

47. Glucksberg H, Storb R, Fefer A, et al. Clinical manifestations of graft versus host disease in human recipients of marrow from HLA-matched sibling donors. Transplantation. 1974;18:295–304.

48. Przepiorka D, Weisdorf D, Martin P, et al. Consensus conference on acute GVHD grading. Bone Marrow Transplant. 1995;15:825–8.

49. Rowlings PA, Przepiorka D, Klein JP, et al. IBMTR severity index for grading acute GVHD: retrospective comparison with Glucksberg grade. Br J Haematol. 1997;97:855–64.

50. Shulmann H, Sullivan KM, Weiden PL, et al. Chronic graft-versus-host disease in man: a clinic pathologic study of 20 long term Seattle patients. Am J Med. 1980;69:204–17.

51. Akpek G, Lee SJ, Flowers ME, et al. Performance of a new clinical grading system for chronic graft-versus-host disease: a multicenter study. Blood. 2003;102:802–9.

52. Storb R, Deeg HJ, Whitehead J, et al. Methotrexate and cyclosporine compared with cyclosporine alone for prophylaxis of acute graft versus host disease after marrow transplantation for leukaemia. N Engl J Med. 1986;314:729–35.

53. Nash RA, Antin JH, Karanes C, et al. A phase III study comparing MTX and Tacrolimus with MTX and CsA for prophylaxis of acute GVHD after marrow transplantation from unrelated donors. Blood. 2000;96:2062–8.

54. Wagner JE, Thompson JS, Carter S, et al. Impact of GVHD prophylaxis on 3-year DFS: results of a multi-centre randomised phase II-III trial comparing T-cell depletion and CsA and MTX/CsA in 410 recipients of unrelated donor bone marrow. Blood. 2002;100:75a–6a.

55. Vogelsang GB. How I treat chronic graft-versus-host disease. Blood. 2001;97:1196–201.

56. Storek J, Dawson MA, Storer B, Stevens-Ayers T, Maloney DG, Marr KA, Witherspoon RP, Bensinger W, Flowers MED, Martin P, Storb R, Appelbaum FR. Boeckh: immune reconstitution after allogeneic marrow transplantation compared with blood stem cell transplantation. Blood. 2001;97:3380–9.

57. Storek J, Viganego F, Dawson MA, Tineke Herremans MMP, Boeckh M, Flowers MED, Storer B, Bensinger WI, Witherspoon RP, Maloney DG. Factors affecting antibody levels after allogeneic hematopoietic cell transplantation. Blood. 2003;1001:3319–24.

58. Shilling HG, McQueen KL, Cheng NW, Shizuru JA, Negrin RS, Parham P. Reconstitution of NK cell recetpor repertoire following HLA-matched hematopoietic cell transplantation. Blood. 2003;101:3730–40.

59. Talvensaari K, Clave E, Douay C, Rabian C, Garderet L, Busson M, Garnier F, Douek D, Gluckman E, Charron D, Toubert A. A Broad T-cell repertoire diversity and an efficient thymic function indicate a favorable long-term immune reconstitution after cord blood stem cell transplantation. Blood. 2002;99:1458–64.

60. Roux E, Dumont-Girard F, Starobinski M, Siegrist CA, Helg C, Chapuis B, Roosnek E. Recovery of immune reactivity after T-cell-depleted bone marrow transplantation depends on thymic activity. Blood. 2000;96:2299–303.

61. Hughes WT, Armstrong D, Bodey GP, et al. 2002 guidelines for the use of antimicrobial agents in neutropenic patients with cancer. Clin Infect Dis. 2002;34:730–51.

62. Marr KA. Epidemiology and outcome of mould infections in hematopoietic stem cell transplant recipients. Clin Infect Dis. 2002;34:909–17.

63. Junghanss C, Marr KA, Carter RA, et al. Incidence and outcome of bacterial and fungal infections following non-myeloablative compared with myeloablative allogeneic hematopoietic stem cell transplantation: a matched control study. Biol Blood Marrow Transplant. 2002;8(9):512–20.

64. Herbrecht R, Denning DW, Patterson TF, et al. Voriconazole *versus* Amphotericin B for primary therapy of invasive aspergillosis. New Engl J Med. 2002;347(6):408–15.

65. Reusser P, Einsele H, Lee J, et al. Randomized multicenter trial of foscarnet versus ganciclovir for pre-emptive therapy of cytomegalovirus infection after allogeneic stem cell transplantation. Blood. 2002;99(4):1159–64.

66. Ljungman P, Ward KN, Crooks BNA, et al. Respiratory virus infections after stem cell transplantation. A prospective study from the Infectious Diseases Working Party of the European Group for Blood and Marrow Transplantation. Bone Marrow Transplant. 2001;28:479–84.

67. Ljungman P, Ribaud P, Eyrich M, et al. Cidofovir for adenovirus infection after allogeneic stem cell transplantation (SCT). A retrospective survey of the Infectious Diseases Working Party of the European Group for Blood and Marrow Transplantation. Bone Marrow Transplant. 2003;31(6):481–6.

68. Martino R, Maertens J, Bretagne S, et al. Toxoplasmosis after hematopoietic stem cell transplantation. A study by the European Group for Blood and Marrow Transplantation Infectious Diseases Working Party. Clin Infect Dis. 2000;31(5):1188–94.

69. Woods WG, Neudorf S, Gold S, et al. A comparison of allogeneic bone marrow transplantation,autologous bone marrow transplantation, and aggressive chemotherapy in children with acute myeloid leukaemia in remission: a report from the Children's Cancer Group. Blood. 2001;97:56–62.

70. Creutzig U, Ritter J, Schellong G, for the AML-BFM Study Group. Identification of two risk groups in childhood acute myelogenous leukemia after therapy intensification in study AML-BFM-83 compared with study AML-BFM-78. Blood. 1990;75:1932–40.

71. Locatelli F, Labopin M, Ortega J, et al. Factors influencing outcome and incidence of long-term complications in children who underwent autologous stem cell transplantation for acute myeloid. Blood. 2003;15(101):1611–9.

72. Schiappe M. Very high risk childhood ALL: results from recent ALL-BFM trials intergroup studies. BMT. 2002;30(suppl 1):S16.

73. Uderzo C, Valsecchi MG, Bacigalupo A, et al. Treatment of childhood acute lymphoblastic leukemia in second remission with allogeneic bone marrow transplantation and chemotherapy: ten-year experience of the Italian Bone Marrow Transplantation Group and the Italian Pediatric Hematology Oncology Association. J Clin Oncol. 1995;13:352–8.

74. Fischer A, Cavazzana-Calvo M, De Saint-Basile G. Naturally occurring primary deficiencies of the immune system. Ann Rev Immunol. 1997;15:93–124.

75. Buckley R. Primary immunodeficiency diseases: dissector of the immunosystem. Immunol Rev. 2002;185:206–19.

76. Candotti F, Notarangelo L, Visconti R. Molecular aspects of primary immunodeficiencies: lessons from cytokine and other signaling pathways. J Clin Investi. 2002;109:1261–9.

77. Antoine C, Muller S, Cant A. Long-term survival and transplantation of haematopoietic stem cells for immunodeficiencies: report of the European experience 1968–1999. Lancet. 2003;361:553–60.

78. Buckley RH, Schiff SE, Schiff RI. Hematopoietic stem-cell transplantation for the treatment of severe combined immunodeficiency. N Engl J Med. 1999;340:508–16.

79. Bertrand Y, Landais P, Friedrich W. Influence of severe combined immunodeficiency phenotype on the outcome of HLA non-identical, T cell depleted bone marrow transplantation: a retrospective European survey from the European group for bone marrow transplantation and the European society for immunodeficiency. J Pediatr. 1999;134:740–8.

80. Guardiola P, Pasquini R, Dokal I, et al. Outcome of 69 allogeneic stem cell transplants for Fanconi anemia using HLA-matched unrelated donors: a study of the European Group for Blood and Marrow Transplantation. Blood. 2000;95:422–9.

81. Gaziev D. Stem cell transplantation for hemoglobinopathies. Curr Opin Pediatr. 2003;15:24–31.

82. Burnett AK. Current controversies: which patients with acute myeloid leukaemia should receive a bone marrow transplantation? – An adult treater's view. Br J Haematol. 2002;118:357–64.

83. Burnett AK, Wheatley K, Goldstone AH, Stevens RF, Hann IM, Rees JH, Harrison G, Medical Research Council Adult and Paediatric Working Parties. The value of allogeneic bone marrow transplant in patients with acute myeloid leukaemia at differing risk of relapse: results of the UK MRC AML 10 trial. Br J Haematol. 2002;118:385–400.

84. Lowenberg B, Downing JR, Burnett A. Acute myeloid Leukaemia. N Engl J Med. 1999;341:1051–62.

85. Suciu S, Mandelli F, de Witte T, et al. Allogeneic compared with autologous stem cell transplantation in the treatment of patients younger than 46 years with acute myeloid Leukaemia (AML) in first complete remission (CR1): an intention-to-treat analysis of the EORTC/GIMEMAAML-10 trial. Blood. 2003 Aug 15;102(4):1232–40.

86. Zittoun RA, Mandelli F, Willemze R, et al. Autologous or allogeneic bone marrow transplantation compared with intensive chemotherapy in acute myelogenous leukaemia. N Engl J Med. 1995;332:217–23.

87. Burnett AK, Goldstone AH, Stevens R, et al. Randomised comparison of addition of autologous bone-marrow transplantation to intensive chemotherapy for acute myeloid leukaemia in first remission: results of MRC AML 10 trial. Lancet. 1998;351:700–8.

88. Anasetti C. Advances in unrelated donor hematopoietic cell transplantation. Haematologica. 2003;88:246–9.

89. Grewal SS, Barker JN, Davies SM, Wagner JE. Unrelated donor hematopoietic cell transplantation: marrow or umbilical cord blood? Blood. 2003;101:4233–44.

90. Rocha V, Cornish J, Sievers EL, et al. Comparison of outcomes of unrelated bone marrow and umbilical cord blood transplants in children with acute Leukaemia. Blood. 2001;97:2962–71.

91. Ruggeri L, Capanni M, Urbani E, et al. Effectiveness of donor natural killer cell alloreactivity in mismatched hematopoietic transplants. Science. 2002;295:2097–100.

92. Ruggeri L, Capanni M, Casucci M, et al. Role of natural killer cell alloreactivity in HLA-mismatched hematopoietic stem cell transplantation. Blood. 1999;94:333–9.

93. Aversa F, Tabilio A, Velardi A, et al. Treatment of high-risk acute Leukaemia with T-cell-depleted stem cells from related donors with one fully mismatched HLA haplotype. N Engl J Med. 1998;339:1186–93.

94. Sebban C, Lepage E, Vernant JP, et al. Allogeneic bone marrow transplantation in adult acute lymphoblastic Leukaemia in first complete remission: a comparative study. French Group of Adult Acute Lymphoblastic Leukaemia. J Clin Oncol. 1994;12:2580–7.

95. Thiebaut A, Vernant JP, Degos L, et al. Adult acute lymphoblastic Leukaemia study testing chemotherapy and autologous and allogeneic transplantation. A follow-up report of the french protocol LALA 87. Hem Onc Clin North Am. 2000;14:1353–66.

96. Avivi I, Rowe JM, Goldstone AH. Stem cell transplantation in adult ALL patients. Best Pract Res Clin Haematol. 2003;15:653–74.

97. Horowitz MM, Messerer D, Hoelzer D, et al. Chemotherapy compared with bone marrow transplantation for adults with lymphoblastic Leukaemia in first remission. Ann Intern Med. 1991;115:13–8.

98. Oh H, Gale RP, Zhang M-J, et al. Chemotherapy vs HLA-identical sibling bone marrow transplants for adults with acute lymphoblastic Leukaemia in first remission. Bone Marrow Transplant. 1998;22:253–7.

99. Dombret H, Gabert J, Boiron JM, et al. Outcome of treatment in adults with Philadelphia chromosome-positive acute lymphoblastic leukemia – results of the prospective multicenter LALA-94 trial. Blood. 2002;100(7):2357–66.

Xenotransplantation 1.0 to 2.0

18

Omar Haque, Daniel Cloonan, Erin E. McIntosh, and Christiane Ferran

18.1 Introduction and Historic Perspective

The shortage of organs for transplantation is the single most important impediment to broad implementation of these life-saving procedures. Numerous efforts to expand the donor pool, including the use of living donors where possible, of extended criteria donor organs, and most recently of machine perfusion to improve organ quality of suboptimal allografts, have somewhat improved the numbers, yet the need is far from being met. In the United States alone, over 113,000 patients were listed for organ transplantation in 2019, with sadly 20 of them dying each day while awaiting transplantation [1].

Omar Haque and Daniel Cloonan equally contributed to this manuscript as first co-authors. Christiane Ferran is last and corresponding author.

O. Haque · D. Cloonan
Department of Surgery, Beth Israel Deaconess Medical Center, Harvard Medical School, Boston, MA, USA
e-mail: ojhaque@bidmc.harvard.edu; dcloonan@bidmc.harvard.edu

E. E. McIntosh
Department of Surgery, Harvard Medical School, Boston, MA, USA

Division of Vascular and Endovascular Surgery, Center for Vascular Biology Research, Beth Israel Deaconess Medical Center, Harvard Medical School, Boston, MA, USA

Utilizing nonhuman tissue to replace a failing organ is not novel, with the first trials dating back to the 1600s [2–4]. In the absence of advanced surgical techniques and of any knowledge of the immunologic response to xenotransplantation, these initial attempts promptly failed. It took over 3 centuries for xenotransplantation to resurface in the 1960s, around the time allotransplantation was also taking off thanks to the recognition of the immunosuppressive properties of steroids and of drugs such as Azathioprine [5]. Several pioneering attempts using kidney xenografts in 1963 [6], heart xenografts in 1964 [7], and liver xenografts in 1969 [8] failed within minutes to days due to hyperacute (HAR) and acute vascular rejection, AKA delayed xenograft rejection (AVR/DXR).

The advent of cyclosporine A (CsA) in 1976 marked a significant turning point for allotransplantation, but also xenotransplantation [9].

C. Ferran (✉)
Department of Surgery, Harvard Medical School, Boston, MA, USA

Division of Vascular and Endovascular Surgery, Center for Vascular Biology Research, Harvard Medical School, Boston, MA, USA

Division of Nephrology, Beth Israel Deaconess Medical Center, Harvard Medical School, Boston, MA, USA

The Transplant Institute, Beth Israel Deaconess Medical Center, Harvard Medical School, Boston, MA, USA
e-mail: cferran@bidmc.harvard.edu

© Springer Nature Switzerland AG 2021
N. Hakim et al. (eds.), *Transplantation Surgery*, Springer Specialist Surgery Series,
https://doi.org/10.1007/978-3-030-55244-2_18

Armed with effective and targeted immunosuppression, hope for the successful clinical utilization of xenografts gained national attention in the case of the famed Baby Fae. Born with a hypoplastic left heart, Baby Fae was operated on in 1984 by Dr. Leonard Bailey and received an ideal size matched baboon cardiac xenograft [10, 11]. Treated with CsA, the baboon heart xenograft functioned for 11 days prior to developing acute rejection that resulted in the patient's death at postoperative day 20 [12].

While no official moratorium was issued in the wake of Baby Fae's death, clinical use of xenografts still came to a halt that was further prompted by the growing success of allografts under CsA-based immunosuppression. The concept of clinical xenotransplantation was revisited in 1992 by Dr. Thomas Starzl, as he was developing tacrolimus as a novel immunosuppressive therapy [13]. Dr. Starzl attempted two baboon liver xenografts. His attempt was met with very limited success, as the first recipient, a 26-year old woman with fulminant liver failure, survived 70 days, while the second, a 62-year old man with hepatitis B cirrhosis, only survived 26 days [14, 15].

Other attempts at xenotransplantation in the following decade, including in Sweden [16], Poland [17], and India [18] faced the same barriers of HAR, AVR, and acute rejection (AR) as well as primary nonfunction [19]. At the molecular level, HAR, which plagued recipients of non-human primate (NHP)—mostly porcine— vascularized xenografts, was linked to preformed antibodies in humans that were directed against galactose alpha1,3-galactoyls (α1,3 Gal) epitopes oligosaccharide motifs expressed on porcine endothelium. Selected for their relatively similar visceral size, short age to maturity, relatively short generational turn over, as well as for obvious ethical and financial considerations, pigs were deemed the ideal species as xenograft donors. Using transgenic technologies, which were revolutionary at the time, a number of groups, including the one led by Dr. David Ayares in 2003, developed a line of alpha1,3-galactose transferase (α1,3GT) knockout pigs [20]. Unable to express α1,3 Gal, these pigs provided xenografts that were markedly less susceptible to HAR, as evidenced in experimental pig to NHP xenotransplantation models and clinically in pig to human xenotransplantation [21].

Unfortunately, with each hurdle crossed, a new barrier presented itself (Fig. 18.1). In the absence of alpha1,3-galactose-mediated HAR, incidence of early AVR/DXR became preeminent [22–24]. Named for its histopathologic similari-

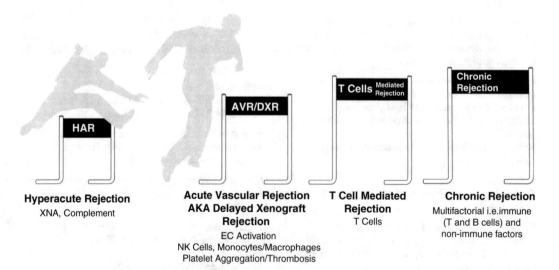

Hyperacute Rejection
XNA, Complement

Acute Vascular Rejection AKA Delayed Xenograft Rejection
EC Activation
NK Cells, Monocytes/Macrophages
Platelet Aggregation/Thrombosis

T Cell Mediated Rejection
T Cells

Chronic Rejection
Multifactorial i.e.immune (T and B cells) and non-immune factors

Fig. 18.1 The Immunological Barriers to Successful Xenotransplantation

ties to acute allograft rejection (AR), AVR is an apparent activation of the xenograft endothelium resulting in vascular inflammation, complement activation, coagulopathy, and inflammatory cytokine release [25–27]. The ability to create a transgenic line of pigs encompassing the genetic modifications (overexpression or KO) required to target all these pathogenic pathways was a titanic, if not impossible, endeavor, considering the limitations of the technology at hand.

The challenges posed by the molecular barriers to successful xenotransplantation were compounded by growing biological concern, namely relating to endogenous retroviruses. Endogenous clinical retroviruses are viruses which have integrated into their host germline DNA, and through a series of mutations ultimately became nonvirulent to their host species [28–30]. Discovery of these viruses in the pig, so called porcine endogenous retroviruses (or PERVs) raised significant concern for a possible trans-species reactivation and infection [31, 32]. In the setting of the potentially devastating infectious consequences that PERVs can cause if xenotransplantation were to proceed, Dr. Fritz Bach and Dr. Harvey Fineberg called for a temporary moratorium until further studies are performed to assess infectious risks to the recipient, and potentially to the general population [33, 34]. As a result, clinical and also much of experimental xenotransplantation was put on hold. Although host PERV infection was demonstrated in initial experimental models of porcine islet cell xenotransplantation [35], ultimately these results could not be repeated or verified with solid organ xenotransplants [36–38]. To date, available data seem to suggest that risks of zoonoses in the setting of xenotransplantation are minimal and manageable [39].

This optimistic view is comforted by the development of revolutionary gene-modifying technologies that have redefined, at the turn of the millennium, modern progress in xenotransplantation.

In the last decade, genetic technologies like CRISPR-Cas9 have opened the doors to multiple gene and gene cassette modifications, allowing the insertion and/or selective deletion of factors to tame xenograft rejection and dysfunction [40].

Targets have not only included alpha1,3-galactose, swine major histocompatibility complexes (MHCs), but also regulators of complement activation, inflammation and coagulation, and ultimately culminated in the inactivation and knockout of PERVs [41–44]. This represents an unprecedented leap forward for xenotransplantation with many potential benefits to come from these advancements. This rebirth of xenotransplantation has not only galvanized the medical and scientific communities, but also led to the burgeoning of at least four major biotechnology companies in Europe, North America, South America, and Asia, whose focus is on genetically modified porcine organs for human xenotransplantation [45–50].

This chapter will review the barriers to xenotransplantation from biochemical to immunologic, emerging technologies for the treatment and modification of xenografts, future directions in xenotransplantation, and, ultimately, provide a realistic assessment of the consequences and cost of this approach on a field of health care unbound by the need for human organ donation.

18.2 Immunological Barriers to Xenotransplantation

Immunological barriers to successful pig-to-primate xenografts result from robust responses of the innate and adaptive immune systems to the xenograft. These responses are characterized by unfettered inflammation predominating at the level of the endothelium of the vascularized xenograft, and by major dysregulation of the coagulation system, leading to a cataclysmic form of thrombotic microangiopathy. It is classically accepted that a porcine xenograft needs to sequentially survive xeno-specific and non-specific immunologic hurdles, which have made success quite elusive. Immunological hurdles to successful xenotransplantation range from very early HAR, to AVR/DXR, followed by classical T-cell-mediated AR, and ultimately chronic rejection (CR), permitted all other barriers are successfully surpassed (Fig. 18.1). We discuss below the molecular culprits driving these events, and describe the genetic and other interventions that may help overcome them.

18.2.1 Hyperacute Rejection: A Vanquished Obstacle

HAR is the first obstacle to successful xenotransplantation. Vascularized organs transplanted from pigs to primates are rejected within minutes to hours after reperfusion as a result of the pre-existing anti-porcine xenoreactive natural antibodies (XNA) present in humans and NHP. XNA recognize and bind specific surface antigens on porcine endothelial cells (EC). Subsequently, EC-bound XNA fix and activate the complement (C) cascade into forming the membrane-attack complex (MAC), which results in EC injury with associated thrombosis, edema, and subsequent consumptive coagulopathy, culminating in rapid, if not immediate, graft failure [51, 52].

The identification over 3 decades ago of a number of oligosaccharide moieties as the prime antigenic epitopes targeted by XNA was a major advance in the field of xenotransplantation [53]. The sugar moiety Gal α1,3-galactose (α1,3 Gal) is the most prominent of these xenoantigens [54]. α1,3Gal is present in most mammals, including New World monkeys, but not in humans or Old World monkeys and apes [54]. This relates to evolutionary genetic events, which occurred 20–30 million years ago in humans and Old World NHP to protect their survival against pathogens [55]. These genetic modifications led to the suppression of the activity of the α1,3Galactosyl transferase (α1,3GT), the key enzyme that catalyzes the formation of α1,3Gal epitopes (Galα1,3Galβ1,4GlcNAc-R) [56]. Consequently, the α1,3Gal structure became highly immunogenic, and triggered a robust humoral immune response in humans [57]. Natural preformed anti-α1,3Gal antibodies are the most abundant natural antibodies, accounting for 1% of immunoglobulins. Generated during neonatal life as a response to α1,3Gal-expressing viruses and microorganisms that colonize the primate's gastrointestinal tract, the vast majority of anti-α1,3Gal XNA are IgM and IgG, with IgA less frequently [58]. However, anti-α1,3Gal IgE can also be detected in certain individuals allergic to meat, or to the therapeutic antibody Cituximab [58]. Anti-α1,3Gal IgM and IgG antibodies are the dominant isotypes that bind to the α1,3Gal moieties expressed on the pig vasculature [20]. Other non-α1,3Gal oligosaccharides, absent in humans, can also elicit XNA. These include N-Glycolylneuraminic acid (Neu5Gc), synthesized by the cytidine monophospho-N-acetylneuraminic acid hydroxylase (CMAH) gene, which is inactive in humans [59]; and also the human SDa blood antigens, synthesized by the beta-1,4-N-acetyl-galactosaminyltransferase 2 (B4GALNT2) [60]. Whether all three enzymes (α1,3GT, CMAH, B4GALNT2), or only the dominant α1,3GT, need to be knocked out in pigs produced for xenotransplantation remains to be seen, especially in light of the other simultaneously targeted pathways to block complement, maintain a healthy, anti-inflammatory and anti-thrombotic endothelium, and resist innate and adaptive immune responses [61–64].

With improved understanding of the molecular basis of HAR, it became evident that elimination of XNA and inhibition of complement activation was the obligate path to overcome this hurdle [65, 66]. For long, the solution remained elusive as a number of therapeutic modalities to deplete XNA in the recipient by plasmapheresis or by immunoaffinity columns, and/or to inhibit complement with cobra venom factor (CVF) or various other inhibitors, remained unsuccessful [52, 67–69]. Inhibition of complement-mediated injury in this context was further confounded by interspecies molecular incompatibilities. Indeed, cell surface-anchored porcine complement-regulatory proteins (CRP) equivalent to human decay accelerating factor (DAF, CD55), membrane cofactor protein (MCP, CD46), complement receptor 1 (CR1) and CD59, whose function is to contain complement-mediated cell damage efficiently protected pig cells against porcine complement, but were ineffective against human complement [66, 70]. In pioneering work, Dalmasso and Bach were the first to introduce human CD55 into porcine EC and show its effectiveness in inhibiting complement-mediated lysis in the presence of human serum [71, 72]. This provided strong proof-of-concept validating this approach to overcome HAR. Technological breakthroughs in the late 80's and early 90's, specifically the advent of transgenesis offered the ideal platform to do that [72, 73]. The first transgenic pigs expressing the human CD55 were generated by White *et al.* in the mid-1990s [74–76]. Their use in pig to primate xenotransplantation models improved HAR, but also obviated the need to express additional human CRP to achieve full benefit. In their current iteration, genetically modified pigs prepped for clinical xenotransplantation express two (CD55/CD46) or three human CRP (CD55/CD46/CD59) [63, 77, 78]. Knockout of the different enzymes catalyzing the production of the xenogeneic oligosaccharides was the obvious second intervention required to block HAR. The generation of KO pigs proved more tedious than transgenic gene overexpression with often random integration. However, with major advancement in cloning and gene-targeting strategies based on homologous recombination, the first α1,3-galactosyltransferase gene-knockout (GTKO) pig was produced in 2003, with initial studies showing prevention of HAR [20]. Again, with the discovery of additional oligosaccharide moieties driving XNA, the current iteration of the donor pig includes additional KO of CMAH (Neu5Gc), and to less extent of B4GALNT2 (SDa) [64, 79]. Importantly, both pigs genetically modified to express human CD55/CD46/CD59 or knocked out for GT/CMAH/B4GALNT2 had normal viability and were fertile.

18.2.2 Acute Vascular Rejection/Delayed Xenograft Rejection: An Endothelial-Centric Tale

Following the successful prevention of HAR, the field was faced with another form of rejection that did not involve T cells or resembled any classical form of allograft rejection, but shared many of the pathologic features of HAR. This form of rejection occurs within days or weeks after transplantation and is referred to as delayed xenograft rejection (DXR) or acute vascular rejection (AVR) [24]. The key pathogenic events driving DXR include the deposition on the graft endothelium of xenoreactive (mostly elicited) antibodies (EXA) and associated binding/activation of complement. This results in an explosive activation of the vascularized graft endothelium. In turn, the acquisition by activated EC of a pro-inflammatory and pro-thrombotic phenotype promotes graft infiltration by activated macrophages and NK cells, which by releasing pro-inflammatory cytokines further amplifies the inflammatory and procoagulant environment. These events culminate in a catastrophic form of thrombotic microangiopathy that ultimately causes graft loss [23, 24, 80]. Unfettered activation of the endothelium and associated change in EC phenotype is the presumed proximal cause of AVR/DXR [23, 24, 81].

Physiologically, a healthy endothelium is paramount to maintaining blood flow and actively preventing thrombosis, detoxifying the organism from reactive oxygen species, and maintaining an appropriate barrier between the blood and the parenchyma of organs [81–83]. These functions are ensured by a number of surface molecules expressed on healthy, non-activated EC. These include: thrombomodulin that binds and activates protein C (aPC), which then binds to protein S (PS) to form one of the most potent anti-coagulant systems of the body [84]; heparan sulfate, which binds antithrombin III to also provide anti-coagulation, the anti-oxidant enzyme superoxide dismutase, and ecto-ATPDase (CD39) that metabolizes ATP into ADP and AMP to inhibit platelet activation and aggregation [85, 86]. Expression and/or activity of these key anti-coagulant and anti-inflammatory molecules is lost or decreased following EC activation—a situation exacerbated by other xeno-specific constraints, notably porcine-human molecular compatibilities of some of these molecules, namely thrombomodulin.

In addition to the loss of built-in protection, the drastic phenotypic change of activated EC is the result of a well-orchestrated transcriptional program that results in the *de novo* expression of a number of molecules (more than 40) that initiate and intensify inflammation and thrombosis

[87]. These proteins include adhesion molecules, such as E-selectin, ICAM-1, VCAM-1 and P-selectin, that facilitate the binding of host mononuclear cells (MNC) to the endothelium and promote bidirectional signaling to further activate EC; pro-thrombotic genes such as tissue factor (the most potent stimulus for coagulation) and plasminogen activator inhibitor 1 (PAl−1), which prevents the dissolution of fibrin clots, and a number of cytokines, including interleukin-1 (IL-1), IL-6, IL-8, MCP-1 and others, that attract host immune cells to the site of the graft [82, 83].

It was evident that the only path to overcome AVR/DXR required inhibiting EC activation, and taming coagulation and thrombosis. By the early 1990s, the field of xenotransplantation moved to achieve this task. This was facilitated by an improved understanding of EC biology that shed light on a few proximal players the targeting of which could influence many of the distal pathogenic effectors of AVR/DXR. The transcription factor nuclear factor kappa B (NF-κB), whose activation results in early gene activation, topped the list of candidates [88–91]. Indeed, most of the genes induced upon EC activation (E-selectin, VCAM-1, ICAM-1, IL-1, IL-6, IL-8, MCP-1, TF, PAI-1) have at least one binding site for NF-κB in their promoters [87, 92–94]. Inhibiting NF-κB, a potent regulator of EC activation, would hinder all aspects of EC activation, independently of the stimulus, including in the context of AVR/DXR.

Briefly, the active DNA binding form of NF-κB is a heterodimer, consisting of members of the NF-κB/Rel family of transcription factors, most prominently canonical NF-κB1 (p50) and RelA (p65) subunits [95, 96]. NF-κB is retained in the cytoplasm of quiescent endothelial cells by association with its inhibitory protein, IκBα. Upon activation of the cell, IκBα is phosphorylated, ubiquitinated, and becomes susceptible to proteolysis, which leads to dissociation from the NF-κB dimer [90]. The release of NF-κB from IκBα in turn allows the active p50-p65 dimer to transmigrate into the nucleus, bind to its target DNA sequence element and activate transcription [97]. In absence of specific small molecule inhib-itors, the obvious choice was to overexpress IκBα, the physiologic inhibitor of NF-κB, or better a phosphorylation-resistant mutant of IκBα. However, data from our laboratory in EC, and from others, showed that inhibition of NF-κB by overexpression of IκBα or knocking down p65/RelA, even if it did inhibit activation, sensitized cells to TNF-mediated apoptosis [98–100]. These data were in keeping with novel evidence that we and others posited, i.e. NF-κB signaling does not only set in motion a pro-inflammatory program, but also an anti-apoptotic program whose function is to promote cell survival in the face of injury [101].

In earlier work, our group made the seminal discovery that a number of NF-κB dependent genes in EC, namely the 7-Zn finger and ubiquitin-editing protein, A20, and the anti-apoptotic Bcl family member, A1/Bfl1, did not only protect EC from apoptotic cell death, but were also as potent as IκBα at inhibiting NF-κB activation [102–105]. These genes immediately became the prime candidates to inhibit NF-κB activation. We demonstrated that their overexpression in EC fully inhibited NF-κB activation in response to a whole gamut of activators, including those relevant to DXR. This was accomplished without sensitizing these cells to TNF-mediated apoptosis, all the while actively protecting EC from apoptosis, and other forms of necrotic cell death, including complement- and NK-mediated cell death [102, 103, 105, 106]. That cytoprotective A20 and A1 require NF-κB for their expression aligns with their intended function as part of a negative feedback loop aimed at preventing inflammation from reaching a certain intensity that would otherwise lead to the demise of the cells. Accordingly, they not only downregulate the expression of proinflammatory proteins, but also their own expression to bring cells back to their basal phenotype [107].

The dual anti-inflammatory and anti-apoptotic functions of A20 and A1 in EC is shared by other anti-apoptotic proteins, namely the prototypic anti-apoptotic Bcl family members, Bcl-2 and Bcl-x_L [108]. However, in contrast to A20, Bcl-2 and Bcl-x_L are different in that they are constitutively expressed in EC, are not induced by proinflammatory cytokines, and do not depend on NF-κB for their expression. This places them in a different category of regulatory molecules from A20 in that they are expressed independently of NF-κB, but can modulate its activation [107]. Exploitation of these genes for the genetic engineering of porcine endothelium to prevent DXR is indirectly supported by some of our earlier work. Long-term survival, despite the return of anti-graft antibodies and complement, in a model of hamster-to-rat heart xenotransplantation treated with cobra venom factor and cyclosporine A associated with increased expression of A20, A20, Bcl-2, Bcl-x$_L$, and hemoxygenase-1 (HO-1) in the xenograft vasculature, specifically EC [101]. Hearts that were rejected either did not express (A20, Bcl) or expressed lower levels (HO-1) of these genes. Bach et al. termed this phenomenon of graft survival despite the return of the offenders, "accomodation" [109, 110]. Remarkably, "accommodated" vessels of long-term surviving heart xenografts were also protected from transplant arteriosclerosis (TA), the pathognomonic feature of chronic allograft rejection, that in contrast was florid in rejecting xenografts whose vasculature did not express the aforementioned genes. This data agrees with related observations in models of vascular allografts, whereby overexpression of A20 and HO1 (or one of its downstream metabolites) also protected from TA [111–116].

Either A20 or any of the Bcl genes could eventually fulfill our aim of protecting the xenograft endothelium and maintaining its barrier and anti-inflammatory, anti-coagulant functions. However, many of A20's attributes, including its cellular distribution—lysosomal as opposed to mitochondrial for Bcl genes—and additional functions qualifying its atheroprotective, renoprotective, β-cell protective, and hepato-regenerative potential, made it one the most attractive candidates for genetic engineering of pigs destined for xenotransplantation [111, 117–132].

For review, A20, discovered as a TNF response gene in human umbilical vein EC [133], is a well-described negative regulator of many inflammatory pathways that culminate in NF-κB activation, as we first reported in EC [102, 134]. A20 also modulates cell survival in a cell type-dependent manner via caspase-dependent and independent mechanisms [106, 133, 135]. The molecular basis for A20-mediated inhibition of NF-κB is not totally resolved, but highly depends on both enzymatic and non-enzymatic ubiquitin editing functions of this versatile molecule [136]. A20 alters ubiquitination and therefore function or level of expression of a number of signaling molecules within the NF-κB pathway, including receptor interacting protein (RIP) kinase, and IKKγ [137, 138]. The latter would capture all NF-κB pathways converging into the signalosome, therefore accounting for the broad NF-κB inhibitory effect of A20, including a wide spectrum of EC activators such as TNF, ROS, the CD40/CD40L dyad, and likely xeno-related offenders [102, 103, 105]. As an increasing number of proteins and biologic processes regulated by ubiquitination is unfolding, we are just starting to grasp the complexity and broad implications of cell- and tissue-specific functions of A20 based on the respective ubiquitome of each cell/tissue [106, 137].

Basal A20 levels are low to undetectable in most cell types. However, its expression is rapidly induced, in a NF-κB dependent manner, in response to a number of danger signals, whether infectious, auto-immune or mechanical [101]. As mentioned earlier, A20 is part of a negative feedback loop aimed at secondarily interrupting inflammation. Regardless of the mechanisms by which A20 terminates inflammatory signals, its dominant role in maintaining homeostasis is emphasized in A20-null mice that develop cachexia and die pre-maturely from uncontrolled severe multi-organ inflammation [135]. This outcome confirms the physiological role A20 plays in modulating inflammation, a central component to many disease processes, including xenograft rejection.

Our laboratory has extensively investigated the functions of A20 in multiple cell types, including EC and vascular smooth muscle cell (SMC). We demonstrated that A20 combines anti-inflammatory and anti-apoptotic functions in EC [102, 103, 106, 139]. In SMC, A20 is anti-inflammatory, but also inhibits SMC proliferation and unexpectedly promotes apoptosis of only the SMC that undergo a phenotypic change from contractile (media) to secretory (neointima) [124]. These functions qualify A20 as an optimal candidate to contain pathologic vascular remodeling, including in atherosclerosis, transplant arteriosclerosis, and, as we previously postulated, xenograft-associated AVR/DXR [132]. In recent years, we uncovered that the atheroprotective effect of A20 goes beyond inhibition of NF-κB inflammatory signals, as A20 also interrupts atherogenic IFNγ signaling by decreasing expression levels of its key intracellular transducer, STAT1, in both EC and SMC [111, 140, 141]. These vascular functions of A20 translate into strong *in vivo* therapeutic benefits. Overexpression of A20 using gene therapy tools resulted in prevention and regression of intimal hyperplasia in a rat carotid model of post-balloon angioplasty [124, 126]. Similarly, A20 overexpression in the aortic arch of diabetic ApoE-KO mice that develop accelerated atherosclerosis significantly reduced atherosclerotic lesions in this *bona fide* model of diabetic vasculopathy [127]. Relevant to the transplantation field, overexpression of A20 in fully mismatched C57BL/6 (H2^b) to BALB/c (H2^d) aorta to carotid artery allografts reduced transplant arteriosclerosis by modulating inflammatory and apoptotic signals, and by remarkably boosting regulatory over pathogenic immune responses, in part through altering the IL-6/TGFβ ratio in the graft [111]. This latter effect of graft-expressed A20 on the alloimmune response agrees with the importance of dampening inflammation as a means to prevent rejection and possibly drive tolerance [112, 142–144].

As mentioned earlier, the promise of A20 as a gene candidate to overcome DXR is reinforced by its many pleiotropic functions in other cell types, including hepatocytes and β cells. Extensive data from our laboratory and others have established the unique hepatoprotective function of A20. Overexpression of A20 in mouse livers protects from chemically-

induced acute fulminant hepatitis [120], lethal and sublethal radical hepatectomy [122, 128], and severe ischemia reperfusion injury [125], all of which captures its "Promethean" qualities that could benefit liver allo and xenografts [131]. Additionally, overexpression of A20 in murine islet grafts improves function and survival of a suboptimal β cell mass and cures diabetes [121]. Akin to vascular allografts, overexpression of A20 in a mouse model of allogeneic islet transplantation transforms the alloimmune response from pathogenic to regulatory, fueling long-term acceptance of these grafts [145]. The first A20 transgenic pig was created in 2009. Even though transgene expression remained moderate, and was limited to skeletal muscle, heart and aortic EC, the authors were still able to validate A20's anti-inflammatory and anti-apoptotic functions [146]. Current iterations of the ideal donor pig consistently include A20.

Besides classical anti-apoptotic genes, other genes that meet the criteria of protecting the endothelium and maintaining its function include two heme-induced molecules, ferritin and HO-1, that function to reduce oxidative damage in an iron-rich environment [147, 148]. In EC, ferritin is induced by heme to protect these cells from the damage incurred by activated neutrophils, and also to inhibit NF-κB activation, although not as effectively as the aforementioned anti-apoptotic genes [149, 150]. Perhaps more potent than ferritin were the many discoveries that showed that HO-1, the rate-limiting enzyme in heme metabolism and whose expression is induced in EC and monocytes in response to stress [151, 152], is a potent "protective" gene whose expression in the vasculature of hamster to heart xenografts is key to the "accommodation" and long-term survival of these grafts [101, 110, 153]. The anti-inflammatory properties of HO-1 depend on the ability of this enzyme to degrade heme to generate bilirubin, free iron, and carbon monoxide (CO). Bilirubin is a potent antioxidant, free iron results in expression of the cytoprotective gene ferritin, and carbon monoxide (CO) at low concentrations inhibits macrophage activation, and NF-κB pro-inflammatory signaling as well as apoptotic responses in EC [154–157]. In addition to HO-1, both bilirubin and CO have been exploited therapeutically to prevent and improve ischemia-reperfusion injury, acute rejection, and transplant arteriosclerosis in animal models of vascularized kidney, heart and lung allografts [114, 115, 152, 158–163]. They have also been highly beneficial experimentally in improving islet graft survival and liver regeneration and repair [129, 164–166]. As for A20, HO-1 tops the list of transgenes that have been overexpressed in the current iteration of the desirable donor pig for xenotransplantation. This will be reviewed in more details under the wish list section.

Disordered coagulation and thrombosis, causing generalized microangiopathy, associated with explosive platelet activation and aggregation is another key pathognomonic feature of DXR. Severe thrombotic microangiopathy still occurrs in swine-to-baboon kidney xenografts despite knock down of α1,3GT or overexpression of human DAF [167]. As stated earlier, the molecular basis of this consumptive coagulopathy, that is particularly severe in liver xenografts, relates to loss of EC-expressed negative regulators of coagulation (thrombomodulin, heparan sulfate and the ectoNTPdase, CD39) [86, 168–170], gain by the activated vasculature of pro-thrombotic attributes (TF), and molecular incompatibilities between the human and the pig coagulation system (thrombomodulin) [171]. Numerous non-genetic based approaches tackling different pathogenic effectors of this cascade, such as infusion of thrombomodulin, administration of apyrase, inhibition of platelet GPIIbIIIa, TF knock down using silencing RNA or development of a PSGL1-targeted CD39 molecule that homes to the endothelial-platelet microenvironment, have shown some beneficial effect in support of their choice as valid targets for the genetic engineering of the desired pig donor for xenotransplantation [172–176]. Transgenic pigs expressing human thrombomodulin were among the first animals to be generated. Other targets including CD39, or Tissue factor Pathway Inhibitor (TFPI) are also being considered [62].

18.2.3 Beyond DXR: The Adaptive Immune Response

As the hurdles of HAR and DXR are surmounted, the xenograft has to face the wrath of the adaptive immune response. Mounting evidence suggests that a number of patients on transplant waitlists can still have circulating xenoreactive antibodies that bind to antigens on porcine cells even from donors where α1,3GT, CMAH, B4GALNT2 have been knocked out (triple KO). On further analysis, these antibodies were anti-HLA antibodies from pre-sensitized patients cross-reacting with class I swine leukocyte antigen (SLA) class I [177]. Accordingly, SLA class I was deemed an obvious target for genome editing in xenotransplantation. A number of SLA class I knockout donor pigs were created for future use in xenotransplantation [61, 177, 178]. Pre-sensitized patients with humoral immunity toward HLA class II molecules may also show cross-reactivity with SLA class II molecules of the xenograft [179]. In that case, site-specific epitope mutagenesis may be attempted in order to decrease binding of these antibodies to pig cells [180]. Based on the above, screening patients for xenoreactive antibody is extremely important when evaluating their individual risk benefit. In the absence of any detectable xenoreactive antibody, one can expect that the only next hurdle that needs to be controlled is that of a classic T-cell-mediated acute cellular rejection [181–184].

Human T-cell responses to porcine xenografts is well documented. This xenograft counterpart of the T-cell-mediated rejection response seen in allografts is reportedly more robust than the one encountered in allografts [185]. Both the direct and indirect pathway of antigen presentation appear to be involved in these anti-pig xenograft responses. However, accumulating *in vivo* evidence from pig-to-primate models suggests that this T-cell response can be overcome by immunosuppressive agents applicable to allotransplantation. However, and in order to achieve reasonable survival, the immunosuppressive regimen that needs to be implemented is often much heavier. Prolonged survival of porcine heart, kidney, or islet xenografts, derived from donors genetically modified to subdue XNA and complement attack, received a combinatorial immunosuppressive protocol that included anti-CD4 and anti-CD8 T-cell depletion, co-stimulation blockade with anti-CD154 or CTLA4-Ig, mycophenolic acid, cyclosporine A, tacrolimus, and steroids [186, 187]. Experience-based learning as the field cautiously progresses demonstrates that the need to efficiently target CD4 T-cells and provide strong co-stimulation blockade is critical in xenotransplantation [187–190]. Obviously, high infectious and oncogenic risks that associate with such potent immunosuppressive regimens are not compatible with acceptable clinical risks. A significant effort has been devoted to the pursuit of tolerance of xenografts through genetic manipulations of the immune system or other means to achieve mixed hematopoietic chimerism [182, 183, 191, 192]. Here again, tolerance has proven to be much more difficult to achieve in xeno than in allo-transplantation. As the field keeps learning, the issue of molecular incompatibilities between pigs and primates was identified as a potential route cause for the difficulty to tolerize. In a recent paper, Tena et al. showed that the difficulty to achieve mixed hematopoietic chimerism in a pig-to-NHP xenograft combination related to the rapid clearance of porcine hematopoietic stem cells by primate macrophages as a result of the ineffectiveness of porcine CD47, which usually blocks phagocytosis, to transduce the required inhibitory signals through the primate regulatory protein alpha [193]. Accordingly, genetic engineering of porcine cells to express human CD47 prolonged transient chimerism, and survival in a pig-to-baboon skin xenograft model [193].

Which genetic modifications will be required to mitigate the T-cell xeno response and prevent acute rejection (AR), and possibly chronic rejection (CR), or even achieve tolerance is still being resolved. However, thanks to a better understanding of the molecular basis for the formidable immunological barriers to xenotransplantation, including through greater appreciation of the role of molecular incompatibilities, and to the ever-growing technical revolutions in gene editing,

one can be cautiously optimistic that clinical translation will soon be looming, if not already happening, at least for skin and islets [194, 195].

18.3 Revolutionary Technologies Breaking the Barriers

Interest for xenotransplantation over the last decades progressed in phases which paralleled technological breakthroughs that reignited the hopes of the medical and the scientific communities in its success. These ranged from major discoveries enabling modifications of the pig genome to derail rejection and improve compatibility, to engineering prowess that led to the development of a number of devices for *ex vivo* perfusion of organs to improve viability and permit delivery of drugs and gene therapies. In this section, we will briefly review some of these technologies, chief of which being the medical revolution brought upon by the CRISPR/Cas9 based technique that enabled, for the first time, simultaneous multiplex genome editing, the engine that reignited the field of xenotransplantation [196, 197].

18.3.1 Genetic Modifications: Transgenesis and Targeted Disruption

A transgenic animal is an animal whose genome has been deliberately modified by input from another organism with the intended consequence of altering the phenotype of the recipient organism [74]. The term "transgenesis" was first coined by J.W. Gordon and F.H. Ruddle in 1981, as they successfully demonstrated integration, even if random, and stable germ line transmission of genes injected into the mouse pronuclei of fertilized eggs [198]. Transmitted through the germ line, every cell, including germ cells, contain the same modified genetic material that becomes an inheritable trait. In addition to microinjection of DNA material into fertilized eggs, two other methodologies based on retrovirus-mediated gene transfer [199], and embryonic stem cell-mediated gene transfer [200] were also successful in achieving the same outcome. The possibility to insert the foreign DNA under a given cell-type specific promoter and in cassettes with built-in regulatory systems, such as tetracycline or tamoxifen, further empowered this technology by enabling the restriction of transgene expression to certain cell types and by switching it on or off on-demand [201–203].

First successful in mice, these techniques were later adapted to large animals, including pigs for xenotransplantation. The world's first transgenic pig was produced in 1995 at Cambridge University to express human DAF/CD55. CD55 expression favorably compared to normal controls and was able to overcome HAR [74–76]. A 6.5 kilobase minigene for human DAF was microinjected into porcine fertilized ova. Over 2/3 of the pigs transcribed the DAF message, but the amount of protein expressed in different tissues varied from pig to pig and from tissue to tissue in a given pig. DAF transgenic pigs developed normally and had no major side-effects, including as related to reproductive ability. With the success of DAF, pigs were generated to express the 2 other key CRP i.e. human CD46 (membrane cofactor protein) and CD59 (membrane inhibitor of reactive lysis, MIRL), and were equally as effective in reducing HAR and prolonging the survival of pig-to-NHP xenotransplants [204–206]. However, triple transgenic pigs expressing all 3 human CRP (CD46, CD55, and CD59) more effectively resisted the complement attack than double transgenic (CD55 and CD59) or mono-transgenic animals [207, 208].

Transgenic pigs were also created to improve the disordered coagulation, consumptive coagulopathy, and EC dysfunction that associate with DXR. These included key human regulators of coagulation and thrombosis, including human thrombomodulin (TM), TFPI, and CD39 whose function does not transcend species [209–212]. A transgenic pig expressing human TM, together with CD46, achieved long xenograft survival (945 days) in a heterotopic pig-to-NHP cardiac xenotransplantation model [209, 210]. Beyond gain of function, transgenic expression of siRNA against pro-coagulant molecules has also been implemented to inhibit consumptive coagulopathy of DXR. Niemann et al. used siRNA to knock down the porcine tissue factor (TF) gene, which decreased its expression by 94.1%, increased coagulation time, and decreased clotting compared with matched control animals [175]. On the EC front, transgenic pigs expressing A20, HO-1, as well as an inhibitor of TNF, have also been generated and shown to protect cells against inflammation and apoptosis [146, 213, 214]. *In vivo*, transgene expression was limited to some cells and organs, hence optimization may be required before we can gauge the full impact of these protective genes on DXR and beyond on xenograft survival and function.

In contrast to gain of function, knockout of pig genes deleterious to the success of xenotransplantation, namely the different enzymes required to produce glycans or SLA Class I molecules, has initially proven more difficult to achieve. While Capecchi et al. developed the methodology for creating targeted alterations in the mouse genome in the late 80's [215], the creation of KO pigs has been much more challenging. Difficulty came from the lack of identifiable embryonic stem cells (ES) in the pig, which would preclude using homologous recombination to create targeted gene deletion. Hence, the first attempts to reduce expression of $\alpha 1,3$Gal in pigs used an indirect strategy whereby pigs were rather made transgenic for H-transferase in order to reduce cell surface carbohydrates [216]. However, after many failures, a first success came in 2003 when the first pigs with a KO in $\alpha 1,3$GT (GTKO) were created using homologous recombination to delete a single copy of $\alpha 1,3$GT, followed by back breeding to homozygosity [20]. This process took almost three years to complete. As molecular biology techniques evolved, including through the discovery of zinc finger nucleases (ZFN), and transcription activator-like effector nucleases (TALEN), it became easier to produce homozygous KO cells in a single reaction and to generate KO pigs within 5–6 months [196, 217]. These techniques enabled the creation of biallelic KO pigs to eliminate more xenoantigens by knocking down 2 of the enzymes involved in the production of cell

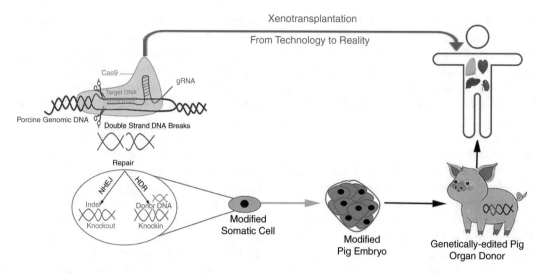

Fig. 18.2 A Schematic Representation of the CRISPR/Cas9 Gene Editing Tool

surface xenogeneic glycans [64, 79]. Finally, the true medical revolution came from the introduction in 2013 of the Clustered Regularly Interspaced Short Palindromic Repeats/CRISPR-associated protein 9 (CRISPR/Cas9) gene editing technology. This technology fueled a medical revolution in the field of xenotransplantation, but also in medicine in general. CRISPR/Cas9 not only facilitated the timely creation of multiple concurrent homozygous gene deletions, but also the introduction of many other genes stacked together in one expression cassette. KO pigs were created with simultaneous KO of the 3 enzymes that produce cell surface xenogeneic glycans in addition to SLA class I KO.

18.3.2 Gene Editing: The CRISPR/Cas 9 Medical Revolution

The CRISPR/Cas9 system is a breakthrough gene editing technology that allows targeted and precise modification of the genome of a living organism through DNA insertion, deletion, replacement, or modification (Fig. 18.2).

The CRISPR/Cas9 system was originally identified in bacteria and archaea as a form of adaptive immunity [218]. CRISPRs are a family of specialized regions of DNA with two dis-

tinct qualities: repeated nucleotide sequences and spaces. They are the result of bacteria capturing snippets of DNA from invading viruses and utilizing this genetic material to create CRISPR arrays. These enable the bacteria to better respond and target the viral DNA if faced with a second insult [219–223]. These sequences are recognized by Cas9, a dual RNA-guided DNA endonuclease enzyme that functions as a pair of molecular scissors, cutting DNA at specific locations in a genome. From studies that deciphered how these immune systems function in bacteria, scientists realized the technological potential of the RNA-guided DNA cleaving enzyme, Cas9, for genome engineering. The guide RNA binds to DNA at a pre-designed sequence and directs the Cas9 protein to the desired segment that needs to be cut. Once the DNA is cut, the cell's natural repair mechanisms are initiated and can change the genome in two ways. One is a simple repair mechanism that brings the two ends together (non-homologous end joining, NHED). The second repair mechanism utilizes a short strand of DNA as a template to fill the gap with a sequence of nucleotides [224]. Scientists can modify this strand of DNA to their choosing, and as a result, introduce any gene or correct any genetic mutation [225].

Relevant to xenotransplantation, CRISPR/ Cas9 offers several advantages over previous site-specific nucleases. The Cas9 endonuclease has the ability to associate with multiple guide RNAs and, hence, permits simultaneous targeting of several loci within a single transfection. This is ideal in the setting of xenotransplantation as it allowed for the efficient combination of multiple genetic KO on a single cell, and also overexpression of several protective genes stacked in a single expression cassette. This has been highly instrumental in creating pigs, where all 3 enzymes GGTA1/CMAH/B4GalNT2, and SLA Class I have been knocked out, and all 3 CRP (CD46, CD55, CD59) have been overexpressed together with human thrombomodulin and anti-inflammatory/cytoprotective A20 and HO-1 [61, 63, 223, 226].

While widely approved in xenotransplantation, CRISPR/Cas9 gene editing faces many ethical concerns when it comes to its application to modify the human genome. Currently, most of its use for therapeutic purposes is limited to somatic cells (cells that are not egg or sperm cells) for fear of opening the door to unethical applications such as selective breeding aimed at enhancing some human traits, or introducing genetic mutations [227].

18.3.3 Cloning: Worth Revisiting?

Cloning is the process of creating genetically identical organisms, either naturally or artificially. Over 2 decades ago, the idea of therapeutic cloning was deemed pertinent to xenotransplantation, as it could generate organs on a large scale [228]. In 1996, Dolly the sheep became the world's most famous clone. She was the first mammal to be cloned from an adult cell instead of an embryo—a major scientific breakthrough [229]. Soon after, the first pig was cloned in 2000 with the hope that this technology will help advance xenotransplantation [230]. This was soon followed by the cloning of Xena, a pig created by scientists in Japan, as a platform that can be exploited to provide organs for human trans-

plantation [231]. In contrast to Dolly, Xena was cloned by microinjecting genetic material from fetal-pig skin cells into eggs devoid of their own genetic material. This method increases selectively and, hence, has the potential to yield precise genetic modifications, a plus over transgenesis. However, all these efforts came to a stall as concerns over PERV infections increased. With the advent of CRISPR/Cas9, the field of xenotransplantation has shied away from cloning. However, new advances in this field, particularly related to decreasing the risk of telomere shortening and aging [232, 233], may eventually bring back this technology that could offer the advantage of accelerating and scaling up production of the optimally engineered pig donor for xenotransplantation.

18.3.4 Ex vivo Perfusion Systems to Deliver Gene Therapies

Ex-vivo perfusion (EVP) is an alternative to the current standard of static cold storage (SCS) and aims to address the current organ shortage by improving the function of marginal grafts, and extending the preservation time of procured grafts [234–238]. The underlying principle behind EVP is elegant in its simplicity. The graft vascular inflow and outflow are cannulated and a specific perfusate consisting of oxygen, nutrients, and metabolic substrates is circulated through the organ, washing out metabolic waste and supporting cellular function. When placed on the pump at 35–38 °C, known as normothermic machine perfusion (NMP), the graft has an opportunity to undergo normal physiologic function and recover from injury incurred before (donor after cardiac death) and during procurement—all prior to transplantation [239].

In addition to resuscitating marginal organs, preventing cold ischemia-related injury, assessing allograft viability pre-transplant and extending the preservation time of procured grafts, EVP is also ideal as a platform for targeted interventions in the field of xenotransplantation, specifically the delivery of gene therapies. Recent work in *ex vivo* liver perfusion provides the unique opportunity for both analysis and therapeutic intervention on donor organs. Perfusing porcine xenografts with human or nonhuman primate blood provides an efficient, high fidelity model to study initial interspecies cellular interactions after xenotransplantation, including post-transplant thrombocytopenia and ischemia-reperfusion injury [240, 241]. Beyond its use as a tool to evaluate whether any given genetic manipulation of pigs delivered the anticipated outcome, *ex vivo* perfusion of xenografts could be ideal for *ex vivo* genetic manipulation of the organ. This approach could broaden the choice or level of expression of the transgene to candidates that would be beneficial for the recipient, but are not compatible with porcine physiology, and therefore, would hamper viability of the donor pig. EVP could be the new route for expanding our "wish list" of genes to create the perfect donor pig for xenotransplantation.

18.4 The Wish List: A Recipe to Build the Pyramid 2.0

In the current era of genetic technologies which empower us to selectively modify donor xenografts with relative ease, the focus has changed from singular gene targets to minimize HAR to complex multigene cassettes that maximize graft compatibility, resistance to immune attacks, and function. This begs the obvious question: what will it take to make the "optimal" pig? The ideal xenograft will not only need to overcome the immediate immunological hurdles, as outlined above, but also to support the physiological function of both the recipient and the donor. In this section, we review what major changes have been made, and also what additional alterations will serve as vital steps in transforming the quest for the perfect pig from fiction to reality (Fig. 18.3).

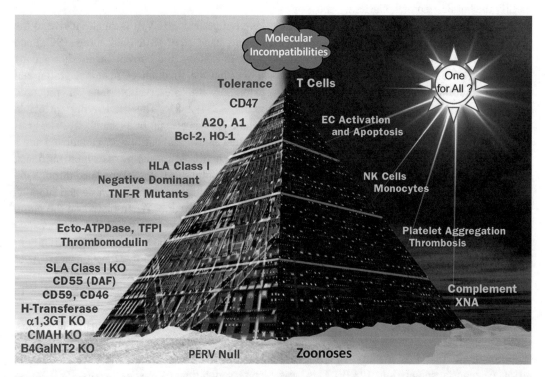

Fig. 18.3 A Minimalist List for the Genetic Engineering of the Optimal Pig for Xenotransplantation. Incremental building of the Pyramid: a balancing act between offend-ers and genetic solutions, based on combining overexpression of protective genes and knockout of deleterious ones

Elimination of zoonotic infectious agents is of critical importance, given the risk they pose not only to the xenograft recipient, but to society at large. Given the recipient's immunosuppressed state to tolerate the xenograft, prevention of infection by porcine pathogens took high priority at the turn of the twenty-first century [39, 242]. The sterile conditions and selective treatment of donor pigs in addition to a number of porcine pathogens not being transmittable to NHP and humans have resulted in zoonoses being a less significant barrier than originally thought, including PERV [243, 244]. Neither burn patients who had received porcine skin grafts as a temporary bridge, nor patients who received porcine corneal implants or more recently recipients of islet xenografts in New Zealand had any evidence of PERV transmission [244, 245]. However, as concern and controversy about PERV transmission remained, scientists reverted to CRISPR/Cas9 gene editing to successfully inactivate PERV in pigs, burying (as depicted in our scheme) this issue as an impediment to clinical xenotransplantation [246]. PERV KO pigs are healthy and breed well.

Along with eliminating or reducing the threat of zoonoses, one of the foremost modifications for the ideal pig xenograft donor are ones that would overcome HAR. As discussed earlier, this issue has already been resolved thanks to the generation of pigs with targeted deletion of α1,3galactosyltransferase (α1,3GT), the enzyme responsible for the expression of the dominant xenoantigenic surface glycan, α1,3galactose, that is recognized by preformed XNA (GTKO pigs), and of CMAH and B4GALNT2, the enzymes that synthesize the non-Gal glycans that are recognized by XNA. Pigs with KO of two or all three of these enzymes have been created. However, we still do not know whether these triple KO animals are necessary, or if the KO of dominant α1,3GT would be sufficient, especially when combined with SLA class I KO, and the overexpression of human CRPs, regulators of coagulation, and anti-inflammatory/anti-apoptotic genes [61–64].

Another key pathogenic effector of HAR and also of AVR/DXR, is complement-dependent cytotoxicity (CDC). As discussed earlier, complement binds XNA and gets activated, which results in the formation of the membrane-attack complex (MAC) and cytotoxicity. In the context of xenotransplantation, damage is aggravated by pig-NHP molecular incompatibilities, whereby porcine CRPs, whose function is to dampen complement activation and toxicity, are ineffective on NHP and human complement. Accordingly, the first pig that was genetically modified for xenotransplantation was made to express human CD55/DAF, a CRP that limits both the classical and alternative pathways of complement activation. Cardiac xenografts from GTKO and CD55 transgenic pigs prevented HAR and improved survival of pig-to-NHP cardiac [247], kidney [248] and liver [249, 250] xenografts. Pigs expressing two other CRPs, CD46 and CD59, were also created, so were pigs expressing two or all three CRPs [204–206]. Triple transgenic porcine xenografts expressing all 3 human CRPs (CD46, CD55, and CD59) resisted better the complement attack than double transgenic (CD55 and CD59) or mono-transgenic animals [207, 208]. These modifications do not only benefit HAR, but also DXR, which is associated with elicited post-transplant xenoreactive antibodies.

With HAR in the rearview mirror, a major obstacle impeding successful xenotransplantation became post-transplant thrombocytopenia and consumptive coagulopathy. Most severe in liver xenografts, consumptive coagulopathy and thrombocytopenia often result in a diffuse hemorrhagic microangiopathy that ultimately causes xenograft failure and recipient death [251]. As detailed earlier, the molecular basis of this disastrous situation is multi-factorial and combines activation-induced loss of EC-associated anticoagulant and anti-thrombotic molecules (thrombomodulin, CD39), which is further aggravated by molecular incompatibilities between pig and human/NHP (thrombomodulin and TFPI), in addition to a net gain by the activated and injured EC of pro-thrombotic and pro-coagulant molecules in part through *de novo* transcription of TF, and exposure/release of multimeric von Willebrand Factor. This improved knowledge of the sequence of events and the molecular players involved in xenograft-associated coagulopathy greatly informed which genes would best inhibit this process. Pigs genetically engineered to express human thrombomodulin were created first and showed great success in terms of normalizing the human/NHP coagulation system, and therefore, minimizing the severity of post-transplantation consumptive coagulopathy and micoangiopathy [210]. Additional choices include pigs genetically engineered to express in their vasculature human TFPI or CD39, a *bona fide* inhibitor of platelet activation and aggregation [209–212, 252]. To day, all pigs that have shown some success in xenotransplantation have been modified to genetically express one of these 3 molecules, and we still do not know whether combining two or all three of them would show greater benefit. This could certainly be checked thanks to the CRISPR/Cas9 technology that has facilitated our ability to implement multiple genetic modifications at once. With porcine xenografts overcoming these early hurdles, the complex issue of AVR/DXR became next to tackle.

One of the pathological features of AVR/DXR that was recognized early on relates to the infiltration of the xenograft by recipient natural killer (NK) cells and monocytes, the first line of cellular response of the innate immune system. Monocytes can differentiate into macrophages and dendritic cells, which serve three functions, all of which are injurious to the graft: phagocytosis, cytokine production, and antigen presentation [253]. Activated NK cells equally unleash their cytokine storm and their MHC Class I-independent cytotoxicity to further aggravate injury [254, 255]. Importantly, heightened *in situ* production of TNF by activated monocytes and of IFNγ by activated NK cells, greatly amplifies EC activation and the associated thrombogenic phenotype. One of the suggested solutions to this problem is to create a transgenic pig expressing an inhibitor of TNF—for example, a truncated form of the human p55 TNF-receptor (TNF-R1) or a human soluble TNF-R1-Fc chimeric molecule that capture TNF and block its signaling in EC [256, 257]. A transgenic pig expressing soluble TNF-R1-Fc has been created, but failed to

pass the test of time as pigs expressing central inhibitors of inflammation such as A20 or HO-1 took precedent. The same can be said for the pursuit of inhibitors of IFNγ signaling. Other options included expressing human HLA-E or β2 microglobulin, two known negative regulators of NK cytotoxicity [258].

Another salient pathological feature of DXR, but also of HAR, is centered around functional and/or physical loss of the anti-inflammatory and anti-coagulant endothelial barrier. As discussed earlier, all immunologic and inflammatory insults associated with early xenograft rejection coalesce around injury to the integrity of the endothelium. We had posited over 20 years ago, that blockade of EC activation and prevention of apoptosis will have the most wide-ranging beneficial effects on xenograft survival. As knowledge in vascular biology progressed, so has the recognition that this could be achieved by tackling the two dominant signaling pathways that fuel the majority of EC's phenotypic switch: i.e. NF-κB and IFNγ signaling pathways [81, 93, 259, 260]. Our laboratory and others accumulated significant evidence showing that these tasks can be safely achieved by tapping into the vessel's built-in physiologic response to injury, i.e. the so-called "protective" genes whose upregulation in response to injury, whether immune, inflammatory, metabolic, or mechanical, serves to protect the integrity of the endothelium and restore its physiologic functions as an anti-coagulant and anti-inflammatory barrier [107]. Two of these "protective" molecules top this list, A20 and HO-1, followed by A1, Bcl2 and BclxL, whose functions were detailed earlier. Remarkably, when expressed at sufficient levels, these multifunctional genes not only inhibit NF-κB activation and (at least for A20) atherogenic IFNγ signaling, but also protect EC from apoptosis and other forms of cell death, including complement-mediated and NK-induced cytotoxicity, and also potentially sway the immune response from pathogenic to regulatory [81, 107, 111, 261]. Building what we termed a "superprotected" endothelium that expresses sufficient levels of A20 and/or HO-1 preempt a phenotypic change of the EC and protect them from death. Based on the biology, one can argue that if efficient, this kind of intervention can have far-reaching therapeutic effects in terms of permitting xenograft survival. It is our hypothesis that by intervening at the apex of the pyramid with "star" genes such as A20 or HO-1, one would necessarily impact other aspects of DXR and of the adaptive T-cell immune response. For instance, it is well-established that systemic inflammation precedes disordered coagulation in the setting of xenotransplantation [262]. Therefore, inhibition of inflammatory responses by A20 or HO-1 could by reducing inflammation decrease the list of gene modifications required to limit the consumptive coagulopathy and microangiopathy of DXR. In another optimistic perspective, one may postulate that expression of genes such as A20 or HO-1 in the graft would also positively influence the type of T-cell immune response and, therefore, facilitate other tolerogenic interventions, keeping the organ healthy and away from the shades of death (Fig. 18.3). The first A20 transgenic pig was created in 2009. Even though transgene expression remained moderate—limited to skeletal muscle, heart, and aortic EC—this study was still able to validate A20's anti-inflammatory and anti-apoptotic functions [146]. Both A20 and HO-1 are consistently part of the list of genes modified in the current iterations of pigs created for xenotransplantation [61, 63, 213, 226].

Last, but not least, on the "wish list" are modifications that could help achieve tolerance and inhibit T-cell-mediated rejection. Immune tolerance is the prevention of an immune response to a particular antigen or tissue. However, if T-cell-mediated rejection to a xenograft can be diminished by modification of the organ, and the need for immunosuppression could be reduced. This would greatly decrease the oncogenic and infectious risks associated with heavy immunosuppressive regimens [263], a highly desirable outcome as we progress towards clinical xenotransplanation [31, 182, 184, 264].

Current tolerogenic protocols include complex manipulations to achieve mixed chimerism and thymic transplantation strategies that were successful in pig-to-baboon models [31, 184,

264]. However, with the appeal of modern technologies that enable multiplex genetic manipulations, the field is exploring novel avenues to manipulate the donor organ as an easier way to drive tolerance. Creation of transgenic pigs expressing human CD47 to suppress elements of the macrophage and T-cell responses is one approach that has already been implemented with some degree of success [193]. Other manipulations to modulate MHC class II expression and reduce inflammation by expressing genes such as A20 and/or HO-1 could also help achieve this very purpose [112].

As xenograft survival increases, it remains to be seen whether with all these genetic manipulations if vascularized xenografts will still suffer chronic rejection, much like allografts. Here again, the hope is that an injury-resistant endothelium would temper the incidence and severity of transplant arteriosclerosis, a pathognomonic feature of chronic rejection in vascularized allografts.

In summary, our optimal minimalistic view of the 2.0 winning recipe, as supported by solid *in vitro* and *in vivo* evidence to convince the regulatory authorities, for the "safest" pig donor includes (1) triple KO of the enzymes synthesizing xenogeneic carbohydrates, and (2) KO of SLA class I, as well as expression of (3) two or three human CRPs (CD46, CD55, CD59), (4) two or three human regulators of coagulation (thrombomodulin, TFPI, CD39), (5) two human anti-apoptotic and anti-inflammatory molecules (A20, HO-1), and (6) immunoregulatory molecules such as human CD47 (Fig. 18.3). Although many alternative genetic modifications could be made to an organ-source pig, we believe that any given list should be as minimalistic as possible, at least for the initial trials in kidney, heart and islet transplantation, before moving to more challenging organs such as liver and lung.

As of today, thanks to the use of donor pigs with different sets of genetic modifications, treatment of the recipient with a variety of immunosuppressive regimens, including co-stimulation blockade molecules such as CTLA4Ig/anti-CD40 mAb, and the many advantages of novel preservation and isolation methods, the survival of a pig-to-NHP hetero-topic heart reached 945 days [209, 265], of orthotopic life-sustaining hearts reached 195 days [266], of kidney xenografts reached 435 days [186, 187, 267], and of islet xenografts reached over 600 days [268]. This progress in islet xenotransplantation is quite commanding and likely to further improve thanks to the current technological advances in encapsulation methods that decrease the risks associated with the implantation of islet grafts in the liver [269]. Additional breakthroughs have also been reported in the difficult field of liver xenografts with a first-time survival rate of 29 days, a true milestone in the effort to bridge patients while they await for an allograft to become available [270]. Now, the field is getting ready for clinical trials cautioned by regulatory agencies and an international consensus. The first clinical trial in New Zealand using encapsulated porcine islet xenografts to treat 14 diabetic patients suffering from hypoglycemia unawareness confirmed the microbiological safety of these xenografts [36]. Following these safety studies, the field is eagerly awaiting the results of efficacy trials for islet xenografts (https://clinical-trials.gov/ct2/show/NCT03162237) [271], and also for next for kidney and heart xenografts.

18.5 The Road Ahead: Persistent Challenges and Cautionary Notes

Despite the optimism that is rightfully driven by current experimental data and initial clinical trials, one needs to be mindful of the remaining challenges, both technical and fundamental. For all its transformative potential, CRISPR/Cas9 gene editing still has a number of limitations. For instance, one unanswered question pertains to the expression level and tissue distribution of transgenes. As an example, A20 expression in most of the transgenic pigs remains limited to a few organs. Accordingly, a kidney xenograft may not have sufficient or any expression.

Another cloud that still hangs over the success of many xenografts is that of molecular incompatibilities between pigs and humans. This issue needs to remain part of the conversation as we strive to create the ideal pig (Fig. 18.3). Molecular incompatibilities are defined as fundamental physiologic differences in the biologic architecture between two different organisms. In the context of xenotransplantation, these incompatibilities have been mostly assessed in the context of immune regulation (complement regulatory proteins, CD47), and of coagulation (thrombomodulin, TFPI, CD39). However, as the field progresses, new molecular incompatibilities, specifically as related to proteins that are key for organ function, are likely to emerge. While porcine insulin is totally functional and has for the longest time been used for the treatment of diabetic patients, the number of proteins manufactured in the liver to support homeostasis of the whole organism might not be as interchangeable. Additionally, they may not be as amenable to genetic manipulations without hampering the viability of the donor pig. We remain optimistic that technological advances to enable controlled and cell-type specific expression or KO of some genes will likelyovercome some of these potential limitations.

Final cautionary notes that cannot be ignored pertain to persistent ethical concerns with using animals for therapeutic purposes. This concern is somewhat tempered by the widespread practice of mass production of genetically modified animals for food. The other elephant in the room is that of cost, which should be reviewed in light of the current health care costs of chronic illnesses, and associated loss of productivity.

Acknowledgments Dr. Ferran is supported by NIH grants R01HL086741, R01 HL 021796 and R21EB024308, as well as by the JDRF grant 2 SRA-2017-343. Dr. McIntosh is the recipient of an NRSA fellowship from the NIH/NHLBI funded T32 training grant 5 T32 HL07733. Dr. Haque is supported by the American Liver Foundation (2019 Hans Popper Memorial Postdoctoral Research Fellowship) and the American College of Surgeons (Grant number 1123-39991 scholarship endowment fund). Dr. Cloonan is the recipient of an NRSA fellowship frpm the NIH/NIAID funded T32 training grant AI 007529.

References

1. Organ Procurement and Transplantation Network. U.S. Department of Health and Human Services. 2019. Available at: https://optn.transplant.hrsa.gov/data/.
2. Goldwyn RM. History of attempts to form a vagina. Plast Reconstr Surg. 1977;59:9–329.
3. Van Haeseker B. Meekeren and his account of the transplant of bone from a dog into the skull of a soldier. Plast Reconstr Surg. 1991;88:173–4.
4. Elgood C. Safavid surgery, analecta medicao-historica. Oxford: Pergamon Press; 1966.
5. Deschamps JY, Roux FA, Sai P, Gouin E. History of xenotransplantation. Xenotransplantation. 2005;12:91–109.
6. Hitchcock CR, Kiser JC, Telander RL, Seljeskog EL. Baboon renal grafts. JAMA. 1964;189:934–7.
7. Hardy JD, et al. Heart transplantation in man developmental studies and report of a case. JAMA. 1964;188:1132–40.
8. Starzl TE. Orthotopic heterotransplantation. Experience in hepatic transplantation, vol. 408. Philadelphia: W.B. Saunders Co; 1969.
9. Borel J, Feurer C, Gubler H. Biological effects of cyclosporine A: a new antilymphocyte agent. Agents Actions. 1976;6:468.
10. Cifarelli PS. Baby fae. West J Med. 1985;142:401–2.
11. Jonasson O, Hardy MA. The case of Baby Fae. JAMA. 1985;254:3358–9.
12. Bailey LL, Nehlsen-Cannarella SL, Concepcion W, Jolley WB. Baboon-to-human cardiac xenotransplantation in a neonate. JAMA. 1985;254:3321–9.
13. Warty V, et al. FK506: a novel immunosuppressive agent. Characteristics of binding and uptake by human lymphocytes. Transplantation. 1988;46:453–5.
14. Starzl TE, et al. Baboon-to-human liver transplantation. Lancet. 1993;341:65–71.
15. Starzl TE, et al. The biological basis of and strategies for clinical xenotransplantation. Immunol Rev. 1994;141:213–44.
16. Bengtsson A, Svalander CT, Molne J, Rydberg L, Breimer ME. Extracorporeal ("ex vivo") connection of pig kidneys to humans. III Studies of plasma complement activation and complement deposition in the kidney tissue. Xenotransplantation. 1998;5:176–83.
17. Czaplicki J, Blonska B, Religa Z. The lack of hyperacute xenogeneic heart transplant rejection in a human. J Heart Lung Transplant. 1992;11:393–7.
18. Gnanapragasam M. Christian perspectives in medical ethics. Bioethics in India. Proceedings of the international bioethics workshop in madras: biomanagement of biogeoresources, 16–19 January 1997, Chennai: University of Madras, 1997. (1997).
19. Cooper DKC, Ekser B, Tector AJ. A brief history of clinical xenotransplantation. Int J Surg. 2015;23:205–10.
20. Phelps CJ, et al. Production of alpha 1,3-galactosyltransferase-deficient pigs. Science. 2003;299:411–4.
21. Cooper DK, et al. Alpha1,3-galactosyltransferase gene-knockout pigs for xenotransplantation: where do we go from here? Transplantation. 2007;84:1–7.
22. Bach FH, et al. Modification of vascular responses in xenotransplantation: inflammation and apoptosis. Nat Med. 1997;3:944–8.
23. Bach FH, et al. Barriers to xenotransplantation. Nat Med. 1995;1:869–73.
24. Bach FH, Winkler H, Ferran C, Hancock WW, Robson SC. Delayed xenograft rejection. Immunol Today. 1996;17:379–84.
25. Bush EL, et al. Coagulopathy in alpha-galactosyl transferase knockout pulmonary xenotransplants. Xenotransplantation. 2011;18:6–13.
26. Leventhal JR, et al. The immunopathology of cardiac xenograft rejection in the guinea pig-to-rat model. Transplantation. 1993;56:1–8.
27. Ramcharran S, Wang H, Hosiawa K, Kelvin D, Zhong R. Manipulation of cytokines as a novel approach to overcome xenotransplant rejection. Transplant Rev. 2005;19:213–20.
28. Akiyoshi DE, et al. Identification of a full-length cDNA for an endogenous retrovirus of miniature swine. J Virol. 1998;72:4503–7.
29. Meije Y, Tonjes RR, Fishman JA. Retroviral restriction factors and infectious risk in xenotransplantation. Am J Transplant. 2010;10:1511–6.
30. Wang SR, Chang JT, Lin MS, Chiang CY, Chang HY. Establishing the reactivity of monoclonal antibodies against porcine endogenous retrovirus envelope protein. Intervirology. 2004;47:93–101.
31. Yamada K, et al. Marked prolongation of porcine renal xenograft survival in baboons through the use of alpha1,3-galactosyltransferase gene-knockout donors and the cotransplantation of vascularized thymic tissue. Nat Med. 2005;11:32–4.
32. Stoye JP, Le Tissier P, Takeuchi Y, Patience C, Weiss RA. Endogenous retroviruses: a potential problem for xenotransplantation? Ann N Y Acad Sci. 1998;862:67–74.
33. Bach FH, et al. Uncertainty in xenotransplantation: individual benefit versus collective risk. Nat Med. 1998;4:141–4.
34. Bach FH, Fineberg HV. Call for moratorium on xenotransplants. Nature. 1998;391:326.
35. van der Laan LJ, et al. Infection by porcine endogenous retrovirus after islet xenotransplantation in SCID mice. Nature. 2000;407:90–4.
36. Wynyard S, Nathu D, Garkavenko O, Denner J, Elliott R. Microbiological safety of the first clinical pig islet xenotransplantation trial in New Zealand. Xenotransplantation. 2014;21:309–23.
37. Elliott RB, Garkavenko O, Escobar L, Skinner S. Concerns expressed about the virological risks of xenotransplantation. Xenotransplantation. 2002;9:422–4.

38. Switzer WM, et al. Lack of cross-species transmission of porcine endogenous retrovirus infection to nonhuman primate recipients of porcine cells, tissues, or organs. Transplantation. 2001;71:959–65.

39. Fishman JA. Infectious disease risks in xenotransplantation. Am J Transplant. 2018;18:1857–64.

40. Cowan PJ, Hawthorne WJ, Nottle MB. Xenogeneic transplantation and tolerance in the era of CRISPR-Cas9. Curr Opin Organ Transplant. 2019;24:5–11.

41. Nunes Dos Santos RM, et al. CRISPR/Cas and recombinase-based human-to-pig orthotopic gene exchange for xenotransplantation. J Surg Res. 2018;229:28–40.

42. Yang L, et al. Genome-wide inactivation of porcine endogenous retroviruses (PERVs). Science. 2015;350:1101–4.

43. Niu D, et al. Inactivation of porcine endogenous retrovirus in pigs using CRISPR-Cas9. Science. 2017;357:1303–7.

44. Ekser B, Li P, Cooper DKC. Xenotransplantation: past, present, and future. Curr Opin Organ Transplant. 2017;22:513–21.

45. Ross MJ, Coates PT. Using CRISPR to inactivate endogenous retroviruses in pigs: an important step toward safe xenotransplantation? Kidney Int. 2018;93:4–6.

46. Jarvis L. eGenesis launches to overhaul transplants. Chem Eng News. 2017;95:12.

47. Week B. Mayo Clinic and United Therapeutics collaborate on lung restoration center. 2015;138.

48. News HP. Revivicor Inc submits patent application for tissue products derived from animals lacking any expression of functional alpha 1,3 galactosyltransferase. Global IP News. 2016 October;18

49. Wang Y. Findings from Y. Wang and Colleagues Update Understanding of Xenotransplantation (Xenotransplantation in China: Present status). Biotech Week. 2019;416.

50. Alexion. Alexion: EC Orphan drug status for soliris in prevention of graft rejection. RTTNews. 2014 Apr 23.

51. Butler JR, et al. The fate of human platelets exposed to porcine renal endothelium: a single-pass model of platelet uptake in domestic and genetically modified porcine organs. J Surg Res. 2016;200:698–706.

52. Cooper DKC, Ekser B, Tector AJ. Immunobiological barriers to xenotransplantation. Int J Surg. 2015;23:211–6.

53. Bird GW, Roy TC. Human serum antibodies to melibiose and other carbohydrates. Vox Sang. 1980;38:169–71.

54. Galili U, Clark MR, Shohet SB, Buehler J, Macher BA. Evolutionary relationship between the natural anti-Gal antibody and the Gal alpha 1–3Gal epitope in primates. Proc Natl Acad Sci USA. 1987;84:1369–73.

55. Galili U. Natural anti-carbohydrate antibodies contributing to evolutionary survival of primates in viral epidemics? Glycobiology. 2016;26:1140–50.

56. Galili U, Shohet SB, Kobrin E, Stults CL, Macher BA. Man, apes, and Old World monkeys differ from other mammals in the expression of alpha-galactosyl epitopes on nucleated cells. J Biol Chem. 1988;263:17755–62.

57. Bouhours D, Pourcel C, Bouhours JE. Simultaneous expression by porcine aorta endothelial cells of glycosphingolipids bearing the major epitope for human xenoreactive antibodies (Gal alpha 1-3Gal), blood group H determinant and N-glycolylneuraminic acid. Glycoconj J. 1996;13:947–53.

58. Galili U. Anti-Gal: an abundant human natural antibody of multiple pathogeneses and clinical benefits. Immunology. 2013;140:1–11.

59. Byrne GW, McGregor CGA, Breimer ME. Recent investigations into pig antigen and anti-pig antibody expression. Int J Surg. 2015;23:223–8.

60. Byrne G, Ahmad-Villiers S, Du Z, McGregor C. B4GALNT2 and xenotransplantation: a newly appreciated xenogeneic antigen. Xenotransplantation. 2018;25:e12394.

61. Fischer K, et al. Viable pigs after simultaneous inactivation of porcine MHC class I and three xenoreactive antigen genes GGTA1, CMAH and B4GALNT2. Xenotransplantation. 2020;27:e12560.

62. Kwon DJ, et al. Generation of alpha-1,3-galactosyltransferase knocked-out transgenic cloned pigs with knocked-in five human genes. Transgenic Res. 2017;26:153–63.

63. Fischer K, et al. Efficient production of multi-modified pigs for xenotransplantation by 'combineering', gene stacking and gene editing. Sci Rep. 2016;6:29081.

64. Lutz AJ, et al. Double knockout pigs deficient in N-glycolylneuraminic acid and galactose alpha-1,3-galactose reduce the humoral barrier to xenotransplantation. Xenotransplantation. 2013;20:27–35.

65. Sandrin MS, et al. Enzymatic remodelling of the carbohydrate surface of a xenogenic cell substantially reduces human antibody binding and complement-mediated cytolysis. Nat Med. 1995;1:1261–7.

66. Zhou H, Hara H, Cooper DKC. The complex functioning of the complement system in xenotransplantation. Xenotransplantation. 2019;26:e12517.

67. Kroshus TJ, et al. Antibody removal by column immunoabsorption prevents tissue injury in an ex vivo model of pig-to-human xenograft hyperacute rejection. J Surg Res. 1995;59:43–50.

68. Kroshus TJ, et al. Complement inhibition with an anti-C5 monoclonal antibody prevents acute cardiac tissue injury in an ex vivo model of pig-to-human xenotransplantation. Transplantation. 1995;60:1194–202.

69. Kroshus TJ, Bolman RM 3rd, Dalmasso AP. Selective IgM depletion prolongs organ survival in an ex vivo model of pig-to-human xenotransplantation. Transplantation. 1996;62:5–12.

70. Dalmasso AP. The complement system in xenotransplantation. Immunopharmacology. 1992;24:149–60.

71. Dalmasso AP, Vercellotti GM, Platt JL, Bach FH. Inhibition of complement-mediated endothelial cell cytotoxicity by decay-accelerating factor. Potential for prevention of xenograft hyperacute rejection. Transplantation. 1991;52:530–3.

72. Pinkert CA, Kooyman DL, Dyer TJ. Enhanced growth performance in transgenic swine. Biotechnology. 1991;16:251–8.

73. Pursel VG, et al. Genetic engineering of livestock. Science. 1989;244:1281–8.

74. Cozzi E, White DJ. The generation of transgenic pigs as potential organ donors for humans. Nat Med. 1995;1:964–6.

75. Rosengard AM, et al. Tissue expression of human complement inhibitor, decay-accelerating factor, in transgenic pigs. A potential approach for preventing xenograft rejection. Transplantation. 1995;59:1325–33.

76. White DJ, et al. The control of hyperacute rejection by genetic engineering of the donor species. Eye (Lond). 1995;9(Pt 2):185–9.

77. Cooper DKC, et al. Justification of specific genetic modifications in pigs for clinical organ xenotransplantation. Xenotransplantation. 2019;26:e12516.

78. Pan D, et al. Progress in multiple genetically modified minipigs for xenotransplantation in China. Xenotransplantation. 2019;26:e12492.

79. Burlak C, et al. Reduced binding of human antibodies to cells from GGTA1/CMAH KO pigs. Am J Transplant. 2014;14:1895–900.

80. Platt JL. New directions for organ transplantation. Nature. 1998;392:11–7.

81. Bach FH, et al. Endothelial cell activation and thromboregulation during xenograft rejection. Immunol Rev. 1994;141:5–30.

82. Cotran RS, Pober JS. Cytokine-endothelial interactions in inflammation, immunity, and vascular injury. J Am Soc Nephrol. 1990;1:225–35.

83. Pober JS, et al. The potential roles of vascular endothelium in immune reactions. Hum Immunol. 1990;28:258–62.

84. Bouwens EA, Stavenuiter F, Mosnier LO. Mechanisms of anticoagulant and cytoprotective actions of the protein C pathway. J Thromb Haemost. 2013;11(Suppl 1):242–53.

85. Platt JL, et al. Release of heparan sulfate from endothelial cells. Implications for pathogenesis of hyperacute rejection. J Exp Med. 1990;171:1363–8.

86. Robson SC, et al. Loss of ATP diphosphohydrolase activity with endothelial cell activation. J Exp Med. 1997;185:153–63.

87. Collins T, Palmer HJ, Whitley MZ, Neish AS, Williams AJ. A common theme in endothelial activation Insights from the structural analysis of the genes for E-selectin and VCAM-1. Trends Cardiovasc Med. 1993;3:92–7.

88. Traenckner EB, Baeuerle PA. Appearance of apparently ubiquitin-conjugated I kappa B-alpha during

89. Traenckner EB, et al. Phosphorylation of human I kappa B-alpha on serines 32 and 36 controls I kappa B-alpha proteolysis and NF-kappa B activation in response to diverse stimuli. EMBO J. 1995;14:2876–83.

90. Baeuerle PA, Baltimore D. I kappa B: a specific inhibitor of the NF-kappa B transcription factor. Science. 1988;242:540–6.

91. Hoffmann A, Levchenko A, Scott ML, Baltimore D. The IkappaB-NF-kappaB signaling module: temporal control and selective gene activation. Science. 2002;298:1241–5.

92. Whitley MZ, Thanos D, Read MA, Maniatis T, Collins T. A striking similarity in the organization of the E-selectin and beta interferon gene promoters. Mol Cell Biol. 1994;14:6464–75.

93. Read MA, Whitley MZ, Williams AJ, Collins T. NF-kappa B and I kappa B alpha: an inducible regulatory system in endothelial activation. J Exp Med. 1994;179:503–12.

94. Ferran C, et al. Inhibition of NF-kappa B by pyrrolidine dithiocarbamate blocks endothelial cell activation. Biochem Biophys Res Commun. 1995;214:212–23.

95. Hoffmann A, Baltimore D. Circuitry of nuclear factor kappaB signaling. Immunol Rev. 2006;210:171–86.

96. Li N, Karin M. Signaling pathways leading to nuclear factor-kappa B activation. Methods Enzymol. 2000;319:273–9.

97. Baeuerle PA, Baltimore D. Activation of DNA-binding activity in an apparently cytoplasmic precursor of the NF-kappa B transcription factor. Cell. 1988;53:211–7.

98. Soares MP, et al. Adenovirus-mediated expression of a dominant negative mutant of p65/RelA inhibits proinflammatory gene expression in endothelial cells without sensitizing to apoptosis. J Immunol. 1998;161:4572–82.

99. Beg AA, Baltimore D. An essential role for NF-kappaB in preventing TNF-alpha-induced cell death. Science. 1996;274:782–4.

100. Van Antwerp DJ, Martin SJ, Kafri T, Green DR, Verma IM. Suppression of TNF-alpha-induced apoptosis by NF-kappaB. Science. 1996;274:787–9.

101. Bach FH, et al. Accommodation of vascularized xenografts: expression of "protective genes" by donor endothelial cells in a host Th2 cytokine environment. Nat Med. 1997;3:196–204.

102. Cooper JT, et al. A20 blocks endothelial cell activation through a NF-kappaB-dependent mechanism. J Biol Chem. 1996;271:18068–73.

103. Ferran C, et al. A20 inhibits NF-kappaB activation in endothelial cells without sensitizing to tumor necrosis factor-mediated apoptosis. Blood. 1998;91:2249–58.

104. Stroka DM, Badrichani AZ, Bach FH, Ferran C. Overexpression of A1, an NF-kappaB-inducible

anti-apoptotic bcl gene, inhibits endothelial cell activation. Blood. 1999;93:3803–10.

105. Longo CR, et al. A20 protects from CD40-CD40 ligand-mediated endothelial cell activation and apoptosis. Circulation. 2003;108:1113–8.

106. Daniel S, et al. A20 protects endothelial cells from TNF-, Fas-, and NK-mediated cell death by inhibiting caspase 8 activation. Blood. 2004;104:2376–84.

107. Bach FH, Hancock WW, Ferran C. Protective genes expressed in endothelial cells: a regulatory response to injury. Immunol Today. 1997;18:483–6.

108. Badrichani AZ, et al. Bcl-2 and Bcl-XL serve an anti-inflammatory function in endothelial cells through inhibition of NF-kappaB. J Clin Invest. 1999;103:543–53.

109. Bach FH, Turman MA, Vercellotti GM, Platt JL, Dalmasso AP. Accommodation: a working paradigm for progressing toward clinical discordant xenografting. Transplant Proc. 1991;23:205–7.

110. Lin Y, et al. Accommodated xenografts survive in the presence of anti-donor antibodies and complement that precipitate rejection of naive xenografts. J Immunol. 1999;163:2850–7.

111. Siracuse JJ, et al. A20-Mediated Modulation of Inflammatory and Immune Responses in Aortic Allografts and Development of Transplant Arteriosclerosis. Transplantation. 2012;93:373–82.

112. Ferran C. The graft unveils its secrets: provocative therapeutic leads to protected vascularized allografts. Transpl Immunol. 2002;9:135–6.

113. Avihingsanon Y, et al. Expression of protective genes in human renal allografts: a regulatory response to injury associated with graft rejection. Transplantation. 2002;73:1079–85.

114. Sato K, et al. Carbon monoxide generated by heme oxygenase-1 suppresses the rejection of mouse-to-rat cardiac transplants. J Immunol. 2001;166:4185–94.

115. Otterbein LE, et al. Carbon monoxide suppresses arteriosclerotic lesions associated with chronic graft rejection and with balloon injury. Nat Med. 2003;9:183–90.

116. Kunter U, et al. Expression of A20 in the vessel wall of rat-kidney allografts correlates with protection from transplant arteriosclerosis. Transplantation. 2003;75:3–9.

117. Grey ST, Arvelo MB, Hasenkamp W, Bach FH, Ferran C. A20 inhibits cytokine-induced apoptosis and nuclear factor kappaB-dependent gene activation in islets. J Exp Med. 1999;190:1135–46.

118. Grey ST, Arvelo MB, Hasenkamp WM, Bach FH, Ferran C. Adenovirus-mediated gene transfer of the anti-apoptotic protein A20 in rodent islets inhibits IL-1 beta-induced NO release. Transplant Proc. 1999;31:789.

119. Grey ST, Lock J, Bach FH, Ferran C. Adenovirus-mediated gene transfer of A20 in murine islets inhibits Fas-induced apoptosis. Transplant Proc. 2001;33:577–8.

120. Arvelo MB, et al. A20 protects mice from D-galactosamine/lipopolysaccharide acute toxic lethal hepatitis. Hepatology. 2002;35:535–43.

121. Grey ST, et al. Genetic engineering of a suboptimal islet graft with A20 preserves beta cell mass and function. J Immunol. 2003;170:6250–6.

122. Longo CR, et al. A20 protects mice from lethal radical hepatectomy by promoting hepatocyte proliferation via a p21waf1-dependent mechanism. Hepatology. 2005;42:156–64.

123. Longo C, et al. A20 protects the liver from lethal ischemia reperfusion injury by promoting hepatocyte proliferation, survival and function. Am J Transplant. 2006;6(suppl 2):248.

124. Patel VI, et al. A20, a modulator of smooth muscle cell proliferation and apoptosis, prevents and induces regression of neointimal hyperplasia. FASEB J. 2006;20:1418–30.

125. Ramsey HE, et al. A20 protects mice from lethal liver ischemia/reperfusion injury by increasing peroxisome proliferator-activated receptor-alpha expression. Liver Transpl. 2009;15:1613–21.

126. Damrauer SM, et al. A20 inhibits post-angioplasty restenosis by blocking macrophage trafficking and decreasing adventitial neovascularization. Atherosclerosis. 2010;211:404–8.

127. Shrikhande GV, et al. O-glycosylation regulates ubiquitination and degradation of the anti-inflammatory protein A20 to accelerate atherosclerosis in diabetic ApoE-null mice. PLoS One. 2010;5:e14240.

128. Damrauer SM, et al. A20 modulates lipid metabolism and energy production to promote liver regeneration. PLoS One. 2011;6:e17715.

129. Wang H, Ferran C, Attanasio C, Calise F, Otterbein LE. Induction of protective genes leads to islet survival and function. J Transp Secur. 2011;2011:141898.

130. da Silva CG, et al. A20 promotes liver regeneration by decreasing SOCS3 expression to enhance IL-6/STAT3 proliferative signals. Hepatology. 2013;57:2014–25.

131. da Silva CG, Cervantes JR, Studer P, Ferran C. A20 – an omnipotent protein in the liver: prometheus myth resolved? Adv Exp Med Biol. 2014;809:117–39.

132. McGillicuddy FC, et al. Translational studies of A20 in atherosclerosis and cardiovascular disease. Adv Exp Med Biol. 2014;809:83–101.

133. Opipari AW Jr, Boguski MS, Dixit VM. The A20 cDNA induced by tumor necrosis factor alpha encodes a novel type of zinc finger protein. J Biol Chem. 1990;265:14705–8.

134. Shembade N, Harhaj EW. Regulation of NF-kappaB signaling by the A20 deubiquitinase. Cell Mol Immunol. 2012;9:123–30.

135. Lee EG, et al. Failure to regulate TNF-induced NF-kappaB and cell death responses in A20-deficient mice. Science. 2000;289:2350–4.

136. Heyninck K, Beyaert R. A20 inhibits NF-kappaB activation by dual ubiquitin-editing functions. Trends Biochem Sci. 2005;30:1–4.

137. Wertz IE, et al. De-ubiquitination and ubiquitin ligase domains of A20 downregulate NF-kappaB signalling. Nature. 2004;430:694–9.

138. Skaug B, et al. Direct, noncatalytic mechanism of IKK inhibition by A20. Mol Cell. 2011;44:559–71.
139. Ferran C, Stroka DM, Badrichani AZ, Cooper JT, Bach FH. Adenovirus-mediated gene transfer of A20 renders endothelial cells resistant to activation: a means of evaluating the role of endothelial cell activation in xenograft rejection. Transplant Proc. 1997;29:879–80.
140. Moll HP, et al. A20 regulates atherogenic interferon (IFN)-gamma signaling in vascular cells by modulating basal IFNbeta levels. J Biol Chem. 2014;
141. Moll HP, et al. A20 haploinsufficiency aggravates transplant arteriosclerosis in mouse vascular allografts: implications for clinical transplantation. Transplantation. 2016;100:e106–16.
142. Matzinger P. Tolerance, danger, and the extended family. Annu Rev Immunol. 1994;12:991–1045.
143. Anderson CC, et al. Testing time-, ignorance-, and danger-based models of tolerance. J Immunol. 2001;166:3663–71.
144. Matzinger P. The danger model: a renewed sense of self. Science. 2002;296:301–5.
145. Zammit NW, et al. A20 as an immune tolerance factor can determine islet transplant outcomes. JCI Insight. 2019;4.
146. Oropeza M, et al. Transgenic expression of the human A20 gene in cloned pigs provides protection against apoptotic and inflammatory stimuli. Xenotransplantation. 2009;16:522–34.
147. Balla J, Jacob HS, Balla G, Nath K, Vercellotti GM. Endothelial cell heme oxygenase and ferritin induction by heme proteins: a possible mechanism limiting shock damage. Trans Assoc Am Phys. 1992;105:1–6.
148. Otterbein LE, Soares MP, Yamashita K, Bach FH. Heme oxygenase-1: unleashing the protective properties of heme. Trends Immunol. 2003;24:449–55.
149. Vercellotti GM, et al. H-ferritin ferroxidase induces cytoprotective pathways and inhibits microvascular stasis in transgenic sickle mice. Front Pharmacol. 2014;5:79.
150. Berberat PO, et al. Heavy chain ferritin acts as an antiapoptotic gene that protects livers from ischemia reperfusion injury. FASEB J. 2003;17:1724–6.
151. Otterbein LE, Choi AM. Heme oxygenase: colors of defense against cellular stress. Am J Physiol Lung Cell Mol Physiol. 2000;279:L1029–37.
152. Katori M, Busuttil RW, Kupiec-Weglinski JW. Heme oxygenase-1 system in organ transplantation. Transplantation. 2002;74:905–12.
153. Soares MP, et al. Expression of heme oxygenase-1 can determine cardiac xenograft survival. Nat Med. 1998;4:1073–7.
154. Soares MP, Bach FH. Heme oxygenase-1 in organ transplantation. Front Biosci. 2007;12:4932–45.
155. Soares MP, Bach FH. Heme oxygenase-1: from biology to therapeutic potential. Trends Mol Med. 2009;15:50–8.
156. Soares MP, et al. Modulation of endothelial cell apoptosis by heme oxygenase-1-derived carbon monoxide. Antioxid Redox Signal. 2002;4:321–9.
157. Brouard S, et al. Carbon monoxide generated by heme oxygenase 1 suppresses endothelial cell apoptosis. J Exp Med. 2000;192:1015–26.
158. Akamatsu Y, et al. Heme oxygenase-1-derived carbon monoxide protects hearts from transplant associated ischemia reperfusion injury. FASEB J. 2004;18:771–2.
159. Yamashita K, et al. Biliverdin, a natural product of heme catabolism, induces tolerance to cardiac allografts. FASEB J. 2004;18:765–7.
160. McDaid J, et al. Heme oxygenase-1 modulates the allo-immune response by promoting activation-induced cell death of T cells. FASEB J. 2005;19:458–60.
161. Neto JS, et al. Protection of transplant-induced renal ischemia-reperfusion injury with carbon monoxide. Am J Physiol Renal Physiol. 2004;287:F979–89.
162. Katori M, Anselmo DM, Busuttil RW, Kupiec-Weglinski JW. A novel strategy against ischemia and reperfusion injury: cytoprotection with heme oxygenase system. Transpl Immunol. 2002;9:227–33.
163. Tsuchihashi S, Fondevila C, Kupiec-Weglinski JW. Heme oxygenase system in ischemia and reperfusion injury. Ann Transplant. 2004;9:84–7.
164. Wang H, et al. Donor treatment with carbon monoxide can yield islet allograft survival and tolerance. Diabetes. 2005;54:1400–6.
165. Lee SS, et al. Heme oxygenase-1, carbon monoxide, and bilirubin induce tolerance in recipients toward islet allografts by modulating T regulatory cells. FASEB J. 2007;21:3450–7.
166. Kuramitsu K, et al. Carbon monoxide enhances early liver regeneration in mice after hepatectomy. Hepatology. 2011;53:2016–26.
167. Shimizu A, et al. Thrombotic microangiopathic glomerulopathy in human decay accelerating factor-transgenic swine-to-baboon kidney xenografts. J Am Soc Nephrol. 2005;16:2732–45.
168. Kaczmarek E, et al. Identification and characterization of CD39/vascular ATP diphosphohydrolase. J Biol Chem. 1996;271:33116–22.
169. Enjyoji K, et al. Targeted disruption of cd39/ATP diphosphohydrolase results in disordered hemostasis and thromboregulation. Nat Med. 1999;5:1010–7.
170. Imai M, et al. Modulation of nucleoside [correction of nucleotide] triphosphate diphosphohydrolase-1 (NTPDase-1)cd39 in xenograft rejection. Mol Med. 1999;5:743–52.
171. Cowan PJ, d'Apice AJ. The coagulation barrier in xenotransplantation: incompatibilities and strategies to overcome them. Curr Opin Organ Transplant. 2008;13:178–83.
172. Wang L, Jiang R, Sun XL. Recombinant thrombomodulin of different domains for pharmaceutical, biomedical, and cell transplantation applications. Med Res Rev. 2014;34:479–502.

173. Koyamada N, et al. Apyrase administration prolongs discordant xenograft survival. Transplantation. 1996;62:1739–43.

174. Lesnikoski BA, et al. Inhibition of platelet GPIIbIIIa prolongs survival of discordant cardiac xenografts. Transplant Proc. 1996;28:703.

175. Ahrens HE, et al. siRNA mediated knockdown of tissue factor expression in pigs for xenotransplantation. Am J Transplant. 2015;15:1407–14.

176. Sashindranath M, et al. Development of a novel strategy to target CD39 antithrombotic activity to the endothelial-platelet microenvironment in kidney ischemia-reperfusion injury. Purinergic Signal. 2017;13:259–65.

177. Martens GR, et al. Humoral reactivity of renal transplant-waitlisted patients to cells from GGTA1/CMAH/B4GalNT2, and SLA class I knockout pigs. Transplantation. 2017;101:e86–92.

178. Reyes LM, et al. Creating class I MHC-null pigs using guide RNA and the Cas9 endonuclease. J Immunol. 2014;193:5751–7.

179. Ladowski JM, et al. Swine leukocyte antigen class II is a xenoantigen. Transplantation. 2018;102:249–54.

180. Ladowski JM, et al. Examining the biosynthesis and xenoantigenicity of class II swine leukocyte antigen proteins. J Immunol. 2018;200:2957–64.

181. Ladowski J, Martens G, Estrada J, Tector M, Tector J. The desirable donor pig to eliminate all xenoreactive antigens. Xenotransplantation. 2019;26:e12504.

182. Sykes M. IXA honorary member lecture, 2017: the long and winding road to tolerance. Xenotransplantation. 2018;25:e12419.

183. Sachs DH, Sykes M, Greenstein JL, Cosimi AB. Tolerance and xenograft survival. Nat Med. 1995;1:969.

184. Yamada K, Sykes M, Sachs DH. Tolerance in xenotransplantation. Curr Opin Organ Transplant. 2017;22:522–8.

185. Scalea J, Hanecamp I, Robson SC, Yamada K. T-cell-mediated immunological barriers to xenotransplantation. Xenotransplantation. 2012;19:23–30.

186. Adams AB, et al. Xenoantigen deletion and chemical immunosuppression can prolong renal xenograft survival. Ann Surg. 2018;268:564–73.

187. Kim SC, et al. Long-term survival of pig-to-rhesus macaque renal xenografts is dependent on CD4 T cell depletion. Am J Transplant. 2019;19:2174–85.

188. Schroder PM, et al. The past, present, and future of costimulation blockade in organ transplantation. Curr Opin Organ Transplant. 2019;24:391–401.

189. Higginbotham L, et al. Pre-transplant antibody screening and anti-CD154 costimulation blockade promote long-term xenograft survival in a pig-to-primate kidney transplant model. Xenotransplantation. 2015;22:221–30.

190. Samy KP, Butler JR, Li P, Cooper DKC, Ekser B. The role of costimulation blockade in solid organ and islet xenotransplantation. J Immunol Res. 2017;2017:8415205.

191. Barth RN, et al. Xenogeneic thymokidney and thymic tissue transplantation in a pig-to-baboon model: I. Evidence for pig-specific T-cell unresponsiveness. Transplantation. 2003;75:1615–24.

192. Sablinski T, et al. Pig to monkey bone marrow and kidney xenotransplantation. Surgery. 1997;121:381–91.

193. Tena AA, et al. Prolonged survival of pig skin on baboons after administration of pig cells expressing human CD47. Transplantation. 2017;101:316–21.

194. Yamamoto T, Iwase H, King TW, Hara H, Cooper DKC. Skin xenotransplantation: historical review and clinical potential. Burns. 2018;44:1738–49.

195. Sykes M, Sachs DH. Transplanting organs from pigs to humans. Sci Immunol. 2019;4.

196. Butler JR, Ladowski JM, Martens GR, Tector M, Tector AJ. Recent advances in genome editing and creation of genetically modified pigs. Int J Surg. 2015;23:217–22.

197. Li P, et al. Efficient generation of genetically distinct pigs in a single pregnancy using multiplexed single-guide RNA and carbohydrate selection. Xenotransplantation. 2015;22:20–31.

198. Gordon JW, Ruddle FH. Integration and stable germ line transmission of genes injected into mouse pronuclei. Science. 1981;214:1244–6.

199. Jaenisch R. Germ line integration and Mendelian transmission of the exogenous Moloney leukemia virus. Proc Natl Acad Sci USA. 1976;73:1260–4.

200. Gossler A, Doetschman T, Korn R, Serfling E, Kemler R. Transgenesis by means of blastocyst-derived embryonic stem cell lines. Proc Natl Acad Sci USA. 1986;83:9065–9.

201. Saez E, No D, West A, Evans RM. Inducible gene expression in mammalian cells and transgenic mice. Curr Opin Biotechnol. 1997;8:608–16.

202. Burcin MM, O'Malley BW, Tsai SY. A regulatory system for target gene expression. Front Biosci. 1998;3:c1–7.

203. Blau HM, Rossi FM. Tet B or not tet B: advances in tetracycline-inducible gene expression. Proc Natl Acad Sci USA. 1999;96:797–9.

204. Murakami H, et al. Transgenic pigs expressing human decay-accelerating factor regulated by porcine MCP gene promoter. Mol Reprod Dev. 2002;61:302–11.

205. Fodor WL, et al. Expression of a functional human complement inhibitor in a transgenic pig as a model for the prevention of xenogeneic hyperacute organ rejection. Proc Natl Acad Sci USA. 1994;91:11153–7.

206. Diamond LE, et al. A human CD46 transgenic pig model system for the study of discordant xenotransplantation. Transplantation. 2001;71:132–42.

207. Zhou CY, et al. Transgenic pigs expressing human CD59, in combination with human membrane cofactor protein and human decay-accelerating factor. Xenotransplantation. 2005;12:142–8.

208. Wu G, et al. Coagulation cascade activation triggers early failure of pig hearts expressing human

complement regulatory genes. Xenotransplantation. 2007;14:34–47.

209. Mohiuddin MM, Reichart B, Byrne GW, McGregor CGA. Current status of pig heart xenotransplantation. Int J Surg. 2015;23:234–9.

210. Miwa Y, et al. Potential value of human thrombomodulin and DAF expression for coagulation control in pig-to-human xenotransplantation. Xenotransplantation. 2010;17:26–37.

211. Petersen B, et al. Pigs transgenic for human thrombomodulin have elevated production of activated protein C. Xenotransplantation. 2009;16:486–95.

212. Wheeler DG, et al. Transgenic swine: expression of human CD39 protects against myocardial injury. J Mol Cell Cardiol. 2012;52:958–61.

213. Yeom HJ, et al. Generation and characterization of human heme oxygenase-1 transgenic pigs. PLoS One. 2012;7:e46646.

214. Yan JJ, et al. Beneficial effects of the transgenic expression of human sTNF-alphaR-Fc and HO-1 on pig-to-mouse islet xenograft survival. Transpl Immunol. 2016;34:25–32.

215. Mansour SL, Thomas KR, Capecchi MR. Disruption of the proto-oncogene int-2 in mouse embryo-derived stem cells: a general strategy for targeting mutations to non-selectable genes. Nature. 1988;336:348–52.

216. Costa C, et al. Transgenic pigs designed to express human CD59 and H-transferase to avoid humoral xenograft rejection. Xenotransplantation. 2002;9:45–57.

217. Yang H, Wu Z. Genome editing of pigs for agriculture and biomedicine. Front Genet. 2018;9:360.

218. Wiedenheft B, Sternberg SH, Doudna JA. RNA-guided genetic silencing systems in bacteria and archaea. Nature. 2012;482:331–8.

219. Jinek M, et al. A programmable dual-RNA-guided DNA endonuclease in adaptive bacterial immunity. Science. 2012;337:816–21.

220. Bosley KS, et al. CRISPR germline engineering – the community speaks. Nat Biotechnol. 2015;33:478–86.

221. Doudna JA, Charpentier E. Genome editing. The new frontier of genome engineering with CRISPR-Cas9. Science. 2014;346:1258096.

222. Makarova KS, et al. Evolution and classification of the CRISPR-Cas systems. Nat Rev Microbiol. 2011;9:467–77.

223. Cong L, et al. Multiplex genome engineering using CRISPR/Cas systems. Science. 2013;339:819–23.

224. Knott GJ, Doudna JA. CRISPR-Cas guides the future of genetic engineering. Science. 2018;361:866–9.

225. Sternberg SH, Doudna JA. Expanding the Biologist's toolkit with CRISPR-Cas9. Mol Cell. 2015;58:568–74.

226. Fischer K, Kind A, Schnieke A. Assembling multiple xenoprotective transgenes in pigs. Xenotransplantation. 2018;25:e12431.

227. Brokowski C, Adli M. CRISPR ethics: moral considerations for applications of a powerful tool. J Mol Biol. 2019;431:88–101.

228. Kfoury C. Therapeutic cloning: promises and issues. Mcgill J Med. 2007;10:112–20.

229. Hodgson J. Dolly opens a farm full of possibilities. Nat Biotechnol. 1997;15:306.

230. Betthauser J, et al. Production of cloned pigs from in vitro systems. Nat Biotechnol. 2000;18:1055–9.

231. Onishi A, et al. Pig cloning by microinjection of fetal fibroblast nuclei. Science. 2000;289:1188–90.

232. Vogel G. In contrast to Dolly, cloning resets telomere clock in cattle. Science. 2000;288:586–7.

233. van der Berg JP, Kleter GA, Kok EJ. Regulation and safety considerations of somatic cell nuclear transfer-cloned farm animals and their offspring used for food production. Theriogenology. 2019;135:85–93.

234. van Smaalen TC, Hoogland ER, van Heurn LW. Machine perfusion viability testing. Curr Opin Organ Transplant. 2013;18:168–73.

235. Rubbini M. Perfusion machines for liver transplantation: technology and multifunctionality. Updat Surg. 2014;66:101–8.

236. Nasralla D, et al. A randomized trial of normothermic preservation in liver transplantation. Nature. 2018;557:50–6.

237. Messer S, Ardehali A, Tsui S. Normothermic donor heart perfusion: current clinical experience and the future. Transpl Int. 2015;28:634–42.

238. Ceresa CDL, et al. Transient cold storage prior to normothermic liver perfusion may facilitate adoption of a novel technology. Liver Transpl. 2019;25:1503–13.

239. Marecki H, et al. Liver ex situ machine perfusion preservation: a review of the methodology and results of large animal studies and clinical trials. Liver Transpl. 2017;23:679–95.

240. Cimeno A, et al. N-glycolylneuraminic acid knockout reduces erythrocyte sequestration and thromboxane elaboration in an ex vivo pig-to-human xenoperfusion model. Xenotransplantation. 2017;24.

241. LaMattina JC, et al. Pig-to-baboon liver xenoperfusion utilizing GalTKO.hCD46 pigs and glycoprotein Ib blockade. Xenotransplantation. 2014;21:274–86.

242. Fishman JA. Infection in xenotransplantation: opportunities and challenges. Curr Opin Organ Transplant. 2019;24:527–34.

243. Denner J, Scobie L, Schuurman HJ. Is it currently possible to evaluate the risk posed by PERVs for clinical xenotransplantation? Xenotransplantation. 2018;25:e12403.

244. Scobie L, et al. Long-term IgG response to porcine Neu5Gc antigens without transmission of PERV in burn patients treated with porcine skin xenografts. J Immunol. 2013;191:2907–15.

245. Choi HJ, et al. Long-term safety from transmission of porcine endogenous retrovirus after pig-to-non-human primate corneal transplantation. Xenotransplantation. 2017;24.

246. Morozov VA, et al. No PERV transmission during a clinical trial of pig islet cell transplantation. Virus Res. 2017;227:34–40.

247. McGregor CG, et al. Human CD55 expression blocks hyperacute rejection and restricts complement activation in Gal knockout cardiac xenografts. Transplantation. 2012;93:686–92.

248. Iwase H, et al. Immunological and physiological observations in baboons with life-supporting genetically engineered pig kidney grafts. Xenotransplantation. 2017;24.

249. Ekser B, Markmann JF, Tector AJ. Current status of pig liver xenotransplantation. Int J Surg. 2015;23:240–6.

250. Ekser B, et al. Genetically-engineered pig-to-baboon liver xenotransplantation: histopathology of xenografts and native organs. PLoS One. 2012;7:e29720.

251. Ezzelarab M, et al. Thrombocytopenia after pig-to-baboon liver xenotransplantation: where do platelets go? Xenotransplantation. 2011;18:320–7.

252. Lin CC, et al. Atorvastatin or transgenic expression of TFPI inhibits coagulation initiated by anti-nonGal IgG binding to porcine aortic endothelial cells. J Thromb Haemost. 2010;8:2001–10.

253. Mannon RB. Macrophages: contributors to allograft dysfunction, repair, or innocent bystanders? Curr Opin Organ Transplant. 2012;17:20–5.

254. von Albertini M, Ferran C, Brostjan C, Bach FH, Goodman DJ. Membrane-associated lymphotoxin on natural killer cells activates endothelial cells via an NF-kappaB-dependent pathway. Transplantation. 1998;66:1211–9.

255. Goodman DJ, Von Albertini M, Willson A, Millan MT, Bach FH. Direct activation of porcine endothelial cells by human natural killer cells. Transplantation. 1996;61:763–71.

256. Cho B, et al. Generation of soluble human tumor necrosis factor-alpha receptor 1-Fc transgenic pig. Transplantation. 2011;92:139–47.

257. Ferran C, et al. Expression of a truncated form of the human p55 TNF-receptor in bovine aortic endothelial cells renders them resistant to human TNF. Transplant Proc. 1996;28:618–9.

258. Weiss EH, et al. HLA-E/human beta2-microglobulin transgenic pigs: protection against xenogeneic human anti-pig natural killer cell cytotoxicity. Transplantation. 2009;87:35–43.

259. Neish AS, et al. Endothelial interferon regulatory factor 1 cooperates with NF-kappa B as a transcriptional activator of vascular cell adhesion molecule 1. Mol Cell Biol. 1995;15:2558–69.

260. Tellides G, Pober JS. Interferon-gamma axis in graft arteriosclerosis. Circ Res. 2007;100:622–32.

261. Matzinger P. An innate sense of danger. Semin Immunol. 1998;10:399–415.

262. Ezzelarab MB, et al. Systemic inflammation in xenograft recipients precedes activation of coagulation. Xenotransplantation. 2015;22:32–47.

263. Zhao Y, Li XC. Transplant tolerance: is it really free of concerns? Trends Immunol. 2007;28:376–7.

264. Yamamoto S, et al. Vascularized thymic lobe transplantation in a pig-to-baboon model: a novel strategy for xenogeneic tolerance induction and T-cell reconstitution. Transplantation. 2005;80:1783–90.

265. Mohiuddin MM, et al. Chimeric 2C10R4 anti-CD40 antibody therapy is critical for long-term survival of GTKO.hCD46.hTBM pig-to-primate cardiac xenograft. Nat Commun. 2016;7:11138.

266. Langin M, et al. Consistent success in life-supporting porcine cardiac xenotransplantation. Nature. 2018;564:430–3.

267. Yamamoto T, et al. Life-supporting kidney xenotransplantation from genetically-engineered pigs in baboons: a comparison of two immunosuppressive regimens. Transplantation. 2019.

268. Shin JS, et al. Long-term control of diabetes in immunosuppressed nonhuman primates (NHP) by the transplantation of adult porcine islets. Am J Transplant. 2015;15:2837–50.

269. Hu S, de Vos P. Polymeric approaches to reduce tissue responses against devices applied for islet-cell encapsulation. Front Bioeng Biotechnol. 2019;7:134.

270. Schmelzle M, et al. Increased plasma levels of microparticles expressing CD39 and CD133 in acute liver injury. Transplantation. 2013;95:63–9.

271. Hering BJ, et al. First update of the International Xenotransplantation Association consensus statement on conditions for undertaking clinical trials of porcine islet products in type 1 diabetes – executive summary. Xenotransplantation. 2016;23:3–13.

Anesthesia for Organ Transplantation

19

Amanda Milligan, Andrew Nath, Nick Pace, and Neil Logan

19.1 Preoperative Assessment

Extensive preoperative assessment of the patient will have taken place by the transplant team, a multidisciplinary team dedicated to investigation and optimization of patients preoperatively. This chapter focuses on the preoperative assessment by the anesthetist prior to theatre, and describes important aspects of the history, examination and investigations that influence anesthetic technique and drug choice.

As with all patients undergoing surgery the anesthetist assesses them before the procedure and collates the evidence to plan perioperative care. They may also have been part of the work-up team. Past medical history is noted systematically, including associated complications, and any changes in symptoms or physiological state, for example a reduced exercise tolerance, which will instigate further investigations pre-operatively. Airway assessment is important in any preoperative visit, particularly investigating for any indications for a rapid sequence induction (RSI).

Predictable comorbidities, such as diabetes and cardiovascular disease, are well known and these are likely to have been well investigated and treated before the patient reaches the transplant list. Each patient will also have predictable morbidity associated with their underlying pathological process, and for this reason they are cared for by specialist transplant teams. Generally, they are high risk patients undergoing major surgery and careful planning cannot be underestimated. Examination of the patient will likely reveal stigmata of the underlying process and/or their comorbid state.

Allergies are documented, particularly any issues with antibiotics and immunosuppressants that may affect the perioperative care or need to veer from protocol.

19.2 Investigations

Extensive investigation is important in patients presenting for transplantation. As part of the referral process and decision making on the patient's appropriateness for transplant they will have had laboratory blood work, imaging, and cardiovascular and respiratory function work up. Depending on their medical history the patient will have had further input from the appropriate specialty, for example endocrinology.

A. Milligan · N. Pace · N. Logan (✉)
NHS Greater Glasgow and Clyde, Queen Elizabeth
University Hospital, Glasgow, Scotland, UK
e-mail: amanda.milligan1@nhs.net;
Neil.Logan@ggc.scot.nhs.uk

A. Nath
NHS Greater Glasgow and Clyde, Golden Jubilee
National Hospital, Clydebank, Scotland, UK
e-mail: a.nath@nhs.net

© Springer Nature Switzerland AG 2021
N. Hakim et al. (eds.), *Transplantation Surgery*, Springer Specialist Surgery Series,
https://doi.org/10.1007/978-3-030-55244-2_19

Optimization of abnormalities, such as anemia, can be made preoperatively, but many patients will still need more up-to-date laboratory investigations and an updated electrocardiogram (ECG) on the day of admission, particularly since many medications can interfere with the patient's biochemistry.

Some patients will be critically unwell, such as those for liver transplant, and may require concomitant resuscitation and life-saving surgery, and investigations such as arterial blood gases will provide further information and point of care coagulation testing perioperatively is also required. Optimization in the critical care area preoperatively may focus on fluid balance and inotropic and/or vasopressor support as a bridge to transplant.

19.3 Preparation of the Patient

Immunosuppressant drugs are sometimes started preoperatively. Liaison between teams is vital to ensure protocols are followed. The surgical brief provides an opportunity to discuss the immunosuppression in addition to ensuring theatre team introductions, the discussion of anticipated surgical and anesthetic events, and to address concerns.

Premedication for anxiolysis may be given in certain circumstances, such as heart transplant patients, but are not routine for other organ transplants. Premedication to treat gastroesophageal reflux/prophylaxis of aspiration of gastric contents is given in at risk patients, and a decision communicated with the preoperative staff regarding which of the patient's usual medications are to be given and fasting time.

Preoperative checks include appropriate consent for the procedure, ensuring adequate blood products are available or have been requested ahead of surgery, and organizing the appropriate postoperative destination, i.e. has a critical care bed been booked for postoperative care.

The anesthetic team should explain the anesthetic risk, postoperative expectation to the patient, including destination and analgesia options, and insertion of invasive lines.

19.4 Intraoperative Considerations

The considerations for each type of transplant surgery are discussed in detail in the relevant section.

General measures include:

- Monitoring; routine monitoring is applied regardless of procedure, invasive monitoring should be considered if indicated, though may be routine in some transplants
- Immunosuppression; already mentioned but is common to all transplants and careful planning is necessary
- Prophylactic antibiotics; local protocols exist for these and with immunosuppression and underlying comorbidities, such as diabetes, these are vital
- Venous-thromboembolism prophylaxis; the stress response to surgery should not be underestimated and the risk of thrombosis in the perioperative period is significant therefore this is part of the perioperative care plan
- Temperature control and pressure area care; hypothermia has significant implications perioperatively and normothermia must be maintained, except for thoracic organ transplantation where hypothermia is targeted. Pressure areas are vulnerable is these patients and long procedures mean careful positioning is paramount

Many centres will have their own protocol for the perioperative care of transplant patients, and a common-sense approach is also required to maintain a balance between adequate anesthesia, analgesia, and cardiovascular stability.

19.5 Postoperative Considerations

Postoperative care is vital to ensure the viability of the newly transplanted graft. Continued optimization of hemodynamic stability and oxygen delivery means the patient must be cared for in the appropriate environment. Most patients will return to the critical care unit postoperatively, either for level 3 or level 2 care depending on organ support requirement. The exception in our institute is renal transplant recipients, who return to the renal ward postoperatively for ongoing care from the medical and surgical teams, unless there is a clear indication for critical care admission.

The anesthetic management of each organ transplant procedure is described in the following sections.

19.6 Heart Transplantation

The anesthetic management of heart transplant patients before, during and after transplantation presents some specific problems for the anesthetist which may influence early and late results.

19.7 Preoperative Management

As increasing the time taken to implant the donor heart affects 1-year mortality, the procedure is carried out as an emergency [1]. However, the transplant program usually ensures that patients are in the "best possible shape". Similarly, the potential "full stomach" rarely occurs because the transplant coordinator should make sure that suitable candidates are getting prepared and fasting. The importance of a coordinated approach and excellent communication between "donor team" and "recipient team" to ensure the optimal timing of the various procedures should not be underestimated.

The patient should be assessed preoperatively by the anesthetist and note made of any previous anesthetic, medical and surgical histories. If the patient is undergoing 're-do' sternotomy, then surgery is more technically challenging, increased time must be allowed for the initial stages of surgery and there is potential for major hemorrhage accessing the mediastinum. Most patients are receiving diuretics and may have low potassium levels whilst other drugs may influence anesthesia; e.g. ACE inhibitors occasionally result in a low systemic vascular resistance dur-

ing cardiopulmonary bypass. In addition to their cardiac disease many patients have reversible impairment of their respiratory, renal and hepatic function and where time allows these should be addressed.

It is necessary to ensure that information from all relevant investigations is available. These include ECG, urea and electrolytes (U + Es), liver function tests (LFTs), full blood count (FBC), coagulation, chest X-ray and tests of cardiac function. Any abnormality should be corrected preoperatively. The patient should be cross-matched for 4 units of concentrated red cells and there should be fresh frozen plasma (FFP) and platelets available, particularly for those with preexisting abnormalities of coagulation, which will be compounded by cardiopulmonary bypass. Most of these patients would have been assessed regularly by cardiologists and there should be recent angiograms and echocardiograms to estimate the residual cardiac function. Patients are usually on optimum medical therapy and although "sick" there is rarely if ever any reason for cancellation to improve the preoperative status.

Increasing numbers of patents are inpatients in critical care areas and are receiving inotrope infusions pre-operatively to support cardiac function whilst awaiting a donor heart. Internationally, 43% of patients receiving heart transplantation receive Mechanical Circulatory Support (MCS) at the time of transplant. The most commonly used method is Left Ventricular Assist Device (LVAD) support, but other devices that may be in situ are Right sided VADs, Intra-Aortic Balloon Pumps, Extra-Corporeal Membrane Oxygenation (ECMO) and total artificial heart devices [2]. The aim of LVAD support as a bridge to transplant is to improve end organ function, nutritional status and physical fitness to improve survival post-transplant. These patients are usually anti-coagulated, and this should be reversed appropriately prior to surgery. Risks of MCS include clotting factor deficiency, acquired VWD, risk of infections from the device, heparin induced thrombocytopenia, and hemorrhage secondary to anticoagulation [2].

19.8 Intraoperative Management

The principles of anesthesia for other types of cardiac surgery apply and many different anesthetic agents and techniques have been used. The technique of choice varies according to individual transplant centers. There is no evidence that any one technique leads to a better outcome than any other. There is much preparation to be done prior to the arrival of the patient in the anesthetic room (Table 19.1), and transfer to theatre of patients with MCS and inotropic infusions is a challenge requiring careful co-ordination. In order to ensure a timely implantation of the donor heart, effective communication between the organ retrieval and transplant team is vital.

Table 19.1 Set up prior to arrival of patient in anesthetic room

Equipment:	
Infusion pumps—at least 4	
Pressure transducers—at least 3	
CVP line	
Arterial line	
Nasopharyngeal and peripheral temperature probes	
Urinary catheter	
Pulmonary artery catheter (used in some centers)	
Drugs:	
Resuscitation	Atropine
	Calcium chloride
	Metaraminol
	Epinephrine (adrenaline)
Inotropes	Dobutamine
	Norepinephrine (noradrenaline)
	Epinephrine (adrenaline)
	Milrinone (if increased pulmonary artery pressure and possible right ventricular failure)
	Vasopressin
Anesthetic	Remifentanil
	Midazolam
	Rocuronium
	Propofol infusion
Others	Methylprednisolone (500 mg at induction, then before removal of Aortic Cross Clamp)
	Tranexamic acid
	Heparin
	Protamine
	Antibiotics according to local protocol
	Immunosuppressive agents according to local protocol

As mentioned earlier, most patients should have been fasted for 6 h and it can be argued that a rapid sequence induction is not appropriate in a patient group with such poor cardiovascular reserve. In addition to standard monitoring, invasive arterial blood pressure monitoring should be inserted prior to induction of anesthesia. Large bore IV access should be achieved. Some anesthetists insist on a central line being inserted prior to induction, in order to facilitate a timely start to surgery after induction of anesthesia, however others feel this is an unnecessary stress on the patient. The patients are preoxygenated. Indeed, most will come down to theater with oxygen. Once all monitoring is established the patient is induced with high dose opiate (in the author's institution remifentanil target-controlled infusion is used), an IV induction agent ± midazolam. A muscle relaxant is administered, and the trachea is then intubated. Anesthesia is maintained according to local habits with propofol by infusion or with inhalational agents such as sevoflurane. Nitrous oxide is best avoided in view of its cardio-depressant activity and the risk of increasing the size of any air embolus.

The central line and urinary catheter may then be placed if not already in situ. There is variation between centers in the site of placement of the central line, some centers insisting on the left internal jugular vein so that endocardial biopsies may be carried out via the right side. Other centers use the femoral vein for endocardial biopsies. A Swan-Ganz catheter if used would need to be pulled back during the procedure and then re-advanced across a suture line. Therefore, it is not universally used initially. All invasive procedures require strict aseptic techniques in view of the patient's impending immunocompromise.

Blood gases, U + Es, activated clotting time (ACT) and thromboelastography (TEG) are done as a baseline. The cardiopulmonary bypass pump is primed with 1.5 l of crystalloid or colloid and this has a significant dilutional effect when the patient is on bypass. Most anesthetists aim for a hematocrit (HCT) of no less than 20% whilst on bypass. If less than this, concentrated red cells are added to the pump. If the preoperative HCT is less than 30%, the requirement for red cells is almost certain. Tranexamic acid is infused according to local protocols to stabilize clot formation and reduce bleeding [3]. A transesophageal echocardiography probe is inserted, and a comprehensive examination is performed to assist fluid, inotrope and vasoconstrictor therapy, both in the native heart and the allograft post-implantation.

Once the heart and bypass cannulas insertion sites have been prepared, intravenous heparin is administered, and the patient put on cardiopulmonary bypass. When the pump is at full flow, the ventilation from the anesthetic machine may be terminated, however there is some evidence that continuing positive pressure ventilation at low minute ventilation reduces perioperative inflammatory mediator release and improves oxygenation after weaning CPB [4]. It is customary in UK practice to cool the patient during bypass to around 28–32 °C. A mean blood pressure of 40–80 mmHg is aimed for, although these figures are entirely arbitrary, and the blood pressure may be manipulated by altering the rate of the anesthetic agent, by use of an inotropic or pressor agent or, rarely, a vasodilator. The perfusionist usually repeats blood gases and ACT half-hourly while on bypass. Before the removal of the aortic cross clamp in the donor heart it is necessary to re-administer the dose of methylprednisolone. Some centers administer magnesium slowly during bypass to decrease postoperative atrial arrhythmias.

With the anastomoses complete and the patient rewarmed, cardiopulmonary bypass is terminated by first reventilating the patient and then decreasing the flow from the bypass pump while watching the patient's response. Due to the ischemic period from explantation to implantation it is usually necessary to administer inotropes at this point. It is customary to start them or increase them prior to the end of bypass, and they are likely to continue for several days post-operatively. The choice of agent is centre dependent, with no evidence of one regime's superiority [5]; in our institution the first-choice agents are dobutamine and norepinephrine. The new heart is denervated, and as such has an intrinsic rate of 100–120 beats per minute and responds to circulating catecholamines rather than direct autonomic stimulation.

It is normally only able to increase its output by increasing its stroke volume. Conduction abnormalities including complete heart block are common and epicardial pacing wires are routinely placed in our institution, with some patients going on to require permanent pace makers later.

Once the surgeon is satisfied with the integrity of the anastomoses and the patient's cardiovascular stability, systemic anticoagulation is reversed with protamine. Owing to the long period of CPB and inflammatory response to surgery, coagulopathy is common. Coagulation studies, TEG and ACT should be checked, and blood and blood products administered accordingly upon administration of protamine. Once surgery is complete the patient is admitted to the intensive therapy unit (ITU) postoperatively.

19.9 Postoperative Management

Care of this patient group is complex. The patient is intubated and ventilated, has multiple invasive monitoring lines and inotropic infusions, and has potential for multiorgan dysfunction. Due to the large doses of immunosuppressant medication administered, the patient is nursed in isolation.

Bloods and blood gases are checked regularly, with any abnormality corrected. Mediastinal and intercostal drain outputs are monitored as the patient has potential for hemorrhage, coagulopathy and cardiac tamponade. If the risk of bleeding is deemed high, then the chest may be left open to prevent tamponade and closed once the patient is more stable [6]. Echocardiography is performed regularly to monitor ventricular function, guide therapy and to identify signs of primary graft failure. Endocardial biopsy is the most sensitive and specific index of graft rejection and is performed every 5–7 days for the first 4–6 weeks.

Primary graft failure is defined as allograft dysfunction that occurs within the first 24 h following transplantation not attributable to other causes. It is the leading cause of early mortality and has a 2–36% incidence in the early post-op period. Treatment is initially with pharmacotherapy, and then can be escalated to MCS if necessary [6].

Disturbances of cardiac rhythm are common in the early postoperative phase. Supraventricular dysrhythmias are the most common post-operative arrhythmia. These abnormalities respond to treatment with standard antidysrhythmic drugs and cardioversion if necessary, however may be a sign of primary graft failure, and thus should be investigated [6].

There is potential for acute kidney injury postoperatively, potentially making fluid management problematic. Initially, in the face of oliguria, loop diuretics may be needed to prevent volume overloading of the right ventricle, but if this is unsuccessful then RRT should be instituted early to control fluid balance [7].

19.10 Right Ventricular Failure

The right ventricle's (RV's) thin walled structure makes it particularly at risk of failure from the ischemic time after harvest from the donor. In addition, the anterior position of the right coronary ostia makes passage of air bubbles down the right coronary artery more likely, and the donor heart is naïve to the high pulmonary artery pressures of a chronic heart failure patient. The patient is invasively ventilated causing deleterious effects on pulmonary vascular resistance (PVR). The result is a particular vulnerability of the RV to failure post-transplant, and its management is challenging.

Central venous pressure (CVP) can be used to guide RV filling pressure, and TOE can help to assess RV size and function. Flattened appearances of the interventricular septum, increased chamber size and increased tricuspid regurgitation are signs of a volume or pressure overloaded RV.

Initial management includes correcting hypoxia, hypercarbia and acidosis with the aim of lowering PVR and RV afterload. Volume overload can be treated with diuretics and renal replacement therapy if needed. Alongside other more commonly used inotropes to increase contractility, milrinone can be used for its lowering effect on PVR. Nitric oxide can be added to inhaled gases, acting locally as a pulmonary vasodilator with minimal systemic absorption, it also lowers PVR. If these measures fail, then VAD therapy can be considered [3].

19.11 Lung Transplantation

Lung transplantation is, in fact, a group of operative procedures comprising single-lung transplant, bilateral sequential lung transplant, lobar transplant and en-block heart-lung transplantation.

COPD, interstitial lung disease, and bronchiectasis (including cystic fibrosis) are the commonest reason for lung transplantation worldwide (36.5%, 29.7% and 18.5% respectively), with pulmonary hypertension and other less common diseases making up a minority of cases. Bilateral sequential lung transplants make up the majority of transplants. The vast majority (85%) of single lung transplants are performed in patients with COPD or ILD, compared to a greater spread across varying pathologies for bilateral sequential transplants [7].

19.12 Preoperative Management

The patient should be seen preoperatively by the anesthetist and particular attention should be paid to past medical, surgical and anesthetic histories. These patients are often oxygen dependent and are unable to tolerate any exertion. It is necessary to assess their cardiovascular and respiratory systems in some detail with regard to function of the right and left ventricles, the presence or indeed absence of pulmonary hypertension, their exercise tolerance, the degree of impairment they currently suffer, and the possible presence of any other system involvement.

The majority of these patients would have undergone a battery of tests. Pulmonary function tests, exercise tolerance tests, full blood count, urea and electrolytes will have been performed prior to listing. Imaging investigations undertaken may include CT of chest which also allows identification of coronary artery calcification, coronary angiography, transthoracic echocardiography to assess ventricular function and estimation of pulmonary artery pressures, and lung perfusion scanning to assess suitability and site for single lung transplantation. Microbiology can be useful in identifying colonization with drug resistant bacteria [8]. It should always be remembered that the clinical situation may have deteriorated since those assessments.

Caution is advised with premedication in patients with COPD, as one should aim to avoid respiratory compromise, but it may, in fact, be beneficial in patients with pulmonary hypertension. Some centers would advise the use of agents which decrease airway secretions. Virtually all patients should come down to theater with supplemental oxygen.

19.13 Intraoperative Management

There is much preparation involved prior to the patient's arrival in theater (Table 19.2).

The patient is identified in the anesthetic room and routine monitoring (ECG, pulse oximetry) established. An arterial line is placed under local

Table 19.2 Preparation for lung transplantation

Equipment	Double lumen tube
	Transducers—at least 3
	Infusion pumps—at least 2
	CVP line + Swan-Ganz catheter
	20-gauge arterial line
	Urinary catheter
	Core temperature probe
	Transesophageal echo
Drugs:	
Anesthetic	Propofol
	Rocuronium
	Fentanyl/alfentanil/remifentanil
	Midazolam
Resuscitation	Ephedrine
	Metaraminol
	Epinephrine (adrenaline)
Inotropes	Dobutamine
	Norepinephrine (noradrenaline)
	Epinephrine (adrenaline)
	Milrinone
	Nitric Oxide
Miscellaneous	Antibiotics
	Immunosuppressive agents according to local protocol

anesthesia for sampling purposes and for direct measurement of blood pressure. Opinion varies as to whether the Swan-Ganz catheter should be inserted prior to induction. However, it is certainly recommended in view of the severe cardiovascular instability which may be associated with one lung ventilation. It will normally float to the side with preferential perfusion, but its position should be checked intraoperatively and prior to stapling of the pulmonary artery—if necessary it can be pulled back and refloated. If a Swan-Ganz catheter is not used a CVP line should be inserted to aid decisions on fluid replacement. An epidural catheter is frequently inserted prior to induction.

Particular attention should be paid to the possibility of reactive airways and hemodynamic instability at induction of anesthesia due to the effect of anesthetic agents on coronary perfusion pressure and myocardial contractility. Either a right- or left-sided double lumen tube may be employed but a left-sided tube is preferable since it avoids the risk of non-ventilation of the right upper lobe and is usually easier to place. The position of the tube should be checked by fiberoptic scope at this point and again later once the patient has been positioned on the operating table. In cystic fibrosis patients it may be beneficial to insert a single lumen tube initially to enable flexible bronchoscopy and removal of tenacious secretions to air ventilation intra-operatively and reduce bacterial contamination of the new lungs. This can then be changed to a double lumen tube prior to the start of surgery [9, 10]. Where necessary in bilateral sequential lung transplant, the endobronchial lumen of the tube may be retracted at the time of bronchial transection of the second lung while ventilation is continued to the first transplanted lung. A nasogastric tube is usually placed prior to the start of surgery.

It is not uncommon to encounter hypotension following induction due to several factors, including tamponade secondary to overdistension of the lungs and impaired venous return with positive pressure ventilation, decreased right ventricular output due to increased pulmonary vascular resistance, withdrawal of the preexisting circulating catecholamines associated with anxiety, and the effects of the anesthetic agents. The treatment of this hypotension should address its cause and usually includes optimization of volume status, inotropes and minimizing intrathoracic pressure.

Intra-operative transesophageal echocardiography is of use for several reasons. It allows assessment of ventricular and valvular function, identification of cardiac defects that require surgery (e.g. atrial septal defect), patency of vascular anastomoses, identification of the presence of air bubbles, and assessment of volume status [11].

Maintenance of anesthesia is with oxygen in air if tolerated and either inhalational anesthesia or a propofol infusion. Theoretically volatile agents affect hypoxic pulmonary vasoconstriction and may affect ventilation perfusion matching, however long-term outcome has not been proved superior with either method and technique varies from centre to centre [11, 12].

19.14 Intraoperative Problems

Several problems may be predicted intraoperatively.

Following the start of one lung ventilation (OLV) several problems arise due to the significant effects it has on airway pressure, oxygenation and hemodynamic stability. Patients with restrictive disease may require a smaller tidal volume and increased rate while those with obstructive disease may require an increased expiratory phase to decrease air-trapping. It is not unusual to have to manipulate the ventilator settings to try to maintain the patient's oxygenation with reasonable airway pressures. On occasion it may be necessary to institute some form of differential lung ventilation (continuous positive airway pressure or oxygen insufflation to the non-ventilated lung) to minimize intrapulmonary shunting.

Some patients develop cardiac or respiratory instability during the procedure. This may be due to inadequate oxygenation, especially during one lung ventilation, or right ventricular failure after clamping of the pulmonary artery. However, it may also be due to hyperinflation of the lungs and air trapping in COPD patients, this in turn leading to decreased venous return, decreased cardiac output and systemic hypotension. In patients with

COPD it may be necessary to allow the carbon dioxide levels to rise (permissive hypercapnia) [12]. Respiratory acidosis may then become a problem, however.

Right ventricular failure and associated hypotension may become a major problem after the pulmonary artery has been clamped and those with restrictive diseases may require pulmonary vasodilators to reduce pulmonary vascular resistance, an infusion of prostaglandin El has the disadvantage that it also produces systemic vasodilation and arterial hypotension and may worsen oxygenation by increasing intrapulmonary shunting. It may therefore be necessary to use pressor agents to maintain systemic blood pressure. Another option is addition of nitric oxide to inhalational gases. It causes vasodilation of the pulmonary vasculature alone and has no effect on systemic pressure. Despite a lack of evidence on long-term mortality, in some institutions it is considered the drug of choice for the management of pulmonary hypertension. If medical management of cardiovascular instability fails, then mechanical circulatory support (MCS) may be instituted.

Traditionally, heparinization and institution of cardiopulmonary bypass (CPB) has been used for MCS during lung transplantation. Due to high anticoagulation dose and inflammatory response this has been associated with increased blood product administration, increased duration of ventilation and increased duration of ICU stay when compared to no mechanical support. Increasingly, Extra-corporeal Membrane Oxygenation (ECMO) is being used as a method of MCS in these cases. Advantages of its use are a reduction of pulmonary artery pressure aiding right ventricular function, improved gas exchange during one lung ventilation, and the facilitation of gentle reperfusion of the newly implanted lung. There is also evidence of reduced rates of primary graft dysfunction and reduced bleeding post-operatively when compared to CPB [12, 13].

After implantation, the pulmonary artery is slowly unclamped over 10 min, and the lung is recruited and ventilated. There is potential at this stage for cardiovascular instability as cold acidotic products of metabolism, and air emboli are washed into the coronary circulation. TOE is useful at this stage for identification of problems listed previously. A positive end-expiratory pressure of approximately 5–10 cm of water is added to allow adequate oxygenation while keeping the inspired oxygen concentration low. It should also help to minimize alveolar transudate. Occasionally the transplanted lung may exhibit a "pulmonary reimplantation response" which manifests as a low pressure pulmonary edema, poor oxygenation and poor lung compliance. This is now thought to be due to ischemia-reperfusion injury but may also be related to denervation and loss of lymphatic drainage of the transplanted lung. It is occasionally accompanied by pulmonary hypertension and the treatment for this has already been outlined.

19.15 Postoperative Management

Patients are admitted to a single room in the ITU postoperatively. It is customary to change the double lumen endobronchial tube to a single lumen tube at the end of the procedure. Immunosuppressive therapy is continued as per local protocol.

There are several areas of importance in the management of these patients.

19.16 Ventilation

Primary graft dysfunction (PGD) is the commonest cause of post-operative mortality and occurs in 10–57% of patients [10]. Its presentation is analogous to ARDS, and the principles of management are similar.

The aim in all patients is to achieve adequate oxygenation with the lowest inspired oxygen concentration possible and to minimize peak airway pressures, both intra and post-operatively, as this has been shown to reduce rates of PGD. Tidal volumes should be set to 7 ml/kg ideal body weight of the donor if known to avoid over distention and volutrauma, and peak inspiratory pressure should be minimized to less than 30 cmH20 to minimize barotrauma to the newly implanted lungs. MCS is associated with greater incidence of PGD, so bronchoscopic toilet may be beneficial in optimizing ventilation in order to avoid this intervention. The International Society of Heart and Lung Transplant (ISHLT) also recommend cautious use of IV fluids in these patients to optimize gas exchange [8].

The postoperative ventilatory management is impacted upon by the specific procedure performed and the underlying condition. In patients undergoing single-lung transplant for COPD the more compliant native lung will be ventilated preferentially. Long expiratory time to account for obstructive air flow and a lower respiratory rate would be beneficial in this patient group. In patients who have undergone a single-lung transplant for restrictive lung disease, the majority of ventilation occurs in the more compliant newly implanted lung, risking over inflation and ventilator induced lung injury (VILI), and tidal volumes may need to be reduced. Independent lung ventilation using a double lumen endobronchial tube may be employed in these instances, however this requires larger levels of sedations and ECMO or extra-corporeal CO_2 removal strategies may be of benefit [10].

In patients receiving bilateral sequential lung transplantation, the same lung protective ventilation strategies are employed as above. If the allograft is undersized compared to the recipient, then using recipient IBW for TV setting may cause overdistention of the new lungs and so donor size should influence TV choice. If gas exchange is so poor that lung protective ventilation does not meet requirements, then ECMO can be employed to allow satisfactory ventilator settings. Singe cannula VV ECMO techniques allow reduced sedation rates and may be beneficial.

19.17 Hemodynamic Instability

It is essential that preload and afterload are Optimized in these patients. There is debate regarding how much crystalloid can safely be given to these patients without effect on the graft and it is not unusual to administer diuretics to these patients rather than try to give them a fluid load to aid urine output.

Hemorrhage postoperatively is not uncommon, more so in those patients who have required MCS for the procedure. MCS is associated with increased blood transfusion requirements (both concentrated red cells and blood products). Pulmonary hypertension and PGD can influence postoperative recovery and the management of pulmonary hypertension has been discussed. It is prudent to mention that prolonged treatment with nitric oxide may lead to transient methemoglobinemia.

19.18 Analgesia

Thoracotomy pain is said to be one of the most severe types of pain and this in turn can lead to severe respiratory impairment in this group of patients. The provision of postoperative analgesia is complicated by pulmonary denervation, the size of surgical incision and any residual impairment of pulmonary function. Analgesia can be provided by two routes—epidural analgesia and intravenous opiates—either by bolus, infusion or once the patient wakes up, by Patient Controlled Analgesia. Epidural analgesia where possible should be considered the standard form of analgesia for these patients. A thoracic epidural catheter may be sited with the patient awake prior to the start of the procedure assuming there are no contraindications (such as patient refusal, coagulopathy, heparin treatment, sepsis) and may be used both intraoperatively and postoperatively. Each institution usually has its own cocktail of drugs for infusion, but a common regimen is 0.1% L-bupivacaine plus 10 µg of fentanyl per ml infused at between 3 and 8 ml/h. Epidural analgesia decreases the time to extubation and reduces ITU length of stay, resulting in excellent postoperative analgesia when compared to intravenous opioids [14]. In those patients requiring CPB and therefore the use of intraoperative heparin for systemic anticoagulation, epidurals are best avoided in view of the risk of epidural hematoma, although some institutions would dispute this.

19.19 Liver Transplantation

Liver transplantation is the sole definitive treatment for end-stage liver disease [15]. Liver failure may be acute or chronic, with end-stage liver disease (ESLD) related to chronic liver disease the most common indication(s) for liver transplant [16]. The anesthetic considerations in managing such patients is complex and requires meticulous planning, with some nuances in the management between chronic and acute liver failure transplant patients.

Pre-operative assessment in chronic liver disease patients is extensive and involves a multi-disciplinary team approach (for example, hepatologist, transplant surgeon and anesthetist, intensive care physician, transplant coordinator, and other health care professionals, such as psychologist or dietician) before being placed on the transplant list [16]. Acute or fulminant hepatic failure patients require a more truncated, but thorough, work-up prior to potential transplantation.

There are many systemic changes associated with liver disease that make the management of patients with ESLD challenging peri-operatively. Every opportunity should be taken to optimize hematological, biochemical, and physiological parameters where able, and medical co-morbidities such as ischemic heart disease or associated cardiomyopathy. Cardiopulmonary events are the leading cause of non-graft related deaths in liver transplant [16] therefore detailed evaluation of function and physiological reserve of these systems is crucial.

Preoperative assessment includes the investigation and treatment/optimization of:

- Jaundice, hyponatremia, ascites, and pleural effusions
- Diabetes
- Cardiac failure and systemic vasodilation with hypotension
- Renal impairment
- Porto-pulmonary and hepatopulmonary syndromes
- Varices
- Coagulopathy
- Nutritional state and muscle mass

Table 19.3 Investigation protocol examples [17]

Investigations in patients readmitted for elective liver transplant		Patients with fulminant hepatic failure for emergency liver transplant			
FBC	Na	FBC	Na	ABG:	PA catheter data:
PT	K	PT	K	H+	CVP
APTT	Urea	APTT	Urea	$PaCO_2$	RAP
Fibrinogen	Creatinine	Fibrinogen	Creatinine	PaO_2	RVP
	Glucose		Glucose	HCO_3^-	PAP
	LFTs		Lactate	BE	PAOP
	GGT		LFTs	FiO_2	CO
			GGT		SvO_2
					PvO_2
CXR (if new clinical signs or none in the last 3 months)		CXR		Height	
ECG		ECG		Weight	
				ABO group	
				CMV status	
Additional tests depending on individual patient:		Neurological monitoring: Max ICP preoperatively Jugular bulb: Higher O₂ sats/lowest O₂ sats Higher lactate/lowest lactate Intercurrent disease			

Routine investigations (Table 19.3) will vary depending on the nature of transplant, i.e. waiting list transplants or acute transplants in fulminant hepatic failure, and clinical picture of the patient.

Drug handling is altered in liver disease, including drugs of anesthesia and analgesia. The metabolism of drugs used during anesthesia may be altered due to:

- decreased serum albumin and abnormal protein binding
- altered volume of distribution
- decreased hepatic blood flow and extraction ratio
- decreased number of functioning hepatocytes
- altered hepatic biotransformation
- decreased hepatic clearance
- altered pharmacodynamics

The management of general anesthesia is discussed further below.

19.20 Preoperative Management

By nature of end stage liver disease (ESLD) the patient may be critically ill preoperatively, and perhaps encephalopathic. Consent should be sought prior to any cognitive impairment, but there may be a necessity to use appropriate consent forms for patients who are incapacitated.

The case anesthetist will assess the patient preoperatively paying attention to comorbidities and up to date investigations. A full anesthetic history is also taken. If there are abnormalities further intervention is guided by these findings, for example uncorrected coagulopathy. In the event of fulminant hepatic failure, intracranial pressure monitoring may be used peri-operatively; this is routine in our local liver unit for such patients, occasionally jugular bulb oxygen saturation monitoring is used. Critically ill patients may require renal replacement therapy preoperatively and decisions should be made regarding its potential continuation intraoperatively.

Premedication for anxiolysis is not routine but may be considered, for example temazepam orally 1–2 h preoperatively. Gastric acid reduction/prophylaxis of gastric acid aspiration is given: our local unit uses ranitidine orally, if the patient isn't already on a proton pump inhibitor, the night before and morning of surgery.

19.20.1 Blood Products

Blood loss is very variable and cell salvage is used intraoperatively, with the severity of pretransplant liver disease, as calculated using the model for end-stage liver disease (MELD), strongly predictive of the need for peri-operative transfusion support [16]. The number of cross-matched packed red blood cell (PRBC) units requested pre-operatively has decreased with newer surgical techniques, the use of cell salvage, and maintenance of a low central venous pressure intraoperatively. Complex cases or re-transplants are likely to require more consideration regarding cross-match requirements. Preoperative PRBC cross-match is likely to be between 5–10 units with the use of other blood products guided by preoperative coagulation tests, including point of care (POC) coagulation testing, which is repeated perioperatively.

Treatment of coagulopathy is likely to include transfusions of fresh frozen plasma (FFP), platelets, and perhaps cryoprecipitate. There is no consensus on the optimum regime or threshold for treatment, and practice is variable across the continent(s), for example coagulation factor concentrates are used widely in mainland Europe but the United Kingdom generally uses FFP. Our local transplant unit advocates considering pre-thawing of 4 units of FFP to treat intraoperative coagulopathy.

19.21 Intraoperative Management

19.21.1 Pre-induction Preparation

In addition to pre-operative patient assessment and blood product preparation, further planning of the intra-operative management is required before induction of anesthesia.

19.21.1.1 Monitoring and Equipment
Waiting list patients may be hemodynamically stable, and therefore the use of routine monitoring requirements should be used before induction of anesthesia. Additional monitors include peripheral nerve monitoring when neuromuscular blocking drugs are used, and temperature in procedures longer than 30 min.

Invasive arterial blood pressure monitoring may be used pre-induction in unstable or critically unwell patients, the arterial line sited after local anesthetic infiltration. All other access lines will be inserted post induction.

The appropriate number of infusion pumps, a rapid infuser for intravenous fluids and blood products, and cell salvage equipment should be available for all cases. Transesophageal echocardiography (TEE) is used in some centres [15] but may be complicated in those with known esophageal varices.

19.21.1.2 Lines
All large blood vessel access lines are performed aseptically with full surgical scrub by the anesthetist and using real-time ultrasound guided insertion. Below are the lines used in our local transplant unit

- Right internal jugular vein: quad lumen central venous catheter (CVC); 7.5Fr pulmonary artery catheter (PAC); large bore venous access such as the Arrow MAC 2 lumen CVC.
- Left radial artery: 3Fr arterial line for blood sampling
- Right femoral artery: 4Fr arterial line for uninterrupted invasive blood pressure monitoring.
- Percutaneous access to the left internal jugular vein in the (rare) instances where veno-venous bypass is required, for venous return from the pump. The surgical 'piggy-back' technique +/− portal vein-inferior vena cava (IVC) shunt creation means this is usually not required.

19.21.1.3 Drugs
Infusions of vasopressor and inotropic drugs may be made in advance, but the aim of low central venous pressure to minimize surgical blood loss means this may not be routine in every centre. Emergency drugs, such as epinephrine 1:10,000 and 1:100,000 concentrations, are drawn up pre-operatively in 10 ml syringes. Other usual emergency drugs include atropine, glycopyrrolate, and metaraminol.

Drugs for anesthesia are discussed below.

19.21.2 Induction of Anesthesia

Induction of anesthesia is via large bore peripheral venous cannula (PVC). In time-critical transplants the patient may not be adequately fasted, necessitating a rapid sequence induction (RSI) of anesthesia. This means the patient is preoxygenated to denitrogenate the lungs and create an oxygen reserve for consumption during apneic phase between induction and tracheal intubation, and cricoid pressure is used in the UK. Those who are fasted but with risk factors for regurgitation and aspiration of gastric contents, for example those with ascites and increased intra-abdominal pressure, will also need a RSI.

Propofol is widely used. It undergoes extrahepatic metabolism and can be used in those with ESLD. Due to the altered cardiovascular response to stress in those with liver cirrhosis [18] the hypotensive response may be exaggerated.

Muscle relaxant options include suxamethonium and rocuronium, in RSI, and atracurium. Atracurium does not depend on liver metabolism and is used as a continuous infusion intraoperatively in our local unit. There are some reports that suggest using rocuronium during liver transplant appears to be a predictor of primary allograft function; in all patients whose neuromuscular recovery time was >150 min experiencing primary graft dysfunction [19].

The action of many opioids is prolonged in severe liver disease; however, fentanyl metabolism is largely unaffected [15]. Remifentanil undergoes ester hydrolysis in tissue and plasma and its duration of action is unaffected by liver disease. Alfentanil has less cardiovascular side effects than fentanyl or remifentanil, but the dose should be reduced [20, 21].

The endotracheal tube should have a large volume low pressure cuff to avoid mucosal damage during the lengthy procedure.

19.21.3 Maintenance of Anesthesia

Volatile agents are predominantly used in the maintenance of anesthesia; isoflurane is the vapor of choice, with oxygen-air mix carrier gas, up to a minimum alveolar concentration (MAC) of 1.0, because it maintains splanchnic blood flow better than other volatiles [15] and may improve blood supply to the transplanted graft. Lower MAC may be used in encephalopathic patients and guided by intracranial pressure monitoring.

Our local unit also uses a continuous infusion of alfentanil, with or without midazolam, after induction. Other centres may have different protocols.

Ventilation parameters aim to optimize oxygenation and control end tidal carbon dioxide concentrations to a partial pressure of 4–4.5 kPa for neuroprotection.

The patient is carefully positioned, and assessment of pressure areas is essential to maintain skin integrity, which is at significant risk in the critically unwell.

A nasogastric tube is inserted in theatre.

19.21.4 Intra-operative Monitoring, Care, and Management of Complications

The table below summarizes the phases of liver transplant surgery (Table 19.4), and the anesthetic implications:

19.21.4.1 Cardiovascular System and Fluids

Continuous 5 lead ECG monitoring, including ST segment analysis [17], is used throughout as well as routine monitoring. Additionally, continuous display of invasive blood pressure, pulmonary artery pressure and mixed venous oxygen saturation is adopted by our local unit. Less invasive cardiac output monitors may have replaced PACs in some centres, except where there is a significant concern of pulmonary hypertension, however patients with severe porto-pulmonary hypertension at preoperative assessment are unlikely to be transplant candidates [16].

As mentioned above, TEE is increasingly used. This allows ventricular size, function, and filling to be assessed, or detect any thrombus or air embolus in the event of hemodynamic instability.

Table 19.4 Phases of liver transplant surgery

Phase	Surgical component	Anesthetic implications
Pre-anhepatic	Inverse T or extended subcostal incision. Dissection and mobilization of liver and surrounding structures. Identification of the porta hepatis. Division of hepatic artery and bile duct.	Hemorrhage: dissection, varices, adhesions, pre-existing coagulopathy. CVS instability: ascitic drainage and hypovolemia, low SVR, maldistribution of blood to splanchnic circulation Over treatment with fluids and/or blood products may cause splanchnic congestion and exacerbate bleeding.
Anhepatic	Cross clamp of supra- and infra-hepatic vena cava. Portal and hepatic veins divided. Explantation of native liver. New liver transplanted, and caval and portal anastomosis. Potential need for veno-venous shunt (VVS).	No production of clotting factors, worsening coagulopathy, fibrinogen deficiency/fibrinolysis. Absent citrate/lactate metabolism, with increasing levels of both. Progressive hypocalcemia. Metabolic acidosis. Reduced cardiac output; potential VVS to maintain venous return and maintain renal perfusion, reduce splanchnic congestion, and delay metabolic acidosis. Reduced gluconeogenesis. Hemorrhage; surgical cause.
Neo-hepatic	Graft reperfusion and vessel reconstruction. Assessment of graft function: bile production, decreasing lactate, normalizing calcium, improved cardiovascular stability.	Abrupt increase in potassium and hydrogen ion concentration; monitor of dysrhythmias and treat with calcium infusion +/−sodium bicarbonate. Increased preload and cardiac output. Progressive hypotension and decrease in SVR. Post reperfusion syndrome.

Hemodynamic instability may be caused by:

- Hemorrhage
- Cross clamping
- Reperfusion
- Co-existing cardiovascular disease

There is a significant decrease in venous return during cross clamping with sequestration of fluid to the lower limbs and gut, effectively reducing adequate circulating volume, however overzealous administration of resuscitation fluid may cause volume overload and compromise graft function if engorged on reperfusion.

Hypotension in early reperfusion is common, and biochemical abnormalities should be sought and treated. Beyond this the management is small increments of vasoconstrictor or inotrope, such as epinephrine, with an infusion if required.

Due diligence in patients with concomitant cardiovascular disease is required and should be included in the differential diagnosis of hypotension.

The primed rapid transfusion device may be required.

19.21.4.2 Respiratory System

Continuous monitoring of airway pressure and inspired and expired gases is mandatory, with end tidal carbon dioxide targets as previously discussed.

Positive end expiratory pressure may be required if oxygenation is problematic, for example ascites causing diaphragmatic splinting. Positive pressure ventilation may contribute to hypotension secondary to increased intrathoracic pressure and reduced venous return.

Ventilation augmentation to increase minute volume during reperfusion will improve the removal of the increased carbon dioxide production secondary to liver metabolism and wash out of products of ischemia.

19.21.4.3 Renal/Biochemistry/ Metabolic/Hematology

There is no proven strategy for avoiding renal failure, other than optimizing fluid balance, maintaining adequate perfusion pressure, normothermia, and avoiding nephrotoxins [17, 22]. Preoperative jaundice also contributes to the risk of renal failure.

Veno-venous bypass may be used to optimize renal perfusion and reduce venous congestion depending on surgical technique. Patients on RRT preoperatively may need this continued intra-operatively.

Biochemical and hematological derangements are common, particularly acid-base balance, potassium, calcium, hemoglobin, clotting, and platelets, which are monitored regularly.

Our local unit measures arterial blood gases, Na+, K+, ionized Ca++, lactate, and glucose:

– Preoperatively
– Every 30 min after induction
– Immediately after clamping the major veins
– The end of the anhepatic phase
– Release of the venous clamps
– Release of the hepatic artery clamp
– Hourly until closure
– Additional samples as clinically indicated

Hypocalcemia is common due to chelation with unmetabolized citrate. Intravenous infusion is given to avoid hypotension, protect against hyperkalemia, and aid coagulation. Local protocols should be followed.

Metabolic acidosis may be due to poor tissue perfusion, optimized as above. Worsening in the anhepatic phase is common, and immediately post reperfusion, with resolution by a working graft over the next few hours postoperatively. Worsening acidosis with hyperlactatemia postoperatively may indicate poor graft function. Medical management is initiated, and the surgical team consulted.

Hyperkalemia is usually transient on reperfusion and doesn't require treatment. A normal ionized calcium will protect the myocardium after cross clamp release. Routine medical management of clinically significant hyperkalemia is standard. Potassium replacement should be avoided in hypokalemia before the graft is functioning.

Monitoring blood glucose levels will direct appropriate management and patients may rarely require a glucose infusion.

Point of care (POC) coagulation testing, full blood count (FBC), and laboratory coagulation testing is performed preoperatively. Our unit repeat the hemoglobin and POC testing:

– At the end of hepatectomy
– Ten minutes post reperfusion
– Sixty minutes post reperfusion
– End of surgery
– Additional testing if clinically indicated, such as excessive surgical bleeding

Laboratory coagulation tests are sent intraoperatively if significant blood loss.

Hypercoagulability should be avoided, and platelet transfusion avoided unless necessary to reduce the risk of hepatic artery thrombosis.

Close monitoring of blood loss will guide appropriate fluid strategies, and patient identification information should be easily seen for cross checking blood products.

After reperfusion hyperfibrinolysis may occur and variable heparin-like substances are released from the newly perfused graft. This makes the coagulopathy complex and relies on clinical judgement and timely performed coagulation testing, as well as close cooperation with laboratory staff. Antifibrinolytics, such as tranexamic acid, are not routinely used, but may play a role and calcium replacement is also required.

Major hemorrhage treatment:

– Correct hypothermia, acidosis and hypocalcemia
– Cell salvage operative field
– Targets hemoglobin >70 g/L or > 80 g/L if the patient has ischemic heart disease
– Other blood products where indicated by POC test algorithm

Our local unit uses ROTEM:

– Target FIBTEM >8 mm
– FFP used first line for fibrin deficiency
– Cryoprecipitate is second line where: 6 units FFP infused and ROTEM suggests persistent fibrin deficiency; CVP >10 cm H_2O and ROTEM suggests persistent fibrin deficiency; FIBTEM A10 < 5 mm
– Factor concentrates are rarely used

19.21.4.4 Neurology

Continuous ICP monitoring +/− jugular bulb oxygen saturation is used locally in patients with fulminant hepatic failure.

19.21.4.5 Temperature and Pressure Areas

Temperature maintenance is paramount, from the moment the patient arrives in the anesthetic room. Under mattress warmers should be instigated in the anesthetic room before induction and continued intraoperatively. Hot air top blankets are also used away from the surgical field. Fluid warmers, heat and moisture exchangers in the anesthetic circuit and continuous temperature monitoring is used.

Temperature management may differ in fulminant hepatic failure and should be discussed at the surgical brief.

Arms are wrapped in Gamgee and positioned as per team preference in a neutral position to avoid peripheral nerve or nerve plexus injury.

Eyes are taped closed, monitoring leads checked, and final pressure point check made before draping the patient.

19.21.4.6 Infection Prophylaxis

Local protocols exist for antibiotic prophylaxis. These may need re-dosed during the procedure depending on duration.

19.21.4.7 Veno-Venous Bypass

New surgical techniques mean that VVB is less frequently used. The piggyback technique no longer requires this. When it is indicated, the bypass cannulas are sited to decompress the splanchnic circulation, passing through a centrifugal pump before being returned to the patient.

19.21.4.8 Miscellaneous

Air embolism is a complication usually associated with VVB. Management is early recognition and communication to the team/VVB technician, and supportive care.

Citrate toxicity results from high volume blood transfusion with excess circulating citrate not metabolized by the liver. It may lead to hypo-calcemia with associated electrophysiological changes and hypotension. Calcium replacement is the treatment, until the functioning graft is metabolically active.

Post Reperfusion Syndrome (PRS) is an exaggerated hemodynamic compromise post graft perfusion. The mean arterial blood pressure, SVR, and heart rate fall, with increased pulmonary artery pressure and CVP suggesting myocardial depression and vasodilation secondary to biochemical disturbances and hypothermia. Adequate flushing of the liver and VVB may reduce the risk, and active management during the anhepatic phase influences the severity.

Graft non-function is always a possibility, up to 5% of cases [22]. Persistent acidosis, hypoglycemia, worsening coagulopathy and thrombocytopenia, hypotension, renal failure and encephalopathy point to primary graft non-function, a post-transplant emergency. General Considerations can be found in Table below (Table 19.5).

19.22 Postoperative Management

Patients are transferred to the intensive care unit (ICU) postoperatively, with routine and invasive blood pressure monitoring. Postoperative care will follow local protocol and be guided by clinical need. Early extubation is often achievable once all metabolic disturbances have normalized and may improve graft flow due to negative intrathoracic pressure in spontaneous ventilation.

Maintenance postoperative fluids should be via the naso-jejunal tube if able with continuous assessment of coagulopathy and fluid balance, avoiding high CVP to reduce hepatic congestion. An appropriate fluid regime is 1–2 ml/kg/h of crystalloid, and albumin or blood products used if indicated.

Postoperative pain relief is usually patient controlled analgesia since regional techniques are contraindicated in coagulopathy.

Immunosuppression is continued, and the patient is monitored closely to identify any complications early.

Table 19.5 Preoperative preparation for liver transplantation

Veno-venous bypass equipment	
Blood warmer	
Bair hugger	
Cell saver	
Rapid infusion device	
Infusion pumps	
Pressure transducer sets	
Cardiac output module, cable and equipment	
SvO_2 monitor	
Transesophageal echocardiogram	
Point of care coagulation test machine	

Drugs should be drawn up in advance and include:	
Anesthetic	Propofol Suxamethonium/rocuronium/atracurium Fentanyl/alfentanil Ranitidine Vaporizer Midazolam
Miscellaneous	Prophylactic antibiotics: e.g. amoxicillin, gentamicin, metronidazole Immunosuppression: e.g. methylprednisolone Blood products
Resuscitation	Atropine Epinephrine (adrenaline) Norepinephrine (noradrenaline) Calcium chloride Metaraminol lignocaine 1% Sodium bicarbonate
Infusions	Atracurium Fentanyl/alfentanil Epinephrine (adrenaline) Norepinephrine (noradrenaline) Calcium chloride

19.23 Renal Transplantation

Renal transplants are the treatment of choice for end stage renal failure (ESRF) [23]. The procedure is carried out in many centres and are predominantly cadaveric renal transplants. The authors will focus on cadaveric renal transplant, as organ procurement is beyond the scope of this chapter.

Patients receiving renal transplants show an almost immediate improvement in quality of life, morbidity, and mortality compared with dialysis [24]. It provides cheaper care for renal failure than ongoing dialysis but is a complex surgical procedure and the outcomes can be attributable to intraoperative physiological status, thus the anesthetic team contribute significantly to improved clinical outcomes.

The main cause of renal failure in the United Kingdom is diabetes mellitus. Many effects of renal failure impact on anesthetic care, in addition to the impact of the underlying cause.

These patients are high risk, particularly diabetic patients with ESRF [25]. Hypertension is very common, whether cause or effect of renal failure, and may be difficult to control. Accelerated atherosclerosis means that there is significant risk of ischemic heart disease that may be silent, again, particularly in diabetic patients. The incidence of valvular heart disease and left ventricular dysfunction is increased, and autonomic neuropathy is common. However, only irreversible ventricular dysfunction with low cardiac output should be considered a contraindication to transplant, because graft viability is endangered [26].

The sequelae of renal failure pose problems intraoperatively:

- Hypovolemia
- Abnormal electrolytes
- Altered acid-base status
- Reduced drug clearance
- Anemia
- Arterio-venous fistulae and difficult intravenous access, central and peripheral
- Delayed gastric emptying

Patients are usually dialyzed prior to theatre, causing hypovolemia which may be exaggerated by general anesthesia. Serum potassium may be high requiring treatment or monitoring, in addition to dictating neuromuscular blocking drugs. Altered acid-base status affects drug handling and clearance, and reduced doses of drugs may be necessary. Anemia is common but well tolerated, with increased cardiac output and low systemic vascular resistance (SVR) to compensate. The oxyhemoglobin dissociation curve is shifted to the right to facilitate oxygen supply at tissue level.

Blood loss intraoperatively is usually minor unless intraoperative complications arise and compromise the anastomosis. Blood transfusion perioperatively is rare.

19.24 Preoperative Management

A full anesthetic history is mandatory and should then be targeted to issues that are ESRF and patient specific. Particular attention is paid to cardiovascular health, respiratory disease, and exercise tolerance. Any recent changes in symptoms may warrant further investigation as deteriorating cardiac function may be an indication of silent myocardial ischemia.

Dialysis assessment is important. Type and frequency of dialysis and when last dialyzed contributes to clinical care. Anuric patients will be fluid restricted and if recently dialyzed will have significant fluid shifts. Arterio-venous fistulae should be noted and must be protected intraoperatively.

The table documents preoperative investigations (Table 19.6).

Many drugs the patient is taking can alter their biochemistry, such as diuretics, or vasomotor tone, for example angiotensin converting enzyme inhibitors. They may also be on immunosuppression from previous transplants, and if this includes steroids then perioperative cover may be required.

Interrogation of diabetic patients' regime and control, along with current blood sugar level, will guide the need for insulin therapy perioperatively.

Although renal transplantation is an urgent procedure it is seldom an emergency and there is usually time to obtain all the necessary preoperative information and results of investigations.

Table 19.6 Investigations for renal transplant

Laboratory investigations	Non-invasive and imaging
FBC	ECG
Urea & electrolytes	CXR
Creatinine	Echocardiogram
eGFR	
Blood glucose	
HbA1c	
Group & save serum sample	

This also means that abnormal biochemistry can be corrected, and patients can be adequately fasted for theatre. The decision to use a RSI is based on individual patient need.

Premedication is rare but can be given if necessary.

19.25 Intraoperative Management

19.25.1 Surgical Brief

Surgical and anesthetic issues are discussed and planned, including the immunosuppression regime, in our unit. Anti-thymocyte globulin (ATG) is increasingly used in our clinical practice and there have been some adverse reactions secondary to the well-recognized cytokine release syndrome. Due to this we have developed protocols for the initiation of ATG that incorporates pre-infusion paracetamol, chlorphenamine and methylprednisolone, and the ATG is infused over 6 h through an infusion pump.

19.25.2 Monitoring and Equipment

Routine monitoring is initiated in the anesthetic room. Invasive blood pressure monitoring is rare and may impact on future fistula formation.

Intravenous access established, and our local unit advocate a 20 Gauge cannula is sufficient.

19.25.3 Lines

A central venous catheter is usually inserted asleep under aseptic conditions and real time ultrasound guided. The surgical team may request a dialysis central venous catheter as an alternative and this is discussed at the surgical brief. The target CVP is 12–14 cm H_2O, which may require significant volumes of fluid to establish. This optimizes graft perfusion, minimizing the risk of pre-renal hypoperfusion on graft function.

A urinary catheter is inserted when the patient is asleep.

19.25.4 Drugs and Fluids

Emergency drugs to be drawn up include metaraminol, ephedrine, glycopyrrolate, and atropine. Additional drugs, such as epinephrine and norepinephrine should be readily available but seldom need made in advance.

Induction of anesthesia is usually with propofol, but thiopentone can also be used. A recent review of anesthetic practice in our local unit revealed no advantage in using atracurium over rocuronium as the neuromuscular blocker in our clinical practice. Many anesthetists are more familiar with rocuronium, therefore the use of this is supported by our department, and sugammadex is used to reverse the block if required. If a RSI is deemed necessary then caution is exerted using suxamethonium in view of potential increase in potassium concentration, with 1.2 mg/kg of rocuronium an alternative.

Opioid use for induction and intraoperative analgesia is usually fentanyl, but there is increasing use of remifentanil infusions. Post operatively we use fentanyl patient-controlled analgesia (PCA), some units may use morphine or oxycodone.

Prophylactic antibiotics are given as per local protocol and patient allergy status.

Local protocols may exist to direct the type of crystalloid used intraoperatively. In our unit there is mixed practice with variable use of Hartmann's solution and 0.9% saline. The postoperative protocol uses 0.9% saline, some institutes use Plasmalyte [27].

19.25.5 Maintenance

Maintenance of anesthesia is usually by vapor, typically sevoflurane. Isoflurane/Desflurane are alternatives. Remifentanil infusions are replaced by fentanyl bolus at the end of the procedure for post op analgesia.

If ATG is not used, then basiliximab is our alternative. In this instance the timing of methylprednisolone is at the surgeon's discretion but is usually around the time of anastomosis/before removal of cross clamps.

Before the patient is woken the surgical team ultrasound the newly transplanted graft and assess for adequate blood flow.

Once the procedure is complete the muscle relaxation is reversed, and the patient is extubated. It is unusual for the patient to require ICU care postoperatively, and patients usually return to the specialist renal ward once recovered.

19.25.6 Temperature and Pressure Areas

Normothermia is important in the care of renal patients. Hypothermia may affect coagulation and drug metabolism, and postoperative shivering increases oxygen consumption. This increased oxygen requirement may unmask myocardial ischemia in vulnerable patients.

Hot air blankets are used intraoperatively to maintain temperature, and intermittent tympanic or continuous temperature probe monitoring used.

Pressure area care is of particular importance as the patients have fragile skin and may have fistula and dialysis grafts that need padding and protecting throughout the procedure.

19.25.7 Postoperative Analgesia

Regular paracetamol and fentanyl PCA are routine, and wound infiltration with local anesthetic by the surgeons is performed. Non-steroidal anti-inflammatory drugs are contra-indicated. Alternatives include regional anesthesia, for example transversus abdominis plane block, or wound infiltration catheters.

Opioids are metabolized by the liver and excreted by the kidney, therefore our PCA settings are altered, with a longer lock-out time, to account for this.

19.25.8 Complications

Surgical complications are infrequent, but sudden hemorrhage with significant blood loss may occur.

Patient complications are related to comorbidities and biochemical abnormalities, and postoperative blood tests are taken in recovery.

19.26 Postoperative Management

In the postoperative period oxygen is administered routinely. Fluid therapy should be guided by the CVP and urine output closely monitored. Postoperatively, potassium should be checked and appropriately treated.

Once the patient is stable they are returned to a specialist renal ward. Immunosuppressive therapy is continued according to local protocol.

19.27 Pancreatic Transplantation

Successful pancreatic transplant provides durable glycemic control and improves survival for patients with diabetes [28].

There are three types of pancreas transplants:

- Simultaneous pancreas and kidney transplant (SPK), most common
- Pancreas after kidney transplant (PAK), second most common, usually after a living donor renal transplant
- Pancreas transplant alone (PTA)

There are two main indications for pancreas transplants: type 1 diabetes with either severe metabolic complications and/or incapacitating problems with insulin therapy, or an eGFR <20 ml/min/1.73 m^2; some type 2 diabetics, such as non-obese patients, are a minority. Most commonly pancreas transplants are in type 1 diabetes, and the nature of the pancreas transplant depends on the underlying difficulty. Patients with difficulties in insulin therapy or metabolic complications alone but normal or near-normal renal function are considered for PTA, and those with renal failure with or without the option for

living kidney donor are considered for PAK and SPK respectively [28, 29].

Diabetes is a major health problem with a high incidence of vascular and degenerative complications. Additionally, diabetic patients are more at risk of peri-operative complications including infection and poor wound healing. Patient selection is greatly important, and particularly regarding cardiovascular fitness: absolute contraindications to pancreas transplant includes excessive cardiovascular risk, documented by the organ donation and transplant advisory group [29].

In the USA there has been a decline in pancreas transplants over the last decade, which may be accounted for by improved medical care of patients, reduced quality of donors (increased obesity and older donors), and lack of consistent referral of transplant candidates from endocrinologists [28].

19.28 Preoperative Management

The patient will have been extensively reviewed and investigated by the referring and transplant teams when considered for the transplant list. Preoperative anesthetic assessment includes a thorough medical, surgical and anesthetic history, particularly focusing on diabetic control and associated complications.

Of importance to perioperative management:

- ischemic heart disease; increased risk of peri-operative cardiovascular event and surgery is contraindicated in those with myocardial infarction within the last 6 months
- evidence of autonomic neuropathy; risk of labile and difficult to manage intra-operative blood pressure and potential dysrhythmias
- dialysis history and biochemistry; causing hypovolemia or potassium abnormality
- blood glucose level; may require variable rate insulin infusion preoperatively and local protocols should be followed
- peripheral neuropathy; careful positioning in theatre to prevent pressure areas or peripheral nerve damage, and document existing deficits to exclude perioperative nerve damage

Table 19.7 Investigations for pancreas transplants

Bloods	Non-invasive investigations and Imaging
FBC Group and save/cross matched blood according to local guidelines Coagulation screen Urea and electrolytes Creatinine and eGFR Calcium Phosphate LFTs Blood glucose and Hb A1c	ECG Echocardiography if indicated, +/− stress testing
Additionally, preoperative testing should include blood borne virus screen and immunology screening, as per local protocols	CXR Additional imaging such as CT or Ultrasound if required

Airway assessment should be thorough as the incidence of difficult intubation is higher in type 1 diabetics due to atlanto-occipital joint stiffness [30].

Preoperative investigations are detailed in the table below (Table 19.7).

Premedication is not always required and is decided on an individual patient basis.

19.29 Intraoperative Management

The principles outlined can be adopted for all types of pancreas transplantation. They can be adapted to individual patient need and many units will have their own guidelines.

19.29.1 Monitoring and Equipment/ Lines

Routine monitoring is attached in the anesthetic room. Consideration should be given to invasive blood pressure monitoring pre-induction in those with significant autonomic dysfunction but may be sited once anaesthetized. In particularly stable patients it may be considered unnecessary and could impact on future fistula formation, even if the patient is having a SPK or PAK transplant.

Intravenous access established for induction and further invasive lines, such as CVC, are sited asleep in accordance to local policy and clinical need. These are ultrasound guided and performed under aseptic conditions. During SPK it may be necessary to insert a dialysis catheter.

There should be separate venous access for the dextrose/potassium/insulin infusion.

A urinary catheter is inserted once the patient is anaesthetized. A naso-gastric tube is also placed.

19.29.2 Drugs and Fluids

Emergency drugs to be drawn up include metaraminol, ephedrine, glycopyrrolate, and atropine, see Table 19.8. Additional drugs, such as epinephrine and norepinephrine should be readily available but seldom need made in advance.

Induction is usually with propofol, but thiopentone can also be used. Patients post dialysis may need dose adjustment or warmed fluid bolus during induction due to potential hypovolemia and therefore hypotension. Muscle relaxation is achieved with the anesthetist's preferred drug(s), and RSI may be required in those with gastroparesis secondary to autonomic neuropathy. Suxamethonium may be considered if potassium level is normal, and rocuronium 1.2 mg/kg is an alternative.

Opioid use for induction and intraoperative analgesia is usually fentanyl, but remifentanil

Table 19.8 Drugs used in the anesthetic management of pancreas transplant

Anesthetic and analgesic drugs	Propofol/thiopental; anesthetic vapor; atracurium/rocuronium; Morphine/fentanyl; paracetamol
Resuscitation	Ephedrine; metaraminol; atropine; glycopyrrolate; crystalloid fluids and cross matched blood
Miscellaneous	Antibiotics Immunosuppressive agents according to local protocol Insulin/dextrose/potassium infusion(s)

intraoperatively is an alternative. Post operatively the patient is usually given a PCA, which may be fentanyl or morphine depending on renal function and unit preference.

Prophylactic antibiotics are given as per local protocol and patient allergy status.

Crystalloid infusions perioperatively may be guided by unit preference, but a balanced solution is usual, for example Hartmann's solution or Plasmalyte. Postoperative fluid management is in critical care and guided by biochemistry and clinical picture.

19.29.3 Maintenance

Maintenance of anesthesia is usually by vapor anesthetic agents, for example sevoflurane or desflurane. Isoflurane is an alternative, with minimal effect on cerebral blood flow and beneficial effects on renal blood flow [31].

Fentanyl boluses are required throughout the procedure for analgesia or at the end of the procedure for postoperative analgesia if remifentanil infusion is used.

Muscle relaxation is maintained by boluses of neuromuscular blocker and monitored using a peripheral nerve stimulator. This is reversed on completion of the procedure, and the patient is usually extubated and taken to recovery, after which they will be transferred to a critical care area.

Regular blood sugar monitoring is required with adjustment/instigation of insulin infusion as guided by results.

19.29.4 Temperature and Pressure Areas

Normothermia is important in the maintenance of normal metabolism of drugs and maintaining hemostasis. Intermittent monitoring of temperature or temperature probe for continuous monitoring may be used. Hot air blankets are also used, with gaps for surgical access.

Patients may be high cardiovascular risk by nature of their diabetes, and increased oxygen consumption if shivery may cause deleterious cardiovascular effects.

Pressure area care is important due to peripheral neuropathy and compromised peripheral perfusion in abnormal microvascular circulation. Any fistulae or dialysis grafts need protected.

19.29.5 Postoperative Analgesia

Regular paracetamol, no non-steroidal anti-inflammatory drugs, and a PCA are routine. Some centres report the use of epidurals for postoperative analgesia but it is generally avoided/unnecessary. Wound infiltration with local anesthetic by the surgeons is performed; alternatives include regional anesthesia, for example transversus abdominis plane block or rectus sheath blocks depending on incision used, or wound infusion catheters.

Opioids are metabolized by the liver and excreted by the kidney, therefore those with renal impairment may need dose or lock-out time adjusted on their PCA. Acute pain services may be involved.

19.29.6 Complications

Immediate intraoperative surgical complications include hemorrhage, where significant blood loss may occur, for example at the anastomotic site after reperfusion.

Metabolic disturbance may occur with release of arterial cross-clamps after anastomosis is complete: metabolic acidosis from reperfusion is common and may contribute to poor clotting and therefore blood loss; hyperkalemia can contribute to cardiac instability; hypotension is multifactorial with redistribution of blood volume and decreased SVR due to anaerobic metabolites and should be treated with fluid resuscitation and vasopressors and/or inotropic drugs.

After graft reperfusion the pancreatic beta cells begin secreting insulin with 5 min [30] and blood glucose monitoring is essential. The insulin infusion may need stopped because profound hypoglycemia may occur. Blood glucose levels should be monitored every 15 min for the following hour post reperfusion, then every 30 min thereafter for the remainder of the surgery. Good glucose control (between approximately 6–8 mmol/l or 120–150 mg/dl [30, 31] is required to prevent islet cell dysfunction secondary to hyperglycemia and rest the beta cells until the metabolic disturbance from reperfusion has resolved [30].

Patient complications are related to their comorbidities as well as the predictable abnormalities above.

19.30 Postoperative Management

Patients are admitted to critical care postoperatively. This provides close monitoring of metabolic status and glycemic control. Hypoglycemia is a common postoperative problem and may require dextrose infusion.

Postoperative critical care bundles are adopted as per the local unit protocol.

The patient's own medications are reintroduced when able, but gut absorption may be impaired due to postoperative ileus.

19.31 Conclusion

The anesthetic management of patients presenting for organ transplantation is challenging yet rewarding. A thorough knowledge of the pathophysiological and pharmacological derangements associated with the various organ failures is essential. Careful pre-, intra- and postoperative management has a significant role to play in the successful outcome of such operations.

References

1. Durkin C, Buckland M. Cardiopulmonary transplantation: anaesthetic implications. Anaesth Intensive Care. 2015;16(7):581–8.
2. Kwak J, Majewski M, LeVan PT. Heart transplantation in an era of mechanical circulatory support. J Cardiothorac Vasc Anesth. 2018 Feb;32(1):19–31.
3. Nguyen L, Banks DA. Anesthetic management of the patient undergoing heart transplantation. Best Pract Res Clin Anaesthesiol. 2017 Jun;31(2):189–200.
4. Bignami E. Mechanical ventilation during cardiopulmonary bypass. J Cardiothorac Vasc Anesth. 2016 Dec;30(6):1668–75.
5. Vega E, Schroder J, Nicoara A. Postoperative management of heart transplantation patients. Best Pract Res Clin Anaesthesiol. 2017 Jun;31(2):201–13.
6. Costanzo MR, et al. The International Society of Heart and Lung Transplantation Guidelines for the care of heart transplant recipients. J Heart Lung Transplant. 2010 Aug;29(8):914–56.
7. Yusen RD, et al. The registry of the international society for heart and lung transplantation: thirty-third adult lung and heart-lung transplant report-2016; Focus Theme: Primary Diagnostic Indications for Transplant. J Heart Lung Transplant. 2016 Oct;35(10):1170–84.
8. Prabhu M, Valchanov K. Pre-anaesthetic evaluation of the patient with end-stage lung disease. Best Pract Res Clin Anaesthesiol. 2017 Jun;31(2):249–60.
9. Slinger P. Anaesthetic management for lung transplantation. Tx Med. 2012;24:27–34.
10. Barnes L. Mechanical ventilation for the lung transplant recipient. Curr Pulmonol Rep. 2015 Jun;4(2):88–96.
11. Nicoara A, Anderson-Dam J. Anesthesia for lung transplantation. Anesthesiol Clin. 2017 Sep;35(3): 473–89.
12. Hoechter DJ, von Dossow V. Lung transplantation: from the procedure to managing patients with lung transplantation. Curr Opin Anaesthesiol. 2016 Feb;29(1):8–13.
13. Hoechter DJ, et al. Extracorporeal circulation during lung transplantation procedures: a meta-analysis. ASAIO J. 2017 Sep/Oct;63(5):551–61.
14. McLean S, Homeyer P et al. Assessing the benefits of preoperative thoracic epidural placement for lung transplantation. J Cardiothorac Vasc Anesth. 2018.
15. Steadman RH. Anesthesia for liver transplant surgery. Anesthesiol Clin North Am. 2004;22:687–711.
16. Kashimutt S, Kotze A. Anaesthesia for liver transplant. Br J Anaesth Educ. 2017;17(1):35–40.
17. Mayes R, Pollok A. Anaesthetic protocol for liver transplantation, 2nd ed. [pdf]. 2016. Scottish Liver Transplant Unit, Edinburgh Royal Infirmary. Accessed on May 24th 2018. Available from https://www.nhslothian.scot.nhs.uk/Services/A-Z/ScottishLiverTransplantUnit/InformationFofClinicalStaff/Documents/ANAESTHETIC%20PROTOCOL%202016.pdf
18. British Transplantation Society Guidelines. Liver transplantation for patients with non-alcoholic steatohepatitis, 1st ed. 2011 [pdf]. British Transplant Society. Accessed on May 24th, 2018. Available from https://bts.org.uk/wp-content/uploads/2016/09/20_BTS_Liver_Non-alcoholic-1.pdf
19. Marcel RJ, Ramsay MA, Hein HA, Nguyen AT, Ramsay KJ, Suit CT, Miller RD. Duration of rocuronium-induced neuromuscular block during

liver transplantation: a predictor of primary allograft function. Anesth Analg. 1997;84(4):870–4.

20. Drury N. Anaesthesia and liver disease part 1, 2012 [pdf]. World federation of societies of anaesthesiologists, anaesthesia tutorial of the week (270). Accessed May 24th, 2018. Available from http://www.frca.co.uk/Documents/270%20Anaesthesia%20and%20Liver%20disease%20Part%201.pdf

21. Soleimanpour H, Safaris S, Nia KS, Sanaie S, Alavian SM. Opioid drugs in liver disease: a systematic review. Hepatitis Monthly. 2016;16(4):e32636. Published online.

22. Allman KG, Wilson IH. Oxford handbook of anaesthesia. 4th ed. Oxford: Oxford University Press; 2016. p. 563–8.

23. Allman KG, Wilson IH. Oxford handbook of anaesthesia. 4th ed. Oxford: Oxford University Press; 2016. p. 126.

24. Mayhew D, Ridgway D, Hunter JM. Update on the intraoperative management of adult cadaveric renal transplantation. Br J Anaesth Educ. 2016;16(2):53–7.

25. Karan G, Kalbe T, Alcaraz A, Aki FT, Budde K, Humke U, Kleinclauss F, Nicita G, Olsburgh JO, Susal C. Guidelines on renal transplantation. European Association of urology. 2009. Accessed May 24th 2018. Available from http://uroweb.org/wp-content/uploads/27-Renal-Transplant_LRV2-May-13th-2014.pdf

26. Ricaurte L, Vargas J, Lozano E, Diaz L. Anesthesia and kidney transplantation. Transplant Proc. 2013;45:1386–91.

27. Renal Unit at the Edinburgh Royal Infirmary. Anaesthetic protocol. [pdf]. Handbook appendix 4. n.d. Accessed on May 24th, 2018.. Available from http://www.edren.org/media/download_gallery/Appendix4AnaestheticProtocol.pdf

28. Dean PG, Kukla A, Stegall MD, Kudva YC. Pancreas transplantation. Br Med J. 2017;357(j):1321.

29. NHS Blood and Transplant Organ donation and transplantation. Pancreas transplantation: patient selection. 2012. Accessed May 24th, 2018. Available from http://odt.nhs.uk/pdf/advisory_group_papers/PAG/Pancreas_Selection_%20policy.pdf

30. Aniskevich S, Perry DK. Anesthesia for pancreas transplantation. Pancreatic Disord Therapy. 2013;3:122.

31. Pichel AC, Macnab WR. Anaesthesia for pancreas transplantation. Cont Educ Anaesth Crit Care Pain. 2005;5(5):p149–52.

Immunosuppressive Pharmacology

20

Ethan P. Marin and Oscar Colegio

20.1 Introduction

Allogeneic transplantation of solid organs and tissues is complicated by immunological rejection, the process by which the recipient immune system attacks and destroys the allogeneic graft. Understanding the mechanisms by which the rejection occurs, and the development of immunosuppressive therapies to prevent rejection, have been foundational advances critical to the practice of organ transplantation in humans.

In this chapter, we will briefly review the basic structure of the immune system, with a goal of describing the pharmacologic targets for immunosuppression. Subsequently, we will review the major classes of immunosuppressive drugs and their pharmacology. Finally, we will discuss the clinical uses of the drugs in treating a patient with a solid organ transplant.

E. P. Marin (✉)
Department of Medicine, Section of Nephrology, Yale School of Medicine, New Haven, CT, USA
e-mail: Ethan.marin@yale.edu

O. Colegio
Transplant Dermatology Center, Roswell Park Comprehensive Cancer Center, Buffalo, NY, USA
e-mail: oscar.colegio@roswellpark.org

20.2 Overview of Immunosuppressive Drugs in Common Usage: Mechanism, Pharmacokinetics, and Adverse Effects

The T lymphocyte is the major cellular target of most immunosuppressive therapies used in transplantation since it is the central actor in rejection pathways. Therapeutic agents may lead to the destruction of T cells, or to the specific inhibition of T cell activation pathways. Activation of the T cell is known to proceed through several steps, termed Signals 1, 2 and 3 (Fig. 20.1) [1]. Signal 1 is the binding of a cell surface T cell receptor to the molecular complex of a major histocompatibility complex (MHC) protein bound to an antigenic peptide on the surface of an antigen presenting cell (APC). Signaling downstream of the activated T cell receptor involves activation of calcineurin, a phosphatase which de-phosphorylates the transcription factor NFAT. The dephosphorylated NFAT moves from the cytoplasm to the nucleus, where it triggers transcription of several downstream genes including the one encoding IL-2. Signal 2 involves a second set of costimulatory interactions between surface proteins of the APC and the T cell: B7–1 and B7–2 (also known as CD80 and CD86) of the APC and CD28 of the T cell. Signal 2 is necessary for the transmission of Signal 1. In the absence of Signal 2, Signal 1 leads

© Springer Nature Switzerland AG 2021
N. Hakim et al. (eds.), *Transplantation Surgery*, Springer Specialist Surgery Series,
https://doi.org/10.1007/978-3-030-55244-2_20

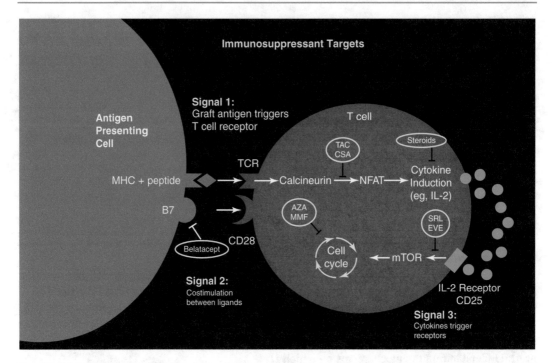

Fig. 20.1 Mechanistic targets of immunosuppressive drugs. Signals 1, 2, and 3 lead to proliferation and activation of T cells. *TAC* tacrolimus, *CSA* cyclosporine, *SRL* sirolimus, *EVE* everolimus, *AZA* azathioprine, *MMF* mycophenolate mofetil

to anergy of the T cell. Signal 3 involves activation of the IL-2 receptor on the T cell by secreted IL-2 in an autocrine and/or paracrine fashion. Downstream signaling from the IL-2 receptor proceeds via the mammalian target of rapamycin (mTOR) complex and culminates in activation of the cell cycle and cellular proliferation. Drugs that interfere with Signals 1, 2 and/or 3 are the backbone of immunosuppressive regimens that allow for successful allotransplantation.

Pharmacologic agents have been developed to inhibit T cell activation *via* disruption of each of the 3 signals described above. Other drugs work by triggering the destruction of T cells and other lymphocytes. This section will discuss drugs in common usage with a review of mechanisms, pharmacokinetics, and relevant adverse effects. The clinical use of these drugs, and the clinical studies that informs their use, will be described in a subsequent section.

Immunosuppressive medications in general entail several class-related risks attributable to inhibition of the immune system. These include primarily increased risk for infection from bacterial, viral and fungal agents, as well as increased rates of malignancy. In particular, kerantinocyte carcinomas (nonmelanomatous skin cancers) are observed to occur at as much as 250-fold increased rates in transplant patients on immunosuppressive therapy relative to the general population [2]. Further, lymphoproliferative disorders occur at significantly higher rates relative to nontransplant patients.

20.2.1 Signal 1 Blockers

Signal 1 is blocked by the calcineurin inhibitors (CNI), cyclosporine and tacrolimus. Each drug binds to a specific intracellular protein (cyclophilin in the case of cyclosporine, and FK506 binding protein in the case of tacrolimus) and then binds and inhibits the phosphatase, calcineurin. Inhibition of calcineurin effectively blocks the transmission of Signal 1 and inhibits T cell activation.

Tacrolimus, first approved by the FDA in 1994, is available as an immediate release oral formulation commonly dosed every 12 h (Prograf) or as an extended release formulation dosed once daily (Astagraf XL and Envarsus XR). Cyclosporine, first approved by the FDA in 1983, is available in unmodified (Sandimmune) and emulsified versions (Neoral); the latter demonstrates more consistent absorption. Both products are dosed every 12 h.

Both CNIs have relatively narrow therapeutic indices, characterized by toxicity at higher serum levels and ineffectiveness at lower serum levels. CNIs thus require routine therapeutic drug level monitoring and customized dosing to achieve target levels. Target levels vary according to patient characteristics, type of organ transplant, immunological risk, institutional preference and other factors. Importantly, both CNIs are metabolized by cytochrome P450 enzyme Cyp3A4/5 and are thus subject to significant changes in rate of metabolism *via* the effects of other drugs or chemicals which induce or inhibit Cyp3A4/5.

CNIs also cause significant adverse effects. Both can cause vasoconstriction manifesting as elevations in serum creatine and hypertension. Prolonged exposure to CNI can lead to chronic renal injury characterized by fibrosis in a striped pattern, along with hyalinosis of small arterioles. CNIs may also cause neurotoxicity characterized both peripherally with tremors and centrally with short term memory loss and seizures. CNI are associated with metabolic effects such as elevated blood sugars, hyperlipidemia, and hypertension. CNI can rarely cause thrombotic microangiopathy, which generally requires cessation of the drug. Both drugs may affect hair patterns: cyclosporine causes hirsutism and hypertrichosis while tacrolimus may lead to hair loss. Cyclosporine also causes gingival enlargement [3].

20.2.2 Signal 2 Blockers

Inhibition of the co-stimulatory Signal 2 is the mechanism of action of a relatively newer class of biologic agents, including belatacept (Nulojix), which was approved by the FDA for use in kidney transplant recipients in 2011. Belatacept is a recombinant fusion protein of the extracellular portion of cytotoxic T-lymphocyte associated antigen 4 (CTLA-4) fused to the Fc portion of human IgG1. It binds to B7 on antigen presenting cells and thus blocks the transmission of Signal 2, which blocks activation of T cells. After initial loading doses, belatacept is given as a monthly IV infusion. Therapeutic drug level monitoring is not required.

Belatacept carries black box warning regarding an increased risk of post-transplant lymphoproliferative disorder (PTLD). Seronegativity for Epstein-Barr virus is a contraindication to belatacept therapy since in increases the risk of PTLD. Additionally, belatacept carries a black box warning against use in liver transplant, due to an increased risk of graft loss and death. Of note, belatacept is associated with lower blood pressures and lipid levels as compared to cyclosporine [4].

20.2.3 Signal 3 Blockers

Several drugs target Signal 3 in different ways. Most direct are the IL-2 receptor antagonists (IL-2RA), of which the only currently available agent is basiliximab (Simulect), a recombinant murine/human IgG antibody that specifically binds the IL-2 receptor alpha chain (also known as CD25) with high affinity. This interaction blocks the activation of the IL-2 receptor by IL-2 and thus inhibits downstream events of IL-2R activation such as cellular proliferation. Basiliximab is typically administered as a 20 mg infusion 2 h prior to reperfusion of the graft at the time of implantation, with a second 20 mg dose given on the fourth day after transplant. The duration of action is 4–6 weeks. Daclizumab (Zenapax) has a similar mechanism of action to basiliximab and was approved by the FDA in 1997. However, it was withdrawn from the market for transplant use as of 2009.

Basiliximab has relatively few adverse effects, although severe acute hypersensitivity reactions have been reported. Rates of infection and malignancy are not substantially higher in patients treated with basiliximab as compared to placebo.

Signaling downstream of IL-2 receptors are mediated by the mTOR complex of proteins. Two inhibitors of mTOR (mTORi) are used in clinical practice, including sirolimus (Rapamune) and everolimus (Zortress). Both inhibit mTOR signaling after complexing first with the FK506-binding protein. Sirolimus is typically dosed once daily, whereas everolimus is dosed every 12 h. Routine monitoring of trough drug levels is recommended, as they predict area under the curve and hence efficacy and toxicity. Both drugs are metabolized by Cyp3A4 enzymes and are susceptible to changes in levels associated with use of inducers and inhibitors of the CYP3A4 system. Common adverse events include hyperlipidemia, and, specifically with sirolimus, hyperglycemia. Both drugs may impair wound healing and should be used with caution in patients with surgical or other wounds. Sirolimus has been associated with worsening proteinuria and may cause focal and segmental glomerulosclerosis. Sirolimus and everolimus have antiviral and anti-malignancy properties.

The cellular proliferation caused by activation of IL-2 receptors (Signal 3) can be reduced by the antimetabolite drugs mycophenolic acid (MPA) and azathioprine, which interfere with purine metabolism and thus impair DNA synthesis. Azathioprine (Imuran) is a prodrug which is metabolized to the active 6-mercaptopurine by glutathione. 6-mercaptopurine is further metabolized by xanthine oxidase and thus cannot be taken with inhibitors of this enzyme, such as allopurinol. Azathioprine is typically dosed daily. It does not require routine therapeutic drug level monitoring, though the levels of metabolites 6-MP and 6-MMP predict toxicity to the bone marrow and liver, respectively. Further, mutations in the enzyme thiopurine S-methyltransferase (TMPT) associated with low enzyme activity predict toxicity; genetic testing before drug initiation may be effective in preventing toxicity [5]. MPA is available as a prodrug, mycophenolate mofetil (MMF; Cellcept), or as enteric coated mycophenolate sodium (Myfortic).

The latter may reduce the upper gastrointestinal adverse effects commonly encountered with MPA, such as dyspepsia. Additional adverse effects include bone marrow suppression and teratogenicity.

MPA inhibits the enzyme inosine monophosphate, which is involved in the *de novo* purine synthesis, thereby inhibiting proliferation of T and B cells almost exclusively. MPA preparations are typically dosed every 12 h, though further divided doses may minimize toxicity in some. Therapeutic drug levels are not measured routinely, as they do not correlate well with area under the curve or efficacy and safety outcomes.

20.2.4 Lymphocyte-Depleting Agents

Several biologic agents have a primary mechanism of action that is independent of blocking Signals 1, 2, and 3. Instead, they trigger the destruction of lymphocytes. These agents comprise antibody preparations which target antigens on immune cells, and lead to destruction of the cells. They are typically long-acting (6–18 months), as significant time is required for metabolism of the drug and reconstitution of the population of the destroyed cells. Repeat usage is often limited by accumulated toxicity. Two of the agents in current use include alemtuzumab and rabbit anti-thymocyte globulin (ATG; Thymoglobulin).

Alemtuzumab (Campath) is a humanized monoclonal antibody produced against CD-52, which is present on T cells as well as some B cells, NK cells, and monocytes. It effectively causes depletion of T cells and other lymphocytes. Adverse effects of alemtuzumab include infusion reactions (which can be avoided via subcutaneous administration) as well as bone marrow toxicity.

Rabbit ATG is a polyclonal antibody preparation prepared from sera of rabbits that have been injected with human thymocytes. It is more effective, and more widely used at present, than a similar product prepared in horses (equine ATG). Rabbit ATG comprises antibodies with reactivities against a variety of antigens found on T cells and other immune cells, and effectively causes lymphodepletion. Rabbit ATG is typically given at a dose of 1.5 mg/kg body weight in 3–7 repeated daily doses. Rabbit ATG has been associated with infusion reactions, including cytokine release syndrome which in characterized by fever, headache, hypotension, and urticaria. Rabbit ATG may also cause hematological abnormalities such as leukopenia and thrombocytopenia, which may limit subsequent doses of thymoglobulin.

20.2.5 Corticosteroids

Corticosteroids (prednisone) are a class of agents that have broad immunosuppressive actions on cells of the immune system which do not fall neatly into a particular signal. When corticosteroids bind the glucocorticoid receptor in the cytoplasm of immune cells, the receptor-ligand complex is translocated to the nucleus where it inhibits the transcription of many genes, including proinflammatory cytokines such as IL-2 (Signal 3), thus limiting T cell proliferation. Further, corticosteroids can reduce the expression of antigen by APCs (Signal 1). Prednisone is typically dosed in a daily regimen and therapeutic drug levels are not measured.

20.3 Clinical Usage of Immunosuppressive Drugs in Transplantation

Modern immunsuppressive therapies in solid organ transplants may be divided into three phases: induction therapies, maintenance therapies, and rejection therapies. Induction treatments are those given at the time of transplant and are intended to rapidly and potently inhibit the immune system at the time of the first exposure to alloantigens. Maintenance regimens, in contrast, are designed for prolonged, routine use to stably suppress rejection and prolong graft survival. Rejection therapies are used specifically when rejections develop. The following section will consider the types of drugs used in each

phase and review common clinical practices and available data from clinical trials. Most of the discussion will center on kidney transplantation, the most common solid organ transplant. Details of agent usage does vary with different organs.

20.3.1 Induction Agents

Induction therapy refers to the use of immunosuppressive drugs given at the time of organ transplantation to potently and rapidly achieve immunosuppression during the initial exposure to alloantigens, which is the time when the risk of acute rejection is greatest. The balance of evidence shows that use of induction reduces the incidence of acute rejection and may prolong graft survival. The Kidney Disease Improving Global Outcomes (KDIGO) group gives the strongest available recommendation to the use of biologic induction agents based on a published base of high quality evidence [6]. Concordantly, data from the Scientific Registry of Transplant Recipients [7] show widespread and growing use of induction agents in the U.S. As recently as 2007, fewer than 80% of adult kidney transplant recipients received induction therapy. However, by 2016 nearly 90% of patients received induction therapy. Induction agents are comprised of either polyclonal or monoclonal antibody preparations which fall into two broad categories based on whether the drug leads to depletion of lymphocytes. Most of the growth in use has been in the lymphocyte depleting agents, which were given to >70% of patients in 2016. Use of non-depleting agents has fallen gradually since 2008.

The main non-depleting induction agent in use currently in the U.S. is basiliximab, which targets the alpha chain of the IL-2 receptor, known as CD25 (see above). Basiliximab was approved by the FDA in 1998 for prevention of rejection in kidney transplant rejection based on 4 key studies. Two of the studies compared basiliximab to placebo, with a 2-drug maintenance regimen (cyclosporine plus corticosteroids) [8, 9]. Both studies reported statistically significant reductions in a composite endpoint of death, graft loss or acute rejection at both 6 and 12 months in patients treated with basiliximab. Both studies also showed significant reductions in biopsy confirmed rejection at 6 and 12 months. Two additional studies compared basiliximab to placebo, with a 3-drug maintenance regimen (cyclosporine, corticosteroids, and either azathioprine or MPA). One of the studies showed significant reductions in a composite of death, graft loss, or acute rejection at 6 months, as well as reductions in biopsy-confirmed rejection at 6 months [10]. The second trial showed similar trends which did not reach statistical significance [11].

An updated Cochrane Review which examined high-quality studies of basiliximab and other IL2R antagonists (IL2RA) was published in 2010 [12]. In this analysis, 32 studies that included a total of 5854 patients showed that, compared with placebo, graft loss was reduced by 25% at 6 months and 1 year. Biopsy proven acute rejection was reduced by 28% at 1 year. In addition, reductions were observed with IL-2RA in both CMV disease (19%) as well as early malignancy (64%) as compared to the used of T cell depleting agents.

The second category of induction agents are those that cause lymphocyte depletion. These agents are antibodies which bind to antigens on primary T cells and other lymphocytes and lead to their subsequent destruction. These agents have a longer duration of action as compared with IL-2RA, as reconstitution of T and B cell population typically requires 6 months or more. The most commonly used of these agents are currently rabbit ATG and alemtuzumab.

Thymoglobulin was approved by the FDA for prevention of acute rejection as induction therapy based on two studies which compared thymoglobulin to IL2RA. Brennan et al., compared thymoglobulin to basiliximab in a randomized, blinded, multicenter study of high risk kidney transplant recipients [13]. The thymoglobulin group displayed reduced acute rejection (15.6% vs. 25.5%, P = 0.02), similar rates of graft loss and delayed graft function, and death. Overall rates of infection were greater with thymoglobulin. A second study compared thymoglobulin to daclizumab, an IL2RA, in patients considered to be at higher risk for rejection. Thymoglobulin

again showed lower rates of acute rejection (15 vs. 27.2%, P = 0.016), however 1-year graft and patient survival were not different [14].

A Cochrane Library meta-analysis of the use of antibody therapies for induction therapy in kidney transplants showed that ATGs (different preparations) as compared to placebo or no induction reduces acute rejection by one third, but does not clearly affect graft or patient survival [15]. ATGs leads to higher rates of leukopenia, thrombocytopenia, and cytomegalovirus (CMV) infections.

Alemtuzumab, a humanized monoclonal anti-CD52 antibody has not been approved by the FDA for use in transplant but has nonetheless been widely used in the transplant community. A meta- analysis of studies comparing alemtuzumab to ATGs in kidney transplantation showed no clear differences in graft survival nor in acute rejection [15]. Interestingly, comparisons of alemtuzumab to no induction did not show clear reduction in acute rejection or all cause graft loss; however these studies generally included steroid withdrawal in the alemtuzumab arm but not the control group [15].

A meta-analysis comparing IL2RA to ATGs in induction (18 studies, >1800 patients) showed reduction in biopsy proven acute rejections in the ATG group, but no difference in graft loss [12]. ATG use lead to higher rates of malignancy and CMV disease.

Interpretation and application of the above studies varies significantly between transplant centers, leading to significant variations in the choice of induction therapy.

20.3.2 Maintenance Immunosuppression

Maintenance immunosuppression is generally started immediately after the transplant and maintained for the life of the graft. Given the variety of available drugs for immunosuppression, numerous different regimens have been devised and studied. Most kidney transplant recipients are maintained on a multidrug regimen that combines drugs of different classes to maximize anti-rejection efficacy while minimizing adverse effects. Common regimens involve combining CNI, antimetabolites, and prednisone. mTORi may be used in place of either CNI or antimetabolites. Belatacept, the Signal 2 coreceptor blocker, may be used in place of a CNI. There is no one clear optimal regimen for every patient and every situation; choice of maintenance immunosuppression is made based on a variety of factors including tolerability, side effect profile, immunologic risk, infectious risk, cost, and other considerations.

20.3.2.1   Calcineurin Inhibitor

Calcineurin inhibitors are generally considered the backbone of immunosuppression maintenance regimens. CNIs are used by >90% of kidney recipients in the U.S [7]. A large meta-analysis of 30 trials (4102 patients) comparing cyclosporine to tacrolimus showed that all primary outcomes favored tacrolimus use [16]. Graft loss and acute rejection were reduced with tacrolimus (by 44 and 31% respectively), and serum creatinine was lower. In contrast, several adverse effects were found to be more pronounced with tacrolimus, including tremor, headache, gastrointestinal disturbances, and hypomagnesemia. The rate of new diabetes was higher with tacrolimus (relative risk of 2.56, 1.86, and 3.86 at 6, 12 and 36 months respectively). Cyclosporine use was associated with more hirsutism, hypertrichosis, and gingival enlargement. In sum, the results showed that for every 100 patients treated with tacrolimus instead of cyclosporine for the first year, 12 patients avoid rejection, 2 avoid graft loss, but 5 additional develop insulin dependent diabetes mellitus. As a result of the superior efficacy, tacrolimus has become by far the most commonly used CNI in the U.S. (>90%) and has largely supplanted cyclosporine, which had revolutionized transplant immunosuppression when introduced a decade earlier.

20.3.2.2   Antimetabolite

A CNI is commonly paired with an antimetabolite in maintenance immunosuppression regimens. The two major antimetabolite drugs used in transplant are azathioprine and MPA. MPA is the newer of the two and was approved by the FDA for the prevention of rejection in kidney transplant in 1995. A meta-analysis of 23 studies which included a total of 3301 patients was recently published, 20 years after FDA approval was granted [17]. The studies all used CNI drugs, with cyclosporine the most common agent. Five of the studies used depleting antibody induction therapy; 5 used induction in only high-risk patients, and 13 did not use antibody induction therapy. The aggregate analyses showed that MPA was superior to azathioprine with regard to graft loss (RR 0.82), death-censored graft loss (RR 0.78), and acute rejection (RR 0.65). There was not a statistically significant difference in mortality nor kidney function. Tissue-invasive CMV disease and GI symptoms were higher with MPA. MPA has been by far the more commonly used antimetabolite in the U.S. for more than a decade; as of 2016, >95% of patients used MPA as compared to <5% using azathioprine [7]. Azathioprine is used commonly in patients who have intolerable adverse effects with MPA or want to become pregnant due to the teratogenicity of MPA.

20.3.2.3   Steroids

Steroids are one of the oldest medications used in transplantation and remain a fundamental part of most immunosuppression regimens. They are commonly used as a high dose "pulse" at the time of transplant, and then chronically at low doses for the life of the allograft. Concern regarding metabolic and other adverse effects has led to evaluation of various strategies to avoid or withdrawal steroid use without increasing rejection or graft loss.

A recent meta-analysis evaluated 48 studies which included a total of 7803 patients in which two different strategies for reducing steroid use were evaluated: discontinuation within 14 days of transplant, or discontinuation later [18]. Overall, acute rejection within 1 year was increased (relative risk 1.77; 95% CI 1.2–2.6) in early steroid withdrawal. However, diabetes mellitus, CMV infections, mortality and graft loss were not statistically different. Confidence in these data is tempered by the low to moderate quality of the studies involved, which frequently were unblinded and/or observed relatively few numbers of events. As a result, steroid-free maintenance regimens remain controversial and are used at different rates at different centers. Overall, steroids are used in approximately 70% of adult kidney transplant recipient in the U.S. at 1 year following transplant [7]. The rate of usage has increased slightly over the past decade.

20.3.2.4 mTOR Inhibitors

The mTORi sirolimus and everolimus have been studied in a variety of contexts, including as substitutes for CNI, and substitutes for antimetabolites at low and high doses of both CNI and mTORi. A large meta-analysis is available encompassing 33 trials of mTORi in different contexts involving 7114 patients [19]. In general, mTORi have been found to be equivalent to comparator drugs with regard to patient and graft survival. mTORi use is generally associated with higher GFR and lower rates of rejection. Evidence of anti-viral and anti-malignancy effects exist; mTORi are often used in patients with skin cancers [20]. However, mTORi use is associated with significant adverse effects including higher rates of dyslipidemia and of bone marrow suppression. Overall, use of mTORi in U.S. kidney transplant recipients is rare and becoming less common over time. Only 1.9% of recipients using them at time of transplant, and 4.9% at 1 year [7].

20.3.2.5 Belatacept

Belatacept, a Signal 2 co-stimulation blocker, was approved by the FDA in 2011 for use in kidney transplant recipients to prevent rejection. Approval was based mainly on two studies which compared two doses of belatacept to cyclosporine in recipients of standard criteria or living donor kidneys [4] or extended criteria kidneys [21]. In both studies, patients received basiliximab induction, and maintenance therapy with MMF and prednisone. Both studies reported that renal function was similar or better in patients receiving belatacept at 12 months. However, the rate of PTLD was also higher. Patients who are seronegative for EBV are contraindicated from receiving belatacept for this reason. The rate and

severity of acute rejection was higher in the belatacept patients who received living or standard criteria donor kidneys. Nonetheless, at 12 months, measured GFR was higher in patients on belatacept who experienced rejections as compared to patients on cyclosporine who did not have rejection. Subsequent meta-analyses of additional studies have reported better GFR, better lipid profiles, lower blood pressure and less diabetes in patients on belatacept as compared to CNIs [22]. Death and graft loss rates were similar. Five year follow ups of the original study participants have reported that the higher GFRs in patients on belatacept relative to cyclosporine are persistent [23, 24]. Belatacept use has been tempered by greater expense, delays in production, and logistical issues related to the requirement for IV infusions.

20.3.3 Treatment of Rejection

Rejection of the allograft can occur due to T cell mediated rejection (TCMR) or by antibody mediated rejection (ABMR), or by a combination of the two. Detailed criteria and classification of the different modes of rejection are defined by the Banff Classification system [25]. When clinically significant rejections occur, they are generally treated with specific immunosuppressive therapies targeted to the mechanism of the rejection, and by modification of subsequent maintenance immunosuppression therapy to prevent future rejection recurrence. As a whole, the evidence supporting different approaches to treating acute rejection are at best, moderate quality [26], and there is a lack of standardized treatments.

20.3.3.1 TCMR

The specific treatment varies by the Banff classification. For TCMR, treatment generally involves pulse methylprednisolone treatment and/or a lymphocyte depleting antibody such as thymoglobulin [26]. Data support the use of lymphocyte depleting antibodies for more severe forms of TCMR. Antibody preparations are also used in rejections that do not respond to initial treatment with pulse steroids.

20.3.3.2 ABMR

For ABMR, therapies are directed toward removal of the donor specific antibody and include plasmapheresis to physically remove the offending antibody. Intravenous immunoglobulin, which has immunomodulatory effects, is commonly given with plasmapheresis and can replace antibodies removed by plasmapheresis. Rituximab, a monoclonal antibody against CD20 which depletes B cells, has also been used in ABMR. However, its effects are uncertain, perhaps since it fails to target the antibody producing plasma cells. Newer therapies are in development for the treatment of ABMR and include protease inhibitors to target plasma cells and IdeS protease, a bacterial enzyme which rapidly and specifically cleaves human IgG [27].

20.4 Concluding Remarks

The development of immunosuppressive medications has been an extraordinary achievement over the past several decades and has paved the way for routine solid organ transplantation in humans. Multiple classes of drugs have been developed to target distinct steps in the activation of T lymphocytes. Synergistic use of this suite of drugs at different stages of the transplant process has made successful prolonged transplantation of solid organs in the absence of significant rejections a routine occurrence. Future challenges include the development of newer agents with equivalent efficacy but fewer adverse effects. Perhaps the most tantalizing goal in transplantation is the identification of methods to induce immune tolerance, a state in which the allograft is tolerated while the immune system retains full function with regards to all other alloantigens. Tolerance would allow for the withdrawal of all immunosuppressive medications. Although much work has been made toward this goal, for the time being the vast majority of transplant patients require chronic immunosuppression.

References

1. Halloran PF. Immunosuppressive drugs for kidney transplantation. N Engl J Med. 2004;351(26):2715–29.

2. Mittal A, Colegio OR. Skin cancers in organ transplant recipients. Am J Transplant. 2017;17(10):2509–30.

3. Ilyas M, Colegio OR, Kaplan B, Sharma A. Cutaneous toxicities from transplantation-related medications. Am J Transplant. 2017;17(11):2782–9.

4. Vincenti F, Charpentier B, Vanrenterghem Y, Rostaing L, Bresnahan B, Darji P, et al. A phase III study of belatacept-based immunosuppression regimens versus cyclosporine in renal transplant recipients (BENEFIT study). Am J Transplant. 2010;10(3):535–46.

5. Hindorf U, Appell ML. Genotyping should be considered the primary choice for pre-treatment evaluation of thiopurine methyltransferase function. J Crohns Colitis. 2012;6(6):655–9.

6. Kidney Disease: Improving Global Outcomes Transplant Work G. KDIGO clinical practice guideline for the care of kidney transplant recipients. Am J Transplant. 2009;9(Suppl 3):S1–155.

7. Hart A, Smith JM, Skeans MA, Gustafson SK, Wilk AR, Robinson A, et al. OPTN/SRTR 2016 annual data report: kidney. Am J Transplant. 2018;18(Suppl 1):18–113.

8. Nashan B, Moore R, Amlot P, Schmidt AG, Abeywickrama K, Soulillou JP. Randomised trial of basiliximab versus placebo for control of acute cellular rejection in renal allograft recipients. CHIB 201 International Study Group. Lancet. 1997;350(9086):1193–8.

9. Kahan BD, Rajagopalan PR, Hall M. Reduction of the occurrence of acute cellular rejection among renal allograft recipients treated with basiliximab, a chimeric anti-interleukin-2-receptor monoclonal antibody. United States Simulect Renal Study Group. Transplantation. 1999;67(2):276–84.

10. Ponticelli C, Yussim A, Cambi V, Legendre C, Rizzo G, Salvadori M, et al. A randomized, double-blind trial of basiliximab immunoprophylaxis plus triple therapy in kidney transplant recipients. Transplantation. 2001;72(7):1261–7.

11. Lawen JG, Davies EA, Mourad G, Oppenheimer F, Molina MG, Rostaing L, et al. Randomized double-blind study of immunoprophylaxis with basiliximab, a chimeric anti-interleukin-2 receptor monoclonal antibody, in combination with mycophenolate mofetil-containing triple therapy in renal transplantation. Transplantation. 2003;75(1):37–43.

12. Webster AC, Playford EG, Higgins G, Chapman JR, Craig J. Interleukin 2 receptor antagonists for kidney transplant recipients. Cochrane Database Syst Rev. 2010;1:CD003897.

13. Brennan DC, Daller JA, Lake KD, Cibrik D, Del Castillo D. Thymoglobulin Induction Study G. Rabbit antithymocyte globulin versus basiliximab in renal transplantation. N Engl J Med. 2006;355(19):1967–77.

14. Noel C, Abramowicz D, Durand D, Mourad G, Lang P, Kessler M, et al. Daclizumab versus antithymocyte globulin in high-immunological-risk renal transplant recipients. J Am Soc Nephrol. 2009;20(6):1385–92.

15. Hill P, Cross NB, Barnett AN, Palmer SC, Webster AC. Polyclonal and monoclonal antibodies for induction therapy in kidney transplant recipients. Cochrane Database Syst Rev. 2017;1:CD004759.

16. Webster AC, Woodroffe RC, Taylor RS, Chapman JR, Craig JC. Tacrolimus versus ciclosporin as primary immunosuppression for kidney transplant recipients: meta-analysis and meta-regression of randomised trial data. BMJ. 2005;331(7520):810.

17. Wagner M, Earley AK, Webster AC, Schmid CH, Balk EM, Uhlig K. Mycophenolic acid versus azathioprine as primary immunosuppression for kidney transplant recipients. Cochrane Database Syst Rev. 2015;12:CD007746.

18. Haller MC, Royuela A, Nagler EV, Pascual J, Webster AC. Steroid avoidance or withdrawal for kidney transplant recipients. Cochrane Database Syst Rev. 2016;8:CD005632.

19. Webster AC, Lee VW, Chapman JR, Craig JC. Target of rapamycin inhibitors (TOR-I; sirolimus and everolimus) for primary immunosuppression in kidney transplant recipients. Cochrane Database Syst Rev. 2006;2:CD004290.

20. Geissler EK. Skin cancer in solid organ transplant recipients: are mTOR inhibitors a game changer? Transplant Res. 2015;4:1.

21. Durrbach A, Pestana JM, Pearson T, Vincenti F, Garcia VD, Campistol J, et al. A phase III study of belatacept versus cyclosporine in kidney transplants from extended criteria donors (BENEFIT-EXT study). Am J Transplant. 2010;10(3):547–57.

22. Masson P, Henderson L, Chapman JR, Craig JC, Webster AC. Belatacept for kidney transplant recipients. Cochrane Database Syst Rev. 2014;11:CD010699.

23. Rostaing L, Vincenti F, Grinyo J, Rice KM, Bresnahan B, Steinberg S, et al. Long-term belatacept exposure maintains efficacy and safety at 5 years: results from the long-term extension of the BENEFIT study. Am J Transplant. 2013;13(11):2875–83.

24. Vincenti F, Blancho G, Durrbach A, Friend P, Grinyo J, Halloran PF, et al. Five-year safety and efficacy of belatacept in renal transplantation. J Am Soc Nephrol. 2010;21(9):1587–96.

25. Haas M, Loupy A, Lefaucheur C, Roufosse C, Glotz D, Seron D, et al. The Banff 2017 Kidney Meeting Report: revised diagnostic criteria for chronic active T cell-mediated rejection, antibody-mediated rejection, and prospects for integrative endpoints for next-generation clinical trials. Am J Transplant. 2018;18(2):293–307.

26. Webster AC, Wu S, Tallapragada K, Park MY, Chapman JR, Carr SJ. Polyclonal and monoclonal antibodies for treating acute rejection episodes in kidney transplant recipients. Cochrane Database Syst Rev. 2017;7:CD004756.

27. Winstedt L, Jarnum S, Nordahl EA, Olsson A, Runstrom A, Bockermann R, et al. Complete removal of extracellular IgG antibodies in a randomized dose-escalation phase I study with the bacterial enzyme IdeS – a novel therapeutic opportunity. PLoS One. 2015;10(7):e0132011.

Machine Perfusion of Human Donor Livers

Maureen J. M. Werner, Vincent E. de Meijer, and Robert J. Porte

Definitions

ATP   Adenosine Triphosphate
ARP   Abdominal Regional Perfusion
AST   Aspartate Aminotransferase
COR   Controlled Oxygenated Rewarming
DAMPs   Danger Associated Molecular Patterns
DBD   Donation after Brain Death
DCD   Donation after Circulatory Death
DHOPE   Dual Hypothermic Oxygenated Machine Perfusion
EAD   Early Allograft Dysfunction
ECD   Extended Criteria Donor
HMP   Hypothermic Machine Perfusion
HOPE   Hypothermic Oxygenated Machine Perfusion
IRI   Ischemia and Reperfusion Injury
MMP   Mid-thermic Machine Perfusion
NMP   Normothermic Machine Perfusion
NRP   Normothermic Regional Perfusion
PNF   Primary Non-function
RCT   Randomized Controlled Trial
ROS   Radical Oxygen Species
SCS   Static Cold Storage
SNMP   Sub-normothermic Machine Perfusion
UW   University of Wisconsin

21.1 Introduction

Machine perfusion technology has been revolutionizing the field of liver transplantation and undergoes rapid clinical implementation. But what is machine perfusion? Why should we implement this? And how can machine perfusion be responsible for increases in the quality and quantity of liver transplants? This chapter will provide an overview of current 'state of the art' of machine perfusion of the liver.

21.2 The History of Machine Perfusion and Its Recent Revival

The concept of *ex-situ* machine perfusion of isolated organs is older than organ transplantation itself. Already in the 1930s Carrel and Lindberg developed a sterile perfusion pump, the 'Lindberg Apparatus', which enabled them to establish prolonged *ex-vivo* metabolic function of isolated organs [1]. In 1968, the first successful machine perfused organ transplantation in humans took place, concerning a kidney after 17 h of machine perfusion [2]. Subsequently, in 1968 Starzl et al. successfully

M. J. M. Werner · V. E. de Meijer · R. J. Porte (✉)
Section of Hepato-Pancreato-Biliary Surgery and
Liver Transplantation, Department of Surgery,
University Medical Center Groningen,
Groningen, The Netherlands
e-mail: m.j.m.werner@umcg.nl;
v.e.de.meijer@umcg.nl; r.j.porte@umcg.nl

© Springer Nature Switzerland AG 2021
N. Hakim et al. (eds.), *Transplantation Surgery*, Springer Specialist Surgery Series,
https://doi.org/10.1007/978-3-030-55244-2_21

transplanted liver grafts which received interim preservation with hypothermic, oxygenated machine perfusion with diluted blood [3]. Nevertheless, in the 1980s the Belzers Wisconsin solution was invented as a suitable static preservation fluid [4]. With this revelation, the golden age of static cold storage (SCS) organ preservation was initiated. Compared to machine perfusion, SCS was a simple, effective, cheap, and transportable alternative, and has been remarkably successful ever since.

21.2.1 Shortage of Suitable Liver Grafts

Over the past decades, with this successful and accessible SCS preservation of liver grafts and the improving outcomes after liver transplantation, the demand for liver grafts has increased worldwide. One of the main limiting factors of liver transplantation nowadays is the severe shortage of suitable donor organs [5]. To overcome this problem, several strategies have been implemented over time, such as domino liver transplantations, splitting of liver grafts and living donor liver transplantation. At present an important and emerging strategy to expand the donor pool is transplanting livers of suboptimal quality derived from high risk donors, or so called extended criteria donors (ECD). ECD liver grafts include steatotic grafts, grafts derived from elderly donors or grafts from donors after circulatory death (DCD). Actually, in the past decade the number of DCD liver transplantations increased fourfold, concerning up to 18% of the liver transplantation in the USA [6] and 30% in some European countries [7]. The major drawback of transplanting these ECD organs is their increased susceptibility to ischemia and reperfusion injury (IRI), with subsequently an increased risk of primary non-function (PNF), early allograft dysfunction (EAD) and postoperative biliary complications. This will be explained in more detail in the continuation of this chapter.

21.2.2 The Mechanism of Ischemia and Reperfusion Injury

In liver transplantation, IRI incorporates the sequence of deleterious processes that appear after temporary deprivation of hepatic oxygenation and nutrient supply during the donation procedure, the preservation period and transplantation procedure [8, 9]. During SCS preservation hypothermia reduces the hepatocellular metabolism. Although a significant reduction in the need for oxygen is established, still there is always some active cellular metabolism present in the liver graft resulting in an oxygen and nutrient debt. Subsequently cellular and mitochondrial disturbances occur, resulting in intracellular depletion of adenosine triphosphate (ATP) and cell swelling by cause of electrolyte shifts. During reperfusion of the liver, the re-oxygenation induces production of toxic radical oxygen species (ROS) and danger associated molecular patterns (DAMPs), which are released by the meanwhile apoptotic and necrotic liver cells. This whole process leads to a disproportionate immune response that is detrimental to organ function [8].

The standard criteria donor liver grafts retain sufficient physiologic reserve capacity to overcome this preservation induced IRI, but ECD grafts appear to be highly susceptible to it. Therefore, especially for ECD grafts machine perfusion is a promising alternative to SCS, to preserve these vulnerable liver grafts under conditions comparable to physiologic conditions to minimize the cascade of IRI and its disastrous effects.

21.3 Timing of Machine Perfusion

The standard procurement technique for livers involves *in-situ* arterial flush following aortic cross-clamping in donation after brain dead (DBD) or after circulatory arrest in DCD. In DBD donors there is enough time for standard organ procurement. For DCD, the procurement of organs is executed with a super-rapid laparotomy and sternotomy with direct arterial cannulation [10], after which the organs are perfused with cold preservation fluid and removed as quickly as possible. After procurement, traditionally the organs will be preserved SCS.

In the past years, for DCD donors there has been growing interest in so called *in-situ* machine perfusion; a technique to restore blood flow after determination of death and before organ procurement, with abdominal regional perfusion using extracorporeal membranous oxygenation devices. Another alternative organ preservation strategy is *ex-situ* machine perfusion, in which the organ is perfused by a machine perfusion device outside of the body. *Ex-situ* as well as *in-situ* machine perfusion will be described in the following section.

21.3.1 *In-Situ* Machine Perfusion

In-situ machine perfusion occurs in the period between determination of death and organ procurement. Nowadays the term abdominal regional perfusion (ARP) is applicable; a technique which restores the circulation to the abdominal organs following circulatory arrest for the purpose of transplantation.

Already in 1997, the concept of using normothermic extracorporeal membranous oxygenation devices in organ donation procedures was first described [11]. In 2002, researchers in Spain clinically implemented this technique in DCD donors. With this new technique their donor pool significantly increased and low rates of PNF, hepatic artery thrombosis and ischemic cholangiopathy were reported [12].

Subsequently, abdominal normothermic regional perfusion (NRP) has also been introduced in France and the United Kingdom. A recent series including 11 liver grafts reported a 1-year graft survival rate of 90% without evidence of post-transplant cholangiopathy. In addition to the liver, this technique may also improve outcomes for DCD kidneys, lungs, and pancreas [13].

In today's NRP procedures, a localized abdominal perfusion circuit is established in the donor, perfusing the organs with oxygenated blood at 37 °C for 2–4 h. With this, essentially converting a DCD retrieval to a DBD type one, a less hasty retrieval is achieved. Using NRP, organ damage and loss due to surgical events may be reduced. NRP may restore cellular energy substrates and improve the quality of ischemic damaged organs. Furthermore, it may offer the ability to assess organ function before transplantation to allow better graft selection [13, 14]. It is envisioned that NRP will increase the yield of retrieved organs per donor and provide better quality organs for the purpose of transplantation, but more experience and further organization is needed.

21.3.2 *Ex-Situ* Machine Perfusion

The concept of *ex-situ* machine perfusion is relatively simple; it provides an environment for the liver graft outside of the body while closely mimicking the physiologic *in-vivo* situation. The liver is connected via its blood vessels to a sterile machine perfusion device and an adjustable continuous flow of perfusate through the liver is generated (Fig. 21.1).

In general, *ex-situ* machine perfusion can be performed at three time points, defined as pre-SCS, post-SCS and preservation machine perfusion as demonstrated in Fig. 21.2 [16].

Pre-SCS incorporates machine perfusion conducted within 3 h after organ procurement followed by a period of SCS. In post-SCS machine perfusion, after a period of SCS the liver is machine perfused prior to organ implantation.

In case of preservation machine perfusion the organ is preserved with machine perfusion during the entire preservation period, from procurement to implantation [17]. However, a short period of SCS is inevitable. During organ procurement and preparation of the organ before connection to the machine the organ is SCS preserved as well as during implantation, to avoid more harmful warm ischemia during the anastomosis time. Preservation machine perfusion is defined as machine perfusion with a SCS duration of less than 3 h, either before or after machine perfusion (Fig. 21.2).

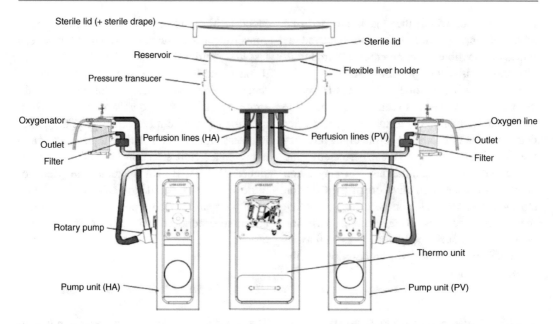

Fig. 21.1 Dual hypothermic machine perfusion in liver transplantation [15]. Systemic drawing of the set-up of dual hypothermic oxygenated machine perfusion. The liver graft can be placed in the reservoir, which can be covered with a transparant lid to maintain a moist and sterile environment. The system is bot pressure and temperature controlled. Two rotatory pumps seperately provide a pulsatile flow to the hepatic artery and a continious flow to the portal vein. The perfusate can be oxygenated by the membrane oxygenators, which also regulate the temperature. Real-time perfusion flow rates and temperatures can be measured and displayed on both pump units

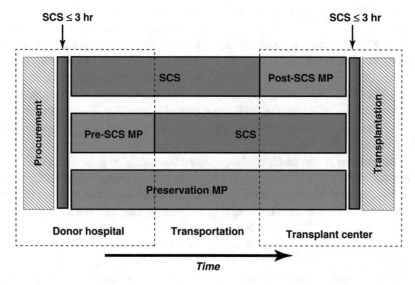

Fig. 21.2 Charts illustrating classification of the timing of machine perfusion [16]. Machine perfusion (MP) conducted within 3 h of organ procurement and followed by a period of static cold storage (SCS) is considered as pre-SCS MP. MP performed after a period of at least 3 h of SCS preservation prior to implantation is considered as post-SCS MP. MP with a SCS duration of less than 3 h, either before or after machine perfusion is defined as preservation machine perfusion

21.4   Types of Machine Perfusion

21.4.1 Overview

As presented in Fig. 21.3, machine perfusion can be subdivided in four categories according to the temperature the perfusion is performed. Based on Van't Hoff's principle (expressed as $Q10 = (K_2 / K_1)^{10/(t2-t1)}$), the rate of metabolism of the liver is depending on the temperature. At hypothermic conditions the liver has a significant reduced metabolism. Machine perfusion therefore can be subdivided in hypothermic machine perfusion (HMP), mid-thermic machine perfusion (MMP), sub-normothermic machine perfusion (SNMP) and normothermic machine perfusion (NMP).

21.4.2 Hypothermic Machine Perfusion

HMP is defined as machine perfusion at temperatures from 0–12 °C [16]. This is the least complex form of machine perfusion and is facilitated by minimal metabolic demands of the liver in hypothermic circumstances. With temperatures of 12 °C and below, the rate of intracellular metabolism and enzymatic reactions decreases to 20% or even less (Fig. 21.3).

HMP is a form of machine perfusion that is typically applied end-ischemic post-SCS. After arrival at the recipient hospital and backtable procurement, the liver graft is connected to the machine by cannulation of both the portal vein and hepatic artery (dual perfusion), or the portal

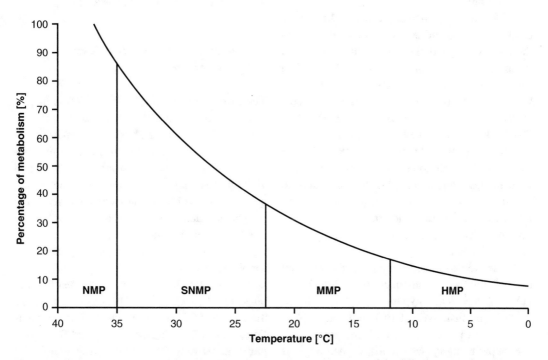

Fig. 21.3 Graphic presentation of the change in rate of metabolism with decreasing temperature [16]. Based on Van't Hoff's principle (expressed as $Q10 = (K_2/K_1)^{10/(t2-t1)}$), this graph demonstrates the significantly reduced metabolism of the liver at hypothermic temperatures. The vertical lines in the graph indicate the lower endpoint of temperature ranges of the different types of machine perfusion proposed. NMP; normothermic machine perfusion (35–38 °C); SMP, sub-normothermic machine perfusion (25–34 °C); MMP, mid-thermic machine perfusion (13–24 °C); HMP, hypothermic machine perfusion (0–12 °C)

vein alone. The liver is than perfused for about 2 to 4 h with a perfusion fluid with or without active, supplemented oxygenation.

Experimental studies have demonstrated end-ischemic HMP as a safe and feasible technique, which restores the hepatocellular energy status and reduces IRI in liver grafts. In 2010 Guarrera et al. first reported successful transplantation of *ex-situ* hypothermic (4–6 °C) machine perfused DBD liver grafts in humans [18]. Dual perfusion with Vasosol perfusion solution (see also paragraph 10.2) with added antioxidants and metabolic substrates was performed via both portal vein and hepatic artery for 3–7 h. Compared to SCS liver grafts, HMP treated livers had a better graft function and attenuated liver injury markers after transplantation.

With these promising results, Dutkowski et al. pretreated DCD liver grafts with hypothermic oxygenated machine perfusion (HOPE) in an attempt to improve graft quality before implantation [19]. Post-SCS, the liver grafts were perfused through the portal vein exclusively for 1 to 2 h with oxygenated (pO2 80–100 kPa) and cooled (10 °C) University of Wisconsin (UW) gluconate solution. HOPE treated livers had lower incidences of EAD, PNF and ischemic cholangiopathy compared to SCS-preserved DCD grafts without HOPE. Graft function and survival, as well as postoperative complications were comparable to DBD controls.

In the Netherlands, van Rijn et al. combined both of the above techniques in a clinical trial [15]. With dual hypothermic oxygenated machine perfusion (DHOPE), oxygenation as well as dual perfusion via both the portal vein and hepatic artery was realized. Although it adds another technical step opposed to portal vein only perfusion, dual perfusion might have additional advantages because bile ducts are mainly depending on arterial blood supply [20]. Additional information about single versus dual perfusion can be found in Sect. 21.6.3. This clinical study suggests that DHOPE is safe and feasible, restores hepatic ATP and reduces reperfusion injury [15].

21.4.3 Mid-thermic and Sub-normothermic Machine Perfusion

MMP is executed at temperatures from 13 to 24 °C and SNMP embraces machine perfusion within a temperature range of 25–34 °C. Both techniques, however, have not been used in human clinical studies thus far. In 2015, Bruinsma et al. demonstrated SNMP in discarded human donor livers offers a viable alternative to conventional SCS, HMP and NMP modalities. SNMP treated liver grafts showed improving function with restoration of tissue ATP levels. A major advance of SNMP is the ability of perfusion with an acellular fluid without an oxygen carrier, since metabolic oxygen demands at 21 °C are met by active oxygenation of the perfusate [21].

21.4.4 Normothermic Machine Perfusion

The overall goal of NMP (35–37 °C) is to preserve human liver grafts *ex-situ* at body temperature simulating a near-physiologic environment by using machine perfusion. Active liver metabolism at 37 °C allows for graft assessment and viability testing prior to transplantation. NMP, however, is a real technically challenge requiring oxygenated dual perfusion via both the hepatic artery and portal vein with perfusate incorporating an adequate oxygen carrier and nutritional supplements.

In 2013, Ravikumar et al. performed the first phase I trial, in which NMP preserved livers were matched to SCS preserved livers. The intervention group comprising both DBD and DCD liver grafts underwent NMP with a red cell–based fluid, after which twenty liver transplantations were executed. NMP appeared to be safe and feasible. Thirty-day graft survival was similar for NMP and SCS, while median peak aspartate aminotransferase (AST) levels and EAD incidence were significantly decreased in the NMP group [22]. Subsequently, the Toronto and Edmonton groups published comparable results from their phase I studies [17, 23, 24].

Currently, several multicenter phase III randomized controlled trials (RCT) comparing NMP with SCS-preservation only are ongoing [25]. The first RCT using NMP as preservation method instead of SCS was recently published by the Consortium for Organ Preservation in Europe, including 121 NMP and 101 SCS preserved liver grafts. For the NMP group, a significant reduction in peak serum AST and EAD incidence were seen [17].

Op den Dries et al. demonstrated the feasibility of end-ischemic NMP by using discarded human donor livers. Discarded liver grafts functioned well during *ex-situ* machine perfusion, with a continuous bile production and normalizing biochemical liver related parameters. Histological examination afterwards confirmed adequate preservation of liver morphology [26]. Subsequently in 2015, the first human liver transplantation using a marginal liver graft resuscitated with end-ischemic NMP was performed. This suboptimal liver graft was initially deemed too high risk and rejected for transplantation, but transplanted after SCS-preservation followed by NMP resuscitation [27]. With the feasibility demonstration of *ex-situ* functional testing of liver grafts, initially discarded ECD liver grafts can be tested for their viability and transplanted if viable, and with that potentially increase the donor pool.

In 2017, based on the presumed synergistic effect of end-ischemic DHOPE and NMP, we designed these two types of machine perfusion in a clinical trial protocol. Nationwide declined high risk donor livers are preserved and transported by SCS, followed by end-ischemic DHOPE (resuscitation phase), controlled oxygenated rewarming (COR; see also Sect. 21.6.4), and subsequent *ex-situ* viability testing during NMP. When meeting the viability criteria at 150 min of NMP (including bile production of ≥10 grams, lactate concentration in perfusate between 0.5–1.7, pH in perfusate between 7.35–7.45, and bile pH >7.45) the livers are transplanted (www.trialregister.nl; NTR5972).

Although until now no RCT has demonstrated an improvement in patient or graft survival or reduction in biliary complications yet, it is nota-

ble that trials with larger numbers and longer term follow-up are required to examine these outcomes.

21.5 Advances of Machine Perfusion

Based on previous experimental studies, machine perfusion has a great potential and offers many advantages and possibilities as compared to or as an adjunct to conventional SCS [12, 19, 25, 28–30]. This technique offers the capability to preserve donor organs while providing them with oxygen and nutrients at various temperatures; the ability to (p)recondition and optimize the function of donor organs, particularly ECD organs, and the possibility of function and viability testing. These concepts will be discussed below in more detail.

21.5.1 Optimal and Prolonged Preservation

Machine perfusion generates a continuous flow with perfusion solution, or perfusate, through the liver graft. The continuous flow supports the endothelial cell function of the graft, while metabolic waste products can be released. Supplementation of oxygen, nutrients, metabolic substrates and other products to the perfusate allow the liver to exert his physiologic metabolic function.

Besides that, like described in Sect. 22.4, temperatures can be regulated during machine perfusion. HMP enables to perfuse the liver graft in a low metabolic state in which the oxygen debt can be restored and graft can be upregulated without any further damage or loss of energy. In NMP a physiological situation is simulated in which the liver can practice its function, including production of hemostatic proteins [31].

A side potential of machine perfusion is the ability for prolonged preservation of the liver. In a recent proof-of-concept study, NMP was used to preserve a human discarded liver graft for 86 h [32]. Another report recently described a successful transplantation of an initially declined human liver after preservation for 26 h, of which 8.5 h with NMP [33]. This raises potential for a more scheduled, or in daytime and prepared transplantation approach, which would be better for both recipient and the surgical team.

21.5.2 (P)reconditioning and Optimization of Liver Graft Function

One of the main advantages of machine perfusion is the opportunity to recondition and optimize liver grafts that have been damaged by warm and subsequently cold ischemia. As previously described, during warm and subsequent cold ischemia ATP stores are rapidly depleted [9, 34]. ATP can be restored during a period of oxygenated HMP prior to implantation of the liver graft [21]. Moreover, the accumulated oxygen and nutrient debts can be restored, and normal repair and regenerative pathways can be re-activated [25]. The liver, with its energy stores and metabolic state replenished, is preconditioned and better prepared for the injurious effects of reperfusion injury after implantation in the recipient [15]. Besides this, in livers with restored ATP the IRI is less conspicuous, probably due to the resuscitation of mitochondria with subsequently a reduction in succinate accumulation, which has been linked to ROS generation after reperfusion.

With new machine perfusion techniques ECD grafts can be (p)reconditioned to potentially alleviate the deleterious effects of IRI at reperfusion.

Notably, cholangiocytes are particularly susceptible to IRI. The most frequent complications after DCD liver transplantation are biliary complications, also known as post-transplant cholangiopathy [9]. Post-transplant cholangiopathy comprises the spectrum of abnormalities of large donor bile ducts, including non-anastomotic biliary strictures, intraductal casts and intrahepatic biloma formation, in the presence of a patent hepatic artery. Non-anastomotic biliary strictures have been reported in up to 30% after DCD liver transplantation, almost three times higher com-

pared to DBD liver transplantation [35]. Van Rijn et al. recently demonstrated that end-ischemic DHOPE reduces histological signs of IRI of bile ducts after DCD liver transplantation [36].

With the increasing incidence of obesity, today 40–60% of donor livers have significant fatty changes (steatosis). The general limit of acceptable donor steatosis is around 30% because steatosis is a known risk factor for increased IRI and poor outcomes after liver transplantation, most importantly PNF [37, 38]. Liver steatosis exacerbates secondary IRI by increased ROS generation, pro-inflammatory immune system activation and impaired ATP production, resulting in hepatic cell necrosis and graft failure upon reperfusion [39]. Besides this, there are indications that steatosis results in endothelial dysfunction [40]. In addition, intracellular lipid droplets may cause ballooning of the hepatocyte leading to an impaired microcirculation, and thus suboptimal flush and perfusion. Machine perfusion has the potential to mitigate the deleterious effects of steatosis [41]. Although clinical experience with defatting is scarce, experimental small-animal studies supplementing defatting cocktails during machine perfusion have shown promising results [42].

21.5.3 Function and Viability Testing

Another major advance of machine perfusion is the ability to test the liver graft for its function and viability. All the more with the usage of ECD liver grafts and their susceptibility to IRI, it remains uncertain which liver graft will develop complications and which one will function properly. The decision to accept or decline a donor liver for transplantation is usually depending on donor past history, laboratory values, ischemia times and intra-operative findings. Machine perfusion may offer a more objective method to distinguish potentially transplantable from 'non-viable' livers, prior to transplantation [43].

During machine perfusion several parameters can be monitored; arterial and portal vascular flow and resistance, as well as bile production. Besides that, immediate analysis of perfusate lactate and glucose can be performed [15]. These data will provide the transplantation team valuable information about the state of the liver.

Like mentioned before, NMP mimics the physiological state of the liver at 37 °C in which the liver is metabolically active, allowing for *ex-situ* real-time assessment of viability prior to transplantation. Lactate concentrations and pH level in perfusate, bile production, and pH level in bile enables the perfusion team to test the liver during perfusion. This is a major advance, which may potentially increase the donor pool as previously discarded ECD liver grafts can be tested for viability and subsequently transplanted if viable.

21.6 Technical Aspects of Machine Perfusion

21.6.1 Machine Perfusion Devices

With the instantaneous development of machine perfusion, several devices for machine perfusion of the liver have been developed. This paragraph provides a brief description of the four most frequently used devices (Table 21.1).

Firstly, the Liver Assist (Organ Assist, Groningen, the Netherlands) device enables pressure-controlled oxygenated perfusion. It consists of two different pump units that provide a pulsatile perfusion of the hepatic artery and continuous flow through the portal vein. Temperature can be set from hypothermic to normothermic conditions using an integrated heater/cooler. It is a mobile device, although not designed for transportation.

Secondly, the OrganOx Metra (Organox, Oxford, UK) device is a fully automated perfusion system, which maintains physiological temperature, flows, pressures, oxygenation and records bile production. It has a robust design for ease of transport and safe storage and includes a self-regulating oxygen supply.

Thirdly, the LifePort Liver Transporter (Organ Recovery systems, Chicago, USA) device is designed to deliver precision controlled perfusion of both the hepatic artery and portal vein. It enables hypothermic perfusion and is supported by redundant preservation systems for safety, dynamic perfusion plus SCS. It's a height-adjustable and mobile device.

Fourthly, the Organ Care System™ Liver (Transmedics, Andover, USA) device is a portable perfusion and monitoring system. The portable console houses all elements of the system, including oxygen supply and a pump that is used to maintain pulsatile flow of warm, nutrient-rich blood to the organ.

21.6.2 Flow Versus Pressure Controlled

Liver machine perfusion devices can be flow- or pressure-controlled and both alternatives have been applied in previously described studies. Pressure-controlled perfusion is considered to be the safest method. During cold preservation, in both SCS and HMP, the sinusoidal endothelial cells are at high risk for injury. In rats, it was demonstrated that increased perfusion pressures resulted in a more complete perfusion, but also in increasing endothelial damage [44]. Furthermore, Fondevila et al. demonstrated in pig livers that high flow rates provoke sinusoidal endothelial injury through overexpression of von Willebrand factor and tumor necrosis factor with subsequent activation of Kupffer- and endothelial cells [45]. Therefore, in HMP pressure-controlled perfusion is a key element to minimize these risks of shear stress, mediator release and sinusoidal damage [30].

21.6.3 Single Versus Dual Perfusion

Machine perfusion of the liver is either performed by single or dual perfusion. With the single perfusion technique, only the portal vein is cannulated whereas in dual perfusion, both hepatic artery and portal vein are cannulated. Single perfusion adds simplicity to the procedure, but can only be applied in hypothermic conditions. Dual perfusion can be applied under hypothermia as well as normothermia.

Advocates of dual perfusion state that perfusion through the hepatic artery emphasizes better

Table 21.1 Overview of the four most frequently used liver machine perfusion devices

Device	Liver assist	OrganOx metra	Organ care system liver	LifePort liver transporter
Circulation	Pressure-controlled	Pressure-controlled	Flow-controlled	Pressure-controlled
Cannulation	Dual & single	Dual	Dual	Dual
Oxygenation	Yes	Yes	Yes	No
Thermic options	Hypothermic & Normothermic	Normothermic	Normothermic	Hypothermic
Transportable	No	Yes	Yes	Yes

oxygen supply to the peribiliary vascular plexus, since it is well known that blood supply to the bile ducts is largely dependent on the hepatic artery. Preservation of the biliary tree is critical, and single portal perfusion may not be sufficient to protect the bile ducts, especially in DCD liver grafts [15, 36]. Moreover, pulsatile arterial perfusion may induce upregulation of biomechnical induced cytoprotective endothelial genes [28]. However, no conclusive studies demonstrating the best hypothermic perfusion route are available yet. For now, both portal vein alone and dual perfusion appear to be equally effective and well tolerated [30].

21.6.4 Controlled Oxygenated Rewarming

A relative new concept in machine perfusion is COR. As previously described, abrupt temperature shifts from hypothermia to normothermia obtained on reperfusion of liver grafts might contribute to reperfusion injury and graft dysfunction after transplantation. Hoyer et al. introduced the COR technique, in which after initial HMP, the temperature was gradually increased to 12 °C, 16 °C, and 20 °C after 30, 45, and 60 min, respectively [46]. Six patients were transplanted with a COR treated liver graft in which, compared to untreated controls, a 50% reduction in peak serum transaminases after transplantation was seen. Six-month graft and patient survival were 100% in the COR group compared to 81 and 85% in the control group. Also Banan et al. suggested, based on a pig study, that a combination of COR and NMP treatment may greatly reduce damage associated with reperfusion by minimizing hepatocellular damage, Kupffer cell activation and sinusoidal endothelial cell dysfunction [47]. The implementation of controlled oxygenated graft rewarming before transplantation has been shown to be a promising measure in clinical routine that warrants further confirmation in randomized controlled trials. As mentioned before, we recently initiated a clinical trial that combines DHOPE, COR and NMP (www.trialregister.nl; NTR5972).

21.7 Machine Perfusion Solution

21.7.1 Oxygenation

Before the 'golden age' of SCS, *ex-situ* machine perfusion of isolated organs was initially performed with diluted blood. Since the reintroduction of machine perfusion numerous perfusion fluids have been developed.

For perfusion solutions, it's important to distinguish between HMP and NMP. As noticed before, at hypothermic temperatures, the rate of metabolisms and enzymatic reactions of the liver grafts are as low as 20%, or even less. With this, the oxygen consumption and need of the liver remains low during machine perfusion. In normothermic conditions, the metabolism of the liver extent from 85% to 100%, with subsequently a serious need for oxygen which cannot be provided by diffusion only. Therefore in NMP, the perfusion fluid requires an adequate oxygen carrier [16].

21.7.2 Perfusion Fluids and Components

Currently, Belzer Machine Perfusion Solution UW (Bridge-to-Life, Northbrook, USA) is the preferred solution for HMP. This is a sterile, isotonic non-pyrogenic solution with an osmolarity of 300 mOsm, sodium and potassium concentration of 100 and 25 mEq/L respectively, and a pH of 7.40.

Another commonly used perfusion solution in HMP is Vasosol (Lifeline Scientific, Chicago, USA), which consist of elements of conventional UW solution with additional vasodilatory and antioxidant components including prostaglandins, nitroglycerin and acetylcysteine. Also mitochondrial stabilizers like alpha-ketoglutarate are constituted [48].

For NMP, a perfusion solution requires a physiological osmolarity and oncotic pressure and an adequate oxygen carrier to deliver oxygen throughout the organ. The golden standard perfusion solution therefore consists of human red blood cells combined with a colloid solution, like fresh frozen plasma [26], Steen solution (XVIVO, Göteborg, Sweden) [23] or gelofusine (B Braun, Melsungen, Germany) [22, 24].

Our group recently developed a NMP perfusion solution that eliminates the need for human blood products. We demonstrated that NMP can effectively be performed by replacing red blood cells with HBOC-201 (Therapeutics LLC, Souderton, USA), a polymerized bovine hemoglobin, and fresh frozen plasma by gelofusine. Perfusing livers with this customized perfusion fluid appeared at least similar to perfusion with red blood cells and fresh frozen plasma. Some of the biomarkers of liver function and injury even suggested a potential superiority of an HBOC-201-based perfusion solution. This opens a perspective for further optimization of NMP solutions [49].

21.7.3 Nutrient and Pharmalogical Supplementation

During the evolution of machine perfusion solutions, several nutrients and pharmacologicals were added to perfusion fluids to (p)recondition and optimize the live grafts. To provide sufficient nutrients for the liver graft, vitamins, glucose, amino acids and trace elements were successfully added to perfusion solutions. To prevent the development of interstitial edema or intracellular contraction, the oncotic and osmotic pressure of perfusion solutions was adjusted by adding sterile H_2O, saline and human albumin. Also sodium bicarbonate can be added for buffering capacity. For NMP broad-spectrum antibiotics were added as prevention for bacterial growth and graft infection under normothermic conditions. Heparin can be added for anticoagulation during machine perfusion [26].

21.8 Machine Perfusion in Practice

Machine perfusion is a technically demanding procedure and requires excellent teamwork. Surgeons, assistants, theatre and scrub nurses, anesthesiologists, and organ perfusionists all need to collaborate closely. In the next paragraphs, a global procedure for machine perfusion is described step by step [50].

21.8.1 Priming the Machine Perfusion Device

Built up the liver perfusion machine following its instructions and add the desired perfusion solution to the sterile machine's tubing circuit. Switch on the perfusion pump(s) and remove all air bubbles from the closed system. Adjust the desired pressures, flows and temperatures and start oxygenation if applicable depending on the type of machine perfusion device that is used. Check the pH and electrolytes of the perfusion fluid and adjust if necessary. In case of NMP, a blood culture should be taken prior to liver perfusion [51].

21.8.2 Donor Liver Procurement and Preparation

The donor liver is procured in the donor hospital using the standard technique of *in-situ* cooling, and is flushed out with cold preservation fluid. In case of dual perfusion, to facilitate cannulation of the artery a segment of the supratruncal aorta should be left attached to the coeliac trunk. The portal vein should be kept as long as possible. The cystic duct should be ligated with a tie and the gall bladder should remain untouched. Also, the usual blood vessel toolkit should be harvested and kept together with the liver graft.

During the whole procedure, maintenance and assurance of sterile technique will be crucial to prevent infections. Therefore cannulation and perfusion must be performed in a location that meets current standards for performing sterile (aseptic) clinical procedures either at the donor hospital or at the transplant center. The liver procurement including dissection of the hepatic artery and portal vein should be performed as usual. In case of dual perfusion, close the distal end of the supratruncal aorta segment and insert the arterial cannula into the proximal end, and secure with a tie. Insert the venous cannula into the portal vein and secure. Depending on the perfusion device, the inferior vena cava should be cannulated or not. In case of NMP, also introduce a silicon catheter in the bile duct and secure to allow intermittent bile sampling. Lastly, flush out the liver via the portal vein cannula to remove the majority of the standard preservation fluid.

21.8.3 Machine Perfusion

Position the liver into the organ chamber according to the manufacturer's instructions. Connect the portal vein cannula to the portal inflow tube of the perfusion device and start portal perfusion. In case of dual perfusion, also connect the arterial cannula to the arterial inflow tube and start arterial perfusion as well. During machine perfusion immediate analysis of blood gas parameters (pO_2, pCO_2, sO_2, HCO_2^- and pH) and biochemical parameters (glucose, calcium, lactate, potassium and sodium) should be performed and adjusted if necessary.

During machine perfusion, accidental decannulation, vessel kinking, interruption of oxygen, power supply or perfusion outside of the target are just some examples of potential device malfunctions that may result in irreversible organ injury. Therefore, the executive center must have a specially trained team which is able to operative the device during preservation and has the ability to safely convert machine preservation to SCS in case of unrecoverable device failure within 10 min of cessation of perfusion.

21.8.4 Viability Testing

In case of NMP, viability testing of the liver during can be assessed with a combination of parameters. First monitor the macroscopic homogeneity of the liver during perfusion to evaluate the quality of the liver. Secondly, monitor the flows during machine perfusion; an initial increase, and subsequent stabilization of the arterial and portal flows indicate stable hemodynamics of the liver. With blood gas analysis of the perfusion fluid,

oxygenation as well as the livers ability of CO_2 extraction can be analyzed. Another indicator for liver function is the quantitative bile production as well as the bile quality. A gradual darkening shade of the bile color should be observed over time. An increase of the total bilirubin and HCO_3 concentration represents and improvement of the produced bile.

Furthermore, stable concentration of hepatic injury markers in the perfusion fluid, such as alanine aminotransferase, potassium and alkaline phosphatase reflects minimal injury of the liver graft.

21.9 Future Perspectives

21.9.1 Ischemia Free Liver Transplantation

The perfect manner to overcome IRI and its disastrous effects is when ischemia could be prevented at all. However, up to now ischemia is an inevitable event of liver transplantation.

Reseachers in China recently developed a new technique of ischemia free organ transplantation [52]. He et al. reported the first case in which a severely steatotic (85–95% fat) liver graft was procured, preserved and implanted under continuous NMP. No ischemia occurred during the procedure. The recipient did not suffer post-reperfusion syndrome or vasoplegia after revascularization of the liver graft and no key pathways of IRI were activated. Liver function tests and histological study revealed minimal injury of the liver and the recipient recovered rapidly after transplantation. Ischemia free organ transplantation seems to be a promising feature in organ transplantation, but more experience and clinical studies are desired.

21.9.2 Extended Machine Perfusion

Like mentioned in Sect. 21.5.1, preservation of a human liver graft extending to 26 h (of which 8.5 h with NMP) with subsequent successful transplantation has been described [33]. Machine perfusion may enable more scheduled liver transplantations. This may provide additional time to further optimize the recipient's condition prior to transplantation. Secondly, the transplantation can be scheduled in daytime, which may theoretically result in a physically better-prepared surgical team. Machine perfusion also offers opportunities for recipients with an expected extended hepatectomy time, including those patients with a history of previous surgery and/or transplantation. Furthermore, if longer machine perfusion remains to be safe and feasible with a portable machine perfusion device longer distances could be bridged between donor and recipient in the future.

21.9.3 Stem Cells and Pharmacologicals

With the emerging experiences of NMP, a new platform for treatment of the liver grafts has emerged. Several techniques were tested in both animal and clinical studies. For example, additional targets, like antiviral medication for viral hepatitis, immune modulation for tolerance induction and gene therapy are under exploration [25].

Rigo et al. explored the feasibility of a pharmacological intervention during NMP by applying human liver stem cells-derived extracellular vesicles on isolated rat livers. At the end of NMP, human liver stem cells-derived extracellular vesicles were incorporated by hepatocytes and histological damage and apoptosis were significantly reduced. Treatment with human liver stem cells-derived extracellular vesicles appeared to be feasible and effectively reduced liver injury during hypoxic NMP [53].

21.10 Conclusions

Machine perfusion is an emerging innovation in liver transplantation that has made the transition to clinical trials. Over the past decade, with several research groups working on machine perfusion various techniques have been explored and implemented. Machine perfusion offers the ability to better preserve donor liver grafts while providing oxygen and nutrients, for reconditioning and optimization of liver grafts, and provides the possibility of liver function and viability testing. Finally, it may extend the duration of *ex-situ* organ storage. With an increasing demand for liver grafts worldwide, machine perfusion promises to be a beneficial alternative preservation method for liver grafts, especially those considered to be of suboptimal quality.

References

1. Carrel A, Lindbergh CA. The culture of whole organs. Science. 1935;81:621–3.
2. Belzer FO, Ashby BS, Gulyassy PF, Powell M. Successful seventeen-hour preservation and transplantation of human-cadaver kidney. N Engl J Med. 1968;278:608–10.
3. Starzl TE, Groth CG, Brettschneider L, Penn I, Fulginiti VA, Moon JB, et al. Orthotopic homotransplantation of the human liver. Ann Surg. 1968;168:392–415.
4. Belzer FO, Glass NR, Sollinger HW, Hoffmann RM, Southard JH. A new perfusate for kidney preservation. Transplantation. 1982;33:322–3.
5. Wertheim JA, Petrowsky H, Saab S, Kupiec-Weglinski JW, Busuttil RW. Major challenges limiting liver transplantation in the United States. Am J Transplant. 2011;11:1773–84.
6. Manyalich M, Nelson H, Delmonico FL. The need and opportunity for donation after circulatory death worldwide. Curr Opin Organ Transplant. 2018;23:136–41.
7. Jochmans I, van Rosmalen M, Pirenne J, Samuel U. Adult liver allocation in Eurotransplant transplantation. 2017;101:1542–1550.
8. van Golen RF, Reiniers MJ, Olthof PB, van Gulik TM, Heger M. Sterile inflammation in hepatic ischemia/reperfusion injury: present concepts and potential therapeutics. J Gastroenterol Hepatol. 2013;28:394–400.
9. de Vries Y, von Meijenfeldt FA, Porte RJ. Posttransplant cholangiopathy: classification, pathogenesis, and preventive strategies. Biochim Biophys Acta. 1864;2018:1507–15.
10. Dominguez-Gil B, Haase-Kromwijk B, Van Leiden H, Neuberger J, Coene L, Morel P, et al. Current situation of donation after circulatory death in European countries. Transpl Int. 2011;24:676–86.
11. Bartlett RH, Gazzaniga AB, Fong SW, Jefferies MR, Roohk HV, Haiduc N. Extracorporeal membrane oxygenator support for cardiopulmonary failure. Experience in 28 cases. J Thorac Cardiovasc Surg. 1977;73:375–86.

12. Fondevila C, Hessheimer AJ, Ruiz A, Calatayud D, Ferrer J, Charco R, et al. Liver transplant using donors after unexpected cardiac death: novel preservation protocol and acceptance criteria. Am J Transplant. 2007;7:1849–55.

13. Minambres E, Suberviola B, Dominguez-Gil B, Rodrigo E, Ruiz-San Millan JC, Rodriguez-San Juan JC, et al. Improving the outcomes of organs obtained from controlled donation after circulatory death donors using abdominal normothermic regional perfusion. Am J Transplant. 2017;17:2165–72.

14. Oniscu GC, Randle LV, Muiesan P, Butler AJ, Currie IS, Perera MT, et al. In situ normothermic regional perfusion for controlled donation after circulatory death-the United Kingdom experience. Am J Transplant. 2014;14:2846–54.

15. van Rijn R, Karimian N, Matton APM, Burlage LC, Westerkamp AC, van den Berg AP, et al. Dual hypothermic oxygenated machine perfusion in liver transplants donated after circulatory death. Br J Surg. 2017;104:907–17.

16. Karangwa SA, Dutkowski P, Fontes P, Friend PJ, Guarrera JV, Markmann JF, et al. Machine perfusion of donor livers for transplantation: a proposal for standardized nomenclature and reporting guidelines. Am J Transplant. 2016;16:2932–42.

17. Nasralla D, Coussios CC, Mergental H, Akhtar MZ, Butler AJ, Ceresa CDL, et al. A randomized trial of normothermic preservation in liver transplantation. Nature. 2018;557:50–6.

18. Guarrera JV, Henry SD, Samstein B, Odeh-Ramadan R, Kinkhabwala M, Goldstein MJ, et al. Hypothermic machine preservation in human liver transplantation: the first clinical series. Am J Transplant. 2010;10:372–81.

19. Dutkowski P, Polak WG, Muiesan P, Schlegel A, Verhoeven CJ, Scalera I, et al. First comparison of hypothermic oxygenated perfusion versus static cold storage of human donation after cardiac death liver transplants: an international-matched case analysis. Ann Surg. 2015;262:764–70.

20. Nishida S, Nakamura N, Kadono J, Komokata T, Sakata R, Madariaga JR, et al. Intrahepatic biliary strictures after liver transplantation. J Hepato-Biliary-Pancreat Surg. 2006;13:511–6.

21. Bruinsma BG, Avruch JH, Weeder PD, Sridharan GV, Uygun BE, Karimian NG, et al. Functional human liver preservation and recovery by means of subnormothermic machine perfusion. J Vis Exp. 2015. https://doi.org/10.3791/52777

22. Ravikumar R, Jassem W, Mergental H, Heaton N, Mirza D, Perera MT, et al. Liver transplantation after ex vivo normothermic machine preservation: a phase 1 (first-in-man) clinical trial. Am J Transplant. 2016;16:1779–87.

23. Selzner M, Goldaracena N, Echeverri J, Kaths JM, Linares I, Selzner N, et al. Normothermic ex vivo liver perfusion using steen solution as perfusate for human liver transplantation: first North American results. Liver Transpl. 2016;22:1501–8.

24. Bral M, Gala-Lopez B, Bigam D, Kneteman N, Malcolm A, Livingstone S, et al. Preliminary single-center Canadian experience of human normothermic ex vivo liver perfusion: results of a clinical trial. Am J Transplant. 2017;17:1071–80.

25. Detelich D, Markmann JF. The dawn of liver perfusion machines. Curr Opin Organ Transplant. 2018;23:151–61.

26. op den Dries S, Karimian N, Sutton ME, Westerkamp AC, Nijsten MW, Gouw AS, et al. Ex vivo normothermic machine perfusion and viability testing of discarded human donor livers. Am J Transplant. 2013;13:1327–35.

27. Perera T, Mergental H, Stephenson B, Roll GR, Cilliers H, Liang R, et al. First human liver transplantation using a marginal allograft resuscitated by normothermic machine perfusion. Liver Transpl. 2016;22:120–4.

28. Burlage LC, Karimian N, Westerkamp AC, Visser N, Matton APM, van Rijn R, et al. Oxygenated hypothermic machine perfusion after static cold storage improves endothelial function of extended criteria donor livers. HPB (Oxford). 2017;19:538–46.

29. Dutkowski P, Schlegel A, de Oliveira M, Mullhaupt B, Neff F, Clavien PA. HOPE for human liver grafts obtained from donors after cardiac death. J Hepatol. 2014;60:765–72.

30. Schlegel A, Dutkowski P. Role of hypothermic machine perfusion in liver transplantation. Transpl Int. 2015;28:677–89.

31. Karangwa SA, Aldemeijer J, Matton APM, Lisman JA, Porte RJ. Production of physiologically relevant quantities of hemostatic proteins during normothermic machine perfusion of human livers. Liver Transplant. 2018.

32. Liu Q, Nassar A, Buccini L, Grady P, Soliman B, Hassan A, et al. Ex situ 86-hour liver perfusion: pushing the boundary of organ preservation. Liver Transpl. 2018;24:557–61.

33. Watson CJ, Randle LV, Kosmoliaptsis V, Gibbs P, Allison M, Butler AJ. 26-hour storage of a declined liver before successful transplantation using ex vivo normothermic perfusion. Ann Surg. 2017;265:e1–2.

34. van Golen RF, van Gulik TM, Heger M. The sterile immune response during hepatic ischemia/reperfusion. Cytokine Growth Factor Rev. 2012;23:69–84.

35. Dubbeld J, Hoekstra H, Farid W, Ringers J, Porte RJ, Metselaar HJ, et al. Similar liver transplantation survival with selected cardiac death donors and brain death donors. Br J Surg. 2010;97:744–53.

36. van Rijn R, van Leeuwen OB, Matton APM, Burlage LC, Wiersema-Buist J, van den Heuvel MC, et al. Hypothermic oxygenated machine perfusion reduces bile duct reperfusion injury after transplantation of donation after circulatory death livers. Liver Transpl. 2018;24:655–64.

37. Schlegel A, Muller X, Dutkowski P. Hypothermic liver perfusion. Curr Opin Organ Transplant. 2017;22:563–70.

38. Chu MJ, Dare AJ, Phillips AR, Bartlett AS. Donor hepatic steatosis and outcome after liver transplantation: a systematic review. J Gastrointest Surg. 2015;19:1713–24.

39. Gehrau RC, Mas VR, Dumur CI, Suh JL, Sharma AK, Cathro HP, et al. Donor hepatic steatosis induce exacerbated ischemia-reperfusion injury through activation of innate immune response molecular pathways. Transplantation. 2015;99:2523–33.

40. Beijert I, Mert S, Huang V, Karimian N, Geerts S, Hafiz EOA, et al. Endothelial dysfunction in steatotic human donor livers: a pilot study of the underlying mechanism during subnormothermic machine perfusion. Transplant Direct. 2018;4:e345.

41. Kron P, Schlegel A, Mancina L, Clavien PA, Dutkowski P. Hypothermic oxygenated perfusion (HOPE) for fatty liver grafts in rats and humans. J Hepatol. 2017; https://doi.org/10.1016/j.jhep.2017.08.028.

42. Nativ NI, Yarmush G, So A, Barminko J, Maguire TJ, Schloss R, et al. Elevated sensitivity of macrosteatotic hepatocytes to hypoxia/reoxygenation stress is reversed by a novel defatting protocol. Liver Transpl. 2014;20:1000–11.

43. Watson CJE, Jochmans I. From "gut feeling" to objectivity: machine preservation of the liver as a tool to assess organ viability. Curr Transplant Rep. 2018;5:72–81.

44. 't Hart NA, der van Plaats A, Leuvenink HG, van Goor H, Wiersema-Buist J, Verkerke GJ, et al. Determination of an adequate perfusion pressure for continuous dual vessel hypothermic machine perfusion of the rat liver. Transpl Int. 2007;20:343–52.

45. Fondevila C, Hessheimer AJ, Maathuis MH, Munoz J, Taura P, Calatayud D, et al. Hypothermic oxygenated machine perfusion in porcine donation after circulatory determination of death liver transplant. Transplantation. 2012;94:22–9.

46. Hoyer DP, Mathe Z, Gallinat A, Canbay AC, Treckmann JW, Rauen U, et al. Controlled oxygenated rewarming of cold stored livers prior to transplantation: first clinical application of a new concept. Transplantation. 2016;100:147–52.

47. Banan B, Xiao Z, Watson R, Xu M, Jia J, Upadhya GA, et al. Novel strategy to decrease reperfusion injuries and improve function of cold-preserved livers using normothermic ex vivo liver perfusion machine. Liver Transpl. 2016;22:333–43.

48. Bae C, Pichardo EM, Huang H, Henry SD, Guarrera JV. The benefits of hypothermic machine perfusion are enhanced with Vasosol and alpha-tocopherol in rodent donation after cardiac death livers. Transplant Proc. 2014;46:1560–6.

49. Matton APM, Burlage LC, van Rijn R, de Vries Y, Karangwa SA, Nijsten MW, et al. Normothermic machine perfusion of donor livers without the need for human blood products. Liver Transpl. 2018;24:528–38.

50. Karimian N, Matton AP, Westerkamp AC, Burlage LC, Op den Dries S, Leuvenink HG, et al. Ex situ normothermic machine perfusion of donor livers. J Vis Exp. 2015. https://doi.org/10.3791/52688

51. Quintini C, Martins P, Shah S, Killackey M, Reed A, Guarrera J, et al. Implementing an innovated preservation technology: The American Society of Transplant Surgeons' (ASTS) standards committee white paper on ex-situ liver machine perfusion. Am J Transplant. 2018; https://doi.org/10.1111/ajt.14945.

52. He X, Guo Z, Zhao Q, Ju W, Wang D, Wu L, et al. The first case of ischemia-free organ transplantation in humans: a proof of concept. Am J Transplant. 2018;18:737–44.

53. Rigo F, De Stefano N, Navarro-Tableros V, David E, Rizza G, Catalano G, et al. Extracellular vesicles from human liver stem cells reduce injury in an ex vivo normothermic hypoxic rat liver perfusion model. Transplantation. 2018;102:e205–10.

Robotics in Transplantation

22

Kiara A. Tulla, Mario Spaggiari,
and Ivo G. Tzvetanov

22.1 Introduction

Minimally invasive surgery has change the landscape of surgical interventions to decrease surgical trauma and improve patient outcomes. It has the known benefits of minimizing locations for surgical site infections, hastening recovery time and improved cosmesis with smaller surgical scars [1]. In transplantation, the incorporation of laparoscopy, first initiated in 1995 [2] improved live donor participation in kidney transplantation, which provided a needed boost in organ availability and concurrently optimal patient outcomes [3]. However, complex procedures such as transplantation have been considered too technically demanding by conventional laparoscopy [4]. The turn of the century saw the introduction of robotics in transplantation with the first transabdominal hand-assisted robotic donor nephrectomy performed at the University of Illinois at Chicago in 2000 [5]. The da Vinci Surgical Robotics System (Intuitive Surgical, Sunnyvale, CA, USA) as the first, and currently only, U.S. Food and Drug Administration (FDA) approved robotics system in practice for live surgical interventions. It continues to provide a computer-assisted device to act as a surrogate manipulator for a surgeon to control small ports and instruments to perform surgical interventions. Some of its advantages are proficient micro-suturing through laparoscopic ports, three-dimensional (3D) high-definition view, and instruments with wrist articulations [6]. Although, the high cost and lack of haptic feedback [7] currently serve as the greatest deterrents of the technology, its ability to provide care to transplant patients who may not receive transplantation because of the risk of surgery on ill obese patients. Thus, this platform can serve to provide equity in transplantation, for the every growing obese diabetic, end stage liver and kidney disease patients. Currently, the greatest application of robotics in transplantation has been in robotic donor nephrectomies and robotic kidney transplantation and to a lesser degree pancreas transplantation and donor hepatectomies for living donor liver transplantation. Here we shed light on the history and progress this technology has provided the transplant community.

22.2 Robotic Hand-Assisted Living Donor Nephrectomy

Living donor kidney transplantation has many known advantages and is the best available treatment for patients with end-stage renal disease (ESRD) [8]. They present with higher quality renal grafts, shorter ischemia time, and the

K. A. Tulla · M. Spaggiari · I. G. Tzvetanov (✉)
Department of Surgery, Division of Transplantation,
University of Illinois at Chicago, Chicago, IL, USA
e-mail: Ktulla@uic.edu; Mspaggia@uic.edu;
itzveta@uic.edu

© Springer Nature Switzerland AG 2021
N. Hakim et al. (eds.), *Transplantation Surgery*, Springer Specialist Surgery Series,
https://doi.org/10.1007/978-3-030-55244-2_22

elective nature of the operation allow for improved patient outcomes. The possibility to provide pre-emptive transplantation before a patient is subject to dialysis has improvement on patient and graft survival [9, 10], but also on patient quality of life [11]. However, these advantages must be balanced in concert with the proper management of patient safety. Donors are healthy individuals exposed to the inherent risk of a surgical intervention without a direct personal benefit.

The introduction of minimally invasive surgery for donor nephrectomies in the mid-1990s was key to boosting the living donation rates [12]. While the open approach with a mini-subcostal incision for live donor nephrectomy reduced morbidity compared to historic controls [13], laparoscopic technique grew as the standard procedure being of its associated improvements in patient recovery [14, 15]. At the same time, that centers with hundreds of laparoscopic donor nephrectomies have been performed since 2000 (Table 22.1), the da Vinci Surgical System has been used in living donor nephrectomies as a logical extension of the widely adapted minimal invasive approach [16] at a more cautious pace. After acquiring experience with robotics in other surgical procedures, the first worldwide transabdominal, hand-assisted robotic donor nephrectomy was performed successfully at the University of Illinois at Chicago in 2000 [5]. Since then, this institution has performed over 1000 robotic donor nephrectomies with excellent outcomes [17].

Table 22.1 Review of current literature of studies conducted in laparoscopic vs robotic donor nephrectomies

Author et al.	Dates	No. of cases
Laparoscopic donor nephrectomies (300+ patients)		
Cooper et al.	1996–2005	1000 Lap
Nogueira et al.	1996–2005	946 Lap
Simforoosh et al.	1997–2011	1510 Lap
Mjoen et al.	1997–2008	244 Lap vs 778 Open
Leventhal et al.	1997–2008	1200 Lap
Carter et al.	1999–2003	361 Lap
Hadijanastassiou et al.	2000–2006	601 Lap vs 1800 Open
Srivastata et al.	2001–2006	380 Lap vs 1000 Open
Kohei et al.	2001–2009	425 Lap (retroperitoneal)
Su et al.	2004	381 Lap
Rajab et al.	1999–2014	1500 Lap
Robotic donor nephrectomies		
Renoult et al.	2002–2004	13 Robotic vs 13 Open
Hubert et al.	2007	38 Robotic
Liu et al.	2012	5 Robotic
Giacomoni et al.	2009–2013	33 Robotic
Bhattu et al.	2014–2015	16 Robotic vs 30 Lap
Horgan (at UIC) et al.	2000–2007	214 Robotic
UIC (unpublished data)	2000–2017	>1000 Robotic

Lap laparoscopic, *UIC* University of Illinois at Chicago

22.2.1 Preoperative Donor Evaluation

The evaluation of potential kidney donors for robotic assisted live kidney donation, does not defer from the accepted guidelines [18]. A multidisciplinary transplant team performs this evaluation of a patient undergoing medium-risk surgery with special attention to characteristics such as medical status, current renal function, comorbidities that can increase the donor's chances of developing renal failure themselves (i.e. diabe-

tes mellitus that is poorly controlled, kidney stones, etc.), and cardiopulmonary health is thoroughly evaluated. Since some individuals donate in their fifties and sixties, if there are points of concern a complete medical work is conducted prior to disallowing donation [19]. Of note, obese donors are not always accepted at many centers, however, out our center patients who are healthy regardless of body mass index (BMI) or prior surgical procedures are considered adequate for donation for a technical perspective. Donors who are obese are encouraged to lose weight prior to date of donation (during evaluation process) as a way to minimize the risks of donation and provided lifestyle education to help improve their health prior to and after donation.

The donor is admitted from home for this operation. Pre-operative instructions include optimization of fluid status the day prior to surgery to maintain optimal renal function. Similarly, intravenous fluids are initiation as soon as the patient is admitted in the pre-procedure area.

22.2.2 Surgical Technique: Left Donor Nephrectomy

After patient is intubated, the donor is positioned either, in right lateral decubitus position for a left nephrectomy or left lateral decubitus position for a right nephrectomy cushioned on a beanbag with axillary roll prior to incision. The patient is adequately fixed to the operative table to prevent instability of the robotic system upon docking and ensuring the donor's safety during the procedure.

Robot-assisted donor nephrectomy is a transabdominal procedure performed with four ports and one 7-cm Pfannenstiel incision for hand assistance and removal of the graft (Fig. 22.1).

A 12-mm laparoscopic port is placed above the umbilicus, close to the midline, at the level of renal hilum. This port is required for the 30-degree robotic camera system. The left mid-clavicular line is appropriate to place the two 8-mm robotic

working ports to achieve good triangulations. They are located proximal and distal, 10–12 cm apart from the camera port. The left lower quadrant is the preferred location to place the last 12-mm port, which is used by the assist to introduce the stapler and provide suction assistance. The patient is placed in Trendelenburg with a minor jack-knife of the table. The robotic system is docked and integrated to the ports, and pneumoperitoneum is achieved with CO_2 to 10 mmHg pressure. The operating surgeon, once the field is prepared, positions him or herself at the robotic console while the bedside surgeon assistant places a hand into the abdomen through the lower abdominal incision (Fig. 22.2).

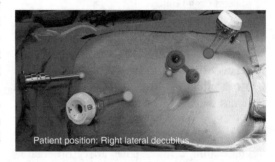

Patient position: Right lateral decubitus

Fig. 22.1 Robotic-Assisted Donor Nephrectomy Port Placement for a Left Nephrectomy: Patient is positioned in the right lateral decubitus position with the head of the patient to the left of the image. Green ports depict robotic arms and camera port. Blue port is assistant port with blue incision depicting assistant hand port

Fig. 22.2 Robotic-Assisted Donor Nephrectomy surgical positioning: At the head of the bed sit the anesthesiologist. The robot is docked on the left side of the bed and anchored to the patient at the appropriate port sites. The lead surgeon is controlling the robot from the console. The assistant surgeon is placed on the right side of the patient near the foot of the bed, with the scrub nurse and surgical table on the right side of the patient

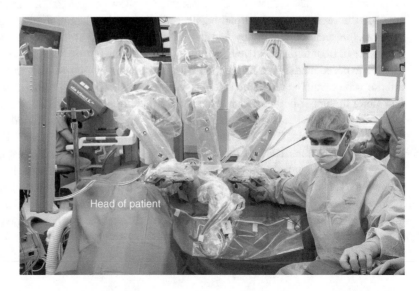

Head of patient

Intra-abdominal dissection begins with the mobilization of the descending and the sigmoid colon. The splenocolic ligament is also partially transected. Once the peritoneum is scored with the electrocautery, the fat plane between the mesentery of the left colon and Gerota's fascia are separated in an atraumatic fashion. This allows bloodless exposure of the anterior surface of the left kidney even in cases with significant intra-abdominal adiposity. To facilitated exposure of the left kidney, occasionally the lower pole of the spleen is freed from its posterior attachments (transect the splenocolic ligament) and the spleen is further mobilized cranially. Furthermore, decreasing tidal volumes may be needed during this phase to restrict movements of the diaphragm to prevent organ injury.

The ureter is identified at the pelvic brim circumferentially dissected along with the gonadal vein using a combination of sharp instrument and finger dissection. As the most distal portion of the ureter is mobilized, care is taken to preserve a generous amount of fat and blood supply to the organ. Once complete, the ureter/gonadal complex is followed superiorly. During this portion of the dissection, a lower polar artery originating from distal abdominal aorta should be identified to prevent unintentional injury of this vessel, which would deprive the ureter sufficient blood supply.

Following the gonadal vein in a proximal direction the operator identifies the renal vein between the retroperitoneal fat pad between the lower medial pole of the kidney and the ureter. The tissue in front of the renal vein is divided and the vein exposed medially to its junction with the inferior vena cava. The left adrenal vein is identified along the upper border of the renal vein. In most of the cases, at least one lumbar vein will join the left renal vein. Precision and care during the isolation and transaction of these veins is of most importance in order to prevent undo harm to the donor. The degrees of freedom the robotic system and instruments provide as well as the 3D vision provide the tools for improved dissection and care compared to conventional laparoscopic instruments. All the veins contributing to the left renal vein are clipped and transected to allow for further skeletonization of the renal vein.

Gerota's fascia is incised superiorly and the adrenal gland is identified and left intact. If a sizable upper polar artery is present, extra care should be taken to preserve this vessel since it could supply 20–30% of the kidney mass. The upper pole of the kidney is then fully mobilized. The assisting surgeon's hand helps to divide the posterior areolar attachments of the kidney bluntly. At this point, the ureter is clipped with two robotic hem-o-lock clips (as distal as possible) and sharply transected right proximal to the clips.

Left renal artery is circumferentially dissected to its origin from the aorta. If multiple arteries are present, every vessel has to be dissected free and followed to their take off from the aorta. When this step is finished, the kidney is only attached by the renal artery and vein.

Before vascular transection, 5000 units of heparin are given intravenously to prevents microcirculatory thrombosis of the graft after arterial transaction. Some surgeons also give a 1 L of fluid bolus, followed by 40 mg of Lasix and 50 g of Mannitol prior to vascular separation, but this practice varies by center.

After 2–3 min, the assistant surgeon beings by advancing the Endo TA stapler through the 12-mm left lower quadrant port with vascular staple load. The utilization of Endo TA stapler allows additional length of the artery that facilitates implantation of the graft. The renal artery is stapled at its origin from the aorta. Recently, the newer da Vinci Xi robot has integrated staplers, which allows the operating surgeon to position and fire the staplers from the console (Fig. 22.3a). Once the staples are in place, the artery is sharply divided with robotic scissors at least 3–4 mm distal from the stapler line (Fig. 22.3b). Subsequently, the renal vein is divided in a similar fashion by the assistant with an Endo GIA vascular stapler (Fig. 22.3c). Immediately after arterial transection, 50 mg of Protamine is given intravenously to reverse the systemic effect of heparin (1 mg Protamine per 100 units of heparin).

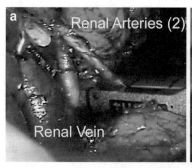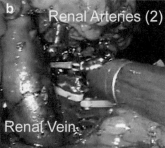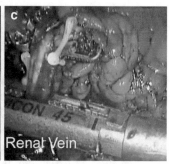

Fig. 22.3 Renal graft vasculature skeletonization. Both the renal arteries (**a**) and veins are exposed. The renal arteries are traversed with endo TA stapler loads and hem- o-lock clips. The renal are then sharply transected with the robotic scissors (**b**). The renal vein is then stapled and divided with an Endo GIA vascular stapler (**c**)

The cavity must be inspected for bleeding once the kidney graft is removed. The arterial and venous stumps are visualized, and the condition of the staple line verified. The renal bed should be inspected for the presence of chylous and lymphatic leak that is addressed with suture ligation if necessary with the robotic platform. At the end of the procedure, the 7 cm incision is closed in layers with fascial closed with 0 PDS and loose approximation of the muscle fibers with 0 Vicryl suture. The two 12-mm port sites are closed with an endo-closure device and 0 Vicryl suture. Skin is closed in the usual fashion.

If the right kidney is to be harvested, the procedure is efficiently performed with the robotic system in contralateral fashion from the one described.

ischemia time with robotic procurement of the grafts is shorter and multiple arteries do not affect the patient outcomes as was once reported in laparoscopy [21]. As a single center, the University of Illinois at Chicago has completed greater than 1000 donor nephrectomies with comparable major complications (using Clavien-Dindo Classification of IIIb or greater [22]) rates to the published values noted in the laparoscopic literature (0.2–7.1%) [23–28]. The procedure has proved to be safe and efficacious even in complex cases of vascular anomalies or obese donors [21]. Although, the adoption of this technique had been limited, it equitable to laparoscopy and can serve as a way for a center to being robotic transplantation and gain experience before performing robotic kidney transplantation.

22.3   Discussion

Minimally invasive donor nephrectomies have revolutionized the volume of live donors and allowed for more patients to obtain the survival benefit of transplantation and fewer years on dialysis. Difficulty with anatomic variations have caused past difficulties with live donation. Over time, the hurdles that affected the utilization of live donation such as vascular compromise due to shorter arterial conduits, ureteral complications due to compromising blood supply and multiple arteries or veins increasing the complexity of the renal transplant and increasing warm ischemia time [20]. Different from laparoscopy, warm

22.4   Robotic-Assisted Kidney Transplantation

The first utilization of the robot in kidney transplantation was performed in France in 2001 [29] however the technique did not use ports, but rather assessed the ability of the robot to perform the surgical sequence. In the late 2000s, after robotic surgery was routinely performed at the University of Illinois at Chicago, the first fully robotic transabdominal kidney transplant was completed in 2009; Giulianotti et al. published a total operative time was 223 min, with warm ischemia time of 50 min [30]. Subsequently, Boggi et al. published their first successful European experience in 2011

[31]. Even if the approach slightly differed from ours, the operative time was 154 min, with 51 min of warm ischemia. Variations in technique were attempted by Doumerc et al. in 2015 [32] where the graft was introduced via a transvaginal approach with a mean operative time was 200 min and warm ischemia time was 55 min. Later, in 2015, the same authors described the first pure robot-assisted approach to living donor kidney transplantation utilizing the transvaginal technique for both donor and recipient surgeries [33]. Despite the encouraging results and pioneering improvements, this technique continues to be cautiously utilized [34].

With the cosmetic promise of the procedure, the technique was utilized in Europe due to increase in patient satisfaction. A collaboration with eight European institutions showed that the RKT could achieve minimal delayed graft function (DGF 4.2%) and wound infections (0.8%), with excellent graft outcomes among the patients selected [35]. However, the approach, at our institution, was initiated to address the detrimental effects wound infections had on graft outcomes [36]. As a reflection of the growing incidence of obesity among the general population, the prevalence of high BMI reached 30–40% among patients on renal replacement therapy [37]. The majority of transplant centers consider BMI $\geq$40 kg/m^2 a contraindication for transplant, and very few centers transplant candidates with BMI above 35 kg/m^2. Oberholzer et al. from our presented a cohort study comparing morbidly obese robotic kidney recipients to the open approach with results showing the advantages and feasibility of the robotic-assisted procedure [34]. This approach gave the opportunity for transplantation to candidates previously rejected due to obesity. Until now our group performed 212 RKT for obese recipients. The robotic system allows minimizing the incision and changing the anatomical location to the upper abdomen, away from contaminated groin area. Applying this technique, we were able to almost completely eradicate the surgical site infection in this high-risk patient population [38] while also providing them a needed survival benefit from restoration of kidney function [39].

All candidates for kidney transplantation undergo a standardized evaluation by multidisciplinary team. These guidelines are currently followed by all transplant centers. Patients are considered for robotic kidney transplantation if they are adults (>18 years old) and have a BMI $\geq$ 30 kg/m^2 at the time of listing (inclusion criteria at our center). We consider significant peripheral vascular disease as a contraindication for the minimally invasive approach.

22.4.1 Surgical Technique: Right-sided Robotic Kidney Transplant

Due to robotic surgery requiring extreme Trendelenburg positioning, with fluid volume redistribution toward the head, in combination with relatively high pneumoperitoneum, especially in obese recipients, ventilation can be seriously affected. Thus, skilled collaboration with the anesthesia, medical and surgical team is of paramount importance to safely complete this high-profile procedure.

After successful intubation and routine perioperative procedures are conduction (immunosuppression administered as needed), the patient is secured in the supine position with both arms tucked. To achieve stable position of the patient to the table, shoulder blocks, large beanbags, and where necessary, silk tape over towels is utilized to provide security on the table with avoidance of pressure points.

After prepping and draping the abdomen, the initial 7-cm upper midline incision, approximately 3–4 cm below the xyphoid process with a GelPort (Applied Medical, Rancho Santa Margarita, CA) device insert. For implantation of the graft to the right external iliac vessels, laparoscopic ports are positioned in the following manner: one 12-mm port for the 30-degree robotic scope is inserted to the right of the umbilicus; two 7-mm robotic ports are inserted, one is placed in the right flank and the other one in the left lower quadrant; 12-mm assistant port is placed on the left side of the umbilicus between the camera and the left lower quadrant robotic port (Fig. 22.4).

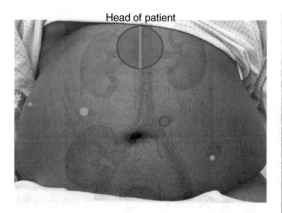

Fig. 22.4 Robotic-Assisted Kidney Transplant Port Placement for a Right-sided Transplant: The patient is positioned supine with head of the patient above the GelPort depicted in the image. Green ports depict robotic arms and camera port. Blue port is assistant port with blue gel port for hand assistance as needed. The target is to triangulate the ports in such a way to have proper visualization of the right iliac fossa, safely dissect, clamp and anastomose the renal artery and vein to the right external iliac vessels when possible. The anatomical location of the arterial and venous supply to the kidney once transplanted is depicted in the image

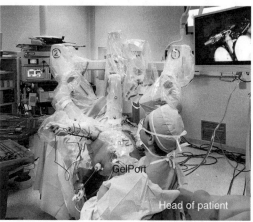

Fig. 22.5 Robotic-Assisted Kidney Transplant surgical positioning: The assistant surgeon positions himself to left side of the patient near the head of the bed. The robot is docked on the right side of the bed. The lead surgeon is controlling the robot from the console. The scrub nurse and surgical table on the left side of the patient

The patient is placed in 30-degree Trendelenburg position with the right-side table up to facilitated gravitational movement of the small bowel and colon away from the right iliac fossa (for implantation to the right external iliac vessels). The robot is docked at the patient's right flank (over anterior superior iliac spine), parallel and slightly diagonal to the recipient body positioning pneumoperitoneum is achieved with CO_2 to 10–12 mmHg pressure. The assisting surgeon is seated on the left site of the operating table, and next to the patient's head (which is covered entirely by the drape). Extra caution is taken to avoid interference with the robotic arms controlled by the surgeon and the endotracheal tube. Vascular suturing can present technical difficulties if appropriate triangulation of the arms and patient positioning is not achieved and maintained by the bedside surgeon (Fig. 22.5).

The cecum is mobilized off the iliac fossa to assist in exposing the right external iliac artery and vein. Importantly, if there is concern for patchy calcifications, manual assessment of the artery by the bedside surgeon is completed to avoid clamp injury and arterial dissection. Two

robotic bulldog clamps are used to clamp the external iliac vein first.

At this point, the kidney graft is introduced into the abdominal cavity by the beside surgeon and oriented to allow for both vascular anastomoses to be completed. We do not perform regional hypothermia as has been described in the past [40, 41], and have found that efficiency with the vascular anastomosis (average warm ischemia time of 40–50 min) maintains excellent patient outcomes.

To begin, the veno-venous anastomosis is performed in an end-to-side fashion with a running a 12-cm double-needle 6-0 Gore-Tex suture with a knot in the middle. Next, the external iliac artery is clamped between robotic bulldogs, and an oval-shaped window is made in the anterior wall of the artery with the use of robotic scissors. The arterial anastomosis is completed in an end-to-side fashion in a running fashion. The knots sutures are anchored avoid complications of the suture slipping, maintaining too much slack, or having the knot fall out. Of note, the needle on this suture is smaller and more malleable, so using fine robotic needled holders in both arms and visual feedback of vital to maintain the curve of the needle intact. The ease of fine vascular suturing allowed by the high-definition 3D vision and wrist-like articulation of the robotic system instruments are the most important advantages for this procedure, which hasten and reduce warm ischemia time. Upon completion of arterial anastomosis, 100 mg of Lasix and 1 g/kg body weight of Mannitol is given intravenously. In some cases, fluid bolus may be required.

After the vascular anastomoses are complete, the clamps on the vein are removed first followed by removal of the arterial clamps. The reperfusion of the organ and hemostasis are visualized. Bleeding points are addressed with single-arm 6-0 Prolene sutures. At this point, the pressure of the pneumoperitoneum is also reduced to ~8 mmHg to minimize possible negative effect of high intraabdominal pressure on graft perfusion and reduce the risk of delayed graft function. Good retraction by the assistant and tenting of the field by the camera port lifting the peritoneal cavity maintains a sufficient visual field. This maneuver also allows for better evaluation to achieve hemostasis due to venous bleeding, which could be obscured by high intraabdominal pressure. Vascular reperfusion is the most critical part of robotic transplantation, since significant vascular and parenchymal bleeding is difficult to control when compared to the open approach. Adequate resuscitation and attention by the anesthesiology team with appropriate resuscitation is of extreme importance.

Adequate reperfusion is verified by a Doppler exam. We routinely introduce 3 mL of systemic indocyanine green (ICG) solution (2.5 mg/mL)

and after one minute utilize the robotic fluorescein camera to evaluated parenchymal perfusion. This gives the providers an excellent opportunity to observe and document the distribution of the dye into the graft as a surrogate for anastomotic patency.

Attention is now turned to the ureteral anastomosis. Diluted methylene blue solution is introduced into the bladder to facilitate localization. The ureter is anastomosed to the bladder with a running 5–0 Monocryl suture. The typical antireflux technique—suturing full thickness of the ureteral wall with the mucosal layer of the bladder—is used. The placement of ureteral stent is optional (surgeon discretion) (Fig. 22.6).

At the end of the procedure, the minilaparotomy is closed with running 0 PDS, and the two 12-mm port sites are closed with an endoclosure device and 0 Vicryl suture. Skin is closed in the usual fashion.

If the kidney is placed in the left iliac fossa, the procedure is efficiently performed with the robotic system in contralateral fashion from the one described.

22.5 Discussion

The initial experiences shared by centers around the world, applying robotics to transplantation, have demonstrated lower surgical complication rates for when kidneys are implanted robotically

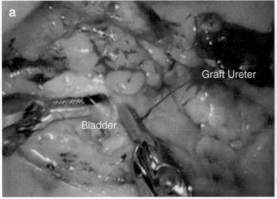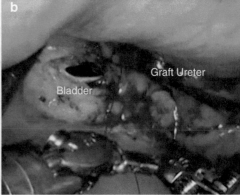

Fig. 22.6 Ureteral anastomosis: The bladder is identified after being filled with methylene blue. Once the bladder is opened with the use of robotic bipolar and robotic scissors the mucosa is identified and 5-0 Monocryl is used to suture (with two needle drivers) the heel of the donor ureter to the lateral opening of the bladder anastomosis (**a** and **b**)

in comparison to similar open transplant cohorts [42, 43]. The technique is efficient and safe, and in our experience provides a way to improve access to transplantation for obese patients denied this life saving procedure at other centers.

Since 2009, the University of Illinois had completed more than 200 robotic-assisted kidney transplants in obese recipients. BMI >30 kg/m^2 has been our only selection criterion, without an upper limit. The mean BMI of the group of patients being 42 kg/m^2, ranging from 28–61 kg/m^2. We reported our early experience in a case-control study [34], where the first 28 robot-assisted kidney transplants were compared to a frequency-matched retrospective cohort of obese recipients who underwent kidney transplantation in the traditional open technique. At 48 months of follow-up, the GFR was 51.5 ± 30.7 ml/min/1.73 m^2 in the robotic group and 51.9 ± 21.8 ml/min/1.73 m^2 in the control group (p = 0.83). The rate of surgical site infections (SSI) was significantly higher in the control group compared with the robotic group (28.6 vs. 0 percent, p = 0.004). At 4 years post-transplant, eight patients in the control group (28.6 percent) experienced graft loss compared with five patients in the robotic group (17.9 percent). Three (37.5 percent) of eight patients who lost the graft in the control group had concomitant SSI. The patient survival at 48 months was 92.5 percent in the robotic group and 92.4 percent in the control group (p = 0.97). Patients transplanted with minimally invasive approach achieved early mobilization, high patient satisfaction, and an excellent long-term graft function were observed.

Our group conducted a study in which the UNOS registry [44] was reviewed for adult living donor kidney transplant recipients with BMI ≥40 kg/m^2 from September 2009 to December 2014. We compared outcomes in RKT versus standard open kidney transplantation at all US centers. Similar patient and graft survival were reported. Renal function, determined by creatinine levels and GFR, was also similar in both groups.

The safety and effectiveness of RKT has only been achieved with the collaboration and experi-ence of the different specialty teams during the entire process of transplantation. By providing excellent kidney graft function and minimizing surgical complications, this surgical technique gives the opportunity to a disadvantaged group of obese patients with ESRD to have improved access to transplantation. Surgeons attempting this procedure require the full armamentarium of robotic surgery skills, including advanced vascular suture techniques.

22.6 Robotic-Assisted Pancreas Transplantation

Despite the advantages in surgical intervention to achieve sustained euglycemia for diabetes mellitus patients, pancreas transplantation has historically had the greatest rate of surgical complications among solid organ transplantation, deterring the utilization of the procedure [45]. As the transplant technique has been mastered, the immunosuppression protocols improved and now the standardization of what is graft survival universalized, the landscape of pancreas transplantation is finally seeing its first increase in recipients in nearly a decade [46]. Type 2 Diabetics are now transplanted more frequently (11.7% in 2016 from 10.5% in 2015) and simultaneous pancreas-kidney transplants account for 76% of all pancreas transplant completed in 2016. However, this is in spite of the dilemma posed by transplanting pancreas transplant candidates who fit the type 2 diabetes mellitus phenotype with metabolic syndrome [47]. These patients in the past, along with obese type 1 diabetics, were frequently denied access because of the increase risk of surgical complications associated with recipient obesity [48–51]. To date, more boundaries in this arena are being challenged to serve the growing obese patient population.

First use of robotics in pancreas transplantation began with robotic in live donor pancreatectomies when live donation was incorporated to boost pancreas transplantation. Horgan et al. [52] reported the first robotic hand-assisted simultaneous nephrectomy and distal pancreatectomy in a living donor. This utilized the robotic system performed the splenic artery and vein isolation down to the celiac trunk and portal vein and division close to the splenic hilum. This early experience would be diverted when live donor pancreatectomies were minimally employed. However, the increased risk of complications such as donor pancreatitis, leaks, and diabetes decreased its utility [53].

After a hiatus, the first robotic pancreas transplants were reported by Boggi et al. [54] using the da Vinci Surgical System. Three transplants—one pancreas alone, one pancreas after kidney, and one simultaneous kidney and pancreas—were performed during this endeavor. The mean warm and cold ischemia times were 30 min and 7.3 h, respectively. Successful robotic control of graft hemorrhage with no need for blood transfusion in one recipient helped prove the platforms feasibility. The introduction of robotics to reduce post-transplant morbidity in these patients would be favorable to boost the recovery of pancreas transplantation nationwide and promote transplantation even in obese candidates. Acquisition of more experience in the future will show whether the application of robotic technique for minimally invasive pancreas transplantation could significantly decrease abdominal wall complications.

All candidates for pancreas transplantation undergo a standardized evaluation by multidisciplinary team. These guidelines are currently followed by all transplant centers with new criteria where patients qualify for transplantation if they have a C-peptide of <2.0 ng/mL or if they have a C-peptide>2.0 ng/mL needed to have a BMI < 30 kg/m^2 (with the BMI cutoff under review by UNOS). Like for our patient who are considered for robotic kidney transplantation, they must be adults who are obese with minimal to no peripheral vascular disease.

22.6.1 Surgical Technique: Left-Sided Robotic Pancreas Transplant

The patient is placed in the supine position to the table on a bean bag and with shoulder supports in the lithotomy position. The knees are lowered to

be in line with abdomen. After prepping and draping the abdomen, a 7-cm midline incision is made 2–3 cm below the xyphoid process and a GelPort (Applied Medical, Rancho Santa Margarita, CA) device is inserted. Once the pneumoperitoneum is achieved, four ports are positioned in the following manner: (1) one 12-mm port is placed supra-umbilical port for the camera, (2) two 8-mm robotic ports are placed one along the left pararectal line some 5 cm below the costal margin and one in the right lower quadrant in the midclavicular line, and (3) one 12-mm assistant port in the right pararectal line around 5 cm below the costal margin (Fig. 22.7). The da Vinci system is placed to the patient's right side. Both right sided robotic and assistant ports are placed in these varied locations from our prior publications [55] because it allows for a simultaneous pancreas-kidney procedure to be completed with 5 ports and 1 hand port.

The patient is placed in 30-degree Trendelenburg position with the left-side table up to facilitated gravitational movement of the small bowel and colon away from the left iliac fossa (for implantation to the left external iliac ves-

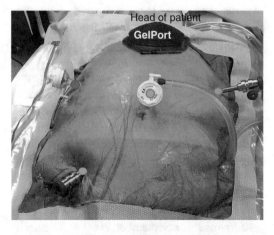

Fig. 22.7 Robotic-Assisted Pancreas Transplant Port Placement for a Left-sided Transplant: The patient is positioned supine with head of the patient superior to the location of the supra-umbilical GelPort. Green ports depict robotic arms and camera port (periumbilical port). Blue port is assistant port with GelPort for hand assistance as needed. The target is to triangulate the ports in such a way to have proper visualization of the left iliac fossa, and to safely dissect, clamp and anastomose the pancreatic arterial and venous inflows as well as pancreatic drainage

sels). The pneumoperitoneum is maintained with CO_2 pressure of 10–12 mmHg. The assisting surgeon is seated on the right-side at the head of the table (which is covered entirely by the drape) (Fig. 22.8).

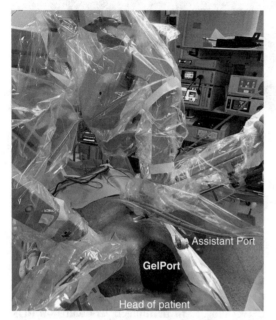

Fig. 22.8 Robotic-Assisted Pancreas Transplant surgical positioning: The assistant surgeon positions himself to right side of the patient near the head of the bed. The robot is docked on the left side of the bed. The lead surgeon is controlling the robot from the console. The scrub nurse and surgical table on the right side of the patient

After mobilization of the descending and sigmoid colon, the retroperitoneum is exposed to identify the common iliac artery and vein. To perform the vascular anastomosis, the iliac artery and vein are encircled (Fig. 22.9a). Due to the inferior-posterior location of the iliac vein, it is cross clamped first. The graft is then introduced into the abdomen with the pancreas head down into the pelvis with the duodenum of the graft facing the bladder. The venous anastomosis is completed in and end-to-side fashion with 6-0 Gore-Tex suture with a knot in the middle. Subsequently, the iliac artery is cross clamped is cross-clamped, and the donor Y arterial conduit (between the donor splenic and superior mesenteric artery) is anastomosed in an end-to-side fashion as well (Fig. 22.9b).

Before vascular reperfusion of the graft, the anesthesia team is warned. Occasionally, significant bleeding can occur during this phase. To reduce the risk of uncontrollable hemorrhage, the back-bench preparation of the donor pancreas is of utmost importance. All dissection that is completed during the cold-phase of procurement with sharp dissection should be suture ligated or tied to prevent reperfusion bleeding. To facilitate the identification of points of bleeding, at the end of the back-bench preparation, custodial solution with methylene blue is infused via the Y arterial conduit. First area to be evaluated is the port vein

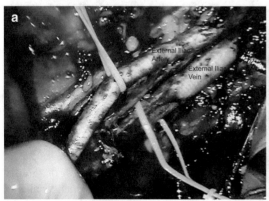
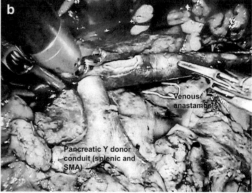

Fig. 22.9 Vascular anastomosis for left-sided pancreas transplant. (**a**) After entering the retroperitoneum of the left iliac fossa, the external iliac artery and vein are encircled with vessel loops. The vein is inferior and posterior to the artery. (**b**) After the venous anastomosis is completed with Gortex suture, the external iliac artery is clamped with robotic bull dogs and the artery is opened with robotic scissors and the Y donor arterial conduit is tailored to allow for adequate blood flow, but limit length which would allow for potential vascular kinking or torsion

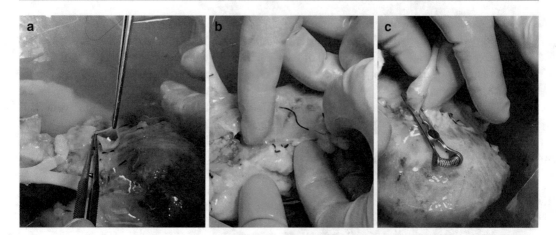

Fig. 22.10 Back bench preparation of pancreas graft for robotic implantation. At the end of the preparation, the graft is infused with custodial solution dyed with methylene blue through the arterial conduit. (**a**) The portal vein is visualized to ensure no defects are noted inside or around the vessel. Subsequently, the parenchyma, especially around the duodenum (**b**) is evaluated for dye leakage, blotting with gauze. Finally, the arterial conduit is evaluated for patency (**c**)

(Fig. 22.10a) to ensure there are no vascular wall defects. Then, attention is turned to the parenchyma and then subsequently to the conduit anastomoses (Fig. 22.10b–c). This sequence, ensures all potential point of bleeding are sutured prior to organ reperfusion. One the organ is re-perfused, clotting agents are placed with some pressure around the graft to control any low flow bleeding. At the same time that hemorrhage is of concern during reperfusion, the release of a large quantities of insulin from the organ implantation can cause severe hypoglycemia, which in combination with blood loss and pneumoperitoneum could lead to hypotension and shock. Therefore, the blood sugar is monitored but minimally treated prior to implantation and reperfusion and upon finishing the anastomosis the glucose is verified and the pneumoperitoneum is reduced (like is advised during the introduction of kidney grafts in robotic assisted kidney transplants).

After the arterial and venous anastomoses are evaluated thoroughly, attention is turned to the exocrine drainage of the pancreas. It is important to find a loop of bowel, preferably early jejunum, that easily reaches the graft duodenum. To achieve a successful enteric drainage, a Roux-en-Y duodenojejunostomy is performed in one of three ways: (1) an end to end EEA stapler anastomosis is achieved (via anvil in the jejunum and stapler fired through the donor duodenum), (2) a hand sewn side to side duodenojejunal anastomosis or (3) a sided to side stapler anastomosis achieved suing a endo GIA stapler to unite a duodenojejunal anastomosis with a hand sewn small defect closure in multiple layers with 4-0 PDS used for the mucosal anastomosis and prolene or vicryl utilized for the external layers (to over sewn). If no small bowel loop reaches to pelvis easily, a duodenocystostomy can be completed via stapler anastomosis (anvil in the bladder).

Doppler exam and systemic ICG (7.5 mg, 3 mL) evaluated via robotic fluorescein camera are concurrently used to evaluate parenchymal perfusion. After all the anastomoses are evaluated for a final time, the robot is undocked, and ports closed. The fascia is closed in the 7 cm GelPort and 12 mm laparoscopic ports in the same fashion as they are described for the robotic kidney transplant.

In the simultaneous pancreas–kidney transplant, the kidney is transplanted in the right iliac fossa, according to the technique previously described for RKT. The port placement is altered slight, such that the assistant port for the pancreas transplant, serves as one of the robotic arms for the kidney transplant and vis-a-versa when possible to utilized only 5 ports (3× 12 mm ports; 2× 8 mm ports) (Fig. 22.11).

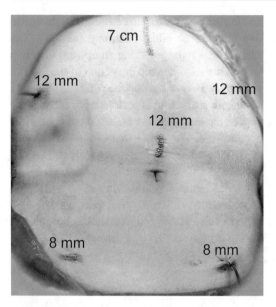

Fig. 22.11 Robotic Simultaneous Pancreas-Kidney Transplant post-transplant scars. The patient received an SPK and the ports that were utilized were 5 total, utilizing the same ports for both parts of the procedure when able. The 7 cm gel port was cranial and the 2× 8 mm ports were caudal on the patient's abdomen

22.7 Discussion

This initial experience showed the safety and feasibility of robotic surgery applied to pancreas transplantation. The graft function observed during follow-up was compatible to standard open pancreas transplants.

After the United Network for Organ Sharing modified its allocation criteria in 2014, where patients with a C-peptide>2.0 ng/mL needed to have a BMI < 28 kg/m² (subsequently increased to BMI of 30), challenges to the BMI cut point have been raised due to the benefit pancreas transplantation has in particular to uremic patients who have ESRD due to diabetes and would fare better with a simultaneous pancreas-kidney transplant [47, 56, 57]. Since 2015, our group at the University of Illinois at Chicago has performed eight fully robotic pancreas transplants. The first and third ones were pancreas alone and all the rest have been simultaneous kidney–pancreas. In all cases the pancreas was transplanted to the left external iliac vessels (pancreas head down), which allowed perfect align-ment of the vascular anastomosis. Three of the cases have required the exocrine drainage to be via a duodenal-cystic anastomosis performed with an EEA stapler inserted across the stump of the graft. Enteric drainage with a duodenojejunal anastomosis has been more recently successful completing a robotically sewn anastomosis over the early use of an EEA stapler. We cannot over-emphasize the importance of diligent harvesting of the pancreatic graft and meticulous backbench preparation to avoid disturbing bleeding after graft reperfusion.

The first 5 patients have had greater than 1 year follow up with all patients, thus far show-ing favorable post-operative outcomes in both the short and long term [58]. All patients have func-tioning grafts (both kidney and pancreas where applicable) and are euglycemic. This approach, because of the decrease in surgical trauma (com-plete laparotomy vs. mini laparotomy with small ports) could provide favorable outcomes for more patients then just obese recipients. Further stud-ies and larger series are necessary before the da Vinci robotic-assisted technique can be considered an alternative approach to the conven-tional open technique.

22.8 Robotic Hand-Assisted Living Donor Hepatectomy

Minimal invasive laparoscopic liver resection has evolved greatly during the past few decades. The experience in minimally invasive liver surgery has been steadily increasing [59] with extensive expansion of laparoscopic liver resections in the east because of the high volume of patients requiring surgical interventions. More than 200 robotic-assisted liver resection cases have been published to date, including living donor right hepatectomy [60–62]. However, as is noted in multiple reviews, authors state that the use of robotics is liver surgery still has many tools to be desired (such as an ultrasonic dissector, argon beam cautery, etc.).

Soubrane et al. reported the first clinical series of pure laparoscopic left lateral sectionectomy for living liver donors [63]. For living donor right hepatectomies, the introduction of laparoscopic surgery can be traced back to 2006, when Koffron et al. first reported using the laparoscopy-assisted method [64].

Due to our extensive institutional experience with major robotic-assisted liver resections [60], we applied this technology to right living lobe donor hepatectomy. Our first case was performed in 2012 by Giulianotti et al. [61] A 53-year-old healthy man, who volunteered to donate the right lobe of his liver to his brother, who had hepatitis C cirrhosis complicated by hepatocellular carcinoma. The liver graft was safely extracted through a lower abdominal incision. Recipient and donor recovered without acute complications.

However, because of the significant morbidity and mortality associated with this procedure, living donor hepatectomy should only be undertaken by experienced surgical teams [65]. Its application in kidney transplantation for both donor and recipients provides a hopeful platform for its utility in hepatic donor surgery in the future. For now, its use in pancreas and liver surgery has been extremely limited, and larger series are needed to address its usefulness in these settings.

Since potential liver donors are relatively young and perfectly healthy, extensive testing, besides the standard liver donor work-up, is rarely needed.

22.8.1 Surgical Technique: Right Lobe Robotic Hepatectomy

The donor was placed in supine semi-lithotomy position and placed in reverse Trendelenburg position was used with some left sided rotation. The patient had 5 laparoscopic ports placed (1 camera port, 3 robotic arms, 1 assistant port) and 1 lower abdominal incision to remove graft as depicted in our previous publication [61].

The robot was docked on the patient's right side. During the initial dissection of live hilum, the gallbladder is removed. After this, the hepatic artery and the right portal vein are dissected free and hepatic duct is localized following preoperative imaging of biliary anatomy (MRCP). The right lobe is retracted along an upward direction to start the retro-hepatic dissection of the inferior vena cava. Before starting the parenchyma transaction, an ultrasound is performed to identify the venous anatomy, and the branching of the middle hepatic vein. The transection of the parenchyma achieved with robotic Harmonic scalpel. The vascular transections are done using Endo-GIA vascular stapler in the following order: (a) right hepatic artery, (b) right portal vein, and (c) right hepatic vein. The blood loss should be minimal during the transection of liver parenchyma.

22.9 Discussion

The patient where this was performed [61] did not require any blood transfusion. The operative time was 480 min, warm ischemia time of 35 minutes, and the estimated blood loss (EBL) was 350 ml. The patient has a hospital length of stay of 8 days with uneventful course. Similarly, Chen et al. [66] also reported a robotic case series (13 cases) with operative time of 590 (353–753) minutes, and short warm ischemia time 9.5 (8–15) minutes. The EBL was minimal, average of 169 (50–500) mL and length of stay was 7 (6–8) days.

Maintaining the central venous pressure relatively low (3–5 mmHg) is of extreme importance. This approach could potentially increase the chance for developing a CO_2 embolism, if a larger hepatic vein is accidentally opened. Maintaining continuous communication and effective collaboration between the anesthesia and surgical teams could not be overemphasized in order to keep the procedure safe.

The main advantages observed with the robotic system, in addition to those previously mentioned, are that it facilitates vascular and biliary dissection all the need of only a smaller sub-umbilical vertical incision for graft extraction. This incision decreases the pain and risk of pulmonary complications associated with upper midline subcostal incisions.

22.10 Conclusion

The utility of robotics in surgery has yet to be fully understood, however, in transplantation, is role is starting to take solid form. The necessary skills, acquired from its adoption in complex general surgery procedures has allowed its introduction in transplantation. The initial experiences are promising. Constant expansion of the knowledge and abilities of the anesthesiologist, surgical, and medical teams, along with the rapid improvement of the robotic technology, continue to challenge the broader application of these minimally invasive approaches to provide optimal patient care. The candidates for solid organ transplantation, with their long-standing complex medical illness and risks with severe immunosuppression, will continue to benefit from the further advancements in surgical techniques.

References

1. Flowers JL, Jacobs S, Cho E, et al. Comparison of open and laparoscopic live donor nephrectomy. Ann Surg. 1997; 226(4):483–9; discussion 489–90.
2. Ratner LE, Ciseck LJ, Moore RG, et al. Laparoscopic live donor nephrectomy. Transplantation. 1995;60(9):1047–9.
3. Eng M. The role of laparoscopic donor nephrectomy in renal transplantation. Am Surg. 2010;76(4):349–53.
4. Rosales A, Salvador JT, Urdaneta G, et al. Laparoscopic kidney transplantation. Eur Urol. 2010;57(1):164–7.
5. Horgan S, Vanuno D, Sileri P, et al. Robotic-assisted laparoscopic donor nephrectomy for kidney transplantation. Transplantation. 2002;73(9):1474–9.
6. Sung GT, Gill IS. Robotic laparoscopic surgery: a comparison of the DA Vinci and Zeus systems. Urology. 2001;58(6):893–8.
7. Herron DM, Marohn M. A consensus document on robotic surgery. Surg Endosc. 2008;22(2):313–25; discussion 311–2.
8. Waterman AD, Morgievich M, Cohen DJ, et al. Living donor kidney transplantation: improving education outside of transplant centers about live donor transplantation – recommendations from a consensus conference. Clin J Am Soc Nephrol. 2015;10(9):1659–69.
9. Horvat LD, Shariff SZ, Garg AX. Global trends in the rates of living kidney donation. Kidney Int. 2009;75(10):1088–98.
10. Kandaswamy R, Kasiske B, Ibrahim H, et al. Living or deceased donor kidney transplants for candidates with significant extrarenal morbidity. Clin Transpl. 2006;20(3):346–50.
11. de Groot IB, Veen JI, van der Boog PJ, et al. Difference in quality of life, fatigue and societal participation between living and deceased donor kidney transplant recipients. Clin Transpl. 2013;27(4):E415–23.
12. Schweitzer EJ, Wilson J, Jacobs S, et al. Increased rates of donation with laparoscopic donor nephrectomy. Ann Surg. 2000;232(3):392–400.
13. Wagenaar S, Nederhoed JH, Hoksbergen AWJ, et al. Minimally invasive, laparoscopic, and robotic-assisted techniques versus open techniques for kidney transplant recipients: a systematic review. Eur Urol. 2017;72(2):205–17.
14. Kok NF, Lind MY, Hansson BM, et al. Comparison of laparoscopic and mini incision open donor nephrectomy: single blind, randomised controlled clinical trial. BMJ. 2006;333(7561):221.
15. Dols LF, Kok NF, d'Ancona FC, et al. Randomized controlled trial comparing hand-assisted retroperitoneoscopic versus standard laparoscopic donor nephrectomy. Transplantation. 2014;97(2):161–7.
16. Horgan S, Benedetti E, Moser F. Robotically assisted donor nephrectomy for kidney transplantation. Am J Surg. 2004;188(4A Suppl):45s–51s.
17. Horgan S, Galvani C, Gorodner MV, et al. Effect of robotic assistance on the "learning curve" for laparoscopic hand-assisted donor nephrectomy. Surg Endosc. 2007;21(9):1512–7.
18. Delmonico F. A report of the Amsterdam forum on the care of the live kidney donor: data and medical guidelines. Transplantation. 2005;79(6 Suppl):S53–66.
19. Giacomoni A, Di Sandro S, Lauterio A, et al. Robotic nephrectomy for living donation: surgical technique and literature systematic review. Am J Surg. 2016;211(6):1135–42.
20. Carter JT, Freise CE, McTaggart RA, et al. Laparoscopic procurement of kidneys with multiple renal arteries is associated with increased ureteral complications in the recipient. Am J Transplant. 2005;5(6):1312–8.
21. Gorodner V, Horgan S, Galvani C, et al. Routine left robotic-assisted laparoscopic donor nephrectomy is safe and effective regardless of the presence of vascular anomalies. Transpl Int. 2006;19(8):636–40.
22. Dindo D, Demartines N, Clavien PA. Classification of surgical complications: a new proposal with evaluation in a cohort of 6336 patients and results of a survey. Ann Surg. 2004;240(2):205–13.
23. Simforoosh N, Soltani MH, Basiri A, et al. Evolution of laparoscopic live donor nephrectomy: a single-center experience with 1510 cases over 14 years. J Endourol. 2014;28(1):34–9.
24. Leventhal JR, Kocak B, Salvalaggio PR, et al. Laparoscopic donor nephrectomy 1997 to 2003: lessons learned with 500 cases at a single institution. Surgery. 2004;136(4):881–90.
25. Hadjianastassiou VG, Johnson RJ, Rudge CJ, et al. 2509 living donor nephrectomies, morbid-

ity and mortality, including the UK introduction of laparoscopic donor surgery. Am J Transplant. 2007;7(11):2532–7.

26. Su LM, Ratner LE, Montgomery RA, et al. Laparoscopic live donor nephrectomy: trends in donor and recipient morbidity following 381 consecutive cases. Ann Surg. 2004;240(2):358–63.

27. Srivastava A, Gupta N, Kumar A. Evolution of the technique of laparoscopic live donor nephrectomy at a single center: experience with more than 350 cases. Urol Int. 2008;81(4):431–6.

28. Mjoen G, Oyen O, Holdaas H, et al. Morbidity and mortality in 1022 consecutive living donor nephrectomies: benefits of a living donor registry. Transplantation. 2009;88(11):1273–9.

29. Hoznek A, Zaki SK, Samadi DB, et al. Robotic assisted kidney transplantation: an initial experience. J Urol. 2002;167(4):1604–6.

30. Giulianotti P, Gorodner V, Sbrana F, et al. Robotic transabdominal kidney transplantation in a morbidly obese patient. Am J Transplant. 2010;10(6):1478–82.

31. Boggi U, Vistoli F, Signori S, et al. Robotic renal transplantation: first European case. Transpl Int. 2011;24(2):213–8.

32. Doumerc N, Roumiguie M, Rischmann P, et al. Total robotic approach with transvaginal insertion for kidney transplantation. Eur Urol. 2015;68(6):1103–4.

33. Doumerc N, Beauval JB, Rostaing L, et al. A new surgical area opened in renal transplantation: a pure robot-assisted approach for both living donor nephrectomy and kidney transplantation using transvaginal route. Transpl Int. 2016;29(1):122–3.

34. Oberholzer J, Giulianotti P, Danielson KK, et al. Minimally invasive robotic kidney transplantation for obese patients previously denied access to transplantation. Am J Transplant. 2013;13(3):721–8.

35. Breda A, Territo A, Gausa L, et al. Robot-assisted kidney transplantation: The European experience. Eur Urol. 2017.

36. Lynch RJ, Ranney DN, Shijie C, et al. Obesity, surgical site infection, and outcome following renal transplantation. Ann Surg. 2009;250(6):1014–20.

37. Kramer HJ, Saranathan A, Luke A, et al. Increasing body mass index and obesity in the incident ESRD population. J Am Soc Nephrol. 2006;17(5):1453–9.

38. Tzvetanov I DBC, Tulla K, Spaggiari M, Gheza F, Di Cocco P, Oberholzer J, Benedetti E. Robotic kidney transplantation in obese recipients: the new standard? Am Transplant Congress, Vol. 18. Seattle, WA, USA, 2018.

39. Krishnan N, Higgins R, Short A, et al. Kidney transplantation significantly improves patient and graft survival irrespective of BMI: a cohort study. Am J Transplant. 2015;15(9):2378–86.

40. Menon M, Sood A, Bhandari M, et al. Robotic kidney transplantation with regional hypothermia: a step-by-step description of the vattikuti urology institute-medanta technique (IDEAL Phase 2a). Eur Urol. 2014;65(5):991–1000.

41. Abaza R, Ghani KR, Sood A, et al. Robotic kidney transplantation with intraoperative regional hypothermia. BJU Int. 2014;113(4):679–81.

42. Tsai MK, Lee CY, Yang CY, et al. Robot-assisted renal transplantation in the retroperitoneum. Transpl Int. 2014;27(5):452–7.

43. Territo A, Gausa L, Alcaraz A, et al. European experience of robot-assisted kidney transplantation: minimum of 1-year follow-up. BJU Int. 2018.

44. Garcia-Roca R, Garcia-Aroz S, Tzvetanov I, et al. Single center experience with robotic kidney transplantation for recipients with BMI of 40 kg/m^2 or greater: a comparison with the UNOS registry. Transplantation. 2017;101(1):191–6.

45. Troppmann C, Gruessner AC, Dunn DL, et al. Surgical complications requiring early relaparotomy after pancreas transplantation: a multivariate risk factor and economic impact analysis of the cyclosporine era. Ann Surg. 1998;227(2):255–68.

46. Kandaswamy R, Stock PG, Gustafson SK, et al. OPTN/SRTR 2016 annual data report: pancreas. Am J Transplant. 2018;18(Suppl 1):114–71.

47. Gruessner AC, Laftavi MR, Pankewycz O, et al. Simultaneous pancreas and kidney transplantation-is it a treatment option for patients with type 2 diabetes mellitus? An analysis of the international pancreas transplant registry. Curr Diab Rep. 2017;17(6):44.

48. Hanish SI, Petersen RP, Collins BH, et al. Obesity predicts increased overall complications following pancreas transplantation. Transplant Proc. 2005;37(8):3564–6.

49. Everett JE, Wahoff DC, Statz C, et al. Characterization and impact of wound infection after pancreas transplantation. Arch Surg. 1994;129(12):1310–6; discussion 1316–7.

50. Humar A, Ramcharan T, Kandaswamy R, et al. The impact of donor obesity on outcomes after cadaver pancreas transplants. Am J Transplant. 2004;4(4):605–10.

51. Sampaio MS, Reddy PN, Kuo HT, et al. Obesity was associated with inferior outcomes in simultaneous pancreas kidney transplant. Transplantation. 2010;89(9):1117–25.

52. Horgan S, Galvani C, Gorodner V, et al. Robotic distal pancreatectomy and nephrectomy for living donor pancreas-kidney transplantation. Transplantation. 2007;84(7):934–6.

53. Tan M, Kandaswamy R, Sutherland DE, et al. Laparoscopic donor distal pancreatectomy for living donor pancreas and pancreas-kidney transplantation. Am J Transplant. 2005;5(8):1966–70.

54. Boggi U, Signori S, Vistoli F, et al. Laparoscopic robot-assisted pancreas transplantation: first world experience. Transplantation. 2012;93(2):201–6.

55. Yeh CC, Spaggiari M, Tzvetanov I, et al. Robotic pancreas transplantation in a type 1 diabetic patient with morbid obesity: a case report. Medicine (Baltimore). 2017;96(6):e5847.

56. Gruessner AC. 2011 update on pancreas transplantation: comprehensive trend analysis of 25,000 cases

followed up over the course of twenty-four years at the International Pancreas Transplant Registry (IPTR). Rev Diabet Stud. 2011;8(1):6–16.

57. Gruessner AC, Gruessner RW. Pancreas Transplantation of US and Non-US Cases from 2005 to 2014 as Reported to the United Network for Organ Sharing (UNOS) and the International Pancreas Transplant Registry (IPTR). Rev Diabet Stud. 2016;13(1):35–58.

58. Spaggiari M, Di Bella C, Di Cocco P, et al. Robotic pancreas transplantation in obese recipients: preliminary results. Am J Transplant. American Transplant Congress. Seattle, WA, USA, 2018. pp. Supp 4.

59. Buell JF, Cherqui D, Geller DA, et al. The international position on laparoscopic liver surgery: The Louisville Statement, 2008. Ann Surg. 2009;250(5):825–30.

60. Giulianotti PC, Coratti A, Sbrana F, et al. Robotic liver surgery: results for 70 resections. Surgery. 2011;149(1):29–39.

61. Giulianotti PC, Tzvetanov I, Jeon H, et al. Robot-assisted right lobe donor hepatectomy. Transpl Int. 2012;25(1):e5–9.

62. Lai EC, Tang CN, Li MK. Robot-assisted laparoscopic hemi-hepatectomy: technique and surgical outcomes. Int J Surg. 2012;10(1):11–5.

63. Soubrane O, Cherqui D, Scatton O, et al. Laparoscopic left lateral sectionectomy in living donors: safety and reproducibility of the technique in a single center. Ann Surg. 2006;244(5):815–20.

64. Koffron AJ, Kung R, Baker T, et al. Laparoscopic-assisted right lobe donor hepatectomy. Am J Transplant. 2006;6(10):2522–5.

65. Barr ML, Belghiti J, Villamil FG, et al. A report of the Vancouver Forum on the care of the live organ donor: lung, liver, pancreas, and intestine data and medical guidelines. Transplantation. 2006;81(10):1373–85.

66. Chen PD, Wu CY, Hu RH, et al. Robotic liver donor right hepatectomy: a pure, minimally invasive approach. Liver Transpl. 2016;22(11):1509–18.

Georgios Vrakas, Annemarie Weissenbacher, and Henk Giele

23.1 Introduction

Vascularized composite allotransplantation (VCA) was initially known as composite tissue allotransplantation (CTA), a term coined by Peacock EE Jr. for transplanting en-block digital flexor tendons and synovial sheaths. However, the term CTA was later changed to VCA in order to avoid confusion with tissue transplants which follow different regulations to organ transplantation [1]. In the last 2 decades, VCAs have marked an emerging era in transplant medicine and are now defined and regulated as organs [2].

Following Peacock's attempt in 1957, which failed due to the absence of immunosuppression, Gilbert R performed the first hand transplant in Ecuador, using the early immunosuppressants (prednisolone and azathioprine) that made renal transplantation feasible. However, this regime wasn't sufficiently potent to avoid early rejection,

G. Vrakas (✉)
University of Maryland, School of Medicine, Baltimore, MD, USA
e-mail: gvrakas@som.umaryland.edu

A. Weissenbacher
Department of Visceral, Transplant and Thoracic Surgery, Medical University of Innsbruck, Innsbruck, Austria
e-mail: annemarie.weissenbacher@i-med.ac.at

H. Giele
Nuffield Departement of Surgery, University of Oxford, Oxford, UK
e-mail: henk.giele2@ouh.nhs.uk

and the transplanted arm was amputated 3 weeks later [3]. This early failure, as well as the failure of experimental animal models, reinforced the consensus that VCA were too immunogenic for successful transplantation, and hindered further attempts for another 30 years.

The modern era of VCA started in Lyon, France in 1998, when Dubernard JM [4] and his team performed the first modern-era hand transplant. Despite its technical and initial success, the recipient struggled psychologically and decided to stop immunosuppression and physiotherapy, leading to rejection and loss of function. This transplant was later amputated. This unfortunate outcome stressed the importance of psychological evaluation and counselling in patient selection. Compliance with immunosuppression and hand therapy is of utmost importance in this challenging field of transplantation. One year later, Breidenbach W and his team in Louisville, performed the first American hand transplant, which remains the longest surviving VCA [5]. Soon afterwards (2000 and 2003), the Lyon and the Innsbruck team [6] performed the first bilateral hand transplants, achieving encouraging sensorimotor recovery and considerably improved quality of life.

In 1998, the same year as the first successful hand transplant but with much less fanfare, Strome M et al. from Cleveland, Ohio performed the first total laryngeal transplantation in a man who had sustained a severe traumatic injury to the larynx and pharynx. They concluded that potential candidates for laryngeal transplantation

© Springer Nature Switzerland AG 2021
N. Hakim et al. (eds.), *Transplantation Surgery*, Springer Specialist Surgery Series,
https://doi.org/10.1007/978-3-030-55244-2_23

include aphonic patients with laryngeal trauma, patients with large benign chondromas requiring laryngectomy, and patients who have undergone laryngectomy for cancer and who remain disease-free after 5 years [7].

In 2003, Levi DM et al. from Miami, reported 8 abdominal wall transplants (AWTx) that facilitated reconstruction and closure of the abdominal compartment in intestinal transplant (ITx) patients with complex abdominal wall defects [8]. Later, the Oxford group reported that the abdominal wall transplant potentially performs a dual role, apart from providing tension-free abdominal closure, the AWTx could be beneficial as an immune modulator and sentinel marker for immunological activity in the host. They found the AWTx a useful tool for timely detection of rejection, possible avoidance of intestinal graft rejection and, more importantly, avoidance of adverse over-immunosuppression in cases of bowel dysfunction not related to graft rejection [9].

The first facial transplant was encouraged by the success of limb transplantation and was performed in 2005, in France, by a team led by Duvauchelle B and Dubernard JM. They transplanted the central and lower face of a brain-dead female donor onto a woman aged 38 years who had suffered traumatic dog bite loss of distal nose, both lips, chin, and adjacent parts of the cheeks [10].

An increasing number of centres have developed multidisciplinary VCA programs and have successfully transplanted a variety of VCAs (e.g. upper limb, face, abdominal wall, trachea, larynx, lower limb, femur, knee joint, peripheral nerves, uterus, penis).

Without doubt, the worldwide success in vascularized composite tissue allotransplantation is the result of both patients and surgeons willing to incur risks to take a novel idea to a practical, functioning reality that enhances the quality of life for a few selected appropriate patients [11].

23.1.1 Upper Limb Transplantation

23.1.1.1 Introduction

Hands are essential for our everyday life. Loss of one hand is, therefore, catastrophic. Loss of both hands debilitating [12]. Prosthetics are the conventional method of treatment for upper limb amputees and can be utilized for amputations from wrist to shoulder. Over the last few years, prosthetics have evolved significantly in terms of voluntary control, complex movement and even sensory feedback. However, patients often reject them because of discomfort, increased weight and limited usefulness [13], as well as deficiencies in social acceptability (aesthetics, self-confidence, other people's opinions, and physical integrity) [14]. The purpose of upper limb transplantation is to achieve better cosmesis (body integrity), durability, sensation and functional interaction through touch and gestures, compared to current prosthetics [15]. The objective in upper limb transplantation is not only technical success, but functional integration.

23.1.1.2 Indications and Patient Selection

Solid organ transplants are life-saving operations, and therefore not subject to the same ethical considerations as VCA, which are predominantly performed to enhance quality of life. Hand transplantation does not obviously prolong life but merely improves quality of life, at the risk of immunosuppression [16]. Therefore, upper extremity transplantation involves weighing the benefit of improved quality of life against the emotional, financial and physical cost of lifelong immunosuppression and the risks of surgery. These are difficult decisions to make, and can vary greatly depending on the extent of disability, the functional demands and expectations of the potential recipient [16]. In addition, the lack of formalized, verified, reliable outcome measures and the absence of long-term results in a large number of patients makes an estimation of the benefit and risk of this surgery difficult. For these reasons, indications for hand transplantation have remained highly individualized to both the recipient and the performing institution. Autonomy, both on the institutional and patient level, remains a priority. There is no established consensus on specific indications for upper extremity transplantation, but as the field continues to grow, so too does the need for an established set of clinical criteria [16, 17].

The American Society for Reconstructive Transplantation (ASRT) has developed a series of criteria and contraindications regarding upper extremity transplantation. These criteria include amputation or irreversible functional loss; however, the amputation or loss of function should be accompanied by medical or functional complications, and demonstrable loss of quality of life as determined by psychological evaluation [16].

23.1.1.3 Surgical Technique

The terms, wrist and distal forearm transplants refer to transplantation at the same level: just proximal to the radiocarpal joint so that enough distal radius and ulna are present within the transplant to achieve adequate osteosynthesis with standard distal radius and forearm plates. Transplantation within the hand itself has been reported as well. For proximal forearm level transplantation, the recipient's stumps and the donor forearms are prepared, simultaneously, by identifying and dissecting neurovascular structures and muscles. Subsequently, radius and ulna bone fixation is performed, followed by revascularization (ulnar and radial artery, two deep and three superficial veins including the cephalic and basilic vein) and reconstruction of muscles, nerves and skin. Bone length is determined by inserting the medial donor epicondyle with the flexor origin to its corresponding site on the recipient's humerus. For muscle reconstruction, a 'piggyback method' can be used to provide corresponding reinnervation of donor musculotendinous flexor and extensor units. In order to ensure reversibility of the procedure, the recipient's muscle remnants medial (M. flexor carpi ulnaris) and lateral (M. extensor carpi radialis longus et brevis, M. brachioradialis) should remain unattached distally, and their nerve supply intact. Conservation of recipient forearm muscle stumps is considered of utmost importance, as they may be required for stimulation of myoelectrical prostheses in case of graft loss (lifeboat procedure). Ulnar and median nerve repairs are made distal to the respective (donor) motor branches. The dorsal extensor muscles are fixed to the recipient

humerus by transosseous sutures. The posterior interosseus nerve is coapted at the supinator level. At the end of surgery, the skin flaps are trimmed and sutured without tension. Distal forearm and hand transplants are simpler in so far that the flexor and extensor activity is provided by the host musculature and tenorraphies are performed distally. Nerve repair is as distal as possible to reduce the regeneration distance particularly for the ulnar motor branch.

As the allografts contain a large quantity of skeletal muscle, known to be more sensitive to ischemia/reperfusion injury than the other structures of the forearm, the principal aim is to keep ischemia time particularly short. This can be achieved by precisely adjusting the time schedules and by having surgical teams simultaneously operating on donor and recipient forearms, and minimising transport time between the two. Perfusion of the grafts with University of Wisconsin preservation solution (500 mL for each side) is only started after all required structures have been identified and prepared at the recipient's stumps [18].

23.1.1.4 Outcomes

Patient survival for isolated upper limb transplantation exceeds 98%, with only one fatality after a bilateral arm transplant in Mexico [19]. The overall allograft survival (107 upper limb allografts in 72 patients), as per the International Registry on Hand and Composite Tissue Transplantation (IRHCTT), is currently calculated at 77.6% (24 limb-losses); however, it is the concomitant hand and face/leg transplants that account for one third of all limb losses and three additional deaths [20, 21]. It should be noted that graft survival surpasses 95% for patients adherent to traditional triple-drug therapy after antibody-based lymphocyte depleting induction therapy [22].

Functional outcomes are highly encouraging, but not consistently reported, in contrast to the transplant occurrence. The main reason for this might be the fact that patients require years to reach maximal function; not to mention that there are no universally agreed outcomes measures (e.g. Carroll, DASH, CFSS, Chen, HTSS) [16, 19]. With the exception of the Hand

Transplant Score System (HTSS), there are no other outcomes measures specifically intended to evaluate hand transplant recipients [23]. Last but not least, the level of transplantation varies greatly from patient to patient, leading to significant functional discrepancy amongst hand transplant recipients [24]. The level of amputation largely determines the outcome however the amputee with some residual hand may have a better outcome if the transplant is electively performed more proximally at distal forearm/wrist level compared to distal forearm level transplantation performed for amputation at the radiocarpal joint [24].

The French group have reported the functional benefits achieved over a mean follow-up period of 7.6 years (range 4–13 years) in 5 bilateral hand transplants [14] (Fig. 23.1). The physical results (motion, strength, sensibility) achieved were considered fair; functional results were considered good, and subjective results considered very good. These results progress dramatically during the first year, significantly during the first three years, or even later especially for sensitivity, then become stable. All patients could perform most daily activities, such as eating, writing, driving, grasping and shaving. The overall results were considered effective and reported as unequalled by any current prosthesis [14].

The Louisville team reported in 2011 their functional outcomes for 6 hand transplants, with all recipients regaining independency in their daily life. Protective sensation was restored in all recipients, while their first patient acquired near-to-normal discrimination (5–9 mm). The other recipients, achieved Carroll Scores ranging from 57–59, that indicate good functional outcomes [25].

In the same year, the Spanish team reported their outcomes after 3 bilateral hand transplants, achieving HTSS scores that indicate good functional outcomes (73.5–79.5) [26].

The Innsbruck team review of their 4 patients, transplanted over 14 years, showed restored protective and discriminative sensation in all patients. HTSS were good or excellent, whereas DASH scores showed great variance. Unilateral and bilateral hand transplant recipients in this cohort evolved similarly with regards to rehabilitation and functional outcomes [27].

The Polish team published their results in 2011 for 7 upper limb transplants in 6 patients though it should be noted that 2 recipients were transplanted at mid- and distal-humeral level. They found that above elbow upper limb transplants were technically easier, given the larger vessels and less structures that had to be repaired (1 bone vs. 2 forearm bones and 2 large muscles vs. 11 flexor and 12 extensor tendons). All patients reported restored protective sensation and 2 recipients with long follow up possessed two-point discrimination [28, 29].

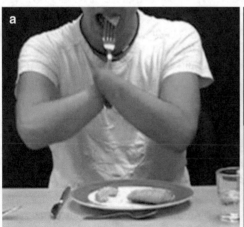 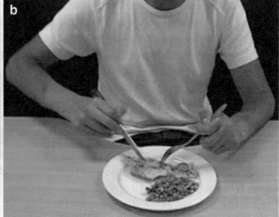

Fig. 23.1 Eating alone before (**a**) and after (**b**) hand transplantation

Johns Hopkins University and the University of Pittsburgh jointly transplanted four bilateral and three unilateral hand/upper extremity allografts in seven patients, including 3 transplants at mid to distal humeral level. All patients achieved good functional outcomes in the early post-transplant period. Functional improvements were faster in the more distal transplants and in those compliant with rehabilitation and immunotherapy. Best overall function was observed in those with more distal transplants and, in specific, in those with more proximal transplants and bilateral transplants. At the time of writing this report, four of the seven recipients had already regained independence in all their daily activities [30, 31].

Breidenbach et al. in their review found that when hand transplantation is limited to patients with single and/or bilateral amputation at the elbow or below, in a medical and social environment where immuno-suppression is available, outcomes are excellent. They showed that mean hand allograft survival was over 5 years, with the longest surviving hand allograft surviving over 15 years. At the time, there were 75 hands transplanted on 52 patients, with a survival rate of 92 percent. They concluded that 5- to 10-year allograft survival is achievable for single or bilateral hand transplants. Moreover, they investigated the impact of the (more frequent) acute rejection episodes on late allograft survival and compared it to the solid organ transplant outcomes. Their analysis demonstrated a statistically significant lower probability of developing chronic rejection for hand transplantation compared with liver, heart, and kidney transplantation [11].

Data collected by the above listed programs are reported to the IRHCTT, which periodically publishes an update of the global experience. According to the latest registry update [19, 32], all reported upper extremity allograft recipients developed protective sensibility, with 91% of them also possessing tactile sensibility and 82% regaining partial discriminative sensibility. Extrinsic motor function was sufficient in all patients to perform grip and pinch actions. Most patients regained independence, enabling independent living and some returned to full-time occupation. Patients with more distal transplants achieved faster sensory and motor function and also, superior discriminatory sensation, whereas more proximal transplants exhibited unreliable recovery of intrinsic function and diminished extrinsic strength as transplantation levels progressed more proximal [19].

23.1.2 Face Transplantation

23.1.2.1 Introduction

Severe congenital deformities or traumatic facial defects can be very challenging to repair with conventional reconstructive techniques, as besides the aesthetic result, it is the expressive function of the face that cannot be adequately restored. Peter Butler, from the Royal Free Hospital in London, was the first surgeon to suggest facial allotransplantation in 2002. However, at the time, it was deemed unwise to proceed without any relevant research [33].

Following the early successes of upper limb transplantation, the first facial transplant, was performed in 2005 by the French team, led by Duvauchelle B and Dubernard JM (Figs. 23.2 and 23.3). They performed a partial facial transplant that included the nose and mouth to a 38 year old recipient woman whose face was mauled by a dog, while she was unconscious. The aesthetic and functional outcome was good and the graft had functioned well for many years, but in 2015 she suffered rejection and loss part of the graft, and a year later she developed immuno-suppression associated complications and died [10, 34]. The first full face transplant, including all intact aesthetic and functional units, was performed in Barcelona in 2010, by a team led by Barret et al. [35] Up to the time of this manuscript, thirty seven facial transplants have been reported worldwide [36].

23.1.2.2 Indications and Patient Selection

As with all VCAs, there is currently no consensus regarding the indications for facial transplantation. Severe facial disfigurement is the obvious indication; however, the definition of this can dif-

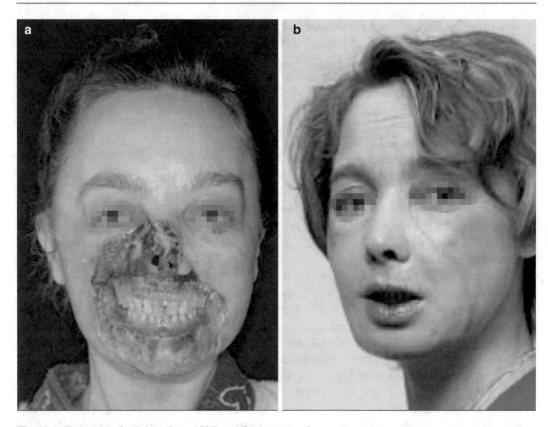

Fig. 23.2 Patient (**a**) after injury (June, 2005) and (**b**) 4 months after surgery

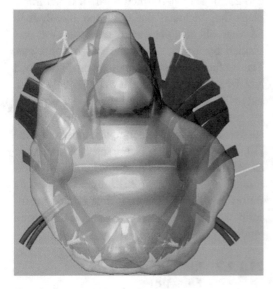

Fig. 23.3 Anatomy of partial allograft with muscles, facial vessels, and motor and sensory nerves that were repaired microsurgically

fer significantly between different centres. Each program is using a different approach and the indications are highly individualized. The main overarching universal guideline is to weigh the aesthetic and functional benefits of conventional restoration against the risks of transplantation and immunosuppression [37].

The Barcelona team considers as absolute indications the complete destruction of the eyelids, including the orbital sphincter, and complete destruction of the lips, including the oral muscle sphincter, as it is not possible to restore the facial muscle sphincters with traditional techniques [38]. Whereas, a French team suggested that the indications for face transplantation should not be based solely on the injury, but instead should include 3 elements: the anatomic deficit, the patient characteristics (including quality of life, health-related quality of life, immunosensitisation, psychosocial support, etc.), as well as the transplantation team experience [39].

Over the years the inclusion criteria keep expanding and, currently, centres consider facial transplantation for previously contraindicated cases. Face transplantation has been performed in HIV positive patients, after self-harm, in the highly sensitized and even in patients with history of malignancy and others. It is still unclear whether facial transplantation should be reserved only for cases where the conventional methods have been tested and failed, or whether it can be used as a first or even 'emergency' operation. An interesting case of 'emergency facial transplant' has been published by the Polish group, who performed the operation in a 31 year old male who had his face amputated in a work accident [40]. Given the small numbers, however, it is difficult to establish widely accepted and precise indications [37, 41, 42].

23.1.2.3 Surgical Technique

Each facial transplant is unique. Preoperative planning is of utmost importance and surgeons need to take into account each individual's craniofacial and orthognathic factors in order to restore normal anatomy. Restoring compromised sensory and motor functions in cases with severe facial defects is of great importance; however, the aesthetic appearance has to be considered as well. Conventional craniofacial surgery planning uses anthropometry and cephalometry and the same principles are applied to facial transplantation in order to maximize allograft function and position. Compared to conventional craniofacial planning, face transplantation is a paradigm shift in reverse order, where composite injury and the subsequent reattachment of the soft tissues in the form of a transplant dictate the osteosynthesis. However, these soft tissue points must be assessed with craniofacial planning and subsequently fixed into proper correlation with the cephalometric landmarks. Precise planning as well as experience with conventional orthognathic movements and surgical correction of congenital syndromes is therefore imperative [43].

Given the complex vascular anatomy as a result of devastating injuries and previous reconstructive attempts, CT angiogram is necessary for preoperative vascular planning. The facial artery is the main pedicle for the facial flap; however, that has to be carefully confirmed.

The facial flaps are retrieved following craniocaudal and lateral-to-medial dissection. The facial nerve branches are dissected medially to the parotid gland and then attached to the recipient ones. The parotid gland is not generally included in the allograft transplantation unless it is used to add bulk. Relevant sensory nerves are coapted [44].

23.1.2.4 Outcomes

The total world face transplantation cohort of 37 patients has 5 deaths and the survival rate is estimated at 86.5% (32/37) [45].

Sensory recovery (thermal and mechanical) is most often achieved by 3 months post transplantation and is frequently an accidental finding during routine biopsies. Full sensory recovery is expected at 8–12 months post transplantation. Semmes-Weinstein, light touch, 2-point discrimination, a calorimetric test and EMG are objective sensory assessment tests to confirm these findings [45]. The operational strategy used to repair sensory nerves differs between centres. Nevertheless, sensory recovery has occurred independent of nerve repair [46].

Motor function is dependent on facial nerve coaptation and is normally restored between 6 and 18 months post transplantation with ongoing improvements over the next few years [47]. Assessment methods include facial muscle re-education program, speech therapy, chewing and swallowing therapy and daily assessment of return of "social" functions of facial mimetics. Also, within the first weeks, patients with a tracheostomy or gastric tube are extubated if possible and gastric tubes are removed. Thus, all patients are able to breath, eat, drink and speak [45, 47].

Active participation of patients in the therapy is very important for motor restoration and given the long recovery time, overall motor results are average compared to the faster sensory recovery. Motor recovery is accelerated when distal nerve repair is done as opposed to proximal isolation of the main trunk of the facial nerve [47]. However, all face transplant recipients were satisfied with functional outcomes and accepted the "new faces" as their own [45].

The aesthetic results of facial transplantation are mostly acceptable (Fig. 23.4). However, there are cases where the recipients now have a 'new deformity', as a result of trauma and reconstructive surgery [47, 48]. These less favourable outcomes could be the result of the technical challenge and complexity to match the facial features of both donor and recipient. However, these outcomes could also be the result of patients' lack of compliance in performing facial exercises, as they get discouraged by the lengthy recovery process [45].

23.1.3 Abdominal Wall

23.1.3.1 Introduction

Abdominal wall transplantation (AWTx) was first described by Levi et al. in 2003 (Fig. 23.5) and has since become increasingly utilized as a technique for primary abdominal closure after isolated intestinal and multivisceral transplantation [8, 49]. Candidates for ITx suffer infrequently from extensive intra-abdominal scarring, sclerosis and damage to the abdominal wall from multiple previous surgical procedures, infections and enterocutaneous fistulas. These result in abdominal domain loss, which in combination with the post reperfusion intestinal oedema and often donor-recipient size mismatch, can make

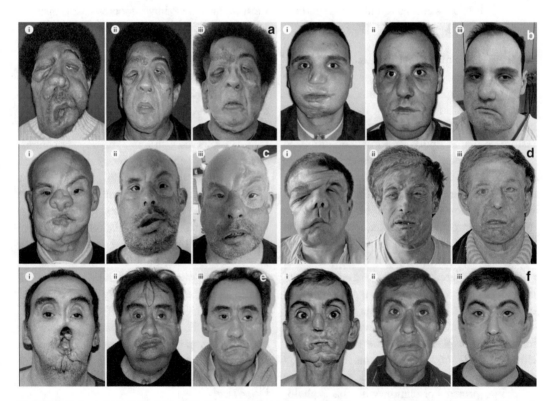

Fig. 23.4 Patients 1 (**a**), 2 (**b**), 3 (**c**), 4 (**d**), 5 (**e**) and 6 (**f**) at inclusion (i), at 1-year post-transplantation (ii), and at maximal follow-up (iii)

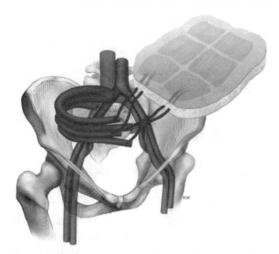

Fig. 23.5 Implantation of abdominal wall composite graft in the recipient

primary closure of the abdominal wall very challenging and sometimes impossible (up to 40%). Tension free closure is crucial to avoid abdominal compartment syndrome and minimize recipient morbidity and AWTx has been utilized by various teams with the intention to achieve primary closure, as it enables a substantial expansion of abdominal domain [9, 50]. The abdominal wall graft can be either partial (vascularised and non-vascularised) or full thickness [49].

An additional benefit of AWTx is the additional information it provides regarding the immunological status of the recipient. The Oxford group based on their experience with simultaneous, same donor, ITx and full thickness AWTx, suggested using the AWTx as a sentinel marker for rejection [9]. Based on the evidence that skin is always the first component to manifest signs of rejection In clinical VCA transplants [22]. Therefore, the enhanced susceptibility and easy visibility of the vascularized skin to rejection provides further benefits in visceral transplant monitoring [50].

23.1.3.2 Indications and Patient Selection

Patients who meet the criteria for ITx with additional major scarring of the anterior abdominal wall and/or loss of abdominal domain have been considered eligible for AWTx, as in terms of abdominal wall reconstruction, as most ITx

recipients are poor candidates for traditional reconstructive techniques, such as tissue advancement or flap closure of the defect [51].

The main issues that are taken into consideration for a simultaneous ITx and AWTx are: (a) underlying primary disease (anatomical or functional short bowel syndrome), (b) loss of abdominal domain (as evaluated by abdominal computed tomography scan), (c) extent of abdominal wall injury (prior surgery or radiotherapy) and (d) quality of abdominal wall (fascia, skin cover, quality of skin, scars, wound healing) [9].

23.1.3.3 Surgical Technique

The Miami group, which pioneered this procedure, used an inverted U incision for the abdominal wall retrieval. Although, this provided a good-sized graft for transplantation, closure of the donor abdominal defect proved very challenging or even impossible. The Oxford Group has used a longitudinal elliptical incision over both rectus abdominis (Fig. 23.6). This leaves the

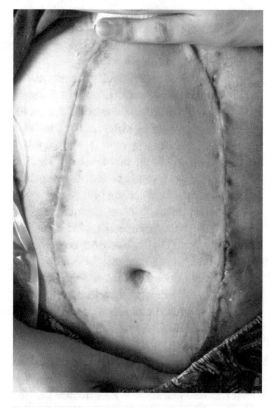

Fig. 23.6 Elliptical abdominal wall transplant

pubic attachment inferiorly and the inferior epigastric vessels entering the deep surface of the graft bilaterally. The vessels are divided with minimal dissection at their origin from the external iliacs with or without a cuff of iliac. The abdominal wall is flushed with UW solution and packed in UW solution in sterile bags and placed in cold storage [49].

The AWTx is implanted after the ITx. Limited bench work is required to prepare the inferior epigastric vessels. The recipient inferior epigastric vessels are dissected from the under surface of the rectus muscles bilaterally and transposed medially, in preparation for anastomosis. The donor abdominal wall is laid in place and attached at the cranial, caudal, and mid-lateral points. End-to-end arterial and venous anastomoses are performed using 10/0 nylon. The abdominal flap is reperfused once the first side is complete. Perfusion and drainage of the entire abdominal wall transplant from one side inferior epigastric artery and vein is sufficient to maintain the entire transplant. However, bilateral arterial and venous anastomoses are performed whenever this is feasible [49].

23.1.3.4 Outcomes

Up to this date, more than 40 full thickness AWTx have been performed worldwide (out of which, 22 by the Oxford group). The AWTx is monitored post operatively by observation of the skin perfusion by colour, temperature, and capillary return, particularly in the first few days. Healing in all AWTx has been reported as normal as native adjacent wound healing [49].

There still remain concerns regarding prolongation of the duration of operation, increased risk of rejection and GVHD. However, recently, the Oxford group has reported that the addition of a VCA probably does not increase the rejection rate. The overall incidence of rejection (intestine and skin) appears to be similar to intestinal transplant patients without abdominal wall transplants (around 30%), but when skin is present rejection is directed predominantly to the skin rather than the intestine [52]. In another study, the same group reported that there is no evidence that the addition of a VCA increases the incidence of

dnDSA formation compared to transplantation of the intestine alone [53]. The immunological effects of combining an abdominal wall transplant with an intestinal transplant remain a matter of ongoing investigation.

23.1.4 Reproductive Organs

23.1.4.1 Uterine Transplantation

Introduction

Uterus transplantation (UTx) is a life enhancing, as well as, a life-giving transplantation and it is the first potential treatment for absolute uterine factor infertility (AUFI). AUFI affects around 1 in every 500 women of fertile age, which on a worldwide base would be around 1.5 million women. For many years, women with AUFI who wanted to become genetic mothers would resort to gestational surrogacy; however, this modality is not widely accessible due to religious, ethical or legal reasons. As a result, adoption would be the only option to achieve motherhood [54]. UTx paves the way for legal, genetic as well as gestational motherhood.

The first UTx from a live donor was performed in Jeddah, Saudi Arabia in 2000. However, the transplanted uterus had to be removed 99 days after the procedure because of acute vascular thrombosis [55]. The first cadaveric UTx was performed in Turkey, but did not result in successful birth. The Gothenburg group, led by Brännström M, group achieved the first live birth post live donor UTx in September 2014, within the first clinical UTx trial, initiated in 2012 in Sweden [56, 57]. Since then another 7 births have been reported from the same clinical trial and recently, the Dallas group announced the first birth in the USA [58].

UTx is the first temporary type of transplantation that has been introduced, as the graft is not intended for lifelong use. The UTx can be removed after one or two babies have been born, as it is important to reduce the potential long-term immunosuppression side-effects. However, the autonomy of the patients should be respected and any future decision to surgically remove the uterus needs to be made in consensus with the recipient and her partner [57].

Indications and Patient Selection

There is a great variety of causes of AUFI and they can be either congenital or acquired. Women lacking the uterus clearly belong to the AUFI group and the uterine absence could be either because of a hysterectomy or congenital uterine agenesis (Mayer-Rokitansky-Küster-Hauser syndrome [MRKHS], 1:4500 women). However, there are women with uterus, albeit with changes in its shape or in its functionality, and they can be either infertile or sub-fertile. Causes of non-functional, but anatomically present uterus are: (i) leiomyomas, (ii) Asherman's syndrome (intrauterine adhesions), (iii) congenital uterine malformations and uterine infertility and (iv) functional dysregulation of the uterus [54]. The field will also most likely expand to individuals that are genetically XY, as transgender male-to-female as well as in women with androgen insufficiency syndrome [59].

Surgical Technique

The open surgical approach has mainly been the standard technique for live donor hysterectomies [57]. Recently robotic-assisted laparoscopic approaches have been performed and may optimize the live donor procedures allowing a faster recovery while reducing the time of surgery (from 10 to 13 h for the open procedure) [60, 61].

Uterus transplantation surgery entails isolation of the uterus with bilateral, long venous, and arterial vascular pedicles. The complexity of the surgery is mostly related to the extensive vascular dissection that includes the distal parts of the internal iliac veins and arteries [57]. The uterine arteries together with the anterior portions of the internal iliac arteries have to isolated, as well as the uterine veins including a segment/patch of the internal iliac vein. Uterine veins, with several connecting branches, could be tightly attached to the ureters and several of the connecting branches must be divided to retrieve the uterus while keeping the donor ureters intact. Venous outflow through the ovarian veins has been considered as an alternative; however, concerns remain about whether the venous outflow using the ovarian veins will be sufficient, especially during pregnancy [61].

In the recipient, through a midline incision, the external iliac vessels are dissected and prepared for anastomosis. The vaginal vault is separated from the bladder and rectum. Sutures, to be used for uterine fixation, are placed bilaterally through the round ligaments, sacrouterine ligaments, and the paravaginal connective tissues. The uterus is brought into the pelvis and end to side vascular anastomoses are performed onto the external iliac vessels (Fig. 23.7). Following reperfusion, the vaginal cuff of the uterus is attached to the recipient's vagina (Fig. 23.8). Attaching the uterus to the round/sacrouterine ligaments, in addition to the paravaginal connective tissues and the bladder peritoneum provides additional structural support. It remains unclear if the vaginal reconstruction in MRKH patients through either dilatation or mucosal reconstruction will impact the surgical procedure [61].

Outcomes

So far, there have been around 40 UTx attempts worldwide and the vast majority of these were live donor procedures [59]. The first UTx attempt, which was performed in Saudi Arabia in 2000, was from an unrelated perimenopausal donor live donor who gave her uterus to a woman that had experienced emergency peripartum hysterectomy. Unfortunately, the transplanted uterus was removed 99 days post-UTx with bilateral uterine vessel thrombosis [55]. The Gothenburg group has been pioneering UTx since 2012 and performed the following 9 live donor cases within the first clinical UTx trial. Out of these 9 cases, 8 were MRKH recipients and one had hysterectomy for cervical cancer. In two of these UTx were removed because of uterine vessel thrombosis and intrauterine abscess [56].

The first live birth post UTx occurred in September 2014 following a UTx from February 2013. This was a MRKH recipient and the donor was a postmenopausal friend. Implantation occurred at the first embryo transfer and the first two trimesters were uncomplicated, apart from one rejection episode. Delivery of a healthy boy

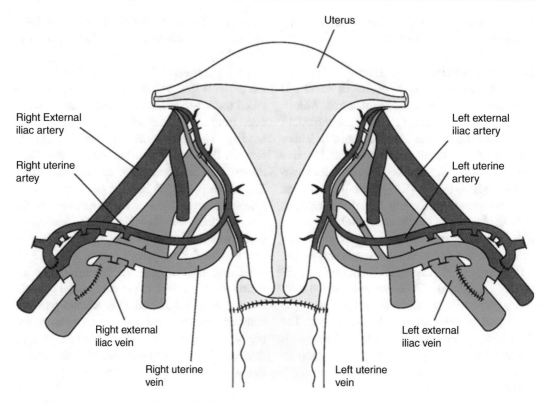

Fig. 23.7 Schematic drawing of the vessel connections of the transplanted uterus

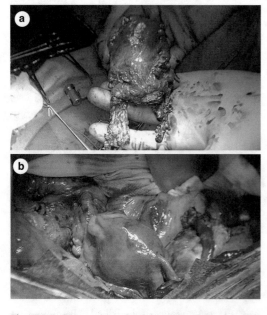

Fig. 23.8 Uterus transplantation procedure (**a**) The uterus with its long vascular pedicles is removed from the donor. (**b**) The uterine graft is revascularised and fixed in the pelvis of the recipient

was achieved by caesarean section at week 31, as the mother became preeclamptic [57]. Between 2014 and 2017, eight healthy children were born from the Swedish clinical UTx trial, with a take-home-baby rate 85% and clinical pregnancy rate of 100% [56].

Following the Swedish trial, more groups developed interest in UTx, with published cases from China, Germany and USA. The Chinese group performed their first donor operation with a robotic assisted laparoscopic approach and used the utero-ovarian veins for venous outflow. The UTx was reported as viable 1 year post transplantation. No pregnancy has been reported yet [60].

The German group reported three UTx attempts, out of which one was terminated straight after the organ retrieval, as attempts to flush the retrieved uterus failed due to extreme resistance of the left uterine artery (UA) and inability to perfuse the right UA. Transplantation was aborted to avoid graft vessel thrombosis or insufficient blood flow during potential pregnancy [62].

In 2016, the Dallas group started the first live donor UTx trial in USA. Five cases have been reported so far, out of which the first 3 suffered early graft loss because of vascular complications, both inflow and outflow [63]. The first healthy baby was delivered in November 2017 following an embryo transfer at 6 months post UTx. The primary reason for this early embryo transfer was the intention to minimize the duration of immunosuppression and its potential side effects [58]. However, as shown by the initial Swedish trial, rejections occurred in the 6–12 month interval at a rate of 57%. Thus, it has been suggested that a wait period of 12 months is recommended [59, 64].

Several other live donor UTx attempts remain unpublished from various teams worldwide. Of special note is the UTx case in Belgrade, Serbia in March 2017, which involved monozygotic twins discordant for MRKH. A mother of three healthy children donated her uterus to her sister with MRKH. Immunosuppression was not used and the embryo transfer after 7 months resulted in pregnancy [59].

Besides live donor UTx, various teams attempted deceased donor UTx and so far there are only three published cases. The first case was performed in Antalya, Turkey in 2011, where a MRKH woman, who had undergone vaginal reconstruction with jejunum segment 2 years previously, received a uterus from a 22-year-old nulliparous brain-dead woman. The entire procedure lasted 8 h: 2 h for allograft procurement, 30 min for transfer from the other hospital, and the remaining time for uterus implantation in the recipient, with bilateral end-to-side anastomosis of the internal iliac vessels of the graft to the external iliac vessels. No live birth has been reported from this case so far [65].

The Cleveland clinic team performed the second deceased donor UTx in February 2016. Unfortunately, the uterus was removed on postoperative day 12 due to a severe candida infection of the graft, which infiltrated the vasculature of the uterus and caused disruption of one of the two arterial anastomoses [66].

The Sao Paolo team performed the third deceased donor UTx case in September 2016 and the first healthy baby from deceased donor UTx was born in December 2017 [67].

23.1.4.2   Penile Transplantation

Introduction
Besides UTx, penile or genitourinary vascularized composite allotransplantation (GUVCA) have been indicative of the need for VCA transplantation, since current reconstructive techniques fail to adequately restore the normal form and function of the penis. Poor cosmetic results, urethral fistulae and/or strictures, and inability to restore erectile function sufficiently as well as a requirement for multiple complex procedures plague conventional genital reconstruction. Especially in soldiers who have suffered limb injury, it is sometimes impossible to use a radial forearm or a pedicled anterolateral thigh for neophalloplasty, because of multiple devastating injuries [68].

The first GUVCA transplant was reported in 2006 by the Guangzhou group for traumatic loss of penis, which unfortunately had to be removed on day 14, because of severe psychological issues [69]. It wasn't until December 2014, that the second transplant took place in South Africa for a patient that lost his penis because of gangrene, following a circumcision ritual. The same team performed another penile transplant in April 2017 [70]. The third GUVCA was performed at Massachusetts General Hospital group in 2016 for a patient with subtotal penectomy for penile cancer [71] and in April 2018, the Johns Hopkins group reported the first total penile and scrotal transplant [72].

Indications and Patient Selection
Current reconstructive options for penile loss or for female-to-male transgender are all autologous tissue based, with or without implant placement for penile rigidity, and they all share the goal of an aesthetically satisfactory and functional phallus, including the ability for standing micturition, tactile and erogenous sensibility and erectile function (sufficient for penetration and possibly

in some cases, insemination). Most limitations of autologous phallopasty techniques come from gender affirmation surgery, where microsurgical free flap reconstruction has become the gold standard, with the radial free flap being the most commonly chosen technique. No ideal technique exists and the patient's reconstructive goals and the extent of urogenital defect determine the method of reconstruction. It has therefore been suggested that GUVCA should be approached as a holistic treatment option, encompassing a series of patient-specific issues, and not as just a single surgical reconstruction procedure [73].

The loss of a penis has profound implications for self-esteem and body image. Besides the psychosocial considerations noted for solid organ and VCA patients, penile candidates should be assessed about their expectations of sexual function, their adaptation to the original condition that contributed to the loss of the penis and their ability to cope with organ rejection or graft loss. Their partner's expectations and receptiveness to the graft are also be important considerations [74].

Surgical Technique

The donor penis is retrieved at the level of the inferior pubic rami. The dorsal penile neurovascular structures are identified and dissected as far proximal as possible before the penis is transected. The team led by van der Werve reported cooling the penis by irrigation with ice cold HTK solution directly into the corpora cavernosa as they found that intra-arterial perfusion via the dorsal penile arteries was not possible because of excessive cannula size [70]. Then the corpora, nerve, and vascular structures were prepared on the bench. The penile stump of the recipient was prepared by excising the distal approximately 0·5 cm of the corpora cavernosa and isolating the urethra and spongiosal stump. Because of previous gangrenous infection, the dorsal penile vessels were obstructed and they therefore resorted to the left inferior epigastric artery, which was re-routed subcutaneously, via a paramedian incision. Nylon 9-0 suture was used for the anastomosis with the right dorsal penile artery. The contralateral dorsal penile artery was similarly

anastomosed to the left superficial external pudendal artery [70]. A 2 mm GEM Microvascular Anastomotic COUPLER ring was used for the anastomosis of the deep dorsal vein of the penis to one of the deep inferior epigastric veins. The vascular clamps were released before the cavernosal and spongiosal anastomoses. Both dorsal nerves were repaired under loupe magnification with a 9-0 nylon epineural suture. The urethra was spatulated and anastomosed with interrupted 3-0 polyglycolic acid sutures. The tunica albuginea of the cavernosal bodies and urethra were sutured in a watertight fashion with interrupted 2-0 polyglycolic acid sutures [70].

Cetrulo et al. began the implantation with a spatulated urethral anastomosis followed by approximation of the corporal bodies which prepared the scaffolding for the delicate neurovascular anastomoses. The cavernosal arteries and deep dorsal vein were anastomosed primarily with standard microsurgical technique. Due to sclerotic recipient dorsal arteries, a vein graft was retrieved from the distal leg and anastomosed end-to-side to the right femoral artery and end-to-end to the right dorsal penile artery. Cadaveric acellular nerve allograft was used to bridge a 2-cm gap between the dorsal penile nerves of the recipient and allograft with standard epineural neurorrhaphies [71].

Research performed by the Johns Hopkins team showed the cavernosal anastomoses may improve later erectile function in the recipient without the requirement for additional surgery to place a penile prosthetic device. Also, use of the external pudendal artery may avoid the complication of penile shaft skin necrosis as this vessel was demonstrated to provide much of the vascularization to this region of the graft [68].

Outcomes

The outcomes are very encouraging from the two published cases, which, first of all, proved the feasibility and potential of GUVCA, as a viable option for restoration of normal external genital appearance and sensation, as well as urinary and sexual function [70, 71].

Complications that have been reported include a fungal infection resulting from the immunosuppression. Phaeohyphomycoses, such as Alternaria spp., are rare opportunistic fungal infections that predominantly affect the skin in immunocompromised patients, particularly those being treated with mycophenolate mofetil. The patient responded well to topical broad spectrum antifungal treatment alone [70]. The patient form MGH had to return to theatres for hematoma evacuation and small wound debridements, and also had an episode of steroid-resistant acute rejection which was treated with 4 days of anti-thymocyte globulin [71].

Increased overall health satisfaction, dramatic improvement of self-image, and significant optimism for the future have been reported and this proves the concept that GUVCA can restore functional defects, as well as improve one's self-image.

23.2 Immunosuppression Protocols

VCA transplantation has adopted the current two-phase induction and maintenance regime protocols from solid organ transplantation.

For induction, most centres depend on polyclonal anti thymoglobulin (ATG) or monoclonal agents such as Basiliximab and Alemtuzumab. Steroids play an important role during induction, maintenance, as well as addressing the rejection episodes. There is a trend towards using Alemtuzumab by different teams. The Louisville group initially used basiliximab for the first 2 patients as induction agent but later used alemtuzumab [25]. The Innsbruck team reported using ATG for the first two out of four cases and alemtuzumab in the next two [27].

Maintenance therapy is widely based on tacrolimus (calcineurin inhibitor), along with mycophenolate mofetil (MMF) (antimetabolite) and also steroids. However, some teams attempt to add an mTor-inhibitor (sirolimus or everolimus) under simultaneous withdrawal or dose reduction of tacrolimus, in order to limit the nephrotoxicity and, also, for its anti-proliferative properties. Topical medications such as tacrolimus and steroid creams sometimes can be utilised to treat acute cutaneous rejection, reversing or preventing superficial skin rejection episodes with minimal systemic effects. The pattern of steroid use is variable in different regimes and the aim of many VCA centres is to withdraw steroids as soon as possible after transplantation due to their side effects.

To favour and justify the risk–benefit equation for VCA transplantation, the risks and complications of long-term immunosuppression have to be carefully balanced against all the potential benefits of these transplants such as, for example, return in motor and sensory function, independence, and improvement in quality of life. Thus, there is an urgent and imminent need to develop novel strategies to minimize or avoid maintenance immunosuppression after VCA [2]. Novel immunosuppressive therapies are looking to induce tolerance and minimize immunosuppression. The "Pittsburgh protocol" is such a novel, donor bone marrow (BM) cell-based treatment protocol, and it was used in 5 hand transplant recipients. Patients were treated with alemtuzumab and methylprednisolone for induction, followed by tacrolimus monotherapy. On day 14, patients received an infusion of donor BM cells isolated from 9 vertebral bodies. The team concluded that this protocol was safe, well tolerated, and allowed upper-extremity transplantation using low-dose tacrolimus monotherapy (trough levels 4–12 ng/ml) [31].

Two VCA-centres published the results after using belatacept, a costimulation blocker, to replace the CNI-based immunosuppression successfully. Cendales et al. from Duke University reported the clinical application of a de novo belatacept-based protocol, transitioned to a CNI-free regimen in a patient after having received hand transplantation [75]. The Innsbruck-team reported their experience with belatacept in four hand-transplanted patients. The goal of this group was not only to protect their VCA-recipients of CNI-triggered side effect, they also used belatacept due to its possible inhibitory effect on the development of donor-specific antibodies. The treatment with belatacept could be successfully applied in three patients but did not work satisfactorily in one who was positive for

CD4 + CD57+ T-cells which are known to be a sign for non-responders to belatacept treatment [76]. Therefore, the implementation of belatacept to replace tacrolimus in hand-transplant recipients can be beneficial but it is important to act with caution and to reflect the immunologic state of the patients at the time of conversion.

Data from the IRHCTT show that 85% of hand transplant recipients experience one or more episodes of acute rejection, [77] which commonly presents as a erythematous maculopapular rash. Monitoring for rejections and managing them is important to have a successful outcome after VCA. In fact, the majority of the hand transplants that have failed, may have had some non-adherence problems in the long-term maintenance of the immunosuppression protocol. The advantages of VCA over solid organ transplants is the skin component, which acts as a visible marker, a 'dynamic canvas', for detecting the rejection pattern [49]. Skin biopsies show initially perivascular lymphocytic infiltration which can progress to epidermolysis. The antibody-mediated rejection is characterised by microvascular injury and tissue destruction. They are detected by immunohistochemical methods. In general, the cell-mediated rejections are treated by increasing the immunosuppressant doses, bolus doses of methyl prednisolone or ATG. The antibody-mediated rejections could be in addition reversed by agents like rituximab, an anti-CD20-antibody, or if resistant to any of the mentioned drug, with alemtuzumab an anti-CD52 antibody. Chronic rejection can be challenging to diagnose; however, it is thought to be associated with intimal hyperplasia [22].

23.3   Conclusion

Over the last 20 years the outcomes and experiences of VCA has ameliorated early concerns, clarified the ethical considerations, stratified the risks, and encouraged an expansion of the indications, and the number of participating centres. There is still much to learn, but the VCA future is bright.

References

1. Peacock EE. Homologous composite tissue grafts of the digital flexor mechanism in human beings. Transplant Bull. 1960 Apr;7:418–21.
2. Azari K, Brandacher G. Vascularized composite allotransplantation. Curr Opin Organ Transplant. 2013 Dec;18(6):631–2.
3. Gilbert R. Transplant is successful with a cadaver forearm. Med Trib Med News. 1964;5:20–3.
4. Dubernard JM, Owen E, Lefrançois N, Petruzzo P, Martin X, Dawahra M, et al. First human hand transplantation. Case report. Transpl Int Off J Eur Soc Organ Transplant. 2000;13(Suppl 1):S521–4.
5. Breidenbach WC, Gonzales NR, Kaufman CL, Klapheke M, Tobin GR, Gorantla VS. Outcomes of the first 2 American hand transplants at 8 and 6 years posttransplant. J Hand Surg. 2008 Sep;33(7):1039–47.
6. Petruzzo P, Badet L, Gazarian A, Lanzetta M, Parmentier H, Kanitakis J, et al. Bilateral hand transplantation: six years after the first case. Am J Transplant Off J Am Soc Transplant Am Soc Transpl Surg. 2006 Jul;6(7):1718–24.
7. Strome M, Stein J, Esclamado R, Hicks D, Lorenz RR, Braun W, et al. Laryngeal transplantation and 40-month follow-up. N Engl J Med. 2001 May 31;344(22):1676–9.
8. Levi DM, Tzakis AG, Kato T, Madariaga J, Mittal NK, Nery J, et al. Transplantation of the abdominal wall. Lancet Lond Engl. 2003 Jun 28;361(9376):2173–6.
9. Gerlach UA, Vrakas G, Sawitzki B, Macedo R, Reddy S, Friend PJ, et al. Abdominal wall transplantation: skin as a sentinel marker for Rejection. Am J Transplant Off J Am Soc Transplant Am Soc Transpl Surg. 2016;16(6):1892–900.
10. Devauchelle B, Badet L, Lengelé B, Morelon E, Testelin S, Michallet M, et al. First human face allograft: early report. Lancet Lond Engl. 2006 Jul 15;368(9531):203–9.
11. Breidenbach WC, Meister EA, Becker GW, Turker T, Gorantla VS, Hassan K, et al. A statistical comparative assessment of face and hand transplantation outcomes to determine whether either meets the standard of care threshold. Plast Reconstr Surg. 2016 Jan;137(1):214e–22e.
12. Grob M, Papadopulos NA, Zimmermann A, Biemer E, Kovacs L. The psychological impact of severe hand injury. J Hand Surg Eur Vol. 2008 Jun;33(3):358–62.
13. Wright TW, Hagen AD, Wood MB. Prosthetic usage in major upper extremity amputations. J Hand Surg. 1995 Jul;20(4):619–22.
14. Bernardon L, Gazarian A, Petruzzo P, Packham T, Guillot M, Guigal V, et al. Bilateral hand transplantation: Functional benefits assessment in five patients with a mean follow-up of 7.6 years (range 4-13 years). J Plast Reconstr Aesthetic Surg JPRAS. 2015 Sep;68(9):1171–83.

15. Khan AA, Diver AJ, Clarke A, Butler PEM. A mathematical risk-benefit analysis of composite tissue allotransplantation. Transplantation. 2007 Dec 15;84(11):1384–90.
16. Elliott RM, Tintle SM, Levin LS. Upper extremity transplantation: current concepts and challenges in an emerging field. Curr Rev Musculoskelet Med. 2014 Mar;7(1):83–8.
17. Hollenbeck ST, Erdmann D, Levin LS. Current indications for hand and face allotransplantation. Transplant Proc. 2009 Mar;41(2):495–8.
18. Schneeberger S, Ninkovic M, Gabl M, Ninkovic M, Hussl H, Rieger M, et al. First forearm transplantation: outcome at 3 years. Am J Transplant Off J Am Soc Transplant Am Soc Transpl Surg. 2007 Jul;7(7):1753–62.
19. Shores JT, Malek V, Lee WPA, Brandacher G. Outcomes after hand and upper extremity transplantation. J Mater Sci Mater Med. 2017 May;28(5):72.
20. Carty MJ, Hivelin M, Dumontier C, Talbot SG, Benjoar MD, Pribaz JJ, et al. Lessons learned from simultaneous face and bilateral hand allotransplantation. Plast Reconstr Surg. 2013 Aug;132(2):423–32.
21. Shores JT, Lee WPA, Brandacher G. Discussion: lessons learned from simultaneous face and bilateral hand allotransplantation. Plast Reconstr Surg. 2013 Aug;132(2):433–4.
22. Petruzzo P, Lanzetta M, Dubernard J-M, Landin L, Cavadas P, Margreiter R, et al. The international registry on hand and composite tissue transplantation. Transplantation. 2010 Dec 27;90(12):1590–4.
23. Lanzetta M, Petruzzo P, Dubernard JM, Margreiter R, Schuind F, Breidenbach W, et al. Second report (1998–2006) of the international registry of hand and composite tissue transplantation. Transpl Immunol. 2007 Jul;18(1):1–6.
24. Shores JT, Brandacher G, Lee WPA. Hand and upper extremity transplantation: an update of outcomes in the worldwide experience. Plast Reconstr Surg. 2015 Feb;135(2):351e–60e.
25. Kaufman CL, Breidenbach W. World experience after more than a decade of clinical hand transplantation: update from the Louisville hand transplant program. Hand Clin. 2011 Nov;27(4):417–21, vii–viii.
26. Cavadas PC, Landin L, Thione A, Rodríguez-Pérez JC, Garcia-Bello MA, Ibañez J, et al. The Spanish experience with hand, forearm, and arm transplantation. Hand Clin. 2011 Nov;27(4):443–53, viii.
27. Hautz T, Engelhardt TO, Weissenbacher A, Kumnig M, Zelger B, Rieger M, et al. World experience after more than a decade of clinical hand transplantation: update on the Innsbruck program. Hand Clin. 2011 Nov;27(4):423–31, viii.
28. Jablecki J, Kaczmarzyk L, Domanasiewicz A, Chelmonski A, Paruzel M, Elsaftawy A, et al. Result of arm-level upper-limb transplantation in two recipients at 19- and 30-month follow-up. Ann Transplant. 2012 Sep;17(3):126–32.
29. Jabłecki J. World experience after more than a decade of clinical hand transplantation: update on the Polish program. Hand Clin. 2011 Nov;27(4):433–42, viii.
30. Shores JT, Brandacher G, Gorantla V, Schneeberger S, Losee J, Lee WPA. A summary of the functional outcomes following transplantation of 8 hands/upper extremities in 5 patients with an innovative cell-based single drug immunotherapy protocol: level 4 evidence. J Hand Surg. 2012 Sep 6;37(8):5.
31. Schneeberger S, Gorantla VS, Brandacher G, Zeevi A, Demetris AJ, Lunz JG, et al. Upper-extremity transplantation using a cell-based protocol to minimize immunosuppression. Ann Surg. 2013 Feb;257(2):345–51.
32. Petruzzo P, Dubernard JM, Lanzetta M The international registry on hand and composite tissue allotransplantation (IRHCTT). Presented at the ASRT meeting in Chicago, November 4th, 2016 2016.
33. Face transplants "on the horizon." 2002 Nov 27 [cited 2018 Sep 9]; Available from http://news.bbc.co.uk/2/hi/health/2516181.stm
34. Lantieri L, Grimbert P, Ortonne N, Suberbielle C, Bories D, Gil-Vernet S, et al. Face transplant: long-term follow-up and results of a prospective open study. Lancet Lond Engl. 2016 Oct 1;388(10052):1398–407.
35. Barret JP, Gavaldà J, Bueno J, Nuvials X, Pont T, Masnou N, et al. Full face transplant: the first case report. Ann Surg. 2011 Aug;254(2):252–6.
36. Sosin M, Rodriguez ED. The face transplantation update: 2016. Plast Reconstr Surg. 2016 Jun;137(6):1841–50.
37. Wo L, Bueno E, Pomahac B. Facial transplantation: worth the risks? A look at evolution of indications over the last decade. Curr Opin Organ Transplant. 2015 Dec;20(6):615–20.
38. Barret JP, Tomasello V. Indications for face transplantation. In: Face trans-plantation. Berlin: Springer; 2015. p. 15–20.
39. Lantieri L. Face transplant: a paradigm change in facial reconstruction. J Craniofac Surg. 2012 Jan;23(1):250–3.
40. Maciejewski A, Krakowczyk Ł, Szymczyk C, Wierzgoń J, Grajek M, Dobrut M, et al. The first immediate face transplant in the world. Ann Surg. 2016 Mar;263(3):e36–9.
41. Cavadas PC, Ibáñez J, Thione A. Surgical aspects of a lower face, mandible, and tongue allotransplantation. J Reconstr Microsurg. 2012 Jan;28(1):43–7.
42. Lantieri L, Hivelin M, Audard V, Benjoar MD, Meningaud JP, Bellivier F, et al. Feasibility, reproducibility, risks and benefits of face transplantation: a prospective study of outcomes. Am J Transplant Off J Am Soc Transplant Am Soc Transpl Surg. 2011 Feb;11(2):367–78.
43. Caterson EJ, Diaz-Siso JR, Shetye P, Junker JPE, Bueno EM, Soga S, et al. Craniofacial principles in face transplantation. J Craniofac Surg. 2012 Sep;23(5):1234–8.
44. Pomahac B, Pribaz JJ, Bueno EM, Sisk GC, Diaz-Siso JR, Chandawarkar A, et al. Novel surgical technique for full face transplantation. Plast Reconstr Surg. 2012 Sep;130(3):549–55.
45. Siemionow M. The decade of face transplant outcomes. J Mater Sci Mater Med. 2017 May;28(5):64.

46. Khalifian S, Brazio PS, Mohan R, Shaffer C, Brandacher G, Barth RN, et al. Facial transplantation: the first 9 years. Lancet Lond Engl. 2014 Dec 13;384(9960):2153–63.

47. Shanmugarajah K, Hettiaratchy S, Butler PEM. Facial transplantation. Curr Opin Otolaryngol Head Neck Surg. 2012 Aug;20(4):291–7.

48. Fischer S, Kueckelhaus M, Pauzenberger R, Bueno EM, Pomahac B. Functional outcomes of face transplantation. Am J Transplant Off J Am Soc Transplant Am Soc Transpl Surg. 2015 Jan;15(1):220–33.

49. Giele H, Vaidya A, Reddy S, Vrakas G, Friend P. Current state of abdominal wall transplantation. Curr Opin Organ Transplant. 2016 Apr;21(2): 159–64.

50. Barnes J, Issa F, Vrakas G, Friend P, Giele H. The abdominal wall transplant as a sentinel skin graft. Curr Opin Organ Transplant. 2016;21(5):536–40.

51. Carlsen BT, Farmer DG, Busuttil RW, Miller TA, Rudkin GH. Incidence and management of abdominal wall defects after intestinal and multivisceral transplantation. Plast Reconstr Surg. 2007 Apr 1;119(4):1247–55; discussion 1256–1258.

52. Vascularised Composite Allografts and Intestinal Transplantation: Does the Skin Component Provide a Pre-Rejection Marker for the Visceral Organ? [Internet]. ATC Abstracts. [cited 2018 Sep 29]. Available from https://atcmeetingabstracts.com/ abstract/vascularised-composite-allografts-and-intes-tinal-transplantation-does-the-skin-component-pro-vide-a-pre-rejection-marker-for-the-visceral-organ/

53. Weissenbacher A, Vrakas G, Chen M, Reddy S, Allan P, Giele H, et al. De novo donor-specific HLA antibodies after combined intestinal and vascularized composite allotransplantation – a retrospective study. Transpl Int Off J Eur Soc Organ Transplant. 2018;31(4):398–407.

54. Dahm-Kähler P, Diaz-Garcia C, Brännström M. Human uterus transplantation in focus. Br Med Bull. 2016 Mar;117(1):69–78.

55. Fageeh W, Raffa H, Jabbad H, Marzouki A. Transplantation of the human uterus. Int J Gynaecol Obstet Off Organ Int Fed Gynaecol Obstet. 2002 Mar;76(3):245–51.

56. Brännström M, Johannesson L, Dahm-Kähler P, Enskog A, Mölne J, Kvarnström N, et al. First clinical uterus transplantation trial: a six-month report. Fertil Steril. 2014 May;101(5):1228–36.

57. Brännström M, Johannesson L, Bokström H, Kvarnström N, Mölne J, Dahm-Kähler P, et al. Livebirth after uterus transplantation. Lancet Lond Engl. 2015 Feb 14;385(9968):607–16.

58. Testa G, McKenna GJ, Gunby RT, Anthony T, Koon EC, Warren AM, et al. First live birth after uterus transplantation in the United States. Am J Transplant Off J Am Soc Transplant Am Soc Transpl Surg. 2018 May;18(5):1270–4.

59. Brännström M. Current status and future direction of uterus transplantation. Curr Opin Organ Transplant. 2018 Oct;23(5):592–7.

60. Wei L, Xue T, Tao K-S, Zhang G, Zhao G-Y, Yu S-Q, et al. Modified human uterus transplantation using ovarian veins for venous drainage: the first report of surgically successful robotic-assisted uterus procurement and follow-up for 12 months. Fertil Steril. 2017;108(2):346-356.e1.

61. Brännström M, Dahm Kähler P, Greite R, Mölne J, Díaz-García C, Tullius SG. Uterus transplantation: a rapidly expanding field. Transplantation. 2018 Apr;102(4):569–77.

62. Brucker SY, Brännström M, Taran F-A, Nadalin S, Königsrainer A, Rall K, et al. Selecting living donors for uterus transplantation: lessons learned from two transplantations resulting in menstrual functionality and another attempt, aborted after organ retrieval. Arch Gynecol Obstet. 2018 Mar;297(3):675–84.

63. Testa G, Koon EC, Johannesson L, McKenna GJ, Anthony T, Klintmalm GB, et al. Living donor uterus transplantation: a single center's observations and lessons learned from early setbacks to technical success. Am J Transplant Off J Am Soc Transplant Am Soc Transpl Surg. 2017 Nov;17(11):2901–10.

64. Mölne J, Broecker V, Ekberg J, Nilsson O, Dahm-Kähler P, Brännström M. Monitoring of human uterus transplantation with cervical biopsies: a provisional scoring system for rejection. Am J Transplant Off J Am Soc Transplant Am Soc Transpl Surg. 2017 Jun;17(6):1628–36.

65. Ozkan O, Akar ME, Ozkan O, Erdogan O, Hadimioglu N, Yilmaz M, et al. Preliminary results of the first human uterus transplantation from a multiorgan donor. Fertil Steril. 2013 Feb;99(2):470–6.

66. Flyckt RL, Farrell RM, Perni UC, Tzakis AG, Falcone T. Deceased donor uterine transplantation: innovation and adaptation. Obstet Gynecol. 2016;128(4):837–42.

67. Soares JM, Ejzenberg D, Andraus W, D'Albuquerque LAC, Baracat EC. First Latin uterine transplantation: we can do it! Clinics. 2016 Nov;71(11):627–8.

68. Szafran AA, Redett R, Burnett AL. Penile transplantation: the US experience and institutional program set-up. Transl Androl Urol. 2018 Aug;7(4):639–45.

69. Hu W, Lu J, Zhang L, Wu W, Nie H, Zhu Y, et al. A preliminary report of penile transplantation. Eur Urol. 2006 Oct;50(4):851–3.

70. van der Merwe A, Graewe F, Zühlke A, Barsdorf NW, Zarrabi AD, Viljoen JT, et al. Penile allotransplantation for penis amputation following ritual circumcision: a case report with 24 months of follow-up. Lancet. 2017 Sep 9;390(10099):1038–47.

71. Cetrulo CL, Li K, Salinas HM, Treiser MD, Schol I, Barrisford GW, et al. Penis transplantation: first US experience. Ann Surg. 2018 May;267(5):983–8.

72. First-Ever Penis and Scrotum Transplant Makes History at Johns Hopkins [Internet]. [cited 2018 Sep 30]. Available from https://www.hopkinsmedicine. org/news/articles/first-ever-penis-and-scrotum-trans-plant-makes-history-at-johns-hopkins

73. Schol IM, Ko DSC, Cetrulo CL. Genitourinary vascularized composite allotransplantation. Curr Opin Organ Transplant. 2017 Oct;22(5):484–9.

74. Jowsey-Gregoire S, Kumnig M. Standardizing psychosocial assessment for vascularized composite allotransplantation. Curr Opin Organ Transplant. 2016;21(5):530–5.
75. Cendales LC, Ruch DS, Cardones AR, Potter G, Dooley J, Dore D, et al. De novo belatacept in clinical vascularized composite allotransplantation. Am J Transplant Off J Am Soc Transplant Am Soc Transpl Surg. 2018 Jul;18(7):1804–9.
76. Grahammer J, Weissenbacher A, Zelger BG, Zelger B, Boesmueller C, Ninkovic M, et al. Benefits and limitations of belatacept in 4 hand-transplanted patients. Am J Transplant Off J Am Soc Transplant Am Soc Transpl Surg. 2017 Dec;17(12):3228–35.
77. Petruzzo P, Dubernard JM. The international registry on hand and composite tissue allotransplantation. Clin Transpl. 2011:247–53.

Index

© Springer Nature Switzerland AG 2021
N. Hakim et al. (eds.), *Transplantation Surgery*, Springer Specialist Surgery Series,
https://doi.org/10.1007/978-3-030-55244-2

Printed in the United States
by Baker & Taylor Publisher Services